Protein Secretion Pathways in Bacteria

Protein Secretion Pathways in Bacteria

Editor: Abrielle Benton

AMERICAN
MEDICAL PUBLISHERS
www.americanmedicalpublishers.com

AMERICAN
MEDICAL PUBLISHERS
www.americanmedicalpublishers.com

Cataloging-in-Publication Data

Protein secretion pathways in bacteria / edited by Abrielle Benton.
p. cm.
Includes bibliographical references and index.
ISBN 979-8-88740-400-4
1. Bacterial proteins. 2. Microbial proteins--Secretion. 3. Proteins--Secretion.
4. Microbial metabolism. 5. Bacteria--Physiology. I. Benton, Abrielle.
QR92.P75 P76 2023
572.36--dc23

American Medical Publishers,
41 Flatbush Avenue,
1st Floor, New York,
NY 11217, USA

ISBN 979-8-88740-400-4 (Hardback)

Contents

Preface

Every book is initially just a concept; it takes months of research and hard work to give it the final shape in which the readers receive it. In its early stages, this book also went through rigorous reviewing. The notable contributions made by experts from across the globe were first molded into patterned chapters and then arranged in a sensibly sequential manner to bring out the best results.

Bacteria are living organisms found ubiquitously in nature and have only one biological cell. They constitute a wide domain of prokaryotic microorganisms. In bacteria, unfolded proteins are transported through the secretion pathways across the cytoplasmic membrane. This transportation consists of three parts, which include a protein targeting component, a motor protein and membrane integrated conducting channel. Bacteria have a range of protein transportation pathways, which are necessary for functions like pathogenicity and viability. Generally, bacterial secretion comprises secretion of unfolded proteins which primarily remain within the cells. In case of gram-negative bacteria, secreted proteins are delivered to inner membrane or the periplasm. The protein can remain in the cell or it is usually transported out of the bacteria via other secretion systems. Klebsiella pneumonia, Yersinia enterocolitica and Vibrio cholerae are the gram-negative bacteria that utilize the secretion system. Gram-positive bacteria that utilize the secretion system include Listeria monocytogenes and Staphylococcus aureus. This book covers in detail some existent theories and innovative concepts on the protein secretion pathways in bacteria. It will provide comprehensive knowledge to the readers.

It has been my immense pleasure to be a part of this project and to contribute my years of learning in such a meaningful form. I would like to take this opportunity to thank all the people who have been associated with the completion of this book at any step.

Editor

1

Delivery of the *Pseudomonas aeruginosa* Phospholipase Effectors PldA and PldB in a VgrG- and H2-T6SS-Dependent Manner

Sarah Wettstadt†*, Thomas E. Wood*†*, Selina Fecht and Alain Filloux**

MRC Centre for Molecular Bacteriology and Infection, Department of Life Sciences, Imperial College London, London, United Kingdom

Correspondence:
Alain Filloux
a.filloux@imperial.ac.uk

The bacterial pathogen *Pseudomonas aeruginosa* uses three type VI secretion systems (T6SSs) to drive a multitude of effector proteins into eukaryotic or prokaryotic target cells. The T6SS is a supramolecular nanomachine, involving a set of 13 core proteins, which resembles the contractile tail of bacteriophages and whose tip is considered as a puncturing device helping to cross membranes. Effectors can attach directly to the T6SS spike which is composed of a VgrG (valine-glycine-rich proteins) trimer, of which *P. aeruginosa* produces several. We have previously shown that the master regulator RsmA controls the expression of all three T6SS gene clusters (H1-, H2- and H3-T6SS) and a range of remote *vgrG* and effector genes. We also demonstrated that specific interactions between VgrGs and various T6SS effectors are prerequisite for effector delivery in a process we called "à la carte delivery." Here, we provide an in-depth description on how the two H2-T6SS-dependent effectors PldA and PldB are delivered *via* their cognate VgrGs, VgrG4b and VgrG5, respectively. We show that specific recognition of the VgrG C terminus is required and effector specificity can be swapped by exchanging these C-terminal domains. Importantly, we established that effector recognition by a cognate VgrG is not always sufficient to achieve successful secretion, but it is crucial to provide effector stability. This study highlights the complexity of effector adaptation to the T6SS nanomachine and shows how the VgrG tip can possibly be manipulated to achieve effector delivery.

Keywords: type VI secretion system, bacterial toxin, phospholipase, VgrG, *Pseudomonas aeruginosa*

INTRODUCTION

The type VI secretion system (T6SS) is a sophisticated protein secretion system that is found in about 25% of Gram-negative bacteria (Bingle et al., 2008). Resembling the contractile tail of bacteriophage (Kanamaru et al., 2002), the T6SS is used by bacteria to drive effector proteins directly into nearby cells, which can be of eukaryotic or prokaryotic nature (Basler et al., 2013). The T6SS is placed onto the bacterial cytoplasmic membrane *via* a membrane complex consisting of TssL, TssM and TssJ proteins (Durand et al., 2012, 2015). The membrane complex is connected to a so-called T6SS baseplate, sitting at the cytosolic side of the inner membrane and made of TssA, TssE, TssF, TssG, TssK, and VgrG (Brunet et al., 2015; Planamente et al., 2016). From the baseplate, the

T6SS sheath is built and polymerizes into the cytoplasm. Composed of TssB and TssC subunits (Leiman et al., 2009), this helical contractile sheath envelops an inner tube, that consists of stacked hexamers of Hcp proteins (Brunet et al., 2014) which are topped by the VgrG spike (Renault et al., 2018). Contraction of the sheath toward the baseplate leads to extracellular release of the VgrG spike and the Hcp tube, where presence of Hcp in the supernatant fraction of bacterial cultures is a standard readout for T6SS activity, since it is a direct measure of a functional T6SS machinery (Pukatzki et al., 2006).

The spike atop the Hcp tube is composed of a trimer of VgrG proteins forming a rigid needle-like structure due to intertwining C-terminal hydrophobic β-sheets (Kanamaru et al., 2002). At the tip of the T6SS VgrG trimer sits a PAAR protein (Shneider et al., 2013) whose conical fold is thought to facilitate the puncturing of target membranes (Browning et al., 2012). One PAAR protein likely binds on top of one VgrG trimer in a way that it interacts with the last β-sheet derived from each VgrG monomer (Shneider et al., 2013).

Pseudomonas aeruginosa contains three T6SS clusters (H1-, H2- and H3-T6SS) each encoding all core T6SS components. The three clusters could be expressed simultaneously (Hachani et al., 2011; Allsopp et al., 2017) while each system delivers different sets of effector proteins into prokaryotic or eukaryotic cells (Russell et al., 2011; Hachani et al., 2014; Jiang et al., 2014; Whitney et al., 2014). Additionally, the *P. aeruginosa* genome contains multiple remote satellite islands, likely acquired *via* horizontal gene transfer, encoding different *vgrG, paar* and effector genes co-regulated with the core T6SS clusters (Jones et al., 2013; Allsopp et al., 2017). Effector genes are usually encoded together with immunity genes allowing the survival of the effector producing strain (Russell et al., 2011) as well as preventing T6SS-dependent intoxication by neighboring sibling cells (MacIntyre et al., 2010).

In some cases, the effector is a covalent extension of a structural component and thus called evolved VgrG-, PAAR-, or Hcp-effector (Ma et al., 2009, 2017; Whitney et al., 2015). If separated, a genetic link between an effector gene and a gene encoding a VgrG-, PAAR-, or Hcp-protein suggests a functional association (Hachani et al., 2014). Indeed, the delivery of many effectors was shown to be dependent on the nearby encoded VgrG, PAAR or Hcp component. In these cases, the effector protein specifically interacts non-covalently with a cognate Hcp hexamer, like Tse2 with Hcp1 in *P. aeruginosa* (Silverman et al., 2013); a PAAR protein, for example TseT with PAAR4 in *P. aeruginosa* (Burkinshaw et al., 2018); or the VgrG spike, as Tle1 with VgrG1 in *Escherichia coli* (Flaugnatti et al., 2015); a concept coined as "à la carte" effector delivery (Hachani et al., 2014). In some instances, the presence of so-called adaptor or chaperone proteins are required to connect effectors to the T6SS spike. These adaptor proteins can be of the DUF4123, DUF1795 or DUF2169 family. The DUF4123 proteins, denoted Tap1 (T6SS adaptor protein 1) from *Agrobacterium tumefaciens* and *Vibrio cholerae* were shown to be required for the recruitment of the effectors Tde1 and TseL, respectively, onto the cognate VgrG1 spikes (Liang et al., 2015; Unterweger et al., 2015; Bondage et al., 2016). DUF1795 proteins were termed Eag proteins and bind to the N-terminal half of PAAR effectors, chaperoning them in the producing cell before recruiting the PAAR effector to the T6SS tip (Diniz and Coulthurst, 2015; Whitney et al., 2015; Quentin et al., 2018). DUF2169 proteins seem to be less prevalent and their involvement in effector delivery has only been shown for Tde2 in *A. tumefaciens* (Bondage et al., 2016).

Pseudomonas aeruginosa encodes the two phospholipases PldA and PldB that were shown to be delivered into prey cells in a T6SS-dependent manner (Russell et al., 2013; Jiang et al., 2014; Boulant et al., 2018). Both effector genes are directly located downstream of two *vgrG* genes and no adaptor gene is encoded in their direct vicinity. This suggests that both effectors are recruited directly to the VgrG spike by a yet undefined mechanism. Here, we elucidated the effector delivery mechanisms of PldA and PldB *via* the T6SS of *P. aeruginosa* and describe an interesting new concept which shows that PldA delivery is not only dependent on one but two VgrG proteins.

MATERIALS AND METHODS

Bacterial Strains and Growth Conditions

Bacterial strains used in this study are described in **Table 1**. *P. aeruginosa* strains were grown in tryptone soy broth (TSB) or LB supplemented with antibiotics where appropriate (streptomycin 2000 $\mu g\ mL^{-1}$, spectinomycin 2000 $\mu g\ mL^{-1}$, carbenicillin 100 $\mu g\ mL^{-1}$, tetracycline 200 $\mu g\ mL^{-1}$) at 37°C with agitation. *E. coli* strains were grown in LB broth supplemented with antibiotics where appropriate (streptomycin 50 $\mu g\ mL^{-1}$, kanamycin 50 $\mu g\ mL^{-1}$, spectinomycin 100 $\mu g\ mL^{-1}$, carbenicillin 50 $\mu g\ mL^{-1}$, tetracycline 15 $\mu g\ mL^{-1}$).

DNA Manipulation

DNA purification was performed using PureLink Genomic DNA mini kit (Life Technologies). Isolation of plasmid DNA was carried out using the QIAprep spin miniprep kit (Qiagen). Restriction endonucleases were used according to the manufacturer's specifications (New England Biolabs or Roche). Oligonucleotides used are listed in **Table 2** and were purchased from Sigma, United Kingdom. The genes or DNA fragments used for the construction of mutator plasmids and deletion mutants were amplified with KOD Hot Start DNA Polymerase (Novagen) as described by the manufacturer with the inclusion of 0.5 M betaine (Sigma). Colony PCR was performed with Taq polymerase (New England Biolabs). DNA sequencing was performed by GATC Biotech.

Construction of *P. aeruginosa* Mutants

Pseudomonas aeruginosa deletion mutants were constructed as described previously (Vasseur et al., 2005) using the suicide plasmid pKNG101 (Herrero et al., 1990; Kaniga et al., 1991). Briefly, to create PAO1Δ*gene-of-interest* (*GOI*), 500-bp DNA fragments of the 5′ (up) and 3′ (down) ends of the target gene were obtained by PCR using PAO1 chromosomal DNA as a template with two pairs of oligonucleotides (Up5′/Up3′ and Down5′/Down3′) (**Table 2**). To create chimeric genes, splicing by overlap extension PCRs was performed. Briefly, approximately 500 bp upstream and downstream of the locus

TABLE 1 | Strains and plasmids used in this work.

Strain or plasmid	Relevant characteristics[a]	Source/References
Strain		
E. coli		
DH5α	F– Φ80*lac*ZΔM15 Δ(*lac*ZYA-*arg*F) U169 *rec*A1 *end*A1 *hsd*R17 (rK–, mK+) *pho*A *sup*E44 λ– *thi*-1 *gyr*A96 *rel*A1	Laboratory collection
CC118(λpir)	Host strain for pKNG101 replication; Δ(*ara-leu*) *araD* Δ*lacX74 galE galK-phoA20 thi-1 rpsE rpoB argE* (Am) *recA1* Rf^R *λpir)*	Laboratory collection
P. aeruginosa		
PAO1	PAO1 wild type strain	Laboratory collection
PAO1 Δ*rsmA*	Deletion in *rsmA* (*PA0905*)	Allsopp et al., 2017
PAO1::*pldA-bla*$_{TEM-1}$	Insertion of *bla*$_{TEM-1}$ before *pldA (PA3487)* STOP codon	Allsopp et al., 2017
PAO1::*pldB-bla*$_{TEM-1}$	Insertion of *bla*$_{TEM-1}$ before *pldB (PA5089)* STOP codon	Allsopp et al., 2017
PAO1 ΔrsmAΔ*pldAtli5a*	Deletion in *rsmA*, *pldA-tli5a* (*PA3487-PA3488*)	This work
PAO1 ΔrsmAΔ*pldAtli5a::lacZ*	Deletion in *rsmA*, *pldA-tli5a PA3487-PA3488*, chromosomal insertion of *lacZ* at *att* site	This work
PAO1 ΔrsmAΔ*pldBtli5b*$_{123}$*::lacZ*	Deletion in *rsmA*, *pldB-tli5b*$_{123}$ (*PA5089-PA5086*), chromosomal insertion of *lacZ* at *att* site	This work
PAO1 ΔrsmAΔ*pldAtli5a* Δ*pldBtli5b*$_{123}$*::lacZ*	Deletion in *rsmA*, *pldA-tli5a PA3487-PA3488*, *pldB-tli5b*$_{123}$ *PA5089-PA5086*, chromosomal insertion of *lacZ* at *att* site	This work
PAO1 Δ*rsmA*Δ*tssE2*	Deletions in *rsmA* and *tssE2* (*PA1657*)	This work
PAO1 Δ*rsmA*Δ*tssK3*	Deletions in *rsmA* and *tssK3* (*PA2363*)	This work
PAO1 Δ*rsmA*Δ*tssE2::pldA-bla*$_{TEM-1}$	Deletions in *rsmA*, *tssE2* and insertion of *bla*$_{TEM-1}$ before *pldA* STOP codon	Allsopp et al., 2017
PAO1 Δ*rsmA*Δ*tssE2::pldB-bla*$_{TEM-1}$	Deletions in *rsmA*, *tssE2* and insertion of *bla*$_{TEM-1}$ before *pldB* STOP codon	This work
PAO1 Δ*rsmA*Δ*tssK3::pldA-bla*$_{TEM-1}$	Deletions in *rsmA*, *tssK3* and insertion of *bla*$_{TEM-1}$ before *pldA* STOP codon	This work
PAO1 Δ*rsmA*Δ*vgrG4b*	Deletions in *rsmA* and *vgrG4b* (*PA3486*)	Allsopp et al., 2017
PAO1 Δ*rsmA*Δ*vgrG4b*Δ*pldBtli5b*$_{123}$	Deletions in *rsmA, vgrG4b PA3486* and *pldB-tli5b*$_{123}$ *PA5089-PA5086*	This work
PAO1 Δ*rsmA*Δ*vgrG4b::pldA-bla*$_{TEM-1}$	Deletions in *rsmA*, *vgrG4b* and insertion of *bla*$_{TEM-1}$ before *pldA* STOP codon	This work
PAO1 Δ*rsmA*Δ*vgrG4b::pldB-bla*$_{TEM-1}$	Deletions in *rsmA*, *vgrG4b* and insertion of *bla*$_{TEM-1}$ before *pldB* STOP codon	This work
PAO1 Δ*rsmA::vgrG4b*^{618}*-vgrG5*^{169}	Deletion in *rsmA* and substitution of gene portion corresponding to *vgrG4b*^{187} with gene portion for *vgrG5*^{169}	This work
PAO1 Δ*rsmA::vgrG4b*^{618}*-vgrG5*^{169} *::pldA-bla*$_{TEM-1}$	Deletion in *rsmA*, insertion of *bla*$_{TEM-1}$ before *pldA* STOP codon, substitution of gene portion corresponding to *vgrG4b*^{187} with gene portion for *vgrG5*^{169}	This work
PAO1 Δ*rsmA*Δ*vgrG4b::vgrG5*^{623}*-vgrG4b*^{187}	Deletions in *rsmA*, *vgrG4b*, substitution of gene portion corresponding to *vgrG4b*^{187} with gene portion for *vgrG5*^{169}	This work
PAO1 Δ*rsmA*Δ*vgrG4b::vgrG5*^{623}*-vgrG4b*^{187}*::pldA-bla*$_{TEM-1}$	Deletions in *rsmA* and *vgrG4b*, insertion of *bla*$_{TEM-1}$ before *pldA* STOP codon, substitution of gene portion corresponding to *vgrG4b*^{187} with gene portion for *vgrG5*^{169}	This work
PAO1 Δ*rsmA*Δ*vgrG4b*Δ*tssE2::vgrG4b*^{618}*-vgrG5*^{169}*::pldA-bla*$_{TEM-1}$	Deletions in *rsmA*, *vgrG4b, tssE2* and insertion of *bla*$_{TEM-1}$ before *pldA* STOP codon and a substitution of gene portion corresponding to *vgrG4b*^{187} with gene portion for *vgrG5*^{169}	This work
PAO1 Δ*rsmA*Δ*vgrG4b*Δ*tssK3::vgrG4b*^{618}*-vgrG5*^{169}*::pldA-bla*$_{TEM-1}$	Deletions in *rsmA*, *vgrG4b, tssK3* and an insertion of *bla*$_{TEM-1}$ before *pldA* STOP codon and a substitution of gene portion corresponding to *vgrG4b*^{187} with gene portion for *vgrG5*^{169}	This work
PAO1 Δ*rsmA*Δ*vgrG4b*Δ*vgrG5*	Deletions in *rsmA*, *vgrG4b* and *vgrG5*	This work
PAO1 Δ*rsmA*Δ*vgrG5*	Deletions in *rsmA* and *vgrG5 (PA5090)*	This work
PAO1 Δ*rsmA*Δ*vgrG5::pldA-bla*$_{TEM-1}$	Deletions in *rsmA* and *vgrG5* and insertion of *bla*$_{TEM-1}$ before *pldA* STOP codon	This work
PAO1 Δ*rsmA*Δ*vgrG5::pldB-bla*$_{TEM-1}$	Deletions in *rsmA* and *vgrG5* and insertion of *bla*$_{TEM-1}$ before *pldB* STOP codon	This work
PAO1 Δ*rsmA*Δ*vgrG5::vgrG4b*^{618}*-vgrG5*^{169}	Deletions in *rsmA* and *vgrG5*, substitution of gene portion corresponding to *vgrG4b*^{187} with gene portion for *vgrG5*^{169}	This work
PAO1 Δ*rsmA*Δ*vgrG5::vgrG4b*^{618}*-vgrG5*^{169}*::pldB-bla*$_{TEM-1}$	Deletions in *rsmA* and *vgrG5,* substitution of gene portion corresponding to *vgrG4b*^{187} with gene portion for *vgrG5*^{169} and insertion of *bla*$_{TEM-1}$ before *pldB* STOP codon	This work

(Continued)

TABLE 1 | Continued

Strain or plasmid	Relevant characteristics[a]	Source/References
PAO1 Δ*rsmA* Δ*TAA*^{vgrG4b}-*ATG*^{pldA}	Deletion in *rsmA,* deletion of STOP codon of *vgrG4b*, 16bp intergenic region and START codon of *pldA*	This work
PAO1 Δ*rsmA* Δ*tssE2* Δ*TAA*^{vgrG4b}-*ATG*^{pldA}	Deletions in *rsmA* and *tssE2,* deletion of STOP codon of *vgrG4b*, 16bp intergenic region and START codon of *pldA*	This work
Plasmids		
pRK2013	Tra$^+$Mob$^+$, Km^R	Laboratory collection
pCR2.1	TA cloning vector, Ap^R, Km^R	Invitrogen
pCR-BluntII-TOPO	Blunt cloning vector, Zeo^R, Km^R	Invitrogen
pKNG101	Suicide vector, *sacB*, Str^R	(39)
pKNG101-*vgrG4b*	pKNG101-*vgrG4b* deletion construct	Allsopp et al., 2017
pKNG101-*vgrG5*	pKNG101-*vgrG5* deletion construct	This work
pKNG101-*pldA-bla*$_{TEM-1}$	pKNG101 deletion construct to fuse *bla*$_{TEM-1}$ to *pldA* gene	This work
pKNG101-*pldB-bla*$_{TEM-1}$	pKNG101 deletion construct to fuse *bla*$_{TEM-1}$ to *pldB* gene	This work
pKNG101- *vgrG5*^{623}-*vgrG4b*^{187}	pKNG101 deletion construct to substitute final 493 bp of *vgrG5* with 564 bp from *vgrG4b*	This work
pKNG101- *vgrG4b*^{621}-*vgrG5*^{169}	pKNG101 deletion construct to substitute final 564 bp of vgrG4b with 493 bp from *vgrG5*	This work
pKNG1010 Δ*TAA*^{vgrG4b}-*ATG*^{pldA}	pKNG101 deletion construct to delete the STOP codon of *vgrG4b*, 16bp intergenic region and START codon of *pldA*	This work
pKNG101-*tssE2*	pKNG101-*tssE2* deletion construct	Allsopp et al., 2017
pKNG101-*tssK3*	pKNG101-*tssK3* deletion construct	Allsopp et al., 2017
pTrc200	Broad host range pVS1 derivative plasmid, *laclq*, *pTrc* promoter, Sm^R/Sp^R	Schmidt-Eisenlohr et al., 1999; Gift from Erh-Min Lai
p *vgrG4b*	pTrc200 producing full length VgrG4b, Sm^R/Sp^R	This work
pBBR1-mcs4	Broad host range vector, with constitutive *PLAC* promoter, Ap^R/Cb^R	Kovach et al., 1995
p *vgrG5*-HA	pBBR1-MCS-4 encoding *vgrG5* with a C-terminal quadruple HA-tag, Ap^R, Cb^R	This work
p *vgrG5*^{628}-HA	pBBR1-MCS-4 encoding *vgrG5*^{628} with a C-terminal quadruple HA-tag, Ap^R, Cb^R	This work
miniCTX::*lacZ*	Mini-CTX1 harboring the *lacZ* with constitutive promoter, Tc^R	Becher and Schweizer, 2000

[a] *Ap^R, ampicillin resistant; Str^R, Streptomycin resistant; Km^R, Kanamycin resistant; Tc^R, Tetracycline resistant, Cb^R carbenicillin resistant, Sp^R spectinomycin resistant.*

of interest was amplified using the internal primers 3′up and 5′down. Two additional primers, 3′down and 5′up, were used that contain complementary sequences to the opposing side of the splice junction and amplified to yield a fusion fragment. Thus, two subsequent overlap extension PCR steps were undertaken, employing an equimolar ratio of the upstream and downstream fragments as the DNA template. The gene fragments were cloned into pCR-BluntII-TOPO (Invitrogen), their sequences confirmed and sub-cloned into pKNG101 suicide vector. The pKNG-derivatives were maintained in the *E. coli* strain CC118λpir and mobilized into *P. aeruginosa* PAK using *E. coli* 1047 carrying the conjugative plasmid pRK2013 (Figurski and Helinski, 1979). Clones, in which double recombination events occurred, resulting in the deletion of *GOI* or fusion to *GOI*, were isolated using counterselection on sucrose plates as previously described (Vasseur et al., 2005). Gene deletion or fusion was verified by PCR using external primers and western blot analysis where appropriate.

Secretion Assay

Secretion assays were performed similarly as previously described (Hachani et al., 2011). Bacterial suspension was diluted from overnight cultures in TSB to OD_{600} of 0.1 and grown at 25°C to an OD_{600} of 4, unless otherwise stated. A bacterial culture sample adjusted to OD_{600} of 1 was harvested by centrifugation and served as the whole cell sample. Simultaneously, 13 mL of culture was centrifuged at 4 000 *g* for 20 min at 4°C to separate the bacterial cells from culture supernatant. 10 ml of the supernatant was transferred into falcon tubes and centrifuged again; 7 mL of the uppermost supernatant was transferred into new tubes and centrifuged. To 1.8 mL supernatant fraction, we added 200 μl trichloroacetic acid to precipitate proteins overnight at 4°C. The protein precipitate was centrifugated at 16 000 *g* for 30 min at 4°C and washed with cold 90% (v/v) acetone before further centrifugation. After removing the supernatant, the washed pellet was air-dried for 30 min and resuspended in 1× Laemmli buffer to an OD_{600} equivalent of 20.

Western Blot Analysis and SDS-PAGE

For SDS-PAGE analysis, cell extracts were loaded onto SDS polyacrylamide gels, migrated and transferred to a nitrocellulose membrane at 3 mA/cm^2. Following transfer, membranes were incubated overnight in blocking buffer (5% milk powder, 0.1% Tween 20 in Tris-buffered saline, pH 8.0). Polyclonal antibodies

TABLE 2 | Oligonucleotides used in this study.

Deleted gene/ Oligonucleotide	Oligonucleotide sequence[a]
vgrG5	
Up5′	ACAGCCATGTGCTCAACG
Up3′	GGTAGGCGTGGCGAACATTCACTGTCC
Down5′	ATGTTCGCCACGCCTACCGGCGCGACG
Down3′	CGCGATGAGGTTGAGGTT
pldAtli5a	
Up5′	GCGATCAAGATGCCGTTGAC
Up3′	TACTTCTTCCTTCTTCTGCAACATGGA TCAGTC
Down5′	CAGAAGAAGGAAGAAGTACTG CCCCGCC
Down3′	TTCTTCACCAGCATCTCGGT
pldBtli5b$_{123}$	
Up5′	CCTGAAGCAGCCGGAACA
Up3′	CCGCAAACCTATCCTCTGCCTCCTCATCC
Down5′	CAGAGGATAGGTTTGCGGTTTGTACAGGT
Down3′	TAGTGATCGAGGCAGGCATG
TAA^{vgrG4b}*-ATG*^{pldA}	
Up5′	CAAGGACCAGAAGAAGCCCTACAA
Up3′	GGCTTCTTCTGGTCCTTGGCC
Gene fusions/ Oligonucleotide	
pldA-bla$_{TEM-1}$	
Up5′	AAGCATCGCACAGCGGCCAGCCT
Up3′	AGGCTGGCCGCTGTGCGATG
Down5′	ATCGCACATGAAAAGGGTTTTGAT
Down3′	TACCTTCGCAGTTTGGCATG
pldB-bla$_{TEM-1}$	
Up5′	CAAGATCGAGGCGCTCGAAG
Up3′	GTCAAAATCTTACGGTGGACGCGG CCAGCCTGGAAG
Down5′	GCATCGCTCAGTCCACCGTTACCAA TGCTTAATCAG
Down3′	ACAGAGCACGGCCCAAAGTC
vgrG5^{623}*-vgrG4b*^{187}	
Up5′	GGCGCCCTGGCACGGATCAAT
Up3′	GTGCCAGGGCGCCGTCGAGGGTG
Down5′	GCCAAGGACTGACAAGGATGAGC
Down3′	TCCTTGTCAGTCCTTGGCCAGT
vgrG4b^{621}*-vgrG5*^{169}	
Up5′	CGGCCCGCAGGTGATGATCAAC
Up3′	TCATCACCTGCGGGCCGCTGATGGC
Down5′	CGCCATGAGCCAAGGACTGAT
Down3′	CTCATGGCGTGGGCTCAT
Amplified gene/ Oligonucleotide	
vgrG4b	
5′	GCATACTCTAGAGTTGATCTGGTTGAGT TCCTTTTC
3′	GCATACGAGCTCTTTTCGAGAAACAGG GGACAG
vgrG5-HA	
5′	atgGTCGACGAATACGCCAGGAACGCAC
3′	tagGCTAGCGCCGCCGCTGTTGATCATCA
vgrG5^{628}	
5′	atgGTCGACGAATACGCCAGGAACGCAC
3′	tagGCTAGCGCCGCCGCTGTTGATCATCA

[a]*Oligonucleotides are presented in the orientation 5′-3′.*

against the C-terminal extension domain of VgrG4b (VgrG4b^C) were used at a dilution of 1:1000, against Hcp2 at 1:1000 (Jones et al., 2013), against LasB 1:1000 (Gift from Romé Voulhoux). Monoclonal anti-Bla$_{TEM-1}$ (BioLegend) and anti-HA antibodies (BioLegend) were used at a dilution of 1:5000. Monoclonal antibodies against the β subunit of RNA polymerase (RpoB, NeoClone) were used at 1:5000. Secondary antibodies conjugated to horseradish peroxidase were used at a dilution of 1:5000. Western blots were developed using Super-Signal West Pico Chemiluminescent Substrate (Pierce) and visualized on a LAS3000 Fuji Imager.

Interbacterial Competition Assays

Interbacterial competition assays were conducted on solid media due to the contact-dependent killing of the T6SS (Hachani et al., 2013). *P. aeruginosa* prey strains contained the Mini-CTX-lacZ plasmid integrated at the *att* site, consequently giving rise to blue colonies on 5-bromo-4-chloro-3-indolyl-D-galactopyranoside (X-gal)-containing media. Overnight cultures in TSB were collected by centrifugation at 8 000 *g* for 3 min before washing twice in 1 ml sterile PBS and normalized to OD_{600} of 3.0. 100 μl of attacker and 100 μl prey strains for a ratio of 1:1 were mixed. This mixture was centrifuged at 8 000 *g* for 3 min and 100 μl supernatant was removed. 5 μl of each competition mix was spotted in duplicates onto LB-agar, the spots dried, and the Petri dish lids secured using parafilm M (Bemis). Competition plates were inverted and incubated at 25°C for 24 h under H2-T6SS-inducive killing conditions (Allsopp et al., 2017).

The input competitions were serially diluted to 10^{-7}, plated on selective media for both attacker and prey (LB agar with 100 μg mL^{-1} X-gal for blue/white differentiation) of *P. aeruginosa* prey/attacker and grown overnight at 37°C to confirm the input ratios. Competition spots were gathered using 5 μl inoculation loops (VWR) and resuspended in 1 mL PBS. The competition output mixture was serially diluted to 10^{-7}, plated on selective media and grown overnight at 37°C similarly, to the input. Both attacker and prey colony forming units were enumerated on both input and output dilution plates. All competition assays were repeated three times unless otherwise stated and the mean colony forming unit (cfu) of surviving prey strains obtained from all experiments was plotted with the standard deviation.

RESULTS AND DISCUSSION

PldA and PldB Are Delivered Into Prey Cells *via* Their Cognate VgrGs and in a H2-T6SS-Dependent Manner

The tandemly organized genes encoding the T6SS effector phospholipase PldA, also known as Tle5a (Russell et al., 2013), and the structural component VgrG4b are upregulated in an *rsmA* mutant and both proteins are secreted by the H2-T6SS in *P. aeruginosa* PAO1 (**Supplementary Figure S1**; Russell et al., 2013; Allsopp et al., 2017). Yet, this genetic link (**Figure 1A**, top panel) suggested PldA to be delivered as a VgrG4b-dependent effector, which we recently demonstrated by monitoring secretion

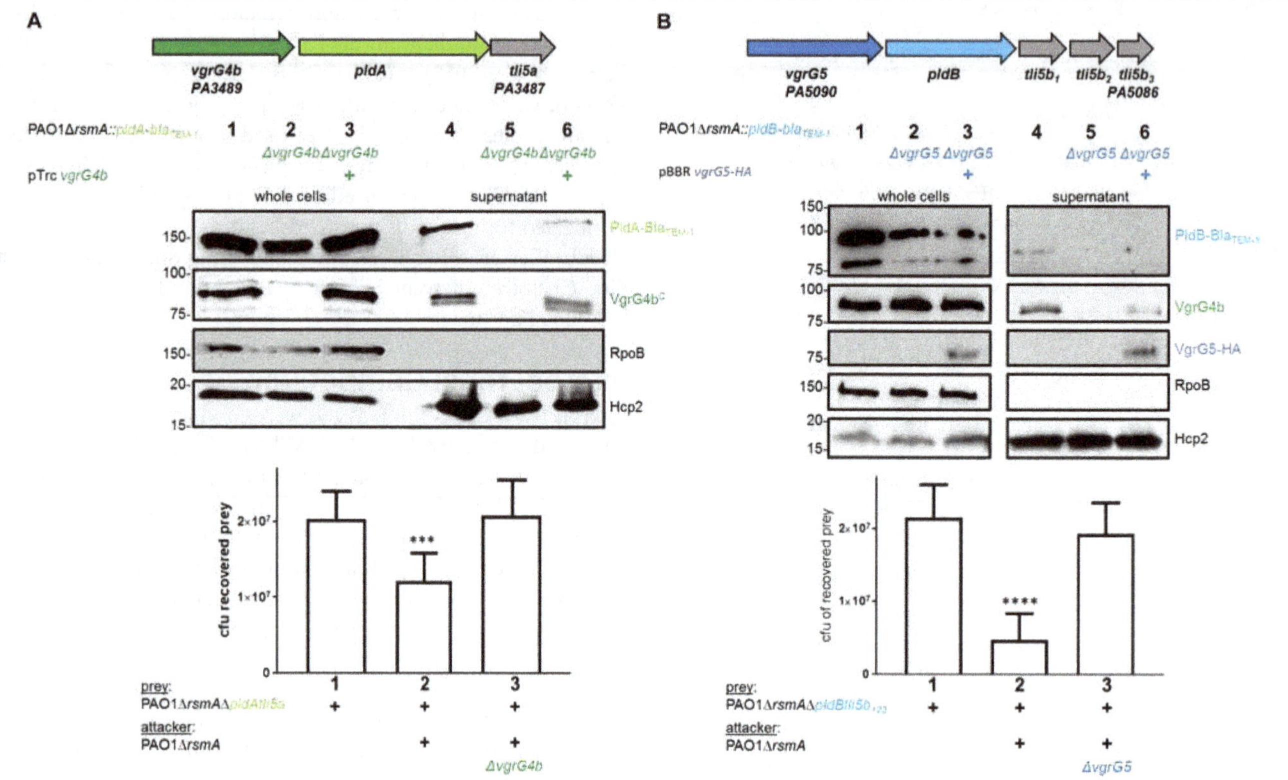

FIGURE 1 | *P. aeruginosa* encodes two phospholipases delivered *via* their cognate VgrGs. **(A)** *vgrG4b* (PA3489, green) is encoded directly upstream of *pldA* (PA3488, bright green). **(B)** *vgrG5* (PA5090, blue) is encoded directly upstream of *pldB* (PA5089, cyan). Second panel: Representative figures of western blots from secretion assays using PAO1 Δ*rsmA* expressing Bla_{TEM-1}-tagged versions of PldA **(A)** or PldB **(B)**. The absence (Δ) of the native *vgrG4b* **(A)** or *vgrG5* **(B)** are indicated. For complementation experiments of the **(A)** *vgrG4b* and **(B)** *vgrG5* mutants, the introduction *in trans* of **(A)** *vgrG4b* (pTrc-*vgrG4b*) and **(B)** *vgrG5* (pBBR1-mcs5-*vgrG5-HA*) are marked with (+). Membranes in **(A)** and **(B)** were revealed, from top to bottom, using antibodies against Bla_{TEM-1}, the C-terminal extension domain of VgrG4b (αVgrG4b^{C}), the HA-tag, RpoB and Hcp2 as indicated on the right. In the bottom panel, bacterial competition outcomes are shown by plots of recovered cfu of prey strains susceptible to PldA delivery, PAO1 Δ*rsmA* Δ*pldAtli5a::lacZ* **(A)**, or PldB delivery, PAO1 Δ*rsmA* Δ*pldBtli5b*$_{123}$*::lacZ* **(B)**, after contact with the attacker strain PAO1 Δ*rsmA* encoding or lacking (Δ) the native *vgrG4b* **(A)** or *vgrG5* **(B)**. Spots were incubated for 24 h at 25 °C in a 1:1 ratio. One-Way ANOVA analysis with Dunnett's multiple comparisons test was conducted on the data set obtained from recovered prey in the absence of an attacker strain with $^{****}p < 0.0001$.

of a chimeric fusion protein PldA-Bla_{TEM-1} (Allsopp et al., 2017). Here, we show that the lack of PldA secretion is solely due to the absence of VgrG4b since PldA release is restored by complementing the *vgrG4b* mutant (**Figure 1A**, middle panel, lane 6). PldA displays antibacterial activity (Russell et al., 2013) and we aimed at elucidating whether VgrG4b would facilitate PldA delivery into neighboring prey cells. We constructed prey strains lacking genes encoding PldA and its immunity Tli5a rendering them susceptible to PldA delivery. When in contact with the parental strain, the prey survival was challenged (**Figure 1A**, lower panel, lane 2), which was not the case when the attacker strain lacked *vgrG4b* (**Figure 1A**, lower panel, lane 3).

Interestingly, *P. aeruginosa* PAO1 produces a second T6SS phospholipase, PldB, also known as Tle5b (Russell et al., 2013), whose corresponding gene is found in a remote locus and downstream of a gene encoding VgrG5 (**Figure 1B**, top panel). To monitor PldB production and secretion using western blot analysis, we engineered a chimeric gene encoding a fusion between PldB and the β-lactamase, Bla_{TEM-1}. Production of the PldB-Bla_{TEM-1} fusion protein is relieved in absence of RsmA (**Supplementary Figure S2**; Allsopp et al., 2017) and we assessed whether PldB delivery is mediated by VgrG5. Remarkably, PldB secretion was abrogated in absence of VgrG5 (**Figure 1B**, middle panel, lane 5), while PldB-mediated killing was abolished when using attacker strains lacking *vgrG5* (**Figure 1B**, bottom panel, lane 3). Complementation of PldB secretion with VgrG5 *in trans* could not be detected (**Figure 1B**, middle panel, lane 6) likely due to low abundance of PldB-Bla_{TEM-1} in complemented cells (lane 3). However, the used VgrG5 construct was functional since it was able to restore VgrG4b secretion, as will be discussed at a later point. Interestingly, secreted PldB-Bla_{TEM-1} was always detected as a smaller band (**Figure 1B**, lane 4) than in the whole cell fraction (lane 1). This is likely to be due to N-terminal processing of the effector as the detected Bla_{TEM-1} domain is fused to the C-terminus of PldB and can still be detected.

A previous study suggested that PldB is delivered into prey cells by the H3-T6SS (Jiang et al., 2014). Here, not only do we show that PldB secretion is dependent on VgrG5, but we observed that VgrG5 secretion is more likely H2-T6SS-dependent. This statement is supported by our analysis

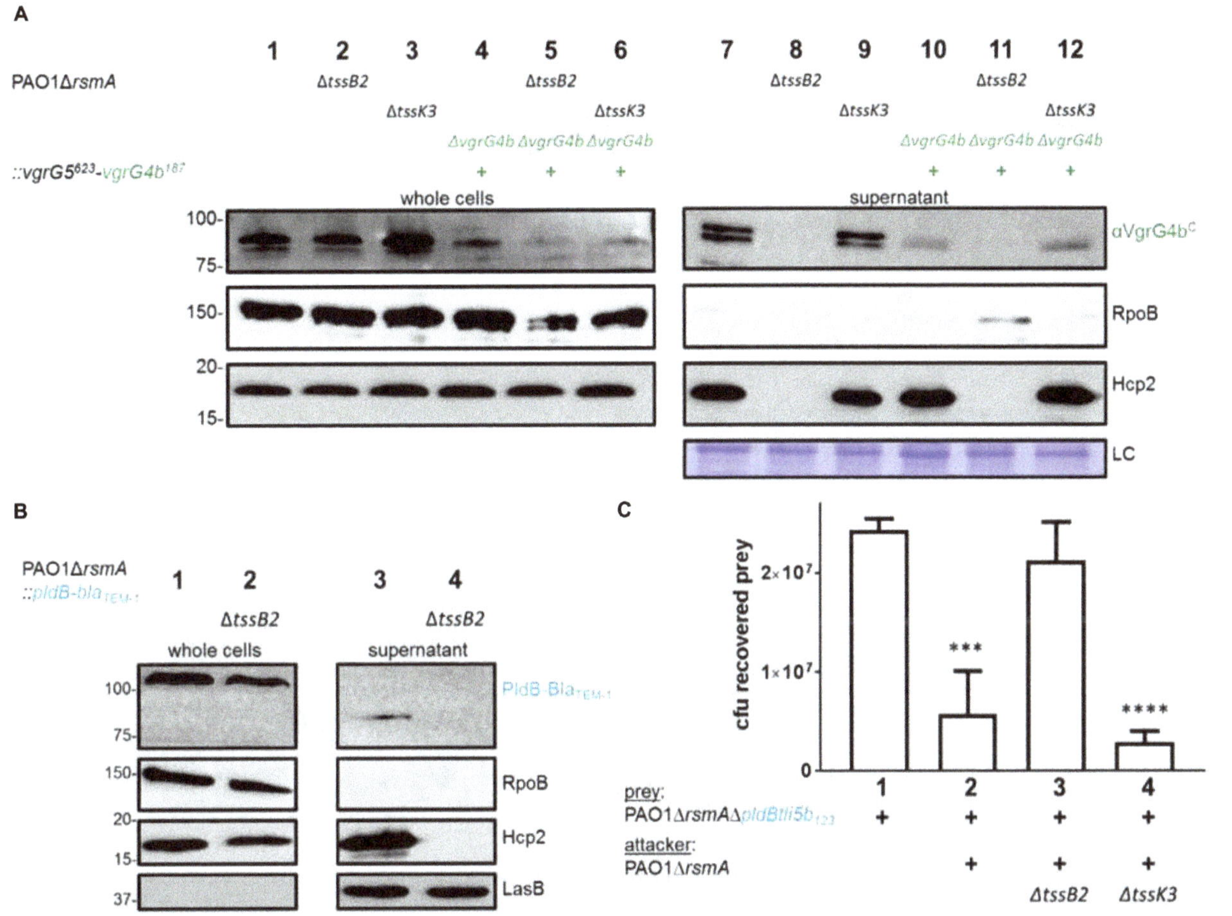

FIGURE 2 | VgrG5 secretion and PldB delivery are H2-T6SS dependent. **(A)** Representative figure of a western blot from a secretion assay using PAO1 Δ*rsmA*. Strains encode native *vgrG4b* or the *vgrG5*^{623}-*vgrG4b*^{187} chimera (+) as well as an active or inactive (Δ) H2-T6SS (Δ*tssB2*) or H3-T6SS (Δ*tssK3*). Antibodies used (from top to bottom) are against VgrG4b^{C}, RpoB and Hcp2 as indicated on the right. A section from a Coomassie gel was included to serve as a loading control (LC) for the supernatant fraction. **(B)** Representative figure of a western blot from a secretion assay using PAO1 Δ*rsmA* expressing a Bla$_{TEM-1}$-tagged version of PldB. Strains produce an active or inactive (Δ*tssB2*) H2-T6SS. Antibodies used (from top to bottom) are against Bla$_{TEM-1}$, RpoB, Hcp2 and LasB as indicated on the right. **(C)** Bacterial competition represented by plots of recovered cfu of prey strain PAO1 Δ*rsmA* Δ*pldBtli5b*$_{123}$*::lacZ* after contact with the attacker strain that encodes a non-functional H2-T6SS (Δ*tssB2*) or H3-T6SS (Δ*tssK3*). As a positive control for PldB-mediated killing, PAO1 Δ*rsmA* was included. Spots were incubated for 24 h at 25 °C in a 1:1 ratio. One-Way ANOVA analysis with Dunnett's multiple comparisons test was conducted on the data set obtained from recovered prey on its own with ****$p < 0.0001$.

of the secretion of a VgrG5^{623}-VgrG4b^{187} chimera (first 623 amino acids of VgrG5, VgrG5^{625} and last 187 aa of VgrG4b, VgrG4b^{187}, **Supplementary Figure S3C**). The VgrG5 portion of the chimera is the core gp27/gp5 domain while the C terminus has been replaced with the C terminus of VgrG4b, which we will describe in further sections. We reasoned that the N-terminal hub domains of the trimeric VgrG spike interact with the top Hcp hexamer of the Hcp tube likely mediating its affiliation to a specific T6SS (Renault et al., 2018). Hence, modifying the C-terminal domain of a VgrG tip protein would have no impact on its affiliation to a specific T6SS. The rationale for using this fusion is that in absence of a VgrG5 antibody we could monitor VgrG5 secretion by western blot analysis using an antibody against the C-terminal domain of VgrG4b. We used PAO1 wild type and mutant strains and showed that the VgrG5^{623}-VgrG4b^{187} chimera is detected in the supernatant of H3-T6SS-inactive (**Figure 2A**, lane 12) but not of H2-T6SS-inactive mutants (**Figure 2A**, lane 11). We further reasoned that if VgrG5 is H2-T6SS-dependent then PldB might also be (**Figure 2B**). We assessed PldB secretion and showed that it was indeed abrogated when using H2-T6SS-inactive mutants (**Figure 2B**, lane 4). Finally, we performed bacterial competition assays (**Figure 2C**) and observed that PldB-mediated killing was only diminished from H2-T6SS inactive attackers (**Figure 2C**, lane 3) but not from those lacking an active H3-T6SS (**Figure 2C**, lane 4).

In all, we demonstrate that VgrG4b and VgrG5 do mediate delivery of their cognate effectors, PldA and PldB, respectively, which agrees with the "à la carte" delivery concept for genetically linked VgrG and cognate T6SS effector. We also showed that these two remote pairs, which are not genetically linked with other core T6SS genes, are H2-T6SS-dependent.

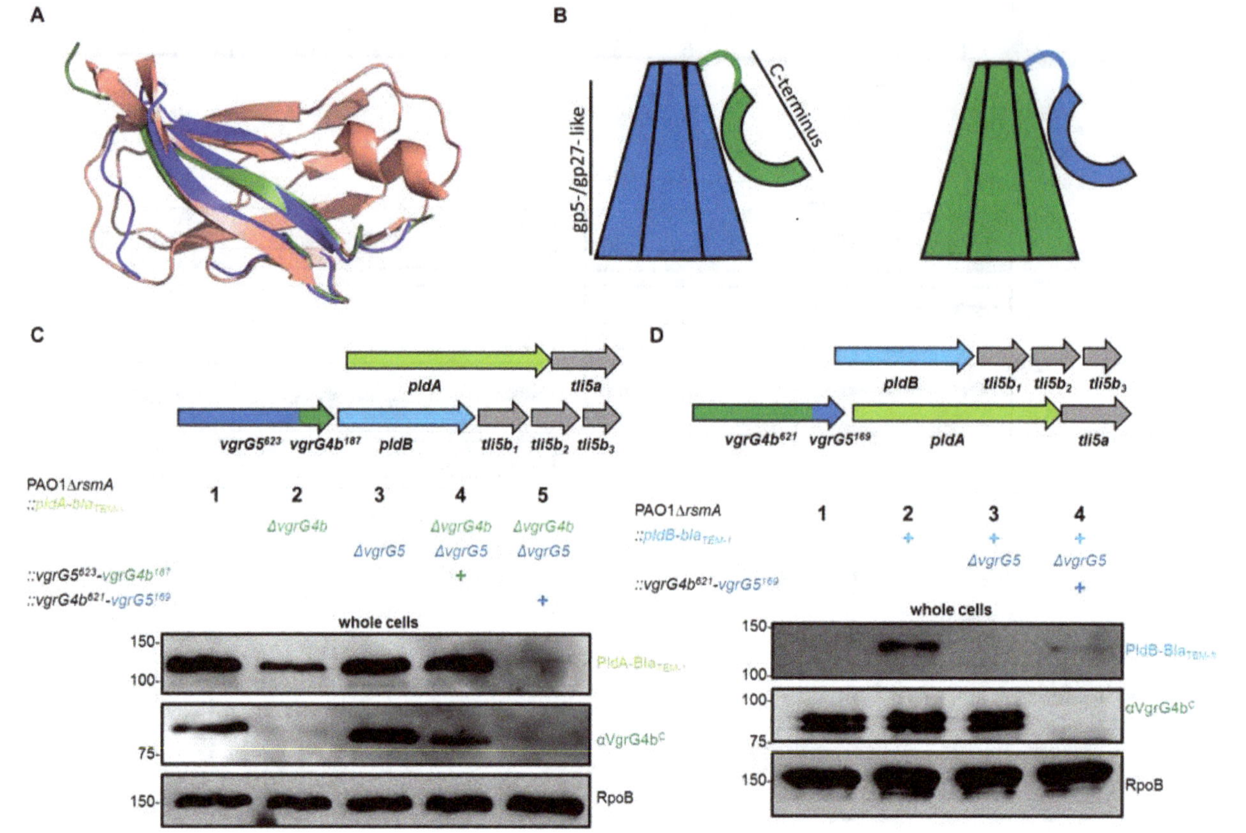

FIGURE 3 | The C-terminal domain of a VgrG specifically stabilizes its cognate effector protein. **(A)** Structural models of the C termini of VgrG4b (green) and VgrG5 (blue) as compared to the transthyretin-like protein from *Salmonella dublin* (red, pdb: 2gpz). **(B)** Schematic of the here used chimerae between VgrG5 (blue) and VgrG4b (green). Highlighted are each the gp5-/gp27-like domains of VgrG4b and VgrG5 as well as the C-terminal domain consisting of the TTR-like domains (aa 648 – 770, see **Supplementary Figure S3** for more details) as shown with an arc form. **(C,D)** Mutant strains carry Bla_{TEM-1}-tagged version of PldA **(C)** or PldB **(D)** as well as the gene clusters as sketched in the top panels and using the color code as in **Figure 1**. **(C)** Strains express one of the following *vgrG* genes: native *vgrG5* (lane 2), native *vgrG4b* (lane 3), *vgrG5*^{623}-*vgrG4b*^{187} chimera (lane 4) or *vgrG4b*^{629}-*vgrG5*^{169} chimera (lane 5). Representative figures of western blots from whole cell fractions of PAO1 Δ*rsmA* derivates as indicated by (+). **(D)** *vgrG4b*^{629}-*vgrG5*^{169} chimera replaces the native *vgrG4b* and the native *vgrG5* gene is deleted. Controls for native effector stability are shown with the parental strains in **(C)** lane 1 and **(D)** lane 2, while the negative controls lack the cognate *vgrG* locus in **(C)** lane 2 or in **(D)** lane 3. Antibodies used (top to bottom) are against Bla_{TEM-1}, VgrG4b^{C} and RpoB as indicated on the right of each panel.

The C-Terminal TTR-Like Domains of VgrG4b and VgrG5 Differ and Are Specific for Recognition of PldA and PldB

Recognition of T6SS effectors by a cognate VgrG could be direct or involve adaptor proteins facilitating the interaction. In *A. tumefaciens* it has been shown that the two VgrGs, VgrG1 and VgrG2, specifically bind and recognize their cognate effectors Tde1 and Tde2 (Bondage et al., 2016). In this case, Tde1 and Tde2 recognition involves two distinct adaptor proteins, Tap1, a DUF4123 protein, and Atu3641, a DUF2169 protein, respectively. The adaptor genes *tap1* and *atu3641* are genetically linked with the cognate effector genes *tde1* and *tde2*, respectively, and the adaptor proteins bind their cognate effectors to recruit them at the C-terminal regions of VgrG1 and VgrG2, respectively (Bondage et al., 2016).

No adaptor genes are located in the vicinity of *pldA* or *pldB* suggesting that the corresponding effectors bind directly to their respective VgrG spikes. Using bioinformatic analysis, we identified transthyretin (TTR)-like folds within the C-terminal domains of both VgrG4b and VgrG5 (**Figure 3A**). Importantly, TTR-like domains within VgrG proteins have been shown to mediate binding of the cognate effector to the VgrG C terminus, as is the case in enteroaggregative *E. coli* and the VgrG1-dependent delivery of Tle1 (Flaugnatti et al., 2015).

The TTR-like domains of VgrG4b and VgrG5 share 25 % sequence identity, while their N-terminal gp5-/gp27-like domains share 69 % identity (**Supplementary Figure S3A**). From these observations, we hypothesized that specificity for PldA and PldB lies within the C-terminal domains of VgrG4b and VgrG5, respectively. To assess this concept, we swapped the C-terminal domains between VgrG4b (the C-terminal 187 amino acids) and VgrG5 (the C-terminal 169 amino acids) as depicted in **Supplementary Figures S3B,C** leading to chimeric VgrG proteins (**Figure 3B**). For VgrG protein detection we used an antibody that specifically recognizes the C terminus of VgrG4b as shown already in **Figure 2A**. As such, from the

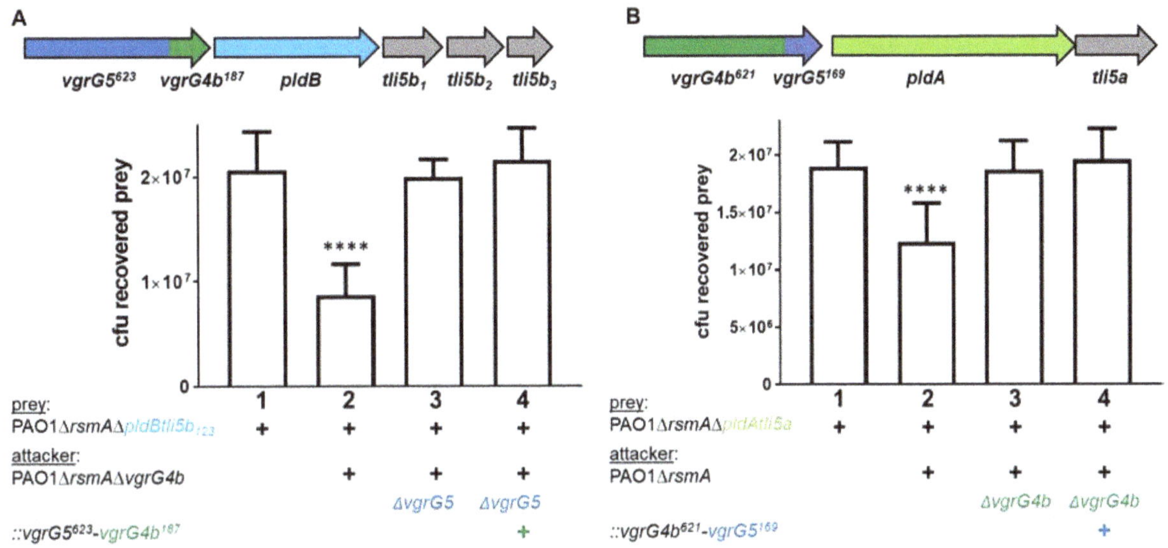

FIGURE 4 | Modifying the VgrG C-terminus abrogates delivery of cognate effectors. The *vgrG* cluster color code is as in **Figure 1**. The mutant strains used carry the gene sequence for **(A)** *vgrG5*^{623}-*vgrG4b*^{187} chimera and **(B)** *vgrG4b*^{621}-*vgrG5*^{169} chimera. Note that mutants in **(A)** encode the N terminal 623 amino acids of VgrG5 (blue) and the last C-terminal 187 amino acids of VgrG4b (+, green, **Supplementary Figure S4B**) and mutants in **(B)** encode the N terminal 621 amino acids of VgrG4b and the last C-terminal 169 amino acids of VgrG5 (+, **Supplementary Figure S4C**). Bottom panels: bacterial competition experiments and plots of recovered cfu of prey strains as described in **Figure 1**. Recovery is after contact with the attacker strain that encodes **(A)** native *vgrG5* or the *vgrG5*^{623}-*vgrG4b*^{187} chimera (+) or **(B)** native *vgrG4b* or the *vgrG4b*^{621}-*vgrG5*^{169} (+). As a positive control for effector-mediated killing, the parental strains were included (lanes 2), while the negative control lacked the cognate *vgrG* (lanes 3). Spots were incubated for 24 h at 25 °C in a 1:1 ratio. One-Way ANOVA analysis with Dunnett's multiple comparisons test was conducted on data set obtained from recovered prey on their own with $^{****}p < 0.0001$.

two chimeric VgrGs, that we engineered, the antibody could detect the VgrG5^{623}-VgrG4b^{187} chimera (**Figure 3C**, lane 4), but not the VgrG4b^{621}-VgrG5^{169} chimera (**Figure 3D**, lane 4). We also used strains that produce Bla$_{TEM-1}$-tagged versions of PldA or PldB (**Figures 3C,D**, upper panels) so that production of these T6SS effectors could be followed with an antibody directed against the Bla$_{TEM-1}$ portion of the chimeric proteins. We performed western blot analysis of whole cell lysates derived from various strains and observed that in absence of VgrG4b, there is a consistent decrease in the amount of the cognate effector PldA (**Figure 3C**, lane 2). A stable PldA protein is only seen in presence of VgrG4b (**Figure 3C**, lanes 1 and 3) or its C-terminal domain (**Figure 3C**, lane 4). Instead, the sole presence of VgrG5 (**Figure 3C**, lane 2) or its C-terminal domain (**Figure 3C**, lane 5) had no stabilizing effect on PldA. On the other hand, the absence of VgrG5 has an even more drastic impact on the abundance of its cognate effector PldB (**Figure 3D**, lane 3). Interestingly, PldB stability was partly restored when the C terminus of the cognate VgrG5 was expressed as part of a VgrG4b chimera (**Figure 3D**, lane 4), which would suggest that the cognate VgrG C terminus is sufficient to help stabilizing the effector.

Here, it is interesting to observe that stability of the T6SS effectors PldA and PldB depends on the C-terminal domains of their cognate VgrGs. On multiple occasions, it has been experimentally validated that T6SS effectors require the presence of cognate T6SS components for their stability. Tse2 from *P. aeruginosa* was shown to be degraded in absence of its receptor Hcp1 (Silverman et al., 2013), while purification of the effector Tde1 from *A. tumefaciens* led to higher yields in presence of its adaptor protein Tap1 (Ma et al., 2014). Furthermore, substrates from other bacterial secretion systems require the presence of dedicated chaperone proteins for stability. For example, the T3SS substrate YopE from *Y. pseudotuberculosis* (Birtalan et al., 2002) as well as the T4SS substrate VirE2 from *A. tumefaciens* (Zhao et al., 2001; Sutherland et al., 2012) require chaperones to connect to the cognate secretion machinery. For PldA and PldB, the C-terminal domains of their cognate VgrGs likely act as chaperone domains.

The mechanism involving specific binding and stabilization of a toxic protein by a secretion component prior to its export likely represents a survival strategy in addition to the presence of cognate immunity proteins. Upon binding of the toxic protein by the secretion component, the cell ensures to rapidly deliver the toxin out of the cell where it can execute its damaging effect. However, when lacking the cognate secretion component, the toxin would accumulate within the cell likely leading to cellular damage. In this case, the cell would trigger degradation of the toxin to quickly prevent deleterious outcomes.

All our results indicate that PldA and PldB are specifically stabilized, and likely chaperoned, by the C-terminal TTR domains of their cognate VgrG proteins. If this were the case, a modified VgrG C-terminal extension domain would jeopardize the cognate effector delivery. We tested this hypothesis and used appropriate *P. aeruginosa* strains producing VgrG4b^{621}-VgrG5^{169} or VgrG5^{623}-VgrG4b^{187} chimera to challenge prey cells susceptible to PldB (**Figure 4A**) or PldA (**Figure 4B**) injection. Note that the susceptibility is conferred by the deletion of appropriate immunity genes, *tli5b*$_{123}$ or *tli5a* in the prey

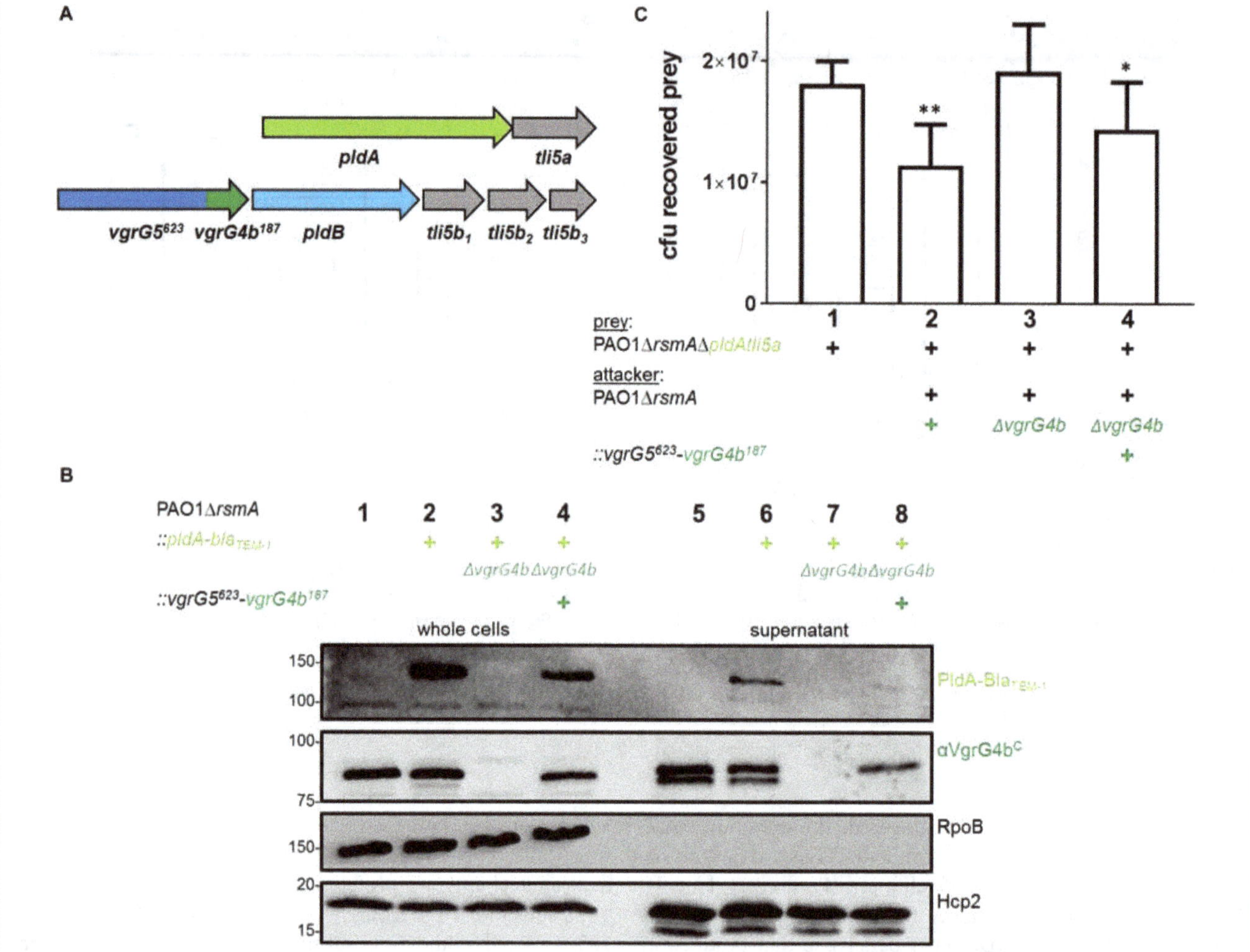

FIGURE 5 | Substitution of the VgrG5 C-terminus with the VgrG4b C-terminus restores PldA delivery. **(A)** Schematic depicting a strain carrying the *vgrG5*^{623}-*vgrG4b*^{187} chimeric gene at the native *vgrG5*. The native *vgrG4b* is deleted. **(B)** Representative figure of a western blot from a secretion assay using PAO1 Δ*rsmA* or PAO1 Δ*rsmA::pldA-bla*$_{TEM-1}$ (+) encoding native *vgrG4b* or the *vgrG5*^{623}-*vgrG4b*^{187} chimera (+). As a control for PldA-Bla$_{TEM-1}$ secretion, the parental strain was included (lane 6), while the negative control lacked the native *vgrG4b* (lane 7). Antibodies used (from top to bottom) are against Bla$_{TEM-1}$, VgrG4b^{C}, RpoB and Hcp2 as indicated on the right. **(C)** Bacterial competition represented by plots of recovered cfu of prey strain PAO1 Δ*rsmA* Δ*pldAtli5a::lacZ* after contact with the attacker strain that encodes native *vgrG4b* or the *vgrG5*^{623}-*vgrG4b*^{187} chimera (+). As a positive control for PldA-mediated killing, PAO1 Δ*rsmA* was included (lane 2), while the negative control lacked *vgrG4b* (lane 3). Spots were incubated for 24 h at 25 °C in a 1:1 ratio. One-Way ANOVA analysis with Dunnett's multiple comparisons test was conducted on data set obtained from recovered prey on their own with ****$p < 0.0001$.

cells. Remarkably, attacker strains with a modified cognate VgrG (**Figure 4**, lanes 4, respectively) failed to outcompete corresponding susceptible prey cells thus confirming that the C-terminal domain of VgrG is instrumental for effector recognition and delivery.

Swapping the C-Terminal TTR-Like Domain to Redirect Effectors to the VgrG Tip

We then sought to exploit the concept of VgrG C-terminal specificity to force PldA to use a VgrG5 vehicle carrying the VgrG4b C terminus, i.e., a VgrG5^{623}-VgrG4b^{187} chimera (**Figure 5A**). Remarkably, PldA was identified in the supernatant fraction of cells expressing VgrG5^{623}-VgrG4b^{187}, which was also secreted (**Figure 5B**, lane 8). We also performed competition assays and showed that cells expressing VgrG5^{623}-VgrG4b^{187} display a competitive advantage toward prey cells lacking the *pldAtli5a* effector-immunity locus, which are thus PldA-sensitive (**Figure 5C**). These results suggest that presence of the C-terminal domain of VgrG4b at the VgrG5 tip is sufficient to adapt VgrG5 for PldA delivery and that it is possible to redirect an effector to a non-cognate VgrG vehicle.

Interdependent VgrG Secretion Compromises the Swapping Specificity Hypothesis

We further aimed to test whether the same concept would hold true to adapt the effector PldB to a non-cognate VgrG

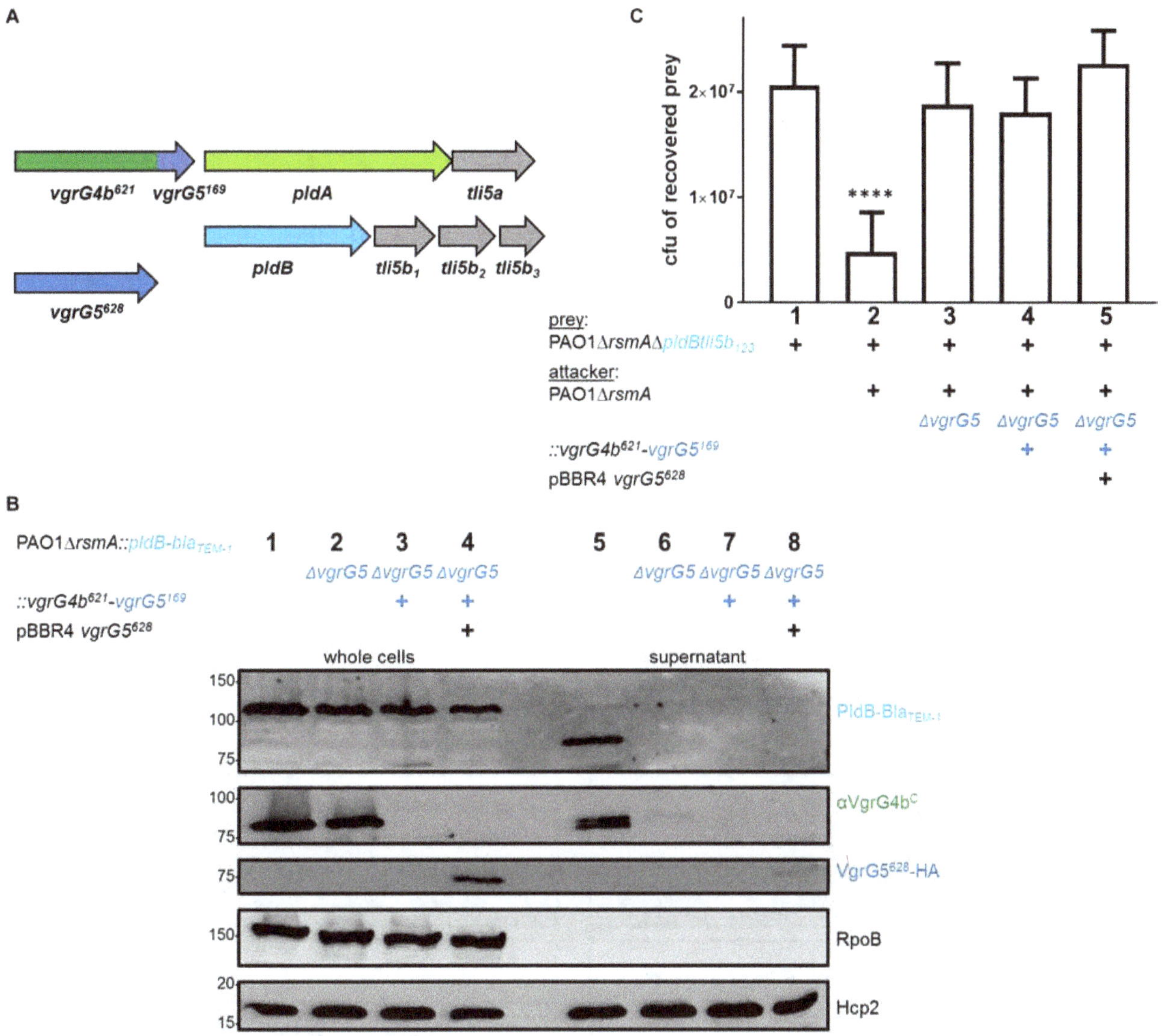

FIGURE 6 | Production of the VgrG5 N-terminus (VgrG5^{628}) does not support PldB secretion. **(A)** Schematic depicting a strain carrying the chimeric gene *vgrG4b*^{629}-*vgrG5*^{169} at the native *vgrG4b* locus and in absence of the native *vgrG5* gene. A construct encoding a quadruple HA-tagged version of VgrG5^{628} is expressed from *pBBR1-mcs4* (pBBR4-*vgrG5*^{628}). **(B)** Representative figure of a western blot of a secretion assay using PAO1 Δ*rsmA::pldB-bla*$_{\text{TEM}-1}$ in presence of the native *vgrG5*, encoding the *vgrG4b*^{629}-*vgrG5*^{169} chimera (+) or carrying pBBR4-*vgrG5*^{628} (+). Antibodies used (from top to bottom) are against Bla$_{\text{TEM}-1}$, VgrG4b^{C}, HA, RpoB and Hcp2 as indicated on the right. **(C)** Bacterial competition represented by plot of recovered cfu of prey strain PAO1 Δ*rsmA* Δ*pldBtli5b*$_3$*::lacZ* after contact with the attacker strain that encoded native *vgrG5* or the *vgrG4b*^{629}-*vgrG5*^{169} chimera (+) or pBBR1-*mcs4 vgrG5*^{628} (+). As a positive control for PldB-mediated killing, PAO1 Δ*rsmA* was included (lane 2), while the negative control lacked the native *vgrG5* locus (lane 3). Spots were incubated for 24 h at 25 °C in a 1:1 ratio. One-Way ANOVA analysis with Dunnett's multiple comparisons test was conducted on data set obtained from recovered prey on their own with $^{****}p < 0.0001$.

vehicle. Indeed, when using the VgrG4b^{621}-VgrG5^{169} chimera to specifically bind and deliver PldB (**Figure 6A**), neither secretion (**Figure 6B**, lane 7) nor delivery into prey cells (**Figure 6C**, lane 4) could be observed. One plausible explanation is that VgrG4b secretion is abolished in absence of VgrG5 (**Figure 6B**, lane 6 and **Figure 1B**, lane 5). This would further impact secretion of the VgrG4b^{621}-VgrG5^{169} chimera as it is expressed in a *vgrG5*-deficient background to avoid cross specificity for the cognate effector PldB. Nevertheless, absence of neither VgrG4b nor VgrG4b^{621}-VgrG5^{169} secretion is due to an inactive H2-T6SS, as Hcp2 is efficiently secreted (**Figure 1B**, lane 5 and **Figure 6B**, lane 6). This result challenged our concept that an effector can be delivered *via* any VgrG vehicle solely by equipping it with the appropriate C-terminal domain.

Since VgrG4b mediates PldA delivery, we hypothesized that VgrG5 absence would thus in turn affect PldA delivery into prey cells, which appeared to be the case (**Figure 7A**, lane 4). A straightforward explanation for VgrG4b secretion being dependent on VgrG5 would be that both might be part of a hetero-trimer. Indeed, in both *P. aeruginosa* and *V. cholerae,*

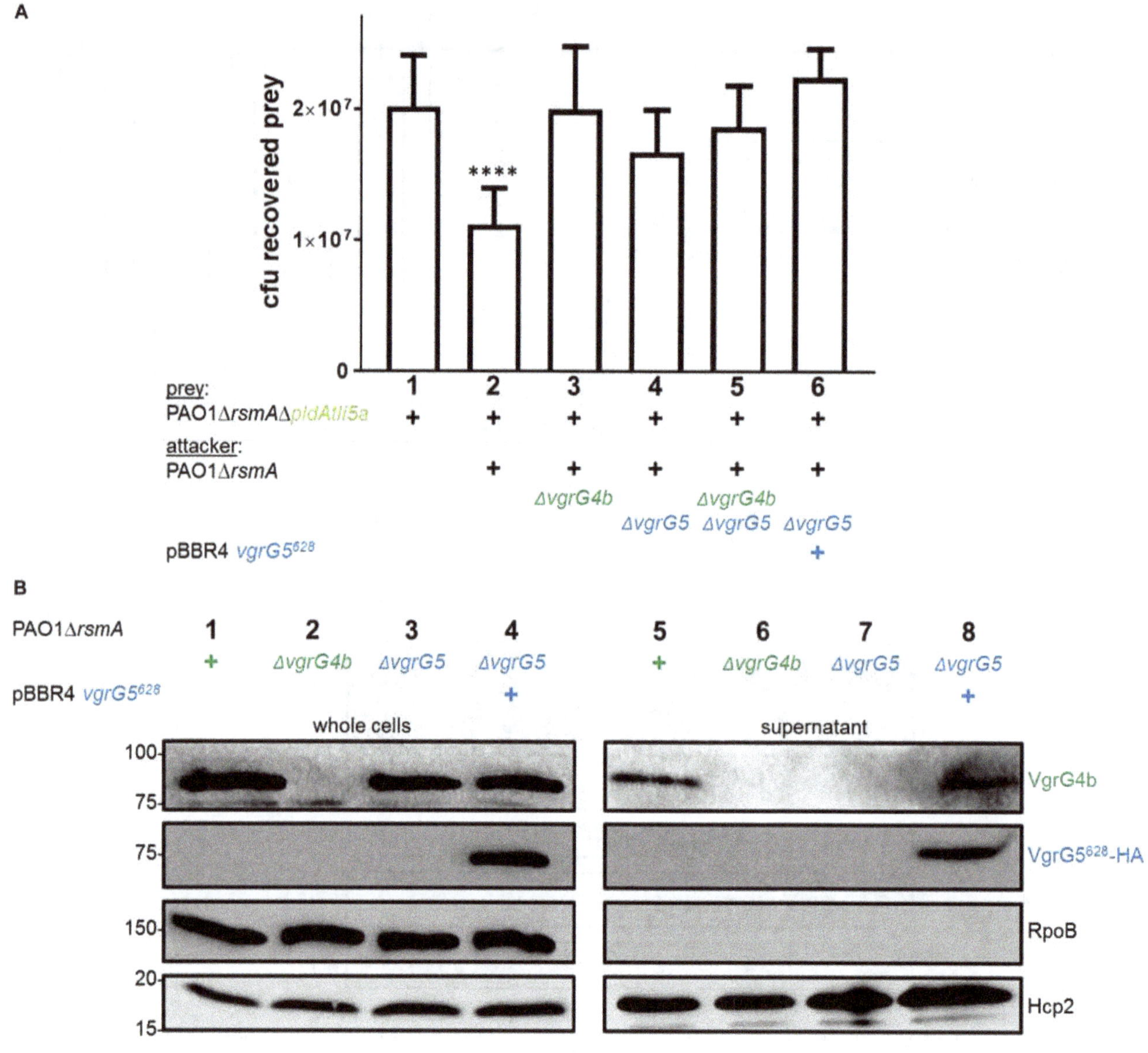

FIGURE 7 | VgrG5 mediates delivery of both PldA and PldB. **(A)** Plots of recovered cfu of prey strains susceptible for PldA delivery upon bacterial competition assays. Prey strains are as described in **Figure 1**. PAO1 Δ*rsmA* attacking strains either lacked (Δ) *vgrG4b*, *vgrG5* or both, or expressed *vgrG5*^{628} *in trans* (+). Spots were incubated for 24 h at 25 °C in a 1:1 ratio. One-Way ANOVA analysis with Dunnett's multiple comparisons test was conducted on the data set obtained from recovered prey on their own with ****$p < 0.0001$. **(B)** Representative figure of western blot from a secretion assay using PAO1 Δ*rsmA*. The absence (Δ) of the native *vgrG5* or *vgrG4b* is shown as well as when expressing an HA-tagged version of *vgrG5*^{628} *in trans* (+). Antibodies (from top to bottom) against the C-terminal portion of VgrG4b (VgrG4b), HA, RpoB and Hcp2 were used as indicated on the right.

it has been suggested that the spike can be made of a hetero-complex of various VgrG proteins (Pukatzki et al., 2007; Hachani et al., 2011). Hence, we investigated whether VgrG4b could be secreted as part of a hetero-trimer with VgrG5. In **Figure 1B**, middle panel, lane 6, we showed that presence of full length VgrG5 is sufficient to restore VgrG4b secretion. Since trimerization of VgrG proteins to a functional spike is mediated by their gp5/gp27-like domains (Spinola-Amilibia et al., 2016), we hypothesized that expression of solely the VgrG5 N-terminal domain (first 628 amino acids, VgrG5^{628}) would suffice to form a functional spike. By performing a secretion assay using a *vgrG5* mutant, we indeed verified that VgrG4b secretion is restored in presence of VgrG5^{628} only (**Figure 7B**, lane 8). This also confirmed that the C terminus of VgrG5 is not required to support VgrG4b secretion.

Since VgrG4b is secreted in presence of VgrG5^{628}, we reasoned that this construct would restore PldA delivery, which was not observed (**Figure 7A**, lane 6). There are potential explanations for this observation. One would be the existence of an effector delivery hierarchy. For example, VgrG5 homotrimer-dependent delivery of PldB might be initially required for subsequent VgrG4b homotrimer-dependent delivery of PldA.

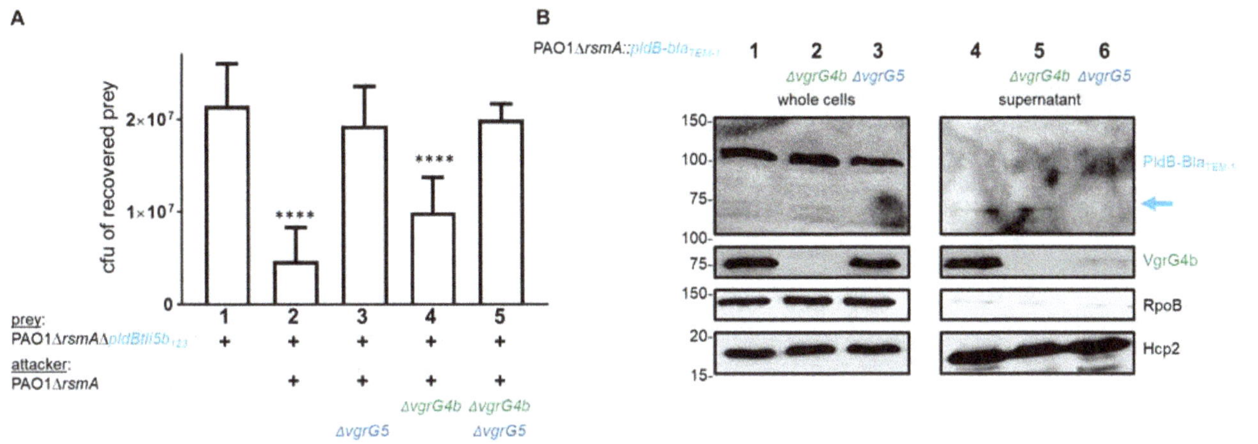

FIGURE 8 | Absence of VgrG4b has no impact on PldB delivery. **(A)** Plots of recovered cfu of prey strains susceptible for PldB delivery upon bacterial competition assays. Prey strains are as described in **Figure 1**. PAO1 Δ*rsmA* attacking strains either lacked (Δ) *vgrG4b*, *vgrG5* or both. Spots were incubated for 24 h at 25°C in a 1:1 ratio. One-Way ANOVA analysis with Dunnett's multiple comparisons test was conducted on the data set obtained from recovered prey on their own with ****$p < 0.0001$. **(B)** Representative figure of a western blot from a secretion assay using PAO1 Δ*rsmA::pldB-bla*$_{TEM-1}$. Strains lack (Δ) native *vgrG4b* or *vgrG5*. The blue arrow on the right indicates the secretion product of PldB-Bla$_{TEM-1}$, which is not visible when *vgrG5* is deleted. Antibodies used (from top to bottom) are against Bla$_{TEM-1}$, VgrG4b^C, RpoB and Hcp2 as indicated on the right.

As such, using the truncated VgrG5^{628} would not suffice to trigger VgrG4b-PldA delivery since PldB was not delivered. We tested this hypothesis by monitoring PldA delivery in absence of PldB (**Supplementary Figure S4**). An attacking strain lacking PldB showed to have the same competitive advantage toward a PldA-lacking strain (lane 5) as the parental strain (lane 2). Hence, the effector hierarchy concept is not fully supported by this observation.

An alternative possibility could be that another T6SS component, such as an adaptor or chaperone, binds the C-terminal domains of VgrG5 and VgrG4b in a VgrG4b-VgrG5 hetero-trimer and thus triggers binding of PldA toward the spike. There is for example evidence suggesting that the chaperone TecT connects the effector TseT to a VgrG4b-VgrG6 hetero-trimer (Burkinshaw et al., 2018). A similar concept could be possible for a VgrG4b-VgrG5-PldA complex. However, the finding that PldA is delivered from a VgrG5^{623}-VgrG4b^{187} chimera lacking the C-terminal domain of VgrG5 (**Figure 5**) is not in full agreement with this hypothesis. Yet it is clear that VgrG5 does not need another VgrG for its secretion and is able to deliver any effector as long as it carries a cognate C-terminal domain, here PldA through the Vgr4b C-terminal domain.

We hypothesized that co-expression of the VgrG5^{628} construct would also facilitate delivery of the VgrG4b^{621}-VgrG5^{169} chimera, which in turn would mediate PldB delivery (**Figure 6A**). However, neither PldB secretion (**Figure 6B**, lane 8) nor PldB-mediated killing (**Figure 6C**, lane 5) could be observed. This result might be explained by the lack of recognition of a cognate PAAR protein, which specifically binds the VgrG tip (Shneider et al., 2013). Here, we starkly modified the PAAR recognition site, which might have rendered this tip unrecognizable for its cognate PAAR protein and thus unsuitable for secretion.

Due to the impact of VgrG5 on PldA delivery, we finally questioned whether VgrG4b would be involved in PldB delivery (**Figure 8**). We challenged PldB-sensitive prey strains with attackers deficient for *vgrG4b*, *vgrG5* or both and observed that VgrG4b absence reduced PldB delivery, while significant killing could still be observed (**Figure 8A**, lane 4). We confirmed these data with a secretion assay demonstrating that PldB is still secreted into the supernatant in VgrG4b absence (**Figure 8B**, lane 5). From these results we conclude that VgrG5 alone suffices for PldB delivery, while PldA delivery depends on both VgrG4b and VgrG5.

VgrG4b Can Deliver PldA When Covalently Linked to the Spike

In the previous sections we made clear that a VgrG spike can recognize its cognate effector likely through specific protein-protein interaction. It is also known that many VgrGs, called "evolved" VgrGs display an effector domain fused at their C terminus (Ma et al., 2009; Sana et al., 2015). We wonder whether there is a rationale behind having the effector fused to the VgrG C terminus versus a protein-protein interaction delivery mode, or whether this is only the result of a fortuitous evolutionary process.

We demonstrated that PldA is delivered as a cargo effector dependent on VgrG4b and here assessed whether delivery is compromised if PldA is covalently linked to the VgrG4b C terminus. Hence, we deleted the STOP codon of *vgrG4b*, the intergenic region and the START codon of *pldA* (**Figure 9A**). Expression of this gene would thus lead to production of one single polypeptide consisting of VgrG4b and PldA, which we could readily detect using western blot analysis (**Figure 9B**, lane 3). The same product was detected in the supernatant fraction of H2-T6SS active strains (**Figure 9B**, lane 7), but not of H2-T6SS inactive strains (**Figure 9B**, lane 8) suggesting that secretion of

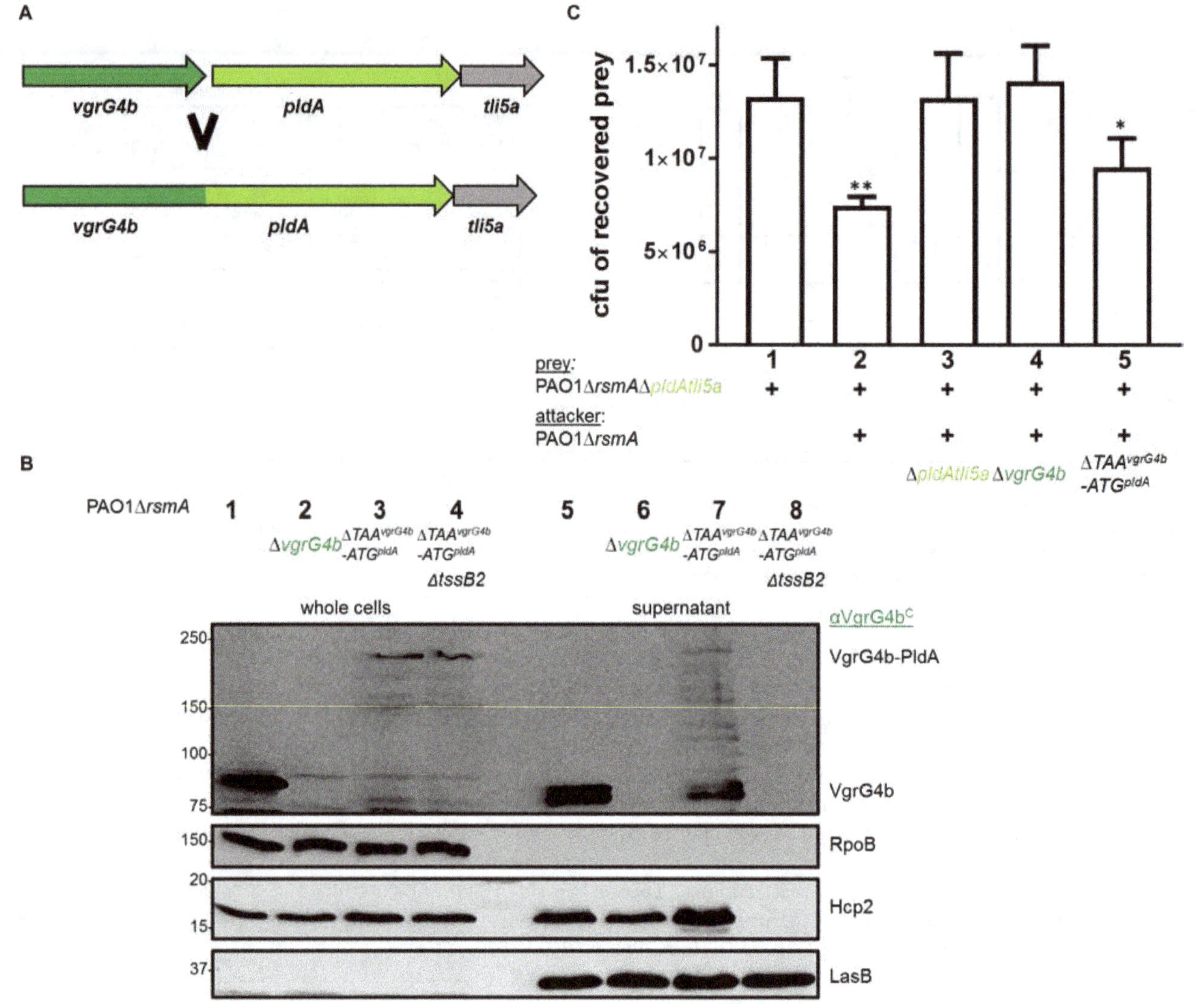

FIGURE 9 | VgrG4b can deliver PldA when fused to its C-terminus. **(A)** The STOP codon of *vgrG4b*, the intergenic region and START-codon of *pldA* were deleted resulting in a single chimeric gene product. **(B)** Representative figure of a western blot from a secretion assay using PAO1 Δ*rsmA* with an active or inactive H2-T6SS (Δ*tssB2*) encoding VgrG4b-PldA (ΔTAA^{vgrG4b}-ATG^{pldA}). As a positive control for VgrG4b secretion, PAO1 Δ*rsmA* (lane 1) was included, while the negative control lacked *vgrG4b* (lane 2). Antibodies used (from top to bottom) are against $VgrG4b^{C}$, RpoB, Hcp2 and LasB, a T2SS substrate (Olson and Ohman, 1992) acting as a loading control for the supernatant, as indicated on the right. **(C)** Bacterial competition represented by plots of recovered cfu of prey strain PAO1 Δ*rsmA* Δ*pldAtli5a*::*lacZ* after contact with the attacker strain encoding WT PldA, WT VgrG4b or the fusion VgrG4b-PldA (ΔTAA^{vgrG4b}-ATG^{pldA}) as indicated. As a positive control for PldA-mediated killing, PAO1 Δ*rsmA* was included (lane 2) while the negative controls lacked *pldAtli5a* (lane 3) or *vgrG4b* (lane 4). Spots were incubated for 24 h at 25 °C in a 1:1 ratio. One-Way ANOVA analysis with Dunnett's multiple comparisons test was conducted on the data set obtained from the recovered prey on its own with *$p < 0.05$ and **$p < 0.01$.

the VgrG4b-PldA fusion remains H2-T6SS-dependent. Note, that additional bands most likely representing VgrG4b degradation products can be detected in the supernatant fraction but to a lesser amount as in the whole cells. This suggests that the artificially evolved VgrG4b-PldA protein becomes prone for proteolysis once secreted into the environment.

We further investigated whether such a fusion could be injected into bacterial prey cells. We challenged PldA-sensitive preys against *P. aeruginosa* strains expressing the VgrG4b-PldA fusion (**Figure 9C**, lane 5) and observed that they are outcompeted to a similar extent as when in competition with the parental strain (**Figure 9C**, lane 2). This led us to conclude that the VgrG4b-PldA fusion protein can be delivered by *P. aeruginosa* both into the extracellular milieu and into neighboring bacteria.

The H2-T6SS Could Be a Core System for the Delivery of Remote VgrG Spikes

We previously showed that *P. aeruginosa* uses its H1-T6SS to deliver at least three different VgrG-dependent antibacterial effectors into target prey cells, namely Tse5, Tse6 and Tse7

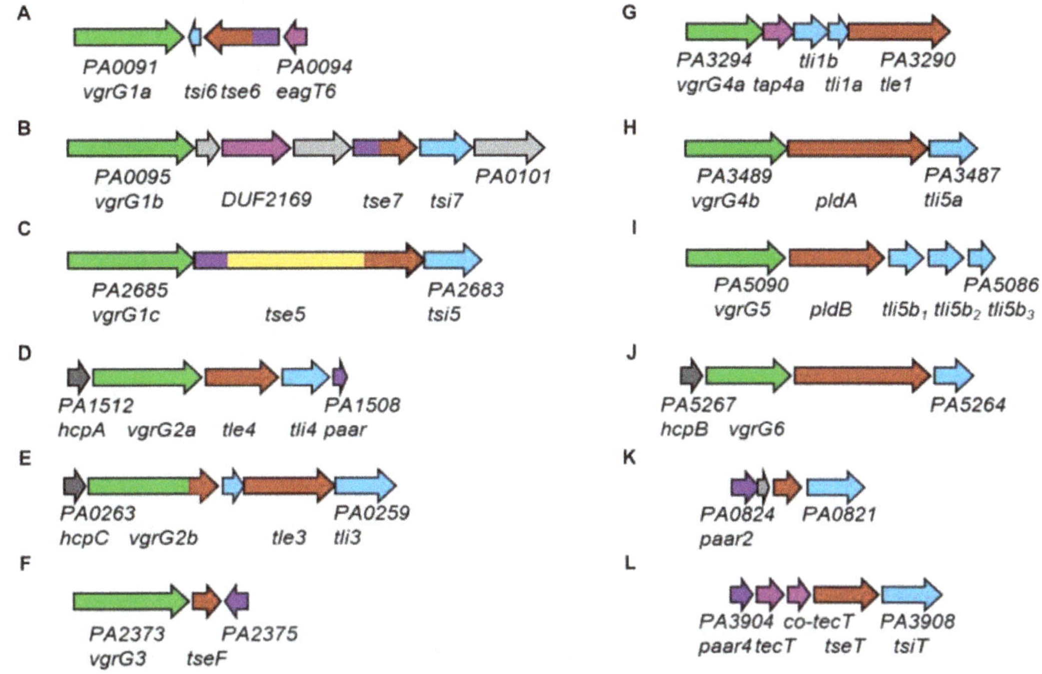

FIGURE 10 | Genomic loci containing *vgrG* or *paar* genes of *P. aeruginosa* PAO1. *vgrG* genes are shown in green, effector genes in red, cognate immunities in cyan, *hcp* genes in dark gray, *paar* genes in purple, *tap* genes in magenta and genes of unknown function in gray. For all examples, the PA numbers of the two outer genes are shown. Effector genes close to their (putative) cognate vgrG or PAAR genes are the following: **(A)** tse6; **(B)** tse7; **(C)** tse5; **(D)** tle4; **(E)** tle3; **(F)** tseF; **(G)** tle1; **(H)** pldA; **(I)** pldB; **(J)** PA5265; **(K)** PA0822; **(L)** tseT.

(Hachani et al., 2014; Pissaridou et al., 2018). All of these effectors are evolved PAARs that interact with their cognate VgrGs, VgrG1c, VgrG1a and VgrG1b (**Figures 10A–C**), respectively, *via* their N-terminal PAAR domains (Shneider et al., 2013; Whitney et al., 2015). In case of the H3-T6SS, information about associated effectors is scarce. In the H3-T6SS cluster, *vgrG3* as well as the effector *tseF* are encoded (**Figure 10F**) and it is proposed that TseF secretion is H3-T6SS-dependent (Lin et al., 2017). Although not experimentally demonstrated, it is likely that considering the genetic linkage, TseF delivery might also be VgrG3-dependent. Previous reports have also suggested that PldB delivery is H3-T6SS-dependent (Jiang et al., 2014), however, here we show that this effector is secreted in a H2-T6SS-dependent fashion and requires the cognate VgrG5.

There is experimental evidence that the H2-T6SS is responsible for delivery of VgrG4b (Allsopp et al., 2017), VgrG5 (this study), VgrG2a and VgrG2b (Sana et al., 2015). We here provide functional evidence, that VgrG4b specifically delivers PldA (**Figure 10H**) and VgrG5 delivers PldB (**Figure 10I**). VgrG2a and VgrG2b are genetically linked to the effector proteins Tle4 (**Figure 10D**) and Tle3 (**Figure 10E**; Jiang et al., 2016), however, their functional links require further investigations. Additionally, VgrG4a, which is encoded on a separate satellite *vgrG* island, is likely affiliated with the H2-T6SS due to a sequence identity of 97% with VgrG4b within the N-terminal gp5/gp27-like domains (Allsopp et al., 2017). Downstream of *vgrG4a*, another effector, Tle1, is encoded (**Figure 10G**), and because of the genetic linkage, most likely delivered in a VgrG4a-dependent manner. VgrG6, encoded on yet another satellite *vgrG* island, is genetically linked to *hcpB* (**Figure 10J**). This might be an indication for its association with the H2-T6SS (Burkinshaw et al., 2018) because the HcpB amino acids sequence is 100 % identical to HcpA and HcpC (Jones et al., 2013), which are genetically linked to genes encoding H2-T6SS spike proteins VgrG2a (**Figure 10D**) and VgrG2b (**Figure 10E**), respectively. Additionally, there is a putative effector gene linked to *vgrG6* whose role has not been studied yet. A remote *paar* cluster (**Figure 10L**) has also been connected to the H2-T6SS, whose gene product PAAR4 mediates delivery of the effector TseT in a TecT, Co-TecT-, VgrG4b- and VgrG6-dependent fashion (Burkinshaw et al., 2018). PAAR2, encoded on yet another orphan island (**Figure 10K**), was shown to be able to functionally replace PAAR4 (Burkinshaw et al., 2018), hence its affiliation with the H2-T6SS is also implicated.

Combining these data and observations, we propose that *P. aeruginosa* uses its H2-T6SS machinery to deliver a multitude of different spikes decorated with various effectors. Interestingly, five (PldA, PldB, Tle3, Tle4 and Tle1) out of seven postulated H2-T6SS-dependent effectors are lipases that have been either experimentally proven (Russell et al., 2013; Jiang et al., 2014, 2016) or proposed due to the presence of the lipase-specific DUF2235 domain. The affiliation of at least five lipases, even though with different substrate specificities (Russell et al., 2013), with one T6SS machinery begs the question of why there would be such effector redundancy. In any case, with such a broad spike repertoire, *P. aeruginosa* has many options for loading its H2-T6SS weapon in order to confer a competitive advantage in a polymicrobial environment. This also mitigates the presumption of the H1-T6SS being the major antibacterial T6SS of *P. aeruginosa* (Hachani et al., 2014; Allsopp et al., 2017) while the H2-T6SS provides *P. aeruginosa* with the versatility to fire various effectors into competing prey cells.

CONCLUSION

The T6SS is a potent bacterial weapon that delivers an arsenal of toxins into eukaryotic and prokaryotic prey cells. All *P. aeruginosa* strains sequenced so far carry three distinct T6SSs, namely H1-, H2- and H3-T6SS, which could act in concert to inject a lethal cocktail of enzymes targeting essential functions in living organisms. Among these are phospholipases, and notably PldA and PldB, which are described in this study and which are considered as trans-kingdom effectors since they challenge the survival of eukaryotic cells as much as bacterial cells. The effector delivery strategy of the T6SS has been shown to be quite variable, and one mode we described here involves an exquisite recognition specificity between the toxin and the cognate T6SS spike, known as a VgrG trimer. The effector specificity lies within the C-terminal domain of a VgrG and we showed that such region in VgrG4b and VgrG5 is a TTR-like domain providing chaperone activity on PldA and PldB, respectively, which is instrumental for efficient secretion of these effectors (**Supplementary Figure S5**). PldA and PldB are encoded remotely from other T6SS core genes but are genetically linked to their cognate VgrG, supporting the concept of *vgrG* islands. As such, the *pldA/vgrG4b* or *pldB/vgrG5* genes, remotely and spread on the entire chromosome, exclusively carry the genes needed to load the T6SS spike (e.g., VgrG/effector or VgrG/Effector/Adaptor) at the tip of the T6SS nanomachine. It thus remains quite elusive on which T6SS core system each of the spike is loaded. Here we showed that both VgrG4b/PldA and VgrG5/PldB are delivered in an H2-T6SS-dependent manner and propose that most *vgrG* island-encoded effectors might actually use the H2-T6SS rather than the H1- or H3-T6SS. It is likely that fitting of the VgrG protein onto the T6SS machine would require specific interactions with the Hcp tube, as was shown recently (Renault et al., 2018). It is thus likely that acquisition of single effectors from other bacterial species by horizontal gene transfer would have to obey a number of rules before they can be fitted on and fired by endogenous T6SSs.

AUTHOR CONTRIBUTIONS

AF and SW conceived the study, participated in its design and coordination and wrote the manuscript. TW engineered the *P. aeruginosa* prey strains and optimized the bacterial killing assay conditions. SW performed most of the experiments and SF contributed to additional experiments. All authors discussed, reviewed and approved the final manuscript.

FUNDING

AF work on T6SS was supported by the MRC grants MR/K001930/1 and MR/N023250/1 and the BBSRC grant BB/I019871/1. SW was supported by the Imperial College President's Scholarship, TW by the Wellcome Trust and Selina Fecht by the Medical Research Council.

ACKNOWLEDGMENTS

We would like to thank Silvia D'Arcangelo for contributing the engineering of the *tssK3* mutant, as well as the parental strains of this study, PAO1 *rsmA*.

REFERENCES

Allsopp, L. P., Wood, T. E., Howard, S. A., Maggiorelli, F., Nolan, L. M., Wettstadt, S., et al. (2017). RsmA and AmrZ orchestrate the assembly of all three type VI secretion systems in *Pseudomonas aeruginosa*. *Proc. Nat. Acad. Sci. U. S. A.* 114, 7707–7712. doi: 10.1073/pnas.1700286114

Basler, M., Ho, B. T., and Mekalanos, J. J. (2013). Tit-for-tat: type VI secretion system counterattack during bacterial cell-cell interactions. *Cell* 152, 884–894. doi: 10.1016/j.cell.2013.01.042

Becher, A., and Schweizer, H. P. (2000). Integration-proficient *Pseudomonas aeruginosa* vectors for isolation of single-copy chromosomal lacZ and lux gene fusions. *Biotechniques* 29, 952.

Bingle, L. E., Bailey, C. M., and Pallen, M. J. (2008). Type VI secretion: a beginner's guide. *Curr. Opin. Microbiol.* 11, 3–8. doi: 10.1016/j.mib.2008.01.006

Birtalan, S. C., Phillips, R. M., and Ghosh, P. (2002). Three-dimensional secretion signals in chaperone-effector complexes of bacterial pathogens. *Mol. cell* 9, 971–980. doi: 10.1016/s1097-2765(02)00529-4

Bondage, D. D., Lin, J. S., Ma, L. S., Kuo, C. H., and Lai, E. M. (2016). VgrG C terminus confers the type VI effector transport specificity and is required for binding with PAAR and adaptor-effector complex. *Proc. Nat. Acad. Sci. U. S. A.* 113, E3931–E3940. doi: 10.1073/pnas.1600428113

Boulant, T., Boudehen, Y. M., Filloux, A., Plesiat, P., Naas, T., and Dortet, L. (2018). Higher prevalence of PldA, a *Pseudomonas aeruginosa* trans-kingdom H2-Type VI secretion system effector, in clinical isolates responsible for acute infections and in multidrug resistant strains. *Front. Microbiol.* 9:2578. doi: 10.3389/fmicb.2018.02578

Browning, C., Shneider, M. M., Bowman, V. D., Schwarzer, D., and Leiman, P. G. (2012). Phage pierces the host cell membrane with the iron-loaded spike. *Structure* 20, 326–339. doi: 10.1016/j.str.2011.12.009

Brunet, Y. R., Henin, J., Celia, H., and Cascales, E. (2014). Type VI secretion and bacteriophage tail tubes share a common assembly pathway. *EMBO Rep.* 15, 315–321. doi: 10.1002/embr.201337936

Brunet, Y. R., Zoued, A., Boyer, F., Douzi, B., and Cascales, E. (2015). The type VI secretion TssEFGK-VgrG phage-like baseplate is recruited to the TssJLM membrane complex via multiple contacts and serves as assembly platform for tail tube/sheath polymerization. *PLoS Genet.* 11:e1005545. doi: 10.1371/journal.pgen.1005545

Burkinshaw, B. J., Liang, X., Wong, M., Le, A. N. H., Lam, L., and Dong, T. G. (2018). A type VI secretion system effector delivery mechanism dependent on PAAR and a chaperone-co-chaperone complex. *Nat. Microbiol.* 3, 632–640. doi: 10.1038/s41564-018-0144-4

Diniz, J. A., and Coulthurst, S. J. (2015). Intra-species competition in *Serratia marcescens* is mediated by type VI secretion Rhs effectors and a conserved effector-associated accessory protein. *J. Bacteriol.* 197, 2350–2360. doi: 10.1128/jb.00199-15

Durand, E., Nguyen, V. S., Zoued, A., Logger, L., Pehau-Arnaudet, G., Aschtgen,

M. S., et al. (2015). Biogenesis and structure of a type VI secretion membrane core complex. *Nature* 523, 555–560. doi: 10.1038/nature14667

Durand, E., Zoued, A., Spinelli, S., Watson, P. J., Aschtgen, M. S., Journet, L., et al. (2012). Structural characterization and oligomerization of the TssL protein, a component shared by bacterial type VI and type IVb secretion systems. *J. Biol. Chem.* 287, 14157–14168. doi: 10.1074/jbc.M111.338731

Figurski, D. H., and Helinski, D. R. (1979). Replication of an origin-containing derivative of plasmid RK2 dependent on a plasmid function provided in trans. *Proc. Nat. Acad. Sci.U. S. A.* 76, 1648–1652. doi: 10.1073/pnas.76.4.1648

Flaugnatti, N., Le, T. T., Canaan, S., Aschtgen, M. S., Nguyen, V. S., Blangy, S., et al. (2015). A phospholipase a anti-bacterial T6SS effector interacts directly with the C-terminal domain of the VgrG spike protein for delivery. *Mol. Microbiol.* 99, 1099–1118. doi: 10.1111/mmi.13292

Hachani, A., Allsopp, L. P., Oduko, Y., and Filloux, A. (2014). The VgrG proteins are "á la carte" delivery systems for bacterial type VI effectors. *J. Biol. Chem.* 289, 17872–17884. doi: 10.1074/jbc.M114.563429

Hachani, A., Lossi, N. S., and Filloux, A. (2013). A visual assay to monitor T6SS-mediated bacterial competition. *J. Vis. Exp.* 73:e50103.

Hachani, A., Lossi, N. S., Hamilton, A., Jones, C., Bleves, S., Albesa-Jove, D., et al. (2011). Type VI secretion system in *Pseudomonas aeruginosa*: secretion and multimerization of VgrG proteins. *J. Biol. Chem.* 286, 12317–12327. doi: 10.1074/jbc.M110.193045

Herrero, M., de Lorenzo, V., and Timmis, K. N. (1990). Transposon vectors containing non-antibiotic resistance selection markers for cloning and stable chromosomal insertion of foreign genes in gram-negative bacteria. *J. Bacteriol.* 172, 6557–6567. doi: 10.1128/jb.172.11.6557-6567.1990

Jiang, F., Wang, X., Wang, B., Chen, L., Zhao, Z., Waterfield, N. R., et al. (2016). The *Pseudomonas aeruginosa* type VI secretion PGAP1-like effector induces host autophagy by activating endoplasmic reticulum stress. *Cell Rep.* 16, 1502–1509. doi: 10.1016/j.celrep.2016.07.012

Jiang, F., Waterfield, N. R., Yang, J., Yang, G., and Jin, Q. (2014). A *Pseudomonas aeruginosa* type VI secretion phospholipase D effector targets both prokaryotic and eukaryotic cells. *Cell Host Microbe* 15, 600–610. doi: 10.1016/j.chom.2014.04.010

Jones, C., Hachani, A., Manoli, E., and Filloux, A. (2013). An *rhs* gene linked to the second type VI secretion cluster is a feature of the *Pseudomonas aeruginosa* strain PA14. *J. Bacteriol.* 196, 800–810. doi: 10.1128/JB.00863-13

Kanamaru, S., Leiman, P. G., Kostyuchenko, V. A., Chipman, P. R., Mesyanzhinov, V. V., Arisaka, F., et al. (2002). Structure of the cell-puncturing device of bacteriophage T4. *Nature* 415, 553–557. doi: 10.1038/415553a

Kaniga, K., Delor, I., and Cornelis, G. R. (1991). A wide-host-range suicide vector for improving reverse genetics in gram-negative bacteria: inactivation of the blaA gene of Yersinia enterocolitica. *Gene* 109, 137–141. doi: 10.1016/0378-1119(91)90599-7

Kovach, M. E., Elzer, P. H., Hill, D. S., Robertson, G. T., Farris, M. A., Roop, R. M. II, et al. (1995). Four new derivatives of the broad-host-range cloning vector pBBR1MCS, carrying different antibiotic-resistance cassettes. *Gene* 166, 175–176. doi: 10.1016/0378-1119(95)00584-1

Leiman, P. G., Basler, M., Ramagopal, U. A., Bonanno, J. B., Sauder, J. M., Pukatzki, S., et al. (2009). Type VI secretion apparatus and phage tail-associated protein complexes share a common evolutionary origin. *Proc. Nat. Acad. Sci. U. S. A.* 106, 4154–4159. doi: 10.1073/pnas.0813360106

Liang, X., Moore, R., Wilton, M., Wong, M. J., Lam, L., and Dong, T. G. (2015).). Identification of divergent type VI secretion effectors using a conserved chaperone domain. *Proc. Nat. Acad. Sci. U. S. A* 112, 9106–9111. doi: 10.1073/pnas.1505317112

Lin, J., Zhang, W., Cheng, J., Yang, X., Zhu, K., Wang, Y., et al. (2017). A *Pseudomonas* T6SS effector recruits PQS-containing outer membrane vesicles for iron acquisition. *Nat. Commun.* 8:14888. doi: 10.1038/ncomms14888

Ma, A. T., McAuley, S., Pukatzki, S., and Mekalanos, J. J. (2009). Translocation of a *Vibrio cholerae* type VI secretion effector requires bacterial endocytosis by host cells. *Cell Host Microbe* 5, 234–243. doi: 10.1016/j.chom.2009.02.005

Ma, J., Pan, Z., Huang, J., Sun, M., Lu, C., and Yao, H. (2017). The Hcp proteins fused with diverse extended-toxin domains represent a novel pattern of antibacterial effectors in type VI secretion systems. *Virulence* 8, 1189–1202. doi: 10.1080/21505594.2017.1279374

Ma, L. S., Hachani, A., Lin, J. S., Filloux, A., and Lai, E. M. (2014). *Agrobacterium tumefaciens* deploys a superfamily of type VI secretion DNase effectors as weapons for interbacterial competition in planta. *Cell Host Microbe* 16, 94–104. doi: 10.1016/j.chom.2014.06.002

MacIntyre, D. L., Miyata, S. T., Kitaoka, M., and Pukatzki, S. (2010). The *Vibrio cholerae* type VI secretion system displays antimicrobial properties. *Proc. Nat. Acad. Sci. U. S. A.* 107, 19520–19524. doi: 10.1073/pnas.1012931107

Olson, J. C., and Ohman, D. E. (1992). Efficient production and processing of elastase and LasA by *Pseudomonas aeruginosa* require zinc and calcium ions. *J. Bacteriol.* 174, 4140–4147. doi: 10.1128/jb.174.12.4140-4147.1992

Pissaridou, P., Allsopp, L. P., Wettstadt, S., Howard, S. A., Mavridou, D. A. I., and Filloux, A. (2018). The *Pseudomonas aeruginosa* T6SS-VgrG1b spike is topped by a PAAR protein eliciting DNA damage to bacterial competitors. *Proc. Nat. Acad. Sci. U. S. A.* 115, 12519–12524. doi: 10.1073/pnas.1814181115

Planamente, S., Salih, O., Manoli, E., Albesa-Jove, D., Freemont, P. S., and Filloux, A. (2016). TssA forms a gp6-like ring attached to the type VI secretion sheath. *EMBO J.* 35, 1613–1627. doi: 10.15252/embj.201694024

Pukatzki, S., Ma, A. T., Revel, A. T., Sturtevant, D., and Mekalanos, J. J. (2007). Type VI secretion system translocates a phage tail spike-like protein into target cells where it cross-links actin. *Proc. Nat. Acad. Sci. U. S. A.* 104, 15508–15513. doi: 10.1073/pnas.0706532104

Pukatzki, S., Ma, A. T., Sturtevant, D., Krastins, B., Sarracino, D., Nelson, W. C., et al. (2006). Identification of a conserved bacterial protein secretion system in *Vibrio cholerae* using the dictyostelium host model system. *Proc. Nat. Acad. Sci. U. S. A.* 103, 1528–1533. doi: 10.1073/pnas.0510322103

Quentin, D., Ahmad, S., Shanthamoorthy, P., Mougous, J. D., Whitney, J. C., and Raunser, S. (2018). Mechanism of loading and translocation of type VI secretion system effector Tse6. *Nat. Microbiol.* 3, 1142–1152. doi: 10.1038/s41564-018-0238-z

Renault, M. G., Zamarreno Beas, J., Douzi, B., Chabalier, M., Zoued, A., Brunet, Y. R., et al. (2018). The gp27-like Hub of VgrG Serves as Adaptor to Promote Hcp Tube Assembly. *J. Mol. Biol.* 430(18 Pt B), 3143–3156. doi: 10.1016/j.jmb.2018.07.018

Russell, A. B., Hood, R. D., Bui, N. K., LeRoux, M., Vollmer, W., and Mougous, J. D. (2011). Type VI secretion delivers bacteriolytic effectors to target cells. *Nature* 475, 343–347. doi: 10.1038/nature10244

Russell, A. B., LeRoux, M., Hathazi, K., Agnello, D. M., Ishikawa, T., Wiggins, P. A., et al. (2013). Diverse type VI secretion phospholipases are functionally plastic antibacterial effectors. *Nature* 496, 508–512. doi: 10.1038/nature12074

Sana, T. G., Baumann, C., Merdes, A., Soscia, C., Rattei, T., Hachani, A., et al. (2015). Internalization of Pseudomonas aeruginosa strain PAO1 into epithelial cells is promoted by interaction of a T6SS effector with the microtubule network. *MBio* 6:e00712. doi: 10.1128/mBio.00712-15

Schmidt-Eisenlohr, H., Domke, N., and Baron, C. (1999). TraC of IncN plasmid pKM101 associates with membranes and extracellular high-molecular-weight structures in *Escherichia coli. J Bacteriol* 181, 5563–5571.

Shneider, M. M., Buth, S. A., Ho, B. T., Basler, M., Mekalanos, J. J., and Leiman, P. G. (2013). PAAR-repeat proteins sharpen and diversify the type VI secretion system spike. *Nature* 500, 350–353. doi: 10.1038/nature12453

Silverman, J. M., Agnello, D. M., Zheng, H., Andrews, B. T., Li, M., Catalano, C. E., et al. (2013). Haemolysin coregulated protein is an exported receptor and chaperone of type VI secretion substrates. *Mol. Cell* 51, 584–593. doi: 10.1016/j.molcel.2013.07.025

Spinola-Amilibia, M., Davo-Siguero, I., Ruiz, F. M., Santillana, E., Medrano, F. J., and Romero, A. (2016). The structure of VgrG1 from *Pseudomonas aeruginosa*, the needle tip of the bacterial type VI secretion system. *Acta. Crystallogr. D Struct. Biol.* 72, 22–33. doi: 10.1107/S2059798315021142

Sutherland, M. C., Nguyen, T. L., Tseng, V., and Vogel, J. P. (2012). The *Legionella* IcmSW complex directly interacts with DotL to mediate translocation of adaptor-dependent substrates. *PLoS Pathog.* 8:e1002910. doi: 10.1371/journal.ppat.1002910

Unterweger, D., Kostiuk, B., Otjengerdes, R., Wilton, A., Diaz-Satizabal, L., and Pukatzki, S. (2015). Chimeric adaptor proteins translocate diverse type VI secretion system effectors in *Vibrio cholerae*. *EMBO J.* 34, 2198–2210. doi: 10.15252/embj.201591163

Vasseur, P., Vallet-Gely, I., Soscia, C., Genin, S., and Filloux, A. (2005). The pel genes of the *Pseudomonas aeruginosa* PAK strain are involved at early and late stages of biofilm formation. *Microbiology* 151, 985–997. doi: 10.1099/mic.0.27410-0

Whitney, J. C., Beck, C. M., Goo, Y. A., Russell, A. B., Harding, B. N., De Leon, J. A., et al. (2014). Genetically distinct pathways guide effector export through the type VI secretion system. *Mol. Microbiol.* 92, 529–542. doi: 10.1111/mmi.12571

Whitney, J. C., Quentin, D., Sawai, S., LeRoux, M., Harding, B. N., Ledvina, H. E., et al. (2015). An interbacterial NAD(P)(+) glycohydrolase toxin requires elongation factor Tu for delivery to target cells. *Cell* 163, 607–619. doi: 10.1016/j.cell.2015.09.027

Zhao, Z., Sagulenko, E., Ding, Z., and Christie, P. J. (2001). Activities of virE1 and the VirE1 secretion chaperone in export of the multifunctional VirE2 effector via an *Agrobacterium* type IV secretion pathway. *J. Bacteriol.* 183, 3855–3865. doi: 10.1128/jb.183.13.3855-3865.2001

2

Super-Resolution Imaging of Protein Secretion Systems and the Cell Surface of Gram-Negative Bacteria

*Sachith D. Gunasinghe [1], Chaille T. Webb [1], Kirstin D. Elgass [2], Iain D. Hay [1] and Trevor Lithgow [1]**

[1] Infection and Immunity Program, Department of Microbiology, Biomedicine Discovery Institute, Monash University, Clayton, VIC, Australia, [2] Monash Micro Imaging, Monash University, Clayton, VIC, Australia

***Correspondence:** Trevor Lithgow trevor.lithgow@monash.edu

Gram-negative bacteria have a highly evolved cell wall with two membranes composed of complex arrays of integral and peripheral proteins, as well as phospholipids and glycolipids. In order to sense changes in, respond to, and exploit their environmental niches, bacteria rely on structures assembled into or onto the outer membrane. Protein secretion across the cell wall is a key process in virulence and other fundamental aspects of bacterial cell biology. The final stage of protein secretion in Gram-negative bacteria, translocation across the outer membrane, is energetically challenging so sophisticated nanomachines have evolved to meet this challenge. Advances in fluorescence microscopy now allow for the direct visualization of the protein secretion process, detailing the dynamics of (i) outer membrane biogenesis and the assembly of protein secretion systems into the outer membrane, (ii) the spatial distribution of these and other membrane proteins on the bacterial cell surface, and (iii) translocation of effector proteins, toxins and enzymes by these protein secretion systems. Here we review the frontier research imaging the process of secretion, particularly new studies that are applying various modes of super-resolution microscopy.

Keywords: protein secretion, outer membrane, lipopolysaccharide, BAM complex

Fluorescence microscopy has proven to be a powerful tool for cell biologists, given the wide array of fluorescent probes available (fluorescent fusion proteins, reactive tags, and fluorescent antibodies) to specifically label and detect sub-cellular components in a cellular context. Together with increasingly higher quality optics, sensitive detectors and coherent light sources, the resolution capacity of fluorescence microscopy has now been extended to generate superior images with finer details than ever before. Until these recent developments, microbiologists were unable to fully capitalize on fluorescence microscopy, since the diffraction limit of light means only objects larger than ~250 nm in lateral dimension and ~500 nm in axial dimension could be resolved: any objects smaller than these limits are merely blurred spots (Patterson et al., 2010). Many of the structures of interest in microbes are much smaller than this classical limit, with bacteria themselves only 1–10 μm in length (Koch, 1996).

The advent of super-resolution microscopy extended the classical limit imposed by conventional light microscopy (Hell, 2007, 2009; Huang et al., 2009, 2010). There are two general classes of super-resolution microscopy. The first class of imaging modalities utilizes spatially patterned fluorescence excitation beams to achieve the sub-diffraction level of resolution. The most notable examples of this technique are stimulated emission depletion (STED) microscopy (Hell and Wichmann, 1994; Klar and Hell, 1999), reversible saturable optical fluorescence transitions (RESOLFT) microscopy (Hell and Wichmann, 1994; Hofmann et al., 2005) and structured illumination microscopy (SIM) (Gustafsson, 2000, 2005).

The second class circumvents the diffraction barrier through actively controlling the fluorescence emitter (fluorescent proteins, antibodies or tags) concentrations by stochastic photo-activation or by stochastic photo-switching (Heilemann et al., 2009; Lippincott-Schwartz and Patterson, 2009; Kamiyama and Huang, 2012), thereby enabling spatio-temporal resolution of emitter localizations. This class includes photoactivation localization microscopy (PALM) (Betzig et al., 2006) and stochastic optical reconstruction microscopy (STORM), collectively known as single molecule localization microscopy (SMLM) (Rust et al., 2006). These techniques are documented to reach 10–25 nm of lateral resolution (Kamiyama and Huang, 2012), a scale that allows visualization of macromolecules in small cellular systems (**Figure 1**).

In order to exploit their environmental niches, bacteria undertake vital tasks such as sensing the external milieu, cell to cell communication, nutrient uptake against concentration gradients, cell-cell warfare and the secretion of macromolecules into the environment. Gram-negative bacteria have a highly evolved cell wall with two membranes composed of a complex array of integral and peripheral proteins, as well as phospholipids and glycolipids. The outer membrane is an asymmetric bilayer, with an inner leaflet of phospholipids and an outer leaflet of lipopolysaccharide (LPS). As discussed herein, we are beginning to appreciate that this asymmetric lipid environment promotes spatial heterogeneity of membrane constituents and impedes the sort of lateral mobility that is common for the proteins integrated in phospholipid bilayers. Super resolution microscopy is being applied to dissect diverse aspects of bacterial cell biology, including membrane protein structure and dynamics (Xie et al., 2008). In this review, we highlight the advances that have been made in understanding spatial-temporal characteristics of bacterial surface proteins, particularly protein secretion systems, that the recent advances in microscopy have allowed. To date, model bacterial systems like *Escherichia coli* and *Caulobacter cresentus* have been the subject for the majority of single molecule localization studies (Gahlmann and Moerner, 2014).

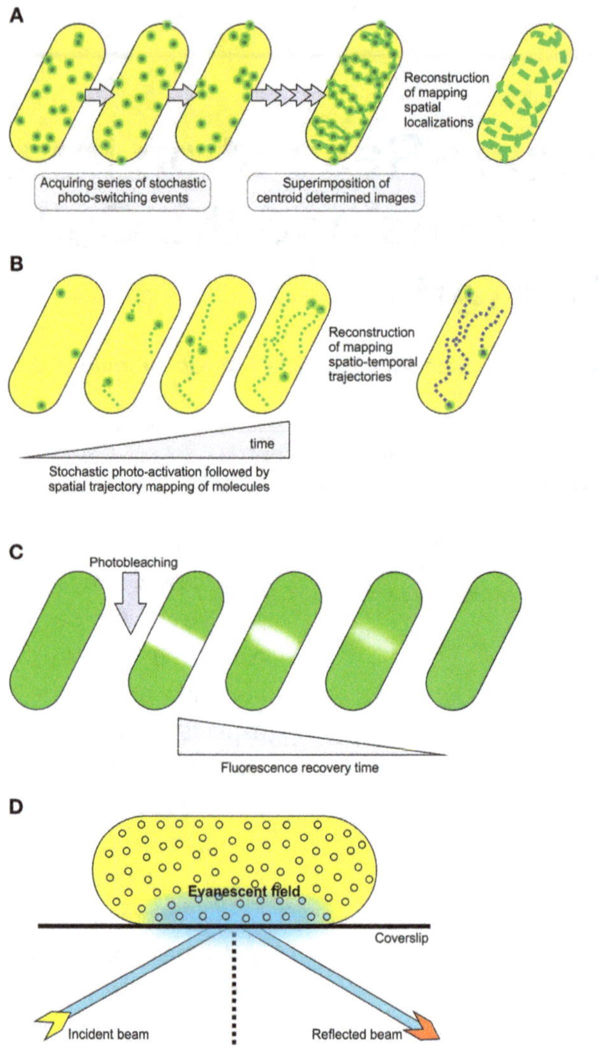

FIGURE 1 | Methods for single molecule localization and tracking. **(A)** STORM and **(B)** PALM super-resolution microscopy, collectively referred to as single molecule localization microscopy methods (SMLM). These modalities utilize stochastic photo-switching or photo-activation of a subset of fluorescence emitters to achieve sub-diffraction resolution of 10–25 nm in lateral dimensions. PALM is well known for live cell imaging and mapping spatiotemporal trajectories of individual fluorescently labeled molecules (Manley et al., 2008). STORM is documented for its use in determining the localized positioning of fluorescently labeled molecules in both live and fixed samples (Kamiyama and Huang, 2012). The mobility of fluorescent fusion proteins in live cells can also be surveyed through **(C)** FRAP and **(D)** TIRF microscopy techniques. In FRAP experiments, a relatively small area within the cell is irreversibly photo-bleached by a high intensity laser beam, followed by subsequent monitoring of the redistribution of non-bleached fluorescence molecules into the photo-bleached region under low laser power. TIRFM relies upon the generation of a rapidly decaying evanescent field at the interface of sample and coverslip to sparsely excite fluorophores, providing a high signal to background noise ratio in single particle tracking studies (Toomre and Bewersdorf, 2010).

FLUORESCENCE IMAGING OF OUTER MEMBRANE STRUCTURE AND BIOGENESIS

Most bacterial outer membrane proteins (OMPs) have a β-barrel architecture (De Geyter et al., 2016; Plummer and Fleming, 2016; Noinaj et al., 2017; Slusky, 2017) and, of these, the channels that allow for selective permeability of small molecules across the outer membrane are referred to as porins (Hancock, 1987). Some of these porins display surface exposed extracellular domains, often simply loops of polypeptide between adjacent β-strands, which none the less provide the means to fluorescently label them for mobility assessment studies on live cells (Gibbs et al., 2004; Spector et al., 2010; Rassam et al., 2015). With the aid of fluorescent recovery after photo-bleaching (FRAP) and single particle tracking using total internal reflection fluorescence microscopy (TIRFM), we are now beginning to understand time-resolved spatial movements of these outer membrane proteins (Gibbs et al., 2004; Spector et al., 2010; Rothenberg et al., 2011; Rassam et al., 2015).

LamB is a trimeric porin responsible for maltose uptake in *E. coli* (Schirmer et al., 1995). LamB also serves as the receptor for certain bacteriophage (Chatterjee and Rothenberg, 2012), and has been extensively studied in terms of diffusion dynamics. Using various labeling techniques and different imaging modalities, LamB mobility has been described using parametric measurements such as the short-time diffusion coefficient. In essence, this quantifies the area a molecule inhabits in a per second measurement. LamB displays a short-time diffusion coefficient of 0.15 - 0.06 $\mu m^2 s^{-1}$, with each molecule therefore being confined to a space of ~20 nm at the outer membrane (Oddershede et al., 2002; Gibbs et al., 2004; Rothenberg et al., 2011). Similar results have come from study of other porins. OmpF, for example, was reported to have short-time diffusion coefficients of 0.006 $\mu m^2 s^{-1}$ (Spector et al., 2010). Similarly, a short-time diffusion coefficient of 0.05 $\mu m^2 s^{-1}$ was reported for the TonB-dependent receptor BtuB, which facilitates cobalamin uptake (Spector et al., 2010). For both OmpF and BtuB, recent work has suggested that their distribution and relative immobility may be due to non-specific, protein-protein interactions (Rassam et al., 2015). OmpA functions to lock the outer membrane to the under-lying peptidoglycan layer, and it had been expected that this feature alone would dictate the relative immobility predicted for OmpA (Samsudin et al., 2016). However, deletion of peptidoglycan binding domain of OmpA, did not affect the diffusion coefficient measurements for the β-barrel domain of OmpA (Verhoeven et al., 2013). These and other studies have led to the understanding that, compared to inner membrane proteins, OMPs generally display orders of magnitude slower diffusion dynamics whether or not they are tethered to other cellular structures (Oddershede et al., 2002; Gibbs et al., 2004; Spector et al., 2010; Rothenberg et al., 2011; Ritchie et al., 2013; Verhoeven et al., 2013; Rassam et al., 2015).

In this emerging paradigm of membrane spatial rigidity, it has become clear that the distribution of LPS is also greatly constrained. By fluorescently labeling LPS via the α-mannose moiety of its O-antigen, distinct helical ribbon-like geometric arrangements were observed for LPS on live *E.coli* (Ghosh and Young, 2005). Very low diffusion coefficients reported by FRAP experiments showed that LPS molecules were practically immobile by comparison with the (already very low) OMP diffusion rates (Mühlradt et al., 1973; Schindler et al., 1980). The current hypothesis is that LPS helical ribbons may represent a geometric arrangement important for staging outer membrane biogenesis. Given the high abundance yet constrained spatial distribution of LPS, it is becoming clear that any model for protein transport into or across the outer membrane will need to take into account this spatial information.

Few studies have yet to directly address the spatio-temporal aspects of the process of β-barrel assembly into the outer membrane. In one, temporal labeling of LamB appearance on the bacterial cell surface has been studied in elegant work, using detailed computational analysis to reconstruct the first spatio-temporal distribution of OMP biogenesis (Ursell et al., 2012). Employing site specific protein labeling strategy using Sfp phosphopantetheinyl transferase to covalently label emergent loops of nascent LamB molecules, the appearance and mobility of LamB molecules was monitored through time-lapse fluorescence microscopy. Inducible pulse-chase expression of LamB revealed an initial emergence of fluorescent punctae which represents a heterogeneous distribution of fluorescent spots per bacterium. The heterogeneous localization of LamB was due to discrete bursts of insertion of new material at discrete sites throughout the outer membrane. This presumably relates to the number and location of active β-barrel assembly machinery (BAM) complexes, which serve to catalyse β-barrel protein assembly into the outer membrane (De Geyter et al., 2016; Plummer and Fleming, 2016; Noinaj et al., 2017). The numbers of these punctae is similar to the number of sites estimated in an early EM-based study that captured porin insertion sites in *Salmonella* Typhimurium using ferritin-conjugated OMP-specific antibodies (Smit and Nikaido, 1978). Importantly, FRAP experiments showed that any laterally measurable movement of the OMPs across the bacterial cell surface was dependent on membrane growth and was not diffusional (Ursell et al., 2012). Since LamB also serves as receptor for several bacteriophage (Hancock and Reeves, 1976), fluorescently labeled λ phage tails have also been used to monitor the endogenous distribution of LamB—without plasmid-borne over-expression—and these studies too find it to be driven by cell growth and elongation (Gibbs et al., 2004).

The process of outer membrane biogenesis also depends on OMP turn-over through generational change in an *E. coli* population. A recent study using covalently modified colicins to fluorescently label two OMPs, BtuB and Cir, elegantly followed this process through TIRFM (Rassam et al., 2015). BtuB and Cir were observed to be clustered together in "OMP islands," huge rafts with an average size of ~ 0.5 μm (hundreds to thousands of proteins molecules would be encompassed in this island, with little or no interstitial lipid present). Unlike the LamB studies, where new material was delivered at points all across the cell surface, Rassam et al. suggested that the insertion of new BtuB and Cir into these rafts was only observed in the mid-cell region (Rassam et al., 2015). Irrespective of the site of new material deposition, computer modeling studies (Wang et al., 2008; Ursell et al., 2012; Rassam et al., 2015) have demonstrated that in either scenario, pre-existent OMPs and LPS will always tend to be forced toward poles, and that cell division will ultimately yield an unequal partitioning of membrane materials to create distinct subpopulations of cells, ones having mixed set of old and new material and others with predominantly or exclusively "young" OMPs. Within a bacterial population this then creates a range of phenotypes in the outer membrane proteome, and a range of adaptive advantages for individual bacteria to survive and replicate in that environment. In various ways, other studies have demonstrated how "older" elements of the other major cell envelope constituents, LPS and peptidoglycan, are also ultimately retained at cell poles (Kato et al., 1990, 2000; De Pedro et al., 2003; Thiem et al., 2007; Thiem and Sourjik, 2008). *In silico* models have predicted this type of protein clustering and binary partitioning of membrane proteins. For example, this temporal positioning has been observed to be important in resolving protein aggregates associated with bacterial cell aging, but is also important in positioning chemoreceptor arrays and regulation of cell division (Janakiraman and Goldberg, 2004;

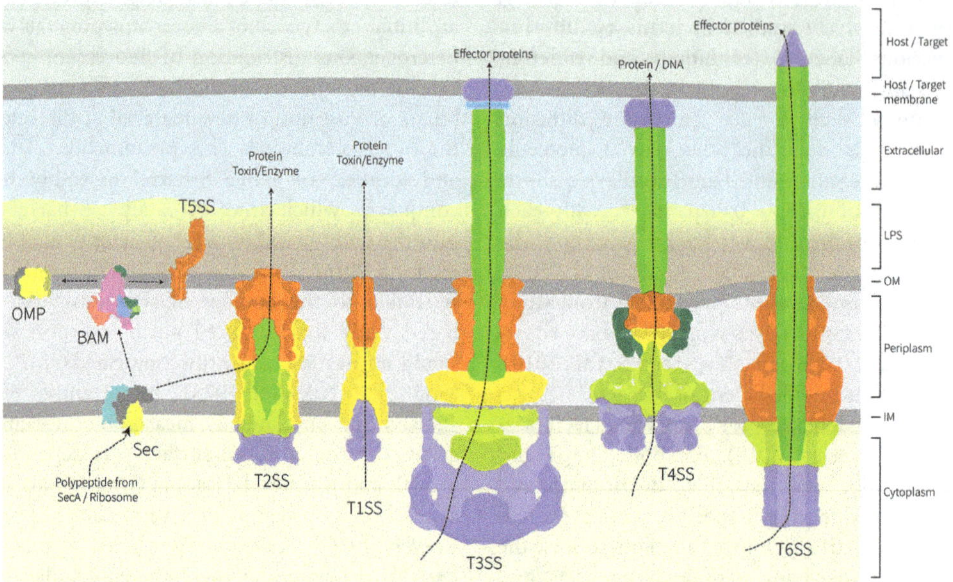

FIGURE 2 | Architecture of the major protein secretion systems found in Gram-negative bacteria. Of the six major protein secretion systems, five span the inner and outer membranes and the periplasm. These nanomachines are thereby trapped in the peptidoglycan layer. The T1SS, T3SS, T4SS, and T6SS collect substrate proteins directly from the cytoplasm for secretion across both membranes, while the T2SS collects substrate proteins from the periplasm with their delivery there being via the Sec translocon (shown) or Tat transport system (not shown). While informed artistic license was taken with the placement, orientation and shape of some proteins/complexes, wherever possible relative structural information was used. The structural data used as a basis in the preparation of this figure are: PDB 1ek9, 5l22, 5mg3, 5d0o, 1mal, 5ksr, 5wq8, 3fpp, 4ksr, 5l22, 3fpp, 4kh3, 4mee; and EMD-2927, EMD-2667, EMD-2567, EMD-1875. The structure and function of these various protein translocation systems are detailed elsewhere in this special volume.

Thiem et al., 2007; Lindner et al., 2008; Thiem and Sourjik, 2008).

FLUORESCENCE-BASED IMAGING OF BACTERIAL SECRETION SYSTEMS

A frontier area of research in bacterial cell biology concerns the assembly and distribution of protein secretion machines. Bacteria have evolved numerous mechanisms to efficiently secrete proteins into the environment and characterization of several protein secretion systems is yielding exciting advances in understanding their structure and function (Dalbey and Kuhn, 2012; Costa et al., 2015). Because these systems are detailed elsewhere in this special edition, we have focused our review on studies where spatial distribution appears to be important either to the biogenesis of the secretion system, or to its function. As highlighted in **Figure 2**, the architecture of these secretion nanomachines can differ from single component systems, to relatively simple systems composed of only 3 subunits, to multicomponent systems containing over 20 protein subunits and spanning all four compartments of the bacterial cell (Dalbey and Kuhn, 2012; Campos et al., 2013; Galán et al., 2014; Ho et al., 2014; Thomas et al., 2014; Trokter et al., 2014; van Ulsen et al., 2014; Zoued et al., 2014; Basler, 2015; Costa et al., 2015; Fan et al., 2016; Notti and Stebbins, 2016).

TYPE 1 SECRETION SYSTEM (T1SS)

Effector proteins secreted through T1SS have been characterized in a number of bacterial pathogens including in uropathogenic *E. coli*, *Bordetella pertussis* and more recently through effector protein RtxA in *Legionella pneumophila* (Brooks et al., 1980; Shrivastava and Miller, 2009; Fuche et al., 2015). Using deletion mutants and fluorescence protein fusion constructs of RtxA (photoactivatable mCherry-RtxA), secretion was monitored through the course of infection. *Legionella* were internalized by host cells into the endoplasmic reticulum-like compartment, the *Legionella*-containing vacuole, where bacterial replication takes place inside the host. With the versatility of genetically-encoded, reactive tags (Halo-tag and SNAP-tag), Barlag et al. imaged subunits of T1SS in *Salmonella enterica* at a nanoscopic level (Barlag et al., 2016). Diffusion coefficients reported for SiiF, the inner membrane component the T1SS were 0.008 $\mu m^2 s^{-1}$ and the secretion machine was confined into 3–4 localized punctae. This very low diffusion coefficient for an inner membrane protein is perhaps predictable, given that T1SS include a TolC-type protein integrated into the outer membrane (Thomas et al., 2014), and in consideration that by spanning the periplasm the T1SS would be trapped within the peptidoglycan meshwork. This peptidoglycan trap would likely apply equally in constraining the movement of other protein secretion systems too (**Figure 2**). Together, these studies illustrate the resourcefulness of fluorescent fusion and enzyme tags and how these can be utilized in super resolution imaging of the secretion machines and their substrates, without altering the functionality of either.

TYPE 2 SECRETION SYSTEM (T2SS)

The T2SS has been identified in a number of bacterial pathogens, and is particularly well known in *Vibrio cholerae* as the system responsible for cholera toxin secretion (Sandkvist et al., 1997; Connell et al., 1998; Lybarger et al., 2009; Sikora et al., 2011). Elements required for the assembly of this T2SS are encoded by the extracellular protein secretion (*eps*) genes (Overbye et al., 1993; Sandkvist et al., 1997; Marsh and Taylor, 1998; Fullner and Mekalanos, 1999) and the localization of fluorescently labeled protein subunits in *V. cholerae* has revealed insight into the assembly and spatial dynamics. Using chromosomal and plasmid borne GFP fusions with the EpsM, EspG and EpsC subunits of the T2SS the subcellular localization of each components was assessed in *Vibrio cholerae* (Lybarger et al., 2009). When chromosomally-expressed (to produce endogenous steady-state levels of protein), GFP-EpsM formed distinct fluorescent foci that were not concentrated at cell poles. Conversely, when plasmid-borne over-expression of GFP-EpsM was instituted, the protein displayed a polar localization.

This discernible effect on protein subcellular localization under differential gene expression is a concern that needs careful consideration. The impact of overexpression on physiologically-relevant vs. non-physiological localizations is equally of concern in studies on other protein secretion systems (and all subcellular structures) too. As mentioned previously, protein aggregates tend to be deposited in polar locations (Janakiraman and Goldberg, 2004; Thiem et al., 2007; Lindner et al., 2008; Thiem and Sourjik, 2008).

Type 4 pili are a locomotional appendage that are ancestrally and structurally related to the T2SS (Peabody et al., 2003). The distribution of T4 pili has been followed using fluorescent protein fusions. An mCherry fusion tag was attached to the BfpB subunit in the Type 4 pili of enteropathogenic *E. coli* (Lieberman et al., 2012). PALM was used to capture single molecule localization events of BfpB-PAmCherry, providing evidence for a largely non-polar distribution pattern in Type 4 pili biogenesis, as is likely in T2SS biogenesis. Conversely, studies in *Pseudomonas aeruginosa* suggest that Type 4 pili biogenesis occurs at sites of cell division: that is, that the nanomachines are pre-installed at what will become a cell pole (after cell division concludes) (Carter et al., 2017). Taken together these exciting studies highlight the complex spatio-temporal scenarios that exist in the cell biology of bacteria, and caution against concluding that what is true in *E. coli* is necessarily true in other bacterial species.

TYPE 3 SECRETION SYSTEM (T3SS)

The T3SS has been identified in several bacterial pathogens including *Yersinia enterocolitica*, *E. coli*, *Shigella flexneri*, and *Salmonella* Typhimurium. While electron microscopy and electron tomography have provided exquisite detail in the structure of these complicated nanomachines (Spreter et al., 2009; Carleton et al., 2013; Radics et al., 2014; Hu et al., 2015, 2017), a number of different fluorescence microscopy imaging studies on live cells have provided in-depth analysis on different stages of T3SS assembly and effector protein secretion into host cells. Time-lapse fluorescence microscopy has monitored the T3SS during *S.* Typhimurium infection of epithelial cells (Schlumberger et al., 2005). A fluorescently-labeled substrate of the T3SS, SipA, was monitored for its emergence into the host cells, and its concomitant depletion from the bacterial cytoplasm. At the event of infection, it was estimated via fluorescence measurements that *S.* Typhimurium was able to deliver $6 \pm 3 \times 10^3$ molecules of SipA to the host cell within 100–600 s, and the effector protein ejection starts ~16–25 s after docking on to the host. In terms of the nanomachine itself, subunits of the T3SS in *S.* Typhimurium have been visualized too (Diepold et al., 2010, 2015; Kudryashev et al., 2015; Notti et al., 2015; Barlag et al., 2016). The diffusion coefficient for SpaS, an inner membrane component of the T3SS, was measured to be $0.055\,\mu m^2 s^{-1}$, which is a similar scale to the diffusion coefficients measured for outer membrane proteins LamB and OmpF. While not directly tested, this level of immobility of the inner membrane elements of the T3SS is consistent with them being constrained in their diffusional movements by the outer membrane components of the nanomachine and the peptidoglycan trap. The same would be true of the T1SS (Barlag et al., 2016), where SiiF is found in the inner membrane but would be constrained in its diffusional movement by its spanning the peptidoglycan and attached to the TolC-homolog SiiC in the outer membrane (Kiss et al., 2007). In these studies, the localization of the T3SS was distributed relatively evenly across the bacterial cell. It would be of great interest to monitor the T3SS distribution in pathogens such as enteropathogenic *E. coli* during the initial events of host cell encounter, when only a single surface of the bacterium engages the epithelial cell surface to initiate pathogen attachment and effacement (Wong et al., 2011; Gaytán et al., 2016). Is there a random engagement of only some T3SS with the host cell? Or does the pathogen control the spatial arrangement of T3SS to ensure maximal engagement on the "host side" of its surface?

TYPE 4 SECRETION SYSTEM (T4SS)

The T4SS functions to transfer proteins and/or DNA in bacterial conjugation encounters or during infection (Ding et al., 2003; Trokter et al., 2014). The Dot/Icm machinery is the T4SS in *Legionella* spp. and is responsible for hundreds of effector proteins throughout the infection cycle (So et al., 2015). Epitope-tagging one of these effectors, LncP, enabled fluorescence imaging of infected macrophages and showed that the protein was secreted from the bacterial cytoplasm by the T4SS and ultimately translocated across a remarkable five membranes in order to be assembled into the mitochondrial inner membrane of the host cell (Dolezal et al., 2012). An equivalent T4SS is found in *Coxiella burnetii*, and has been reported to be exclusively located at one pole of the bacterium (Morgan et al., 2010). It has been suggested that in these species, bacteria-host membrane contact might be required to initiate secretion into the host cell cytoplasm (Voth and Heinzen, 2007). That being the case, a unique localization of the T4SS nanomachines would promote the efficiency of effector protein secretion.

The T4SS has been well characterized in the plant pathogen *Agrobacterium tumefaciens* (Zupan et al., 2000), where it is composed of 12 subunits (Das and Xie, 2000; Ward et al., 2002; Jakubowski et al., 2003; Low et al., 2014; Trokter et al., 2014; Chandran Darbari and Waksman, 2015; Costa et al., 2015) and facilitates the delivery of tumor inducing pTi plasmid to plant cells, causing overproduction of certain plant growth hormones and leading to a resultant tumor (Dessaux et al., 1993). Initial spatial location studies on the T4SS in *A. tumefaciens* suggested that the VirD4 and VirB6 components were located at cell poles (Kumar and Das, 2002; Judd et al., 2005). Using deconvolution fluorescence microscopy and antibodies to specifically label the T4SS in *A. tumefaciens*, multiple clustered regions were observed along the cell periphery, i.e., not at the cell poles, in a majority of bacterial cells (Aguilar et al., 2011). Based on these finding, the authors proposed a lateral attachment model providing a more effective means for contact between pathogen and host during *A. tumefaciens* infection compared to a cell pole mediated attachment.

TYPE 5 SECRETION SYSTEM (T5SS)

There are several sub-types of T5SS, including autotransporters, inverse autotransporters, two-partner secretion systems and others (Fan et al., 2016; Heinz et al., 2016). Fluorescence microscopy studies on autotransporters derived from a variety of bacteria, including AIDA-I from *E. coli*, IcsA and SepA from *Shigella flexneri*, BrkA from *Bordetella pertussis*, and BimA from *Burkholderia thailandensis*, were shown to be directly localized to bacterial cell poles when translocated to the cell surface (Charles et al., 2001; Jain et al., 2006; Lu et al., 2015). Indeed, when IcsA, SepA, and BrkA were expressed in *E. coli* systems, they still migrated to the poles, suggesting that intrinsic features in the autotransporters programmes this polar localization (Jain et al., 2006). Conversely, at least one autotransporter, Ag43, was localized as covering the whole cell surface without any concentration toward poles (Danese et al., 2000; Kjærgaard et al., 2000). It is important to note that none of these studies have addressed where the integration event took place, nor any dynamics of movement of the autotransporters, but rather visualized their steady-state positioning. In addition to the effects of cell division or LPS leading to polar localization, the location at which a protein is translocated across the cytoplasmic membrane, through processes collectively considered as "transertion" (Bakshi et al., 2014; Matsumoto et al., 2015), may be important in determining how a protein achieves polar localization.

TYPE 6 SECRETION SYSTEM (T6SS)

While being the most recently discovered of the major protein secretion systems in Gram-negative bacteria, predictions suggest the T6SS to be present in ~25% of species (Basler et al., 2012). Characterization studies show that the T6SS functions in virulence for several pathogens including *B. thailandensis*, *Pseudomonas aeruginosa*, *Serratia marcescens* and *V. cholerae* (Mougous et al., 2006; Pukatzki et al., 2006, 2007; Schwarz et al., 2014). Structural elucidation of the T6SS from *V. cholerae* revealed startling similarities to bacteriophage tails. In general, T6SSs are assembled to contain a contractible sheath, baseplate and a membrane puncturing spike to mediate effector protein secretion into host cells (Basler et al., 2012; Filloux, 2013). Using a super-folder green fluorescent protein (sfGFP) fusion to VipA, one of the two protein components that makeup the contractile sheath, long straight tubular structures were localized in the cytoplasm extending along the width or length of the bacterium (Basler et al., 2012). Time-lapse fluorescence microscopy revealed these sub-cellular structures were highly dynamic in nature. They assemble at 20–30 s μm^{-1}, rapidly contracted to about 50% from their original length within ≤5 ms, and finally disassembled over a 30–60 s period (Basler et al., 2012). Recent studies using a similar fluorescent protein fusion tag approach captured the baseplate protein TssA joining the sheath component's polymerization in *E. coli* (Zoued et al., 2016).

T6SSs are often used in inter-species warfare, in order to outcompete bacterial neighbors (Hood et al., 2010; MacIntyre et al., 2010; Schwarz et al., 2010; Murdoch et al., 2011; Zoued et al., 2014; Journet and Cascales, 2016). Time-lapse fluorescence microscopy quantitatively demonstrated this antibacterial activity through predator-prey cell dynamics on live cells (Brunet et al., 2013). Co-culturing a pathogenic, "predator" *E. coli* strain expressing TssB-sfGFP (TssB is alternatively known as VipA) and a non-pathogenic, "prey" *E. coli* strain devoid of T6SS expressing fluorescent protein mCherry, showed that only upon contact with the prey was the contraction of the sheath structure triggered in predator cells. Conversely, in *S. marcescens* equivalent experimental strategies showed that the bacteria does not wait to encounter prey (or enemy) cells, but behaves aggressively and fires the T6SS irrespective of any provocation by cell-cell contact (Gerc et al., 2015). These studies again highlight the diverse behaviors that different bacterial species have evolved to deploy against their neighbors and enemies, and provide fascinating insight into the dynamics of how T6SS effector proteins are secreted to target other bacteria.

CONCLUSION

It is early in the application of super resolution microscopy techniques to capture the cellular events in the biogenesis and action of protein secretion systems in bacteria. Already, studies have challenged our preconceptions on bacterial cell envelope organization and protein dynamics. For example, the outer membrane is not a fluid mosaic, but a turgid structure that constrains membrane protein movement. Selective deployment of a protein secretion system is thereby possible at highly precise locations. High resolution imaging modalities will be tremendously useful in answering long-standing questions in bacterial cell biology, such as what mechanisms drive the biogenesis of outer membrane vesicles (Turnbull et al.,

2016), questions which until recently have largely been experimentally intractable. A further example is the extent to which transertion—the coupling of transcription, translation, and translocation—provides a mechanism for highly localized distributions of membrane proteins. This review has indicated the uses for the growing number of versatile fluorescent probes, which can be used in the distinct cellular environments, and how they promise to extend fluorescence microscopy applications even further. Examining host-pathogen interactions, detailing the nanoscale organization of protein secretion systems and studying the dynamic nature of sub-cellular compartments in live bacteria is now possible through super resolution microscopy. In the future, no doubt, these imaging techniques will be applied to understand the cell biology of the grand diversity of bacterial species, beyond characteristic model bacteria.

AUTHOR CONTRIBUTIONS

SG read the literature and wrote the manuscript. CW read the literature and wrote the manuscript. KE read the literature and wrote the manuscript. IH read the literature and wrote the manuscript. TL read the literature and wrote the manuscript.

ACKNOWLEDGMENTS

We thank Dr. Alex Fulcher for comments on the manuscript. SG thanks Dr. Toby Bell for training and critical discussions in single molecule imaging. The authors' work in this area is supported by NHMRC Program Grant 1092262 and the Australian Research Council (ARC; FL130100038). SG is supported by an ARC Laureate Scholarship, IH and CW are ARC Laureate Postdoctoral Fellows, and TL is an ARC Australian Laureate Fellow.

REFERENCES

Aguilar, J., Cameron, T. A., Zupan, J., and Zambryski, P. (2011). Membrane and core periplasmic *Agrobacterium tumefaciens* virulence Type IV secretion system components localize to multiple sites around the bacterial perimeter during lateral attachment to plant cells. *MBio* 2, e00218-e00211. doi: 10.1128/mBio.00218-11

Bakshi, S., Choi, H., Mondal, J., and Weisshaar, J. C. (2014). Time-dependent effects of transcription- and translation-halting drugs on the spatial distributions of the *Escherichia coli* chromosome and ribosomes. *Mol. Microbiol.* 94, 871–887. doi: 10.1111/mmi.12805

Barlag, B., Beutel, O., Janning, D., Czarniak, F., Richter, C. P., Kommnick, C., et al. (2016). Single molecule super-resolution imaging of proteins in living *Salmonella enterica* using self-labelling enzymes. *Sci. Rep.* 6:31601. doi: 10.1038/srep31601

Basler, M., Pilhofer, M., Henderson, G. P., Jensen, G. J., and Mekalanos, J. J. (2012). Type VI secretion requires a dynamic contractile phage tail-like structure. *Nature* 483, 182–186. doi: 10.1038/nature10846

Basler, M. (2015). Type VI secretion system: secretion by a contractile nanomachine. *Philos. Trans. R. Soc. B* 370:20150021. doi: 10.1098/rstb.2015.0021

Betzig, E., Patterson, G. H., Sougrat, R., Lindwasser, O. W., Olenych, S., Bonifacino, J. S., et al. (2006). Imaging intracellular fluorescent proteins at nanometer resolution. *Science* 313, 1642–1645. doi: 10.1126/science.1127344

Brooks, H. J., O'Grady, F., McSherry, M. A., and Cattell, W. (1980). Uropathogenic properties of *Escherichia coli* in recurrent urinary-tract infection. *J. Med. Microbiol.* 13, 57–68. doi: 10.1099/00222615-13-1-57

Brunet, Y. R., Espinosa, L., Harchouni, S., Mignot, T., and Cascales, E. (2013). Imaging type VI secretion-mediated bacterial killing. *Cell Rep.* 3, 36–41. doi: 10.1016/j.celrep.2012.11.027

Campos, M., Cisneros, D. A., Nivaskumar, M., and Francetic, O. (2013). The type II secretion system-a dynamic fiber assembly nanomachine. *Res. Microbiol.* 164, 545–555. doi: 10.1016/j.resmic.2013.03.013

Carleton, H. A., Lara-Tejero, M., Liu, X., and Galan, J. E. (2013). Engineering the type III secretion system in non-replicating bacterial minicells for antigen delivery. *Nat. Commun.* 4:1590. doi: 10.1038/ncomms2594

Carter, T., Buensuceso, R. N., Tammam, S., Lamers, R. P., Harvey, H., Howell, P. L., et al. (2017). The type IVa pilus machinery is recruited to sites of future cell division. *MBio* 8:e02103-16. doi: 10.1128/mBio.02103-16

Chandran Darbari, V., and Waksman, G. (2015). Structural biology of bacterial type IV secretion systems. *Annu. Rev. Biochem.* 84, 603–629. doi: 10.1146/annurev-biochem-062911-102821

Charles, M., Pérez, M., Kobil, J. H., and Goldberg, M. B. (2001). Polar targeting of *Shigella* virulence factor IcsA in *Enterobacteriacae* and *Vibrio*. *Proc. Natl. Acad. Sci. U.S.A.* 98, 9871–9876. doi: 10.1073/pnas.171310498

Chatterjee, S., and Rothenberg, E. (2012). Interaction of bacteriophage λ with its *E. coli* receptor, LamB. *Viruses* 4, 3162–3178. doi: 10.3390/v4113162

Connell, T. D., Metzger, D. J., Lynch, J., and Folster, J. P. (1998). Endochitinase is transported to the extracellular milieu by the eps-encoded general secretory pathway of *Vibrio cholerae*. *J. Bacteriol.* 180, 5591–5600.

Costa, T. R., Felisberto-Rodrigues, C., Meir, A., Prevost, M. S., Redzej, A., Trokter, M., et al. (2015). Secretion systems in Gram-negative bacteria: structural and mechanistic insights. *Nat. Rev. Microbiol.* 13, 343–359. doi: 10.1038/nrmicro3456

Dalbey, R. E., and Kuhn, A. (2012). Protein traffic in Gram-negative bacteria–how exported and secreted proteins find their way. *FEMS Microbiol. Rev.* 36, 1023–1045. doi: 10.1111/j.1574-6976.2012.00327.x

Danese, P. N., Pratt, L. A., Dove, S. L., and Kolter, R. (2000). The outer membrane protein, Antigen 43, mediates cell-to-cell interactions within *Escherichia coli* biofilms. *Mol. Microbiol.* 37, 424–432. doi: 10.1046/j.1365-2958.2000.02008.x

Das, A., and Xie, Y. H. (2000). The *Agrobacterium* T-DNA transport pore proteins VirB8, VirB9, and VirB10 interact with one another. *J. Bacteriol.* 182, 758–763. doi: 10.1128/JB.182.3.758-763.2000

De Geyter, J., Tsirigotaki, A., Orfanoudaki, G., Zorzini, V., Economou, A., and Karamanou, S. (2016). Protein folding in the cell envelope of *Escherichia coli*. *Nat. Microbiol.* 1:16107. doi: 10.1038/nmicrobiol.2016.107

De Pedro, M. A., Schwarz, H., and Koch, A. L. (2003). Patchiness of murein insertion into the sidewall of *Escherichia coli*. *Microbiology* 149, 1753–1761. doi: 10.1099/mic.0.26125-0

Dessaux, Y., Petit, A., and Tempe, J. (1993). Chemistry and biochemistry of opines, chemical mediators of parasitism. *Phytochemistry* 34, 31–38. doi: 10.1016/S0031-9422(00)90778-7

Diepold, A., Amstutz, M., Abel, S., Sorg, I., Jenal, U., and Cornelis, G. R. (2010). Deciphering the assembly of the *Yersinia type* III secretion injectisome. *EMBO J.* 29, 1928–1940. doi: 10.1038/emboj.2010.84

Diepold, A., Kudryashev, M., Delalez, N. J., Berry, R. M., and Armitage, J. P. (2015). Composition, formation, and regulation of the cytosolic c-ring, a dynamic component of the type III secretion injectisome. *PLoS Biol.* 13:e1002039. doi: 10.1371/journal.pbio.1002039

Ding, Z., Atmakuri, K., and Christie, P. J. (2003). The outs and ins of bacterial type IV secretion substrates. *Trends Microbiol.* 11, 527–535. doi: 10.1016/j.tim.2003.09.004

Dolezal, P., Aili, M., Tong, J., Jiang, J. H., Marobbio, C. M., Lee, S. F., et al. (2012). *Legionella pneumophila* secretes a mitochondrial carrier protein during infection. *PLoS Pathog.* 8:e1002459. doi: 10.1371/journal.ppat.1002459

Fan, E., Chauhan, N., Udatha, D. G., Leo, J. C., and Linke, D. (2016). Type V secretion systems in bacteria. *Microbiol. Spectr.* 4:VMBF-0009-2015. doi: 10.1128/microbiolspec.VMBF-0009-2015

Filloux, A. (2013). Microbiology: a weapon for bacterial warfare. *Nature* 500, 284–285. doi: 10.1038/nature12545

Fuche, F., Vianney, A., Andrea, C., Doublet, P., and Gilbert, C. (2015). Functional type 1 secretion system involved in *Legionella pneumophila* virulence. *J. Bacteriol.* 197, 563–571. doi: 10.1128/JB.02164-14

Fullner, K. J., and Mekalanos, J. J. (1999). Genetic characterization of a new type IV-A pilus gene cluster found in both classical and El Tor biotypes of *Vibrio cholerae*. *Infect. Immun.* 67, 1393–1404.

Gahlmann, A., and Moerner, W. (2014). Exploring bacterial cell biology with single-molecule tracking and super-resolution imaging. *Nature Rev. Microbiol.* 12, 9–22. doi: 10.1038/nrmicro3154

Galán, J. E., Lara-Tejero, M., Marlovits, T. C., and Wagner, S. (2014). Bacterial type III secretion systems: specialized nanomachines for protein delivery into target cells. *Annu. Rev. Microbiol.* 68, 415–438. doi: 10.1146/annurev-micro-092412-155725

Gaytán, M. O., Martínez-Santos, V. I., Soto, E., and González-Pedrajo, B. (2016). Type three secretion system in attaching and effacing pathogens. *Front. Cell. Infect. Microbiol.* 6:129. doi: 10.3389/fcimb.2016.00129

Gerc, A. J., Diepold, A., Trunk, K., Porter, M., Rickman, C., Armitage, J. P., et al. (2015). Visualization of the *Serratia* type vi secretion system reveals unprovoked attacks and dynamic assembly. *Cell Rep.* 12, 2131–2142. doi: 10.1016/j.celrep.2015.08.053

Ghosh, A. S., and Young, K. D. (2005). Helical disposition of proteins and lipopolysaccharide in the outer membrane of *Escherichia coli*. *J. Bacteriol.* 187, 1913–1922. doi: 10.1128/JB.187.6.1913-1922.2005

Gibbs, K. A., Isaac, D. D., Xu, J., Hendrix, R. W., Silhavy, T. J., and Theriot, J. A. (2004). Complex spatial distribution and dynamics of an abundant *Escherichia coli* outer membrane protein, LamB. *Mol. Microbiol.* 53, 1771–1783. doi: 10.1111/j.1365-2958.2004.04242.x

Gustafsson, M. G. (2000). Surpassing the lateral resolution limit by a factor of two using structured illumination microscopy. *J. Microsc.* 198, 82–87. doi: 10.1046/j.1365-2818.2000.00710.x

Gustafsson, M. G. (2005). Nonlinear structured-illumination microscopy: wide-field fluorescence imaging with theoretically unlimited resolution. *Proc. Natl. Acad. Sci. U.S.A.* 102, 13081–13086. doi: 10.1073/pnas.0406877102

Hancock, R. (1987). Role of porins in outer membrane permeability. *J. Bacteriol.* 169, 929. doi: 10.1128/jb.169.3.929-933.1987

Hancock, R. E., and Reeves, P. (1976). Lipopolysaccharide-deficient, bacteriophage-resistant mutants of *Escherichia coli* K-12. *J. Bacteriol.* 127, 98–108.

Heilemann, M., Dedecker, P., Hofkens, J., and Sauer, M. (2009). Photoswitches: key molecules for subdiffraction-resolution fluorescence imaging and molecular quantification. *Laser Photon. Rev.* 3, 180–202. doi: 10.1002/lpor.2008 10043

Heinz, E., Stubenrauch, C. J., Grinter, R., Croft, N. P., Purcell, A. W., Strugnell, R. A., et al. (2016). Conserved features in the structure, mechanism, and biogenesis of the inverse autotransporter protein family. *Genome Biol. Evol.* 8, 1690–1705. doi: 10.1093/gbe/evw112

Hell, S. W. (2007). Far-field optical nanoscopy. *Science* 316, 1153–1158. doi: 10.1126/science.1137395

Hell, S. W. (2009). Microscopy and its focal switch. *Nat. Methods* 6, 24–32. doi: 10.1038/nmeth.1291

Hell, S. W., and Wichmann, J. (1994). Breaking the diffraction resolution limit by stimulated emission: stimulated-emission-depletion fluorescence microscopy. *Opt. Lett.* 19, 780–782. doi: 10.1364/OL.19.000780

Ho, B. T., Dong, T. G., and Mekalanos, J. J. (2014). A view to a kill: the bacterial type VI secretion system. *Cell Host Microbe* 15, 9–21. doi: 10.1016/j.chom.2013.11.008

Hofmann, M., Eggeling, C., Jakobs, S., and Hell, S. W. (2005). Breaking the diffraction barrier in fluorescence microscopy at low light intensities by using reversibly photoswitchable proteins. *Proc. Natl. Acad. Sci. U.S.A.* 102, 17565–17569. doi: 10.1073/pnas.0506010102

Hood, R. D., Singh, P., Hsu, F., Güvener, T., Carl, M. A., Trinidad, R. R., et al. (2010). A type VI secretion system of *Pseudomonas aeruginosa* targets a toxin to bacteria. *Cell Host Microbe* 7, 25–37. doi: 10.1016/j.chom.2009.1 2.007

Hu, B., Lara-Tejero, M., Kong, Q., Galan, J. E., and Liu, J. (2017). *In situ* molecular architecture of the *Salmonella* type III secretion machine. *Cell* 168, 1065–1074.e1010. doi: 10.1016/j.cell.2017.02.022

Hu, B., Margolin, W., Molineux, I. J., and Liu, J. (2015). Structural remodeling of bacteriophage T4 and host membranes during infection initiation. *Proc. Natl. Acad. Sci. U.S.A.* 112, E4919–E4928. doi: 10.1073/pnas.15010 64112

Huang, B., Babcock, H., and Zhuang, X. (2010). Breaking the diffraction barrier: super-resolution imaging of cells. *Cell* 143, 1047–1058. doi: 10.1016/j.cell.2010.12.002

Huang, B., Bates, M., and Zhuang, X. (2009). Super-resolution fluorescence microscopy. *Annu. Rev. Biochem.* 78, 993–1016. doi: 10.1146/annurev.biochem.77.061906.092014

Jain, S., van Ulsen, P., Benz, I., Schmidt, M. A., Fernandez, R., Tommassen, J., et al. (2006). Polar localization of the autotransporter family of large bacterial virulence proteins. *J. Bacteriol.* 188, 4841–4850. doi: 10.1128/JB.003 26-06

Jakubowski, S. J., Krishnamoorthy, V., and Christie, P. J. (2003). *Agrobacterium tumefaciens* VirB6 protein participates in formation of VirB7 and VirB9 complexes required for type IV secretion. *J. Bacteriol.* 185, 2867–2878. doi: 10.1128/JB.185.9.2867-2878.2003

Janakiraman, A., and Goldberg, M. B. (2004). Evidence for polar positional information independent of cell division and nucleoid occlusion. *Proc. Natl. Acad. Sci. U.S.A.* 101, 835–840. doi: 10.1073/pnas.0305747101

Journet, L., and Cascales, E. (2016). The type VI secretion system in *Escherichia coli* and related species. *EcoSal Plus* 7:ESP-0009-2015. doi: 10.1128/ecosalplus.ESP-0009-2015

Judd, P. K., Kumar, R. B., and Das, A. (2005). The type IV secretion apparatus protein VirB6 of *Agrobacterium tumefaciens* localizes to a cell pole. *Mol. Microbiol.* 55, 115–124. doi: 10.1111/j.1365-2958.2004.04378.x

Kamiyama, D., and Huang, B. (2012). Development in the STORM. *Dev. Cell* 23, 1103–1110. doi: 10.1016/j.devcel.2012.10.003

Kato, N., Ohta, M., Kido, N., Ito, H., Naito, S., Hasegawa, T., et al. (1990). Crystallization of R-form lipopolysaccharides from *Salmonella minnesota* and *Escherichia coli*. *J. Bacteriol.* 172, 1516–1528. doi: 10.1128/jb.172.3.1516-1528.1990

Kato, N., Sugiyama, T., Naito, S., Arakawa, Y., Ito, H., Kido, N., et al. (2000). Molecular structure of bacterial endotoxin (*Escherichia coli* Re lipopolysaccharide): implications for formation of a novel heterogeneous lattice structure. *Mol. Microbiol.* 36, 796–805. doi: 10.1046/j.1365-2958.2000.01893.x

Kiss, T., Morgan, E., and Nagy, G. (2007). Contribution of SPI-4 genes to the virulence of *Salmonella enterica*. *FEMS Microbiol. Lett.* 275, 153–159. doi: 10.1111/j.1574-6968.2007.00871.x

Kjærgaard, K., Schembri, M. A., Hasman, H., and Klemm, P. (2000). Antigen 43 from *Escherichia coli* induces inter-and intraspecies cell aggregation and changes in colony morphology of *Pseudomonas fluorescens*. *J. Bacteriol.* 182, 4789–4796. doi: 10.1128/JB.182.17.4789-4796.2000

Klar, T. A., and Hell, S. W. (1999). Subdiffraction resolution in far-field fluorescence microscopy. *Opt. Lett.* 24, 954–956. doi: 10.1364/OL.24.000954

Koch, A. L. (1996). What size should a bacterium be? A question of scale. *Annu. Rev. Microbiol.* 50, 317–348. doi: 10.1146/annurev.micro.50.1.317

Kudryashev, M., Diepold, A., Amstutz, M., Armitage, J. P., Stahlberg, H., and Cornelis, G. R. (2015). *Yersinia enterocolitica* type III secretion injectisomes form regularly spaced clusters, which incorporate new machines upon activation. *Mol. Microbiol.* 95, 875–884. doi: 10.1111/mmi.12908

Kumar, R. B., and Das, A. (2002). Polar location and functional domains of the *Agrobacterium tumefaciens* DNA transfer protein VirD4. *Mol. Microbiol.* 43, 1523–1532. doi: 10.1046/j.1365-2958.2002.02829.x

Lieberman, J. A., Frost, N. A., Hoppert, M., Fernandes, P. J., Vogt, S. L., Raivio, T. L., et al. (2012). Outer membrane targeting, ultrastructure, and single molecule localization of the enteropathogenic *Escherichia coli* type IV pilus secretin BfpB. *J. Bacteriol.* 194, 1646–1658. doi: 10.1128/JB. 06330-11

Lindner, A. B., Madden, R., Demarez, A., Stewart, E. J., and Taddei, F. (2008). Asymmetric segregation of protein aggregates is associated with cellular aging and rejuvenation. *Proc. Natl. Acad. Sci. U.S.A.* 105, 3076–3081. doi: 10.1073/pnas.0708931105

Lippincott-Schwartz, J., and Patterson, G. H. (2009). Photoactivatable fluorescent proteins for diffraction-limited and super-resolution imaging. *Trends Cell Biol.* 19, 555–565. doi: 10.1016/j.tcb.2009.09.003

Low, H. H., Gubellini, F., Rivera-Calzada, A., Braun, N., Connery, S., Dujeancourt, A., et al. (2014). Structure of a type IV secretion system. *Nature* 508, 550–553. doi: 10.1038/nature13081

Lu, Q., Xu, Y., Yao, Q., Niu, M., and Shao, F. (2015). A polar-localized iron-binding protein determines the polar targeting of *Burkholderia* BimA autotransporter and actin tail formation. *Cell Microbiol.* 17, 408–424. doi: 10.1111/cmi.12376

Lybarger, S. R., Johnson, T. L., Gray, M. D., Sikora, A. E., and Sandkvist, M. (2009). Docking and assembly of the type II secretion complex of *Vibrio cholerae*. *J. Bacteriol.* 191, 3149–3161. doi: 10.1128/JB.01701-08

MacIntyre, D. L., Miyata, S. T., Kitaoka, M., and Pukatzki, S. (2010). The *Vibrio cholerae* type VI secretion system displays antimicrobial properties. *Proc. Natl. Acad. Sci. U.S.A.* 107, 19520–19524. doi: 10.1073/pnas.1012931107

Manley, S., Gillette, J. M., Patterson, G. H., Shroff, H., Hess, H. F., Betzig, E., et al. (2008). High-density mapping of single-molecule trajectories with photoactivated localization microscopy. *Nat. Methods* 5, 155–157. doi: 10.1038/nmeth.1176

Marsh, J. W., and Taylor, R. K. (1998). Identification of the *Vibrio cholerae* type 4 prepilin peptidase required for cholera toxin secretion and pilus formation. *Mol. Microbiol.* 29, 1481–1492. doi: 10.1046/j.1365-2958.1998.01031.x

Matsumoto, K., Hara, H., Fishov, I., Mileykovskaya, E., and Norris, V. (2015). The membrane: transertion as an organizing principle in membrane heterogeneity. *Front. Microbiol.* 6:572. doi: 10.3389/fmicb.2015.00572

Morgan, J. K., Luedtke, B. E., and Shaw, E. I. (2010). Polar localization of the *Coxiella burnetii* type IVB secretion system. *FEMS Microbiol. Lett.* 305, 177–183. doi: 10.1111/j.1574-6968.2010.01926.x

Mougous, J. D., Cuff, M. E., Raunser, S., Shen, A., Zhou, M., Gifford, C. A., et al. (2006). A virulence locus of *Pseudomonas aeruginosa* encodes a protein secretion apparatus. *Science* 312, 1526–1530. doi: 10.1126/science.1128393

Mühlradt, P. F., Menzel, J., Golecki, J. R., and Speth, V. (1973). Outer membrane of *Salmonella*. *Eur. J. Biochem.* 35, 471–481.

Murdoch, S. L., Trunk, K., English, G., Fritsch, M. J., Pourkarimi, E., and Coulthurst, S. J. (2011). The opportunistic pathogen *Serratia marcescens* utilizes type VI secretion to target bacterial competitors. *J. Bacteriol.* 193, 6057–6069. doi: 10.1128/JB.05671-11

Noinaj, N., Gumbart, J. C., and Buchanan, S. K. (2017). The β-barrel assembly machinery in motion. *Nat. Rev. Microbiol.* 15, 197–204. doi: 10.1038/nrmicro.2016.191

Notti, R. Q., Bhattacharya, S., Lilic, M., and Stebbins, C. E. (2015). A common assembly module in injectisome and flagellar type III secretion sorting platforms. *Nat. Commun.* 6:7125. doi: 10.1038/ncomms8125

Notti, R. Q., and Stebbins, C. E. (2016). The structure and function of type III secretion systems. *Microbiol. Spectr.* 4:VMBF-0004-2015. doi: 10.1128/microbiolspec.VMBF-0004-2015

Oddershede, L., Dreyer, J. K., Grego, S., Brown, S., and Berg-Sørensen, K. (2002). The motion of a single molecule, the λ-receptor, in the bacterial outer membrane. *Biophys. J.* 83, 3152–3161. doi: 10.1016/S0006-3495(02)75318-6

Overbye, L. J., Sandkvist, M., and Bagdasarian, M. (1993). Genes required for extracellular secretion of enterotoxin are clustered in *Vibrio cholerae*. *Gene* 132, 101–106. doi: 10.1016/0378-1119(93)90520-D

Patterson, G., Davidson, M., Manley, S., and Lippincott-Schwartz, J. (2010). Superresolution imaging using single-molecule localization. *Annu. Rev. Phys. Chem.* 61, 345–367. doi: 10.1146/annurev.physchem.012809.103444

Peabody, C. R., Chung, Y. J., Yen, M.R., Vidal-Ingigliardi, D., Pugsley, A. P., and Saier, M. H. (2003). Type II protein secretion and its relationship to bacterial type IV pili and archaeal flagella. *Microbiology* 149, 3051–3072. doi: 10.1099/mic.0.26364-0

Plummer, A. M., and Fleming, K. G. (2016). From chaperones to the membrane with a BAM! *Trends Biochem. Sci.* 41, 872–882. doi: 10.1016/j.tibs.2016.06.005

Pukatzki, S., Ma, A. T., Revel, A. T., Sturtevant, D., and Mekalanos, J. J. (2007). Type VI secretion system translocates a phage tail spike-like protein into target cells where it cross-links actin. *Proc. Natl. Acad. Sci. U.S.A.* 104, 15508–15513. doi: 10.1073/pnas.0706532104

Pukatzki, S., Ma, A. T., Sturtevant, D., Krastins, B., Sarracino, D., Nelson, W. C., et al. (2006). Identification of a conserved bacterial protein secretion system in *Vibrio cholerae* using the *Dictyostelium* host model system. *Proc. Natl. Acad. Sci. U.S.A.* 103, 1528–1533. doi: 10.1073/pnas.0510322103

Radics, J., Konigsmaier, L., and Marlovits, T. C. (2014). Structure of a pathogenic type 3 secretion system in action. *Nat. Struct. Mol. Biol.* 21, 82–87. doi: 10.1038/nsmb.2722

Rassam, P., Copeland, N. A., Birkholz, O., Tóth, C., Chavent, M., Duncan, A. L., et al. (2015). Supramolecular assemblies underpin turnover of outer membrane proteins in bacteria. *Nature* 523, 333–336. doi: 10.1038/nature14461

Ritchie, K., Lill, Y., Sood, C., Lee, H., and Zhang, S. (2013). Single-molecule imaging in live bacteria cells. *Phil. Trans. R. Soc. B* 368:20120355. doi: 10.1098/rstb.2012.0355

Rothenberg, E., Sepúlveda, L. A., Skinner, S. O., Zeng, L., Selvin, P. R., and Golding, I. (2011). Single-virus tracking reveals a spatial receptor-dependent search mechanism. *Biophys. J.* 100, 2875–2882. doi: 10.1016/j.bpj.2011.05.014

Rust, M. J., Bates, M., and Zhuang, X. (2006). Sub-diffraction-limit imaging by stochastic optical reconstruction microscopy (STORM). *Nat. Methods* 3, 793–796. doi: 10.1038/nmeth929

Samsudin, F., Ortiz-Suarez, M. L., Piggot, T. J., Bond, P. J., and Khalid, S. (2016). OmpA: a flexible clamp for bacterial cell wall attachment. *Structure* 24, 2227–2235. doi: 10.1016/j.str.2016.10.009

Sandkvist, M., Michel, L. O., Hough, L. P., Morales, V. M., Bagdasarian, M., Koomey, M., et al. (1997). General secretion pathway (eps) genes required for toxin secretion and outer membrane biogenesis in *Vibrio cholerae*. *J. Bacteriol.* 179, 6994–7003. doi: 10.1128/jb.179.22.6994-7003.1997

Schindler, M., Osborn, M. J., and Koppel, D. E. (1980). Lateral diffusion of lipopolysaccharide in the outer membrane of *Salmonella typhimurium*. *Nature* 285, 261–263. doi: 10.1038/285261a0

Schirmer, T., Keller, T. A., Wang, Y.-F., and Rosenbusch, J. P. (1995). Structural basis for sugar translocation through maltoporin channels at 3.1 angstrom resolution. *Science* 267:512. doi: 10.1126/science.7824948

Schlumberger, M. C., Müller, A. J., Ehrbar, K., Winnen, B., Duss, I., Stecher, B., et al. (2005). Real-time imaging of type III secretion: *Salmonella* SipA injection into host cells. *Proc. Natl. Acad. Sci. U.S.A.* 102, 12548–12553. doi: 10.1073/pnas.0503407102

Schwarz, S., Singh, P., Robertson, J. D., LeRoux, M., Skerrett, S. J., Goodlett, D. R., et al. (2014). VgrG-5 is a *Burkholderia* type VI secretion system-exported protein required for multinucleated giant cell formation and virulence. *Infect. Immun.* 82, 1445–1452. doi: 10.1128/IAI.01368-13

Schwarz, S., West, T. E., Boyer, F., Chiang, W.-C., Carl, M. A., Hood, R. D., et al. (2010). *Burkholderia* type VI secretion systems have distinct roles in eukaryotic and bacterial cell interactions. *PLoS Pathog.* 6:e1001068. doi: 10.1371/journal.ppat.1001068

Shrivastava, R., and Miller, J. F. (2009). Virulence factor secretion and translocation by *Bordetella* species. *Curr. Opin. Microbiol.* 12, 88–93. doi: 10.1016/j.mib.2009.01.001

Sikora, A. E., Zielke, R. A., Lawrence, D. A., Andrews, P. C., and Sandkvist, M. (2011). Proteomic analysis of the *Vibrio cholerae* type II secretome reveals new proteins, including three related serine proteases. *J. Biol. Chem.* 286, 16555–16566. doi: 10.1074/jbc.M110.211078

Slusky, J. S. (2017). Outer membrane protein design. *Curr. Opin. Struct. Biol.* 45, 45–52. doi: 10.1016/j.sbi.2016.11.003

Smit, J., and Nikaido, H. (1978). Outer membrane of gram-negative bacteria. XVIII. Electron microscopic studies on porin insertion sites and growth of cell surface of *Salmonella typhimurium*. *J. Bacteriol.* 135, 687–702.

So, E. C., Mattheis, C., Tate, E. W., Frankel, G., and Schroeder, G. N. (2015). Creating a customized intracellular niche: subversion of host cell signaling by *Legionella* type IV secretion system effectors 1. *Can. J. Microbiol.* 61, 617–635. doi: 10.1139/cjm-2015-0166

Spector, J., Zakharov, S., Lill, Y., Sharma, O., Cramer, W. A., and Ritchie, K. (2010). Mobility of BtuB and OmpF in the *Escherichia coli* outer membrane: implications for dynamic formation of a translocon complex. *Biophys. J.* 99, 3880–3886. doi: 10.1016/j.bpj.2010.10.029

Spreter, T., Yip, C. K., Sanowar, S., Andre, I., Kimbrough, T. G., Vuckovic, M., et al. (2009). A conserved structural motif mediates formation of the periplasmic rings in the type III secretion system. *Nat. Struct. Mol. Biol.* 16, 468–476. doi: 10.1038/nsmb.1603

Thiem, S., Kentner, D., and Sourjik, V. (2007). Positioning of chemosensory clusters in *E. coli* and its relation to cell division. *EMBO J.* 26, 1615–1623. doi: 10.1038/sj.emboj.7601610

Thiem, S., and Sourjik, V. (2008). Stochastic assembly of chemoreceptor clusters in *Escherichia coli*. *Mol. Microbiol.* 68, 1228–1236. doi: 10.1111/j.1365-2958.2008.06227.x

Thomas, S., Holland, I. B., and Schmitt, L. (2014). The type 1 secretion pathway—the hemolysin system and beyond. *Biochim. Biophys. Acta* 1843, 1629–1641. doi: 10.1016/j.bbamcr.2013.09.017

Toomre, D., and Bewersdorf, J. (2010). A new wave of cellular imaging. *Annu. Rev. Cell Dev. Biol.* 26, 285–314. doi: 10.1146/annurev-cellbio-100109-104048

Trokter, M., Felisberto-Rodrigues, C., Christie, P. J., and Waksman, G. (2014). Recent advances in the structural and molecular biology of type IV secretion systems. *Curr. Opin. Struct. Biol.* 27, 16–23. doi: 10.1016/j.sbi.2014.02.006

Turnbull, L., Toyofuku, M., Hynen, A. L., Kurosawa, M., Pessi, G., Petty, N. K., et al. (2016). Explosive cell lysis as a mechanism for the biogenesis of bacterial membrane vesicles and biofilms. *Nat Commun.* 7:11220. doi: 10.1038/ncomms11220

Ursell, T. S., Trepagnier, E. H., Huang, K. C., and Theriot, J. A. (2012). Analysis of surface protein expression reveals the growth pattern of the gram-negative outer membrane. *PLoS Comput. Biol.* 8:e1002680. doi: 10.1371/journal.pcbi.1002680

van Ulsen, P., ur Rahman, S. U., Jong, W. S., Daleke-Schermerhorn, M. H., and Luirink, J. (2014). Type V secretion: from biogenesis to biotechnology. *Biochim. Biophys. Acta* 1843, 1592–1611. doi: 10.1016/j.bbamcr.2013.11.006

Verhoeven, G. S., Dogterom, M., and den Blaauwen, T. (2013). Absence of long-range diffusion of OmpA in *E. coli* is not caused by its peptidoglycan binding domain. *BMC Microbiol.* 13:66. doi: 10.1186/1471-2180-13-66

Voth, D. E., and Heinzen, R. A. (2007). Lounging in a lysosome: the intracellular lifestyle of *Coxiella burnetii*. *Cell. Microbiol.* 9, 829–840. doi: 10.1111/j.1462-5822.2007.00901.x

Wang, H., Wingreen, N. S., and Mukhopadhyay, R. (2008). Self-organized periodicity of protein clusters in growing bacteria. *Phys. Rev. Lett.* 101:218101. doi: 10.1103/PhysRevLett.101.218101

Ward, D. V., Draper, O., Zupan, J. R., and Zambryski, P. C. (2002). Peptide linkage mapping of the *Agrobacterium tumefaciens* vir-encoded type IV secretion system reveals protein subassemblies. *Proc. Natl. Acad. Sci. U.S.A.* 99, 11493–11500. doi: 10.1073/pnas.172390299

Wong, A. R., Pearson, J. S., Bright, M. D., Munera, D., Robinson, K. S., Lee, S. F., et al. (2011). Enteropathogenic and enterohaemorrhagic *Escherichia coli*: even more subversive elements. *Mol. Microbiol.* 80, 1420–1438. doi: 10.1111/j.1365-2958.2011.07661.x

Xie, X. S., Choi, P. J., Li, G. W., Lee, N. K., and Lia, G. (2008). Single-molecule approach to molecular biology in living bacterial cells. *Annu. Rev. Biophys.* 37, 417–444. doi: 10.1146/annurev.biophys.37.092607.174640

Zoued, A., Brunet, Y. R., Durand, E., Aschtgen, M.S., Logger, L., Douzi, B., et al. (2014). Architecture and assembly of the Type VI secretion system. *Biochim. Biophys. Acta* 1843, 1664–1673. doi: 10.1016/j.bbamcr.2014.03.018

Zoued, A., Durand, E., Brunet, Y. R., Spinelli, S., Douzi, B., Guzzo, M., et al. (2016). Priming and polymerization of a bacterial contractile tail structure. *Nature* 531, 59–63. doi: 10.1038/nature17182

Zupan, J., Muth, T. R., Draper, O., and Zambryski, P. (2000). The transfer of DNA from *Agrobacterium tumefaciens* into plants: a feast of fundamental insights. *Plant J.* 23, 11–28. doi: 10.1046/j.1365-313x.2000.00808.x

3

Life After Secretion—*Yersinia enterocolitica* Rapidly Toggles Effector Secretion and can Resume Cell Division in Response to Changing External Conditions

Bailey Milne-Davies, Carlos Helbig, Stephan Wimmi, Dorothy W. C. Cheng†, Nicole Paczia and Andreas Diepold*

Department of Ecophysiology, Max Planck Institute for Terrestrial Microbiology, Marburg, Germany

Correspondence:
Andreas Diepold
andreas.diepold@mpi-marburg.mpg.de

Many pathogenic bacteria use the type III secretion system (T3SS) injectisome to manipulate host cells by injecting virulence-promoting effector proteins into the host cytosol. The T3SS is activated upon host cell contact, and its activation is accompanied by an arrest of cell division; hence, many species maintain a T3SS-inactive sibling population to propagate efficiently within the host. The enteric pathogen *Yersinia enterocolitica* utilizes the T3SS to prevent phagocytosis and inhibit inflammatory responses. Unlike other species, almost all *Y. enterocolitica* are T3SS-positive at 37°C, which raises the question, how these bacteria are able to propagate within the host, that is, when and how they stop secretion and restart cell division after a burst of secretion. Using a fast and quantitative *in vitro* secretion assay, we have examined the initiation and termination of type III secretion. We found that effector secretion begins immediately once the activating signal is present, and instantly stops when this signal is removed. Following effector secretion, the bacteria resume division within minutes after being introduced to a non-secreting environment, and the same bacteria are able to re-initiate effector secretion at later time points. Our results indicate that *Y. enterocolitica* use their type III secretion system to promote their individual survival when necessary, and are able to quickly switch their behavior toward replication afterwards, possibly gaining an advantage during infection.

Keywords: bacterial protein secretion, host-pathogen interaction, regulation of virulence mechanisms, protein translocation, *Yersinia enterocolitica*, enteropathogens

INTRODUCTION

Bacteria use their type III secretion systems (T3SS) in a variety of ways to survive in different environments. The virulence-associated T3SS[1] is a membrane-spanning nanosyringe that is used by various Gram-negative bacteria to export effector proteins into the cytoplasm of eukaryotic host cells, allowing them to modify host cell behavior (Cornelis, 2006; Galán, 2009; Pha, 2016).

[1]In this manuscript, T3SS refers to virulence-associated T3SS. The common "Sct" nomenclature (Hueck, 1998; Portaliou et al., 2016) is used for T3SS components, see (Diepold and Wagner, 2014) for species-specific names.

The T3SS protein complex, commonly named the injectisome, is comprised of an extracellular needle, a series of membrane rings embedding an export apparatus, and several cytosolic components (**Figure 1A**). The needle creates a continuous channel that connects the bacterium to the host cytoplasm with the help of translocator proteins that form a needle tip and a pore within the host cell membrane (Håkansson et al., 1996; Nauth et al., 2018; Park et al., 2018), thus allowing the translocation of effector proteins. The membrane rings anchor the injectisome in the peptidoglycan and the inner and outer membrane, while the export apparatus facilitates the transfer of effectors from the bacterial cytosol through the needle (Kuhlen et al., 2018). The cytosolic components, which shuttle between the cytosol and the injectisome, bind to chaperone-effector complexes and govern the order of secretion (Akeda and Galán, 2005; Lara-Tejero et al., 2011; Diepold et al., 2015). During the assembly and function of the T3SS, three substrate classes are subsequently exported. The early substrates include the needle subunit and a ruler protein that determines the length of the needle. Once the correct needle length is reached, the hydrophilic translocator, classified as intermediate substrate, is exported and assembles a needle tip (Mueller et al., 2005). At this stage, the T3SS is in a standby mode (Enninga and Rosenshine, 2009), and secretion of the late substrates, the pore-forming hydrophobic translocators and the virulence effectors, can be induced, for example by host cell contact.

Pathogens including *Salmonella, Shigella, Pseudomonas*, and *Yersinia* use their T3SS to promote survival and enhance pathogenicity within the host (Büttner, 2012; Deng et al., 2017). In some pathogenic species, such as *Salmonella enterica* and *Pseudomonas aeruginosa*, T3SS are heterogeneously expressed resulting in two subpopulations (Rietsch and Mekalanos, 2006; Sturm et al., 2011; Rundell et al., 2016). The resulting mixed populations can allow bacteria that express the T3SS to promote the survival of their siblings that do not. This is evident for the T3SS encoded by the *Salmonella* pathogenicity island (SPI)-1, where bacteria utilize their T3SS to promote entry into host cells, but also to induce inflammation of the intestinal lumen and remove competition of the intestinal flora (Stecher et al., 2007; Müller et al., 2009; Knodler et al., 2010; Behnsen et al., 2014). The SPI-1-utilizing bacteria display a retarded growth rate, which is a common trait of actively type III-secreting bacteria (Kupferberg and Higuchi, 1958; Mehigh et al., 1989; Fowler and Brubaker, 1994; Sturm et al., 2011). As a result, bacteria that do not express their T3SS outgrow the SPI-1-active population, which can be interpreted as an investment of the SPI-1-active bacteria into increased chances for their genetically identical SPI-1-inactive siblings (Sturm et al., 2011; Diard et al., 2013; Sánchez-Romero and Casadesús, 2018; Weigel and Dersch, 2018).

Yersinia enterocolitica is considered a largely extracellular pathogen that uses its T3SS mainly to prevent phagocytosis, inhibit inflammatory responses and promote dissemination (Navarro et al., 2005; Cornelis, 2006; Galán, 2009; Pha, 2016). Once *Yersinia* are exposed to a temperature of 37°C (e.g., after entering a host organism), they start expressing T3SS components (Skurnik et al., 1984; Lambert de Rouvroit et al., 1992). During infection, *Y. enterocolitica* can come into contact with host cells, such as macrophages, dissociate, and possibly establish contact with further host cells. Contact with a host cell activates the secretion of effectors, called Yops (*Yersinia* outer proteins), by the T3SS (Cornelis, 2002). *In vitro*, this activation can be achieved by the chelation of calcium (Ca^{2+}) from the extracellular environment. Under these conditions, the bacteria begin exporting their effectors and upregulate effector expression (Cornelis et al., 1987; Wiley et al., 2007; Dewoody et al., 2013). In this study, we used strains based on wild-type *Y. enterocolitica* expressing all virulence effectors (MRS40), as well as on a strain lacking the six main virulence effectors YopH,O,P,E,M,T, as well as the aspartate-beta-semialdehyde dehydrogenase gene (ΔHOPEMTasd), which is consequently avirulent, auxotrophic for the cell wall component diaminopimelic acid, and can be analyzed under safety class 1 conditions.

Prior studies have mainly focused on the activation of the T3SS by host cell contact or Ca^{2+} chelation. However, the post-secretion events like deactivation, reestablishment of bacterial division and the possibility of reactivation of the T3SS are likely to play an equally essential role in promoting bacterial survival and pathogenesis within the host. We therefore used a fast and quantitative *in vitro* secretion assay to examine the initiation and termination of type III secretion in *Y. enterocolitica*, monitored the rate of cell growth and division throughout these steps, and assessed whether previously T3SS-active bacteria can initiate further secretion events. Our results show that activation and deactivation occur immediately in response to changing external conditions, and that after secretion, bacteria transition back to division within short time, while remaining able to reactivate their T3SS.

RESULTS

Expression and Assembly of the *Y. enterocolitica* T3SS Is Uniform and Stable Under Different Conditions

Earlier visualizations of T3SS components within *Y. enterocolitica* showed that most bacteria express T3SS, which are localized in a non-random pattern of small patches visible as fluorescent foci at the bacterial surface (Diepold et al., 2010, 2017; Kudryashev et al., 2015). To quantify the fraction of T3SS-positive *Y. enterocolitica*, we analyzed how many bacteria within a population displayed this standard pattern of fluorescence for functional EGFP-labeled versions of a T3SS inner membrane ring protein (SctD), and a cytosolic protein (SctQ) at 37°C. Both under non-secreting conditions (presence of 5 mM Ca^{2+} in the medium) and secreting conditions (chelation of Ca^{2+} by addition of 5 mM EGTA), all or almost all bacteria were T3SS-positive (**Figure 1B, Supplementary Figure 1**). Even after long-term incubation under secreting conditions for 3 h, the vast majority of bacteria (>98%) were T3SS-positive (**Figure 1C**).

Activation Kinetics of the *Y. enterocolitica* T3SS by Ca^{2+} Chelation

The previous results showed that *Y. enterocolitica* populations almost uniformly assemble T3SS injectisomes. We next analyzed

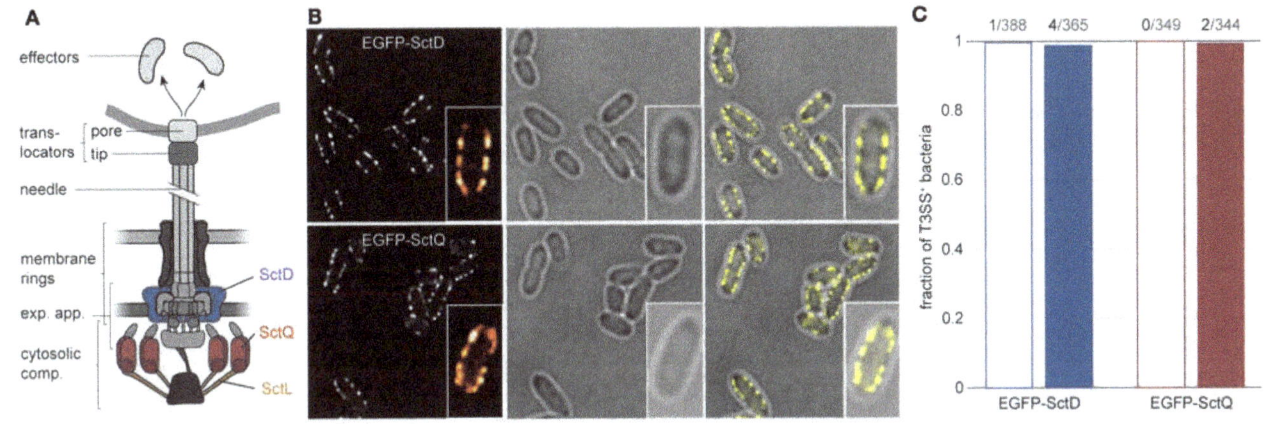

FIGURE 1 | The type III secretion system is expressed in almost all *Y. enterocolitica*, both under secreting and non-secreting conditions. **(A)** Schematic overview of the different substructures of the T3SS (left). Positions of the labeled proteins analyzed in this study are indicated (right). exp. app, export apparatus. **(B)** Micrographs of *Y. enterocolitica* ΔHOPEMTasd expressing EGFP-SctD (top) or EGFP-SctQ (bottom) from their native genetic localization. Three hours after induction of T3SS expression by temperature shift to 37°C under non-secreting conditions, bacteria were subjected to secreting conditions, and imaged. Left, EGFP fluorescence (insets show fluorescence intensity for one enlarged bacterium in ImageJ red-hot coloring scale); center, corresponding phase contrast images; right, overlay. Larger fields of view and images of bacteria under non-secreting conditions are shown in **Supplementary Figure 1**. **(C)** Fraction of bacteria with standard expression and distribution of T3SS (multiple membrane foci) for the indicated fusion protein, 3 h after induction of expression of the T3SS under non-secreting conditions (empty bars) or secreting conditions (filled bars) $n = 344–388$. Numbers on top indicate the number of bacteria that do not display multiple visible T3SS, and the number of analyzed bacteria. Secreting and non-secreting conditions refer to incubation in medium with addition of 5 mM EGTA or $CaCl_2$, respectively.

the activation and deactivation of these injectisomes in more detail, using an improved version of a previously published enzymatic export assay (Diepold et al., 2015), which measures the export of the reporter construct $YopH_{1-17}$-β-lactamase (Charpentier and Oswald, 2004; Marketon et al., 2005). The updated protocol utilizes the pACYC184 plasmid instead of pBAD, which removes background β-lactamase activity (**Supplementary Figure 2A**). The higher signal/noise ratio of the modified assay allowed us to reliably quantify secretion in intervals of down to 5 min, and we confirmed that the enzymatic assay itself is not strongly influenced by the used concentration of $CaCl_2$ or EGTA (**Supplementary Figure 2B**). We therefore were able to quantify the initiation of secretion in *Y. enterocolitica* ΔHOPEMTasd within the first 15 min after Ca^{2+} chelation. Within this time range, secretion is difficult to quantify even in an accumulative standard *in vitro* secretion assay (**Figure 2A**). For the reporter export assay, bacteria were grown at 37°C under non-secreting conditions, allowing for assembly, but not activation of T3SS. Secretion was then activated by resuspension in medium lacking Ca^{2+} and samples were taken every 5 min, and tested for export of the reporter substrate into the supernatant within the following 5 min. The results of the reporter assay clearly show that secretion is fully active at the earliest time range after activation (0–5 min) (**Figure 2B**), suggesting that effector secretion is initiated immediately by Ca^{2+} chelation. To test whether this fast activation of effector secretion impacts the cellular ATP levels, we determined the adenylate energy charge (([ATP]+0.5[ADP])/([ATP]+[ADP]+[AMP])) of wild-type *Y. enterocolitica* ΔHOPEMTasd, incubated under the same conditions, 10 min after activation of the T3SS. We found that the energy charge of the secreting cultures was not significantly decreased in this time range (**Supplementary Figure 3**). In line with these findings, the level of secretion of the reporter substrate remained constant throughout the first 2 h after secretion (**Figure 2B**, **Supplementary Figure 4** and data not shown). Secretion activity in a freshly activated wild-type strain was comparable to that of a SctW (YopN) deletion strain, which is calcium-blind and continuously secretes effectors (**Supplementary Figure 4**), underlining that the level of protein secretion immediately after activation is comparable to the level during ongoing secretion.

T3SS Effector Secretion Ceases Within Minutes After Removal of the Activating Signal

Next, we measured if and how fast the T3SS is inactivated upon reintroduction of Ca^{2+} into the medium. Wild-type *Y. enterocolitica* that had been secreting for 2 h were subjected to non-secreting medium, and the export of the reporter substrate was measured in 10-min intervals afterwards. Already within the first period after Ca^{2+} addition, the export of the reporter strongly dropped compared to the control that was left under secreting conditions (**Figure 3A**, **Supplementary Figure 4**). Based on the amount of exported reporter substrate under non-secreting conditions over time (green bars in **Figure 3A**), deactivation is likely to occur within the first minutes after the removal of the activating signal. Similar to the activation, deactivation of secretion did not increase the energy charge of the bacteria within these time ranges (**Supplementary Figure 3**).

To further investigate the inactivation of secretion, we aimed to determine, which factor, temperature or Ca^{2+} concentration, has a greater effect on the export of different substrate classes.

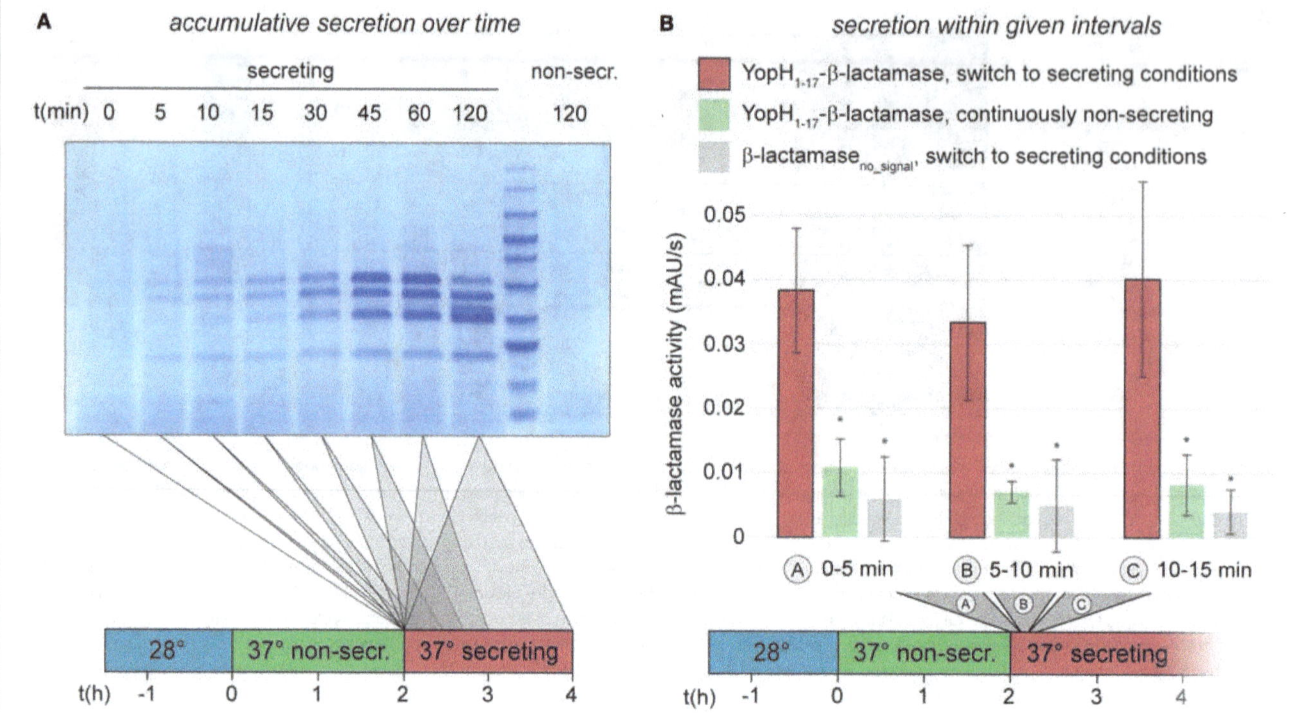

FIGURE 2 | Immediate activation of the T3SS can be measured by an *in vitro* β-lactamase assay. **(A)** Accumulative effector secretion into the culture supernatant during a standard *in vitro* secretion assay using *Y. enterocolitica* MRS40. At the time points indicated (0 min = activation of T3SS secretion by resuspension of bacteria in secreting medium, see also time line at bottom), the culture supernatant of 3×10^9 bacteria was removed and visualized by Coomassie staining of an SDS-PAGE gel. Control (far right), bacteria resuspended in non-secreting medium. **(B)** Quantification of effector export in the indicated time ranges after resuspension of *Y. enterocolitica* ΔHOPEMTasd in secreting medium (see also time line at bottom). Red bars, β-lactamase activity indicative of export of the reporter T3SS substrate $YopH_{1-17}$-β-lactamase; green bars, non-secreting control; gray bars, β-lactamase lacking a T3SS secretion signal under secreting conditions. Error bars indicate standard deviation of the averages of technical triplicates between three biological replicates. $^{*}p < 0.05$ vs. the $YopH_{1-17}$-β-lactamase, switch to secreting conditions, sample (red bars) in a two-tailed homoscedastic *t*-test. Secreting and non-secreting (non-secr.) conditions refer to incubation in medium with addition of 5 mM EGTA or $CaCl_2$, respectively.

We therefore analyzed the export of virulence effectors (YopE and YopM), the needle protein SctF, the hydrophilic translocator SctA (=LcrV), and the ruler protein SctP in a wild-type strain expressing all virulence effectors (MRS40). Cultures were grown in secreting conditions and after 3 h, the previously secreting cultures were exposed to non-secreting or secreting conditions, at 26 or 37°C. Our results show that while export of the virulence effectors was strongly repressed by the addition of Ca^{2+}, they were secreted in the absence of Ca^{2+}, irrespective of the temperature (**Figures 3B,C**). Export of the needle, translocator and ruler protein, in contrast, was more strongly influenced by the temperature than by the Ca^{2+} level, although this effect was not statistically significant for SctF and SctP (**Figures 3B,C**). The resuspension steps used in our protocol do not affect assembled needles, and in all cases, cell lysis was negligible; differences in expression levels cannot explain the observed export phenotype (**Supplementary Figures 5–7**).

Y. enterocolitica Can Resume Growth or Engage in New Secretion Activity After Secretion Has Ended

Having analyzed the activation and deactivation of type III secretion by external signals, we turned our interest to the events after secretion. Specifically, we wanted to find out whether and when post-secretion *Y. enterocolitica* can resume division and/or re-initiate secretion. To answer the first question, we compared the optical culture density of wild-type *Y. enterocolitica* (MRS40) bacteria that had previously been secreting, and were then either kept under secreting conditions, or subjected to non-secreting conditions. Compared to the non-secreting control, secreting bacteria slow down their division (**Figures 4A,B**, "first incubation"). Strikingly, previously secreting bacteria that were subjected to non-secreting conditions resumed division within a short time (**Figures 4A,B**, "second incubation"). This phenotype is linked to T3SS activity, as indicated by the steady division of T3SS-negative ΔSctD bacteria under all tested conditions (**Figures 4A,B**). As expected, constantly secreting bacteria (the "Ca^{2+} blind" ΔSctW (ΔYopN) strain (Yother and Goguen, 1985), **Supplementary Figure 7**) displayed growth curves similar to wild-type under secreting conditions, irrespective of the medium. Similar results were obtained on solid medium, where T3SS-positive bacteria did not divide, and only slightly increased their cell volume, under sustained secreting conditions, in contrast to T3SS-negative bacteria (**Figure 4C, Supplementary Figure 8**). Under non-secreting conditions, both populations displayed a higher rate of growth and division

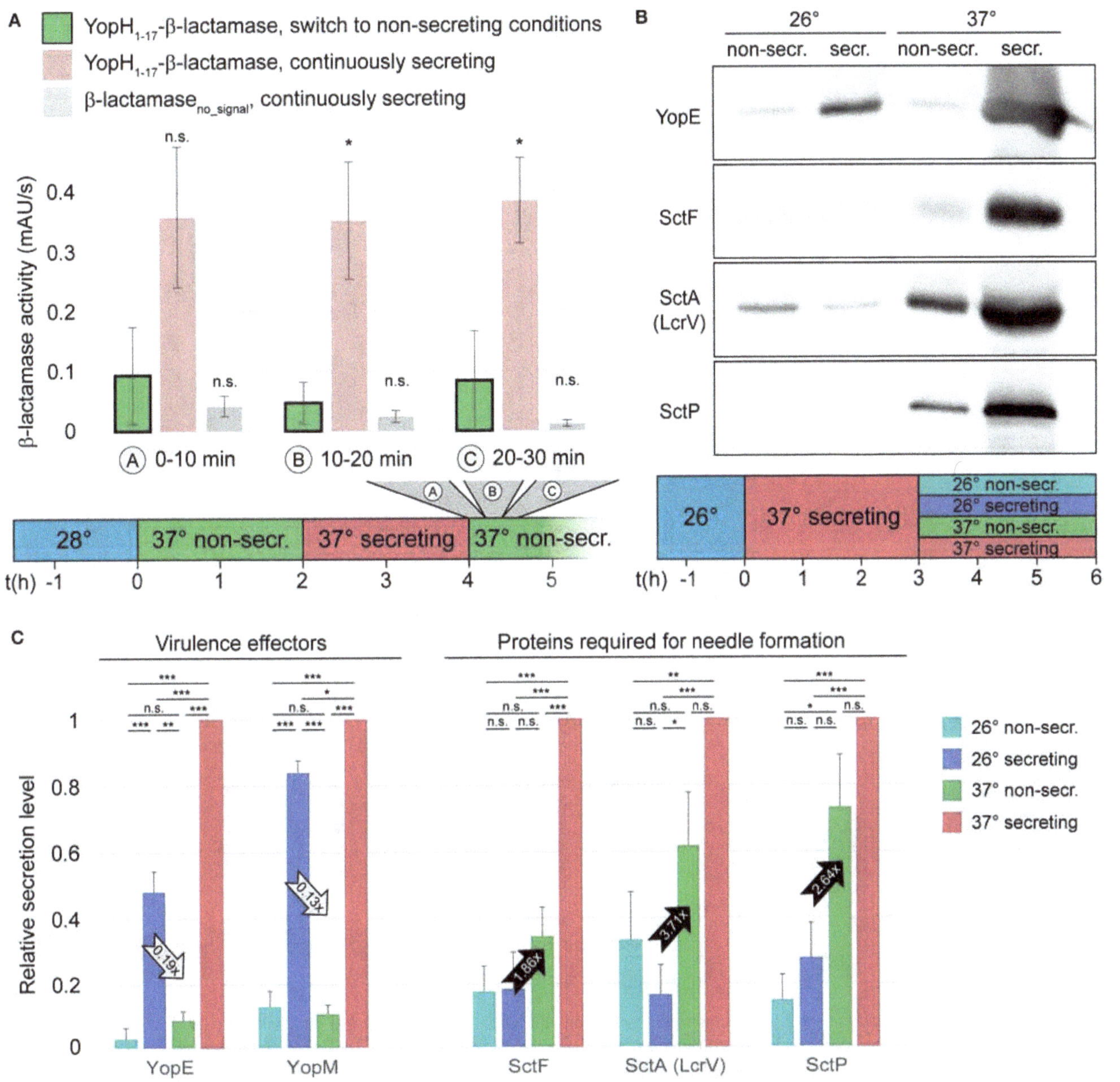

FIGURE 3 | Type III secretion, but not needle formation, is stopped within short time in the absence of activating signal. **(A)** Quantification of effector export in the indicated time ranges after resuspension of *Y. enterocolitica* ΔHOPEMTasd in non-secreting medium (see also time line at bottom). Green bars, β-lactamase activity indicative of export of the reporter T3SS substrate $YopH_{1-17}$-β-lactamase; red bars, secreting control; gray bars, β-lactamase lacking a T3SS secretion signal under secreting conditions. Error bars indicate standard deviation of the averages of technical triplicates between three biological replicates. $^{*}p < 0.05$ vs. the $YopH_{1-17}$-β-lactamase, switch to non-secreting conditions, sample in a two-tailed homoscedastic *t*-test; n.s., difference not statistically significant. **(B)** The export of different substrate classes is influenced differently by the temperature and the external calcium concentration. Wild-type *Y. enterocolitica* expressing all effectors (MRS40) were grown at 26°C for 1.5 h, and subsequently at 37°C under secreting conditions for 3 h. Afterwards, they were resuspended in different conditions, as indicated (top and time line at bottom) for another 3 h. Proteins secreted by 3×10^9 bacteria were separated on an SDS-PAGE gel and analyzed by immunoblot using antibodies against the indicated proteins, the effector YopE, the needle subunit SctF, the hydrophilic translocator SctA (LcrV), and the ruler protein SctP ($n = 4$, image representative). The respective analysis for bacteria directly subjected to the indicated conditions after incubation at 26°C, Coomassie-based analysis of all secreted proteins, and protein expression controls are displayed in **Supplementary Figure 6**. **(C)** Relative secretion levels of indicated virulence effectors (left) and proteins required for needle export (right) under the indicated conditions [see time line in **(B)**]. Secretion levels were quantified by densitometric analysis of the bands for the respective proteins in Coomassie-stained SDS-PAGE gels for YopE and YopM ($n = 3$) and immunoblots for YopE (one additional analysis), SctF, SctA (LcrV), and SctP ($n = 4$ in each case), and normalized to the respective secretion level at 37°C under secreting conditions. Error bars display the standard error of the mean; arrows indicate the difference between the influence of the temperature (28°C, secreting conditions) and calcium levels (37°C, non-secreting conditions) and the ratio of secretion under these conditions. Secreting and non-secreting (non-secr.) conditions refer to incubation in medium with addition of 5 mM EGTA or $CaCl_2$, respectively. $^{*}p < 0.05$, $^{**}p < 0.01$, $^{***}p < 0.001$ in a two-tailed homoscedastic *t*-test; n.s., difference not statistically significant.

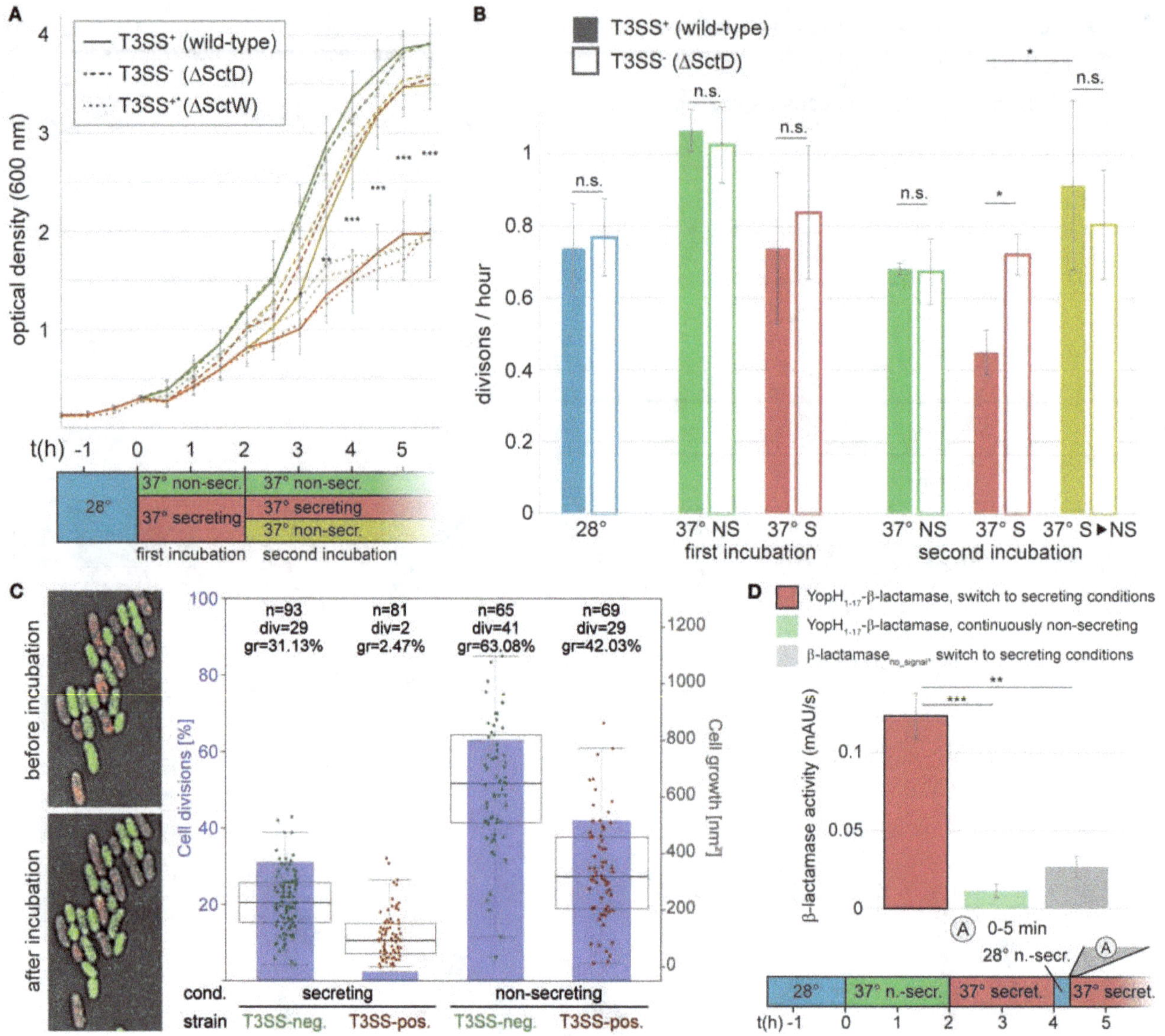

FIGURE 4 | Bacteria can resume division, or engage in another round of secretion after deactivation of secretion. **(A)** Growth curves (optical culture density at 600 nm) of T3SS-positive *Y. enterocolitica* wild-type MRS40 expressing all virulence effectors ($T3SS^+$, continuous lines), T3SS-negative bacteria ($T3SS^-$, dashed lines), and Ca^{2+}-blind constantly secreting bacteria ($T3SS^{+*}$, dotted lines) incubated under the conditions indicated in the time line (bottom). **(B)** Number of bacterial divisions per hour during the different phases, colors as in **(A)**. Filled bars, T3SS-positive bacteria; open bars, T3SS-negative bacteria. Error bars indicate the standard deviation of the averages of technical triplicates between three independent biological replicates. **(C)** Growth and division of T3SS-positive (mCherry-SctL, red) and T3SS-negative (EGFP-SctL ΔSctD, green) *Y. enterocolitica* ΔHOPEMTasd on LB-agarose pads under secreting conditions during the first 2 h of the second incubation period [see **(A)**]. Left, fluorescence micrographs showing growth and division of green (T3SS-negative), but not of red (T3SS-positive) bacteria within the analysis period. Right, quantification of fraction of cell divisions (blue bars and axis on left side) and cell growth (increase in two-dimensional cell area on micrographs) per initial bacterium (box charts and single data points, right axis) for the indicated strains and conditions. Each data point represents a single measurement. The boxes show the median and quartiles (75th and 25th percentile). The whiskers extend 1.5 times the interquartile range until the furthest data point within this range. No standard deviation is displayed. n, number of analyzed bacteria; div, number of bacteria dividing within analysis period; gr, average growth (increase of cell area) within analysis period. Cell growth is statistically significantly different ($p < 0.001$ in a two-tailed homoscedastic *t*-test) for all pairwise comparisons of strains and conditions. **(D)** Quantification of effector export in the indicated time range after resuspension of *Y. enterocolitica* ΔHOPEMTasd in secreting medium after a 15 min incubation in non-secreting medium at 28°C (see time line at bottom). Red bar, β-lactamase activity indicative of export of the reporter T3SS substrate $YopH_{1-17}$-β-lactamase; green bar, non-secreting control; gray bar, β-lactamase lacking a T3SS secretion signal under secreting conditions. Error bars indicate standard deviation of the averages of technical triplicates between three biological replicates. Secreting and non-secreting conditions refer to incubation in medium with addition of 5 mM EGTA or $CaCl_2$, respectively. The incubation steps at 28°C (blue bars) are performed in medium with 5 mM $CaCl_2$. $^*p < 0.05$; $^{**}p < 0.01$; $^{***}p < 0.001$ in a two-tailed homoscedastic *t*-test; n.s., difference not statistically significant. For **(A)**, this statistical analysis applies to the difference between wild-type and ΔSctD under secreting conditions (continuous and dashed red lines), other time points were not statistically significantly different.

(**Figure 4C**, **Supplementary Figure 8**). Taken together, these results indicate that individual *Y. enterocolitica* cells not only can disengage from secretion within a short time, but also quickly resume division in the absence of further stimulating signals.

To determine if *Y. enterocolitica* can also go through repeated cycles of secretion activation and deactivation, we tested the reactivation of secretion in bacteria that had been secreting for 2 h, and where secretion was stopped afterwards by addition of $CaCl_2$. These bacteria were incubated in the presence of Ca^{2+} for 15 min at 28°C to suppress the formation of new injectisomes (**Figure 3B**), and then again subjected to secreting conditions (37°C, absence of Ca^{2+}). The secretion of effectors started within the first 5 min after the renewed incubation under secreting conditions (**Figure 4D**), which shows that type III secretion can be reactivated, and that this occurs within a similarly short time as the initial activation of secretion.

DISCUSSION

Life after secretion—the deactivation of the T3SS, the recovery of division, and possible additional encounters with host cells—is incompletely understood in *Yersinia*, despite the critical role of these events in the infection process. In this study, we therefore explored the kinetics of activation and, most crucially, deactivation of secretion by external cues, as well as the potential of *Y. enterocolitica* to restart division and to re-initiate secretion afterwards. During infection, when *Y. enterocolitica* enter the Peyer's Patches, bacteria may come into contact with immune cells. In this situation, fast initiation of effector export provides essential defense against phagocytosis and inflammatory signals to the immune system (Grosdent et al., 2002; Navarro et al., 2005; Galán, 2009; Pha, 2016; Philip et al., 2016). Such fast activation of type III secretion has indeed been shown for various bacteria (Enninga et al., 2005; Schlumberger et al., 2005; Mills et al., 2008). Following the interaction with the host, however, *Y. enterocolitica* conceivably benefit from stopping effector export, which may allow them to resume division and disseminate within the host (where the bacteria may again face contact with immune cells). To study T3SS activation and deactivation kinetics in a fast, reproducible and quantitative manner, we used an *in vitro* secretion assay for the reporter substrate β-lactamase in *Y. enterocolitica*, fused to the minimal secretion signal for the native *Y. enterocolitica* virulence effector YopH (Sory et al., 1995). Low and high calcium levels, as used in the assay, have been proposed to mimic the intracellular environment within host cells (low Ca^{2+}), and the extracellular host environment (high Ca^{2+}), respectively (Fowler and Brubaker, 1994). Our results show that just like activation of secretion (**Figure 2**), deactivation (**Figure 3A**) occurs immediately when introduced into secreting or non-secreting media, respectively.

The ability of *Y. enterocolitica* to respond quickly to these external stimuli suggests one or several highly sensitive regulation mechanisms. How exactly host cell contact and changes in the environment, such as the Ca^{2+} levels, are sensed, is still unclear. A number of studies, predominantly performed in *Shigella flexneri* and *Pseudomonas aeruginosa*, suggest that the needle tip senses host cell contact (Veenendaal et al., 2007; Roehrich et al., 2013; Armentrout and Rietsch, 2016), and that the signal is transmitted through rearrangements of the needle subunits to the cytosolic interface of the T3SS (Kenjale et al., 2005; Torruellas et al., 2005; Davis and Mecsas, 2006). Other external factors, such as the Ca^{2+} level and factors inducing other T3SS such as Congo Red might also be sensed at the needle tip and be transmitted the same way. However, the composition of the cytosolic complex of the *Y. enterocolitica* T3SS was shown to be influenced by external Ca^{2+} levels in strains lacking SctD (and therefore also not assembling needles), suggesting a direct sensing mechanism (Diepold et al., 2017). The Ca^{2+}-dependent interaction of the ruler SctP and the cytosolic gatekeeper protein SctW in enteropathogenic *E. coli* (EPEC) supports yet another model in which the export of effectors is inhibited as long as a local influx of Ca^{2+} ions occurs through T3SS needles which are not in contact to a host cell (Shaulov et al., 2017).

Notably, in our deactivation experiments, not all substrate classes were affected equally by the Ca^{2+} level. While export of the tested effectors (YopE and YopM) was strongly suppressed upon addition of Ca^{2+}, the export of early and intermediary substrates, required for the formation of new needles, continued, albeit at a lower rate. In contrast, a reduction of the temperature to 26°C at continuous low Ca^{2+} levels strongly decreased the export of early and intermediary substrates, but allowed the continued export of the effectors (**Figure 3B**). This phenotype is most likely not a mere effect of the expression levels of the exported proteins: While the initial expression of all T3SS export substrates is strongly regulated by the temperature, as a consequence of the temperature-dependent expression of the main transcriptional regulator of the T3SS, VirF (Cornelis et al., 1989; Hoe and Goguen, 1993; Böhme et al., 2012), this effect is far less pronounced in a system that has previously been activated by incubation at 37°C under secreting conditions (**Supplementary Figures 6A,B**). This indicates that in the latter case, mRNA and proteins levels are sufficient for continuous effector secretion at low Ca^{2+} levels, even at 26°C. The secretion of the proteins required for needle formation is more strongly repressed at 26°C (although this effect is only statistically significant for SctA=LcrV), suggesting that the inhibition of the secretion of needle-related proteins and effectors are controlled by additional, and different, regulatory pathways. A similar differential regulation of secretion of the different substrate classes has been shown for *P. aeruginosa* (Cisz et al., 2008) and EPEC (Shaulov et al., 2017), suggesting that this mechanism is conserved amongst different T3SS.

Regulating the events after secretion is particularly important for *Y. enterocolitica*, which differ from other pathogens in that they homogeneously express the T3SS when exposed to 37°C (**Figure 1**, **Supplementary Figure 1**), and that the complete population can activate secretion *in vitro* (Wiley et al., 2007). The low fraction of T3SS-negative bacteria even after prolonged *in vitro* secretion (**Figure 1C**), despite the lower replication rate of these bacteria, highlights the important role of T3SS function during infection in *Y. enterocolitica*. What then happens after a bacterium has survived an encounter with an immune cell? Once effector secretion has ceased, *Y.*

enterocolitica benefit from re-initiating faster replication, but have to remain guarded for additional interactions with immune cells. It has been an open question whether re-initiation of replication can be observed *in vitro*, where all injectisomes are activated (Wiley et al., 2007), which might differ from the situation during an infection (Heroven and Dersch, 2014; Avican et al., 2015). We found that *Y. enterocolitica* can quickly resume division when exposed to a non-secreting environment after prior incubation in a secretion-activating environment (**Figures 4A–C**). This recovery (as well as the cessation of growth and division upon secretion initiation) appears independent of the cellular energy levels, which did not significantly drop under secreting conditions within the tested time range in the used effector-less strain (**Supplementary Figure 3**). At this point, renewed contact with host cells, especially immune cells, is possible. We have shown that accordingly, previously secreting *Y. enterocolitica* continue to assemble new needles (**Figure 3B**), and that reactivation of the T3SS is possible and occurs immediately when introduced from non-secreting media back into secreting media (**Figure 4D**). Reestablishing secretion likely allows the bacteria to defend themselves during future interactions with immune cells. Notably, the experiments to investigate the kinetics of secretion start and stop, as well as the re-initiation of growth and division, were performed in an effector-less strain background (ΔHOPEMTasd). The observed effects are therefore independent of any additional regulatory role of the effectors themselves (Dewoody et al., 2013).

Effector translocation into macrophages prevents phagocytosis and inflammation, which both the interacting bacterium and bystanders benefit from. However, the ability to quickly restart growth after interaction with immune cells implies that *Y. enterocolitica* do not sacrifice to combat immune cells in an altogether altruistic manner, but also attempt to increase individual fitness. Other pathogens deviate from this strategy, and utilize their T3SS differently. In the well-studied example of *Salmonella* Typhimurium SPI-1, only a fraction of bacteria express the T3SS, while the remaining bacteria do not express the T3SS. The SPI-1 activity elicits an inflammatory response that reduces competition with established microflora. Due to the inflammation and the decreased growth rate of the population expressing the SPI-1 T3SS genes, the subpopulation not expressing the SPI-1 genes outgrows both the SPI-1-expressing population and competing bacteria (Sturm et al., 2011; Diard et al., 2013; Weigel and Dersch, 2018). The cooperative virulence of *Salmonella* therefore allows for SPI-1 negative bacteria to colonize the intestinal lumen and thus promotes the competitiveness of the population and efficient invasion of the host (Stecher et al., 2007; Müller et al., 2009; Knodler et al., 2010; Ramos-Morales, 2012; Behnsen et al., 2014).

It is currently unclear whether the suppression of growth during secretion is based on the leakage of ions and amino acids, which might be either co-transported with the secreted proteins or passively diffuse through the T3SS during secretion (Fowler and Brubaker, 1994; Fowler et al., 2009), the metabolic burden caused by biosynthesis, assembly and operation of the T3SS (Brubaker, 2005; Sturm et al., 2011; Wilharm and Heider, 2014; Wang et al., 2016), yet unknown specific regulatory mechanisms, or a combination thereof. Wang et al. showed that in the related *Y. pseudotuberculosis*, activation of the T3SS by Ca^{2+} chelation or host cell contact leads to an increased copy number of the virulence plasmid (Wang et al., 2016). A decrease in virulence plasmid copy number upon deactivation of secretion could therefore increase the amount of energy available for growth and division; however, it is unclear whether such an effect could account for the rather quick recovery of growth and division presented in this study (**Figures 4A,C**). Notably, on solid medium, cell growth differs between secreting and non-secreting conditions (addition of 5 mM EGTA or $CaCl_2$, respectively) even for a T3SS-deficient strain (**Figure 4C**), which indicates an additional T3SS-independent effect of calcium or other divalent cations on growth on solid medium. Taken together, the finding that growth and cell division are restored within short time after secretion has ceased is most compatible with a direct effect of ion leakage, or a specific regulatory mechanism.

The results of this study describe important parameters of *Y. enterocolitica*'s life after secretion. They show the ability to stop type III secretion and re-initiate growth and division within short time after the loss of the activating signal, while remaining able to enter another round of secretion, and support the notion that *Y. enterocolitica* applies the T3SS in an individual rather than a purely altruistic manner.

MATERIALS AND METHODS

Bacterial strains and constructs used in this study are listed in **Table 1**.

E. coli Top10 was used for cloning and grown on Luria-Bertani (LB) agar plates or in LB medium at 37°C. Chloramphenicol and streptomycin were used to select for expression and suicide vectors at concentrations of 10 and 50 µg/ml, respectively.

Yersinia enterocolitica strains were grown over night at 28°C in brain heart infusion (BHI) medium containing nalidixic acid (35 µg/ml), and diaminopimelic acid (60 µg/ml) for ΔHOPEMTasd strains. Day cultures were grown in BHI supplemented with nalidixic acid, diaminopimelic acid where required, $MgCl_2$ (20 mM), and glycerol (0.4% v/v). For non-secreting conditions, 5 mM $CaCl_2$ was added to the medium, whereas for secreting conditions, residual Ca^{2+} was chelated by addition of 5 mM EGTA.

Plasmids were constructed using Phusion polymerase (New England Biolabs). Mutators for exchange of genes on the pYV virulence plasmid were created as previously described (Diepold et al., 2011). Inserted sequences were confirmed by sequencing (Eurofin Genomics). *Y. enterocolitica* mutants were generated by allelic exchange, resulting in the exchange of wild-type gene sequences with the mutated gene (Kaniga et al., 1991).

β-Lactamase Assay

ΔHOPEMTasd-based *Y. enterocolitica* were used for the β-lactamase (bla) assays to allow handling in a biological safety level 1 environment. *Y. enterocolitica* harboring pAD626 (pACYC184::YopH$_{1-17}$-bla) or pAD627 (pACYC184::bla) were inoculated from overnight cultures to an optical density at 600 nm (OD_{600}) of 0.10 (0.12 in validation experiment) in

TABLE 1 | Bacterial strains and genetic constructs used in this study.

Strain	Relevant characteristics of virulence plasmid	References
***Y. enterocolitica* strains**		
MRS40	Wild-type pYV plasmid of *Y. enterocolitica* E40 (pYVe40) ΔblaA	Sory et al., 1995
IML421*asd* (ΔHOPEMTasd)	pYVmrs40 $yopO_{\Delta 2-427}$ $yopE_{21}$ $yopH_{\Delta 1-352}$ $yopM_{23}$ $yopP_{23}$ $yopT_{135}$ Δ*asd*	Kudryashev et al., 2013
AD4051	pYVmrs40 Δ*sctD*	Diepold et al., 2010
AD4085	pYViml421asd *egfp-sctQ*	Kudryashev et al., 2013
AD4306	pYViml421asd *egfp-sctD*	Diepold et al., 2015
AD4483	pYViml421asd *egfp-sctL* Δ*sctD*	Diepold et al., 2017
ADTM4521	pYViml421asd *mCherry-sctL*	This study
IM41	pYVmrs40 $sctW_{45}$ (does not encode *sctW=yopN*)	Boland et al., 1996
CH4006	pYViml421asd $sctF_{S5C}$	This study
Plasmid	**Relevant characteristics**	**References**
Plasmids		
pACYC184	Expression vector	New England Biolabs
pKNG101	oriR6K sacBR^{+} oriTRK2 strAB^{+} (suicide vector)	Kaniga et al., 1991
pAD626	pACYC184::$yopH_{1-17}$-*bla* (β-lactamase from pBAD::His-B cloned in-frame with first 17 amino acids of *Y. enterocolitica* yopH)	This study
pAD627	pACYC184::*bla*	This study
pADTM521	pKNG101 *mCh-sctL* (*pamCherry* and flexible linker cloned in-frame at the N-terminus of *sctL*)	Diepold et al., 2017
pCH06	pKNG101 $sctF_{S5C}$ (serine to cysteine point mutation of amino acid 5 in *sctF*)	This study

Strains and constructs used in this study. Y. enterocolitica strains are based on either the wild-type strain MRS40 or the multi-effector knock-out strain ΔHOPEMTasd (IML421asd), which lacks the virulence effectors YopH, YopO, YopP, YopE, YopM, and YopT, and is auxotrophic for diaminopimelic acid as result from a mutation in the aspartate-β-semialdehyde (asd) gene. The knock-out of the virulence effectors and the asd mutation is used for biosafety purposes, allowing these strains to be handled in a biosafety 1 level environment.

non-secreting BHI medium. After shaking incubation at 28°C for 1.5 h, the culture was shifted to 37°C to induce the *yop* regulon. After 2 h (1.5 h in the initial validation experiment) of incubation at 37°C, bacteria were collected (unless stated differently, bacteria were collected by centrifugation (2,400 g, 4 min, 37°C), and resuspended in an equal amount of fresh medium pre-warmed to 37°C throughout the protocol), and resuspended in secreting BHI medium. Over the next 15 min, the activation kinetics analysis was performed (see below). To determine the deactivation kinetics, cultures were incubated for 2 h at 37°C in secreting medium and were then collected and resuspended in non-secreting medium. Over the next 30 min, the deactivation kinetics analysis was performed (see below). To determine the reactivation kinetics, cultures were incubated in the secreting medium for 2 h at 37°C and were then collected and resuspended in non-secreting medium pre-warmed to 28°C. Cultures were incubated at 28°C for 15 min, collected and resuspended in secreting medium at 37°C, where the reactivation kinetics analysis was performed.

Samples for the kinetics analysis of activation, deactivation, and reactivation of secretion were treated as follows: after resuspension, 400–800 μl samples were removed from the culture at the indicated time points (0, 5, 10 min for activation; 0, 10, 20 min for deactivation; 0 min for reactivation), collected, resuspended in fresh medium as indicated and incubated in a table top shaking incubator at 37°C, 800 rpm for 5 min (activation and reactivation) or 10 min (deactivation). After this incubation, bacteria were removed by centrifugation (16,000 g, 2 min), and the supernatant was stored at room temperature until all samples of one experiment were collected. For each sample, 100 μl supernatant were added to a Sarstedt TC-Platte 96 well plate in triplicates. 10 μl/well of β-lactamase substrate solution (10 μM Nitrocefin (Merck) in phosphate buffered saline) were added. β-lactamase activity was quantified by the increase in absorbance at 483 nm, caused by β-lactamase catalyzed hydrolysis of Nitrocefin, for 40 rounds of 30 s each at 30°C using a Tecan Infinite 200 Pro photometer. The results are averages of β-lactamase activity, determined by linear regression within the linear range of the absorbance, of three independent experiments that were run in technical triplicates for each experiment.

The initial validation assay was performed as described above with the following modifications: 200 μl supernatant was added to a Sarstedt TC-Platte 96 well plate in triplicates, and 20 μl/well of β-lactamase substrate solution (20 μM Fluorocillin Green 495/525 (Life Technologies in 0.1 M Tris-HCl pH 7.5) was added. β-lactamase activity was quantified by the increase in fluorescence caused by β-lactamase catalyzed hydrolysis of the substrate, measured at 495 ± 5 nm excitation and 525 ± 10 nm emission for 30 rounds every 30 s using a Tecan Infinite 200 Pro photometer. The result is the increase of fluorescence over time of one experiment that was run in a technical triplicate.

In vitro Secretion Time Course

Yersinia enterocolitica (MRS40) were selected for the *in vitro* secretion assay to compare the effector export over time. *Y. enterocolitica* were grown as stated above for the β-lactamase assay. At each indicated time point (0, 5, 10, 15, 30, 45, 60, and 120 min secreting; 120 min non-secreting) following activation,

2 ml of culture samples were taken for further analysis (see secretion analysis).

Growth Curve Experiment

Yersinia enterocolitica MRS40, AD4051 (ΔSctD), and IM41 (ΔSctW=YopN) cultures for growth curve experiments were inoculated from overnight cultures to an OD_{600} of 0.12 in non-secreting BHI medium. After incubating at 28°C for 1.5 h, the culture was divided in three parts and collected (2,400 g, 4 min, 37°C). The pellet was then resuspended in either non-secreting medium (one part) or secreting medium (two parts), both pre-warmed at 37°C, to induce the *yop* regulon. The cultures were incubated at 37°C for 2 h, and collected again (2,400 g, 4 min, 37°C). One previously secreting culture was resuspended in secreting medium and the second was resuspended in non-secreting medium; the previously non-secreting culture was resuspended in fresh non-secreting medium, all pre-warmed at 37°C. Cultures were incubated at 37°C for 3.5 h. Throughout the experiment, the optical density at 600 nm wavelength (OD_{600}) of all cultures was measured every 30 min in a 1:3 dilution. The number of divisions per time for each culture was determined using the OD_{600} values for −1.5 h and 0 h (28°C), 0 h and 2 h (first incubation), and 2 h and 4 h (second incubation).

Secretion Analysis

Culture samples were centrifuged (20,000 g, 5 min, 4°C) and 1.8 ml of the supernatant (SN) was collected. SN proteins were precipitated using trichloroacetic acid 10% (w/v) final for 24–48 h at 4°C. Proteins were separated on 4–20% gradient SDS-PAGE gels (BioRad). Samples were normalized to contain the proteins secreted by 0.4 OD units of bacteria (the equivalent of 0.4 ml culture at an OD_{600} of 1). Secreted proteins were stained with "Instant Blue," Coomassie-based staining solution (Expedeon). Immunoblots were carried out using rabbit polyclonal primary antibodies against *Y. enterocolitica* SctP (MIPA57, 1:3000), YopE (MIPA73, 1:1000), SctA (LcrV) (MIPA220, 1:2000), or SctF (MIPA223, 1:1000), goat anti-rabbit secondary antibodies conjugated to horseradish peroxidase (Dako, 1:5000), and ECL chemiluminescent substrate (Pierce).

Fluorescence Microscopy—Visualization of Growth Under Secreting and Non-secreting Conditions

Yersinia enterocolitica AD4483 (ΔHOPEMTasd EGFP-SctL ΔSctD) (Diepold et al., 2017) and ADTM4521 (ΔHOPEMTasd mCherry-SctL) cultures for microscopy were inoculated from overnight cultures to an OD_{600} of 0.15 in secreting medium. Cultures were incubated at 28°C for 1.5 h and then shifted to 37°C for 2 h. Next, 750 μl of each culture were centrifuged (2,400 g, 3 min), and resuspended in 100 μl of either secreting or non-secreting medium for both strains. 2 μl of resuspended culture were spotted on preheated (37°C) agarose pads containing 1.5% (w/v) low melting agarose, LB, nalidixic acid (35 μg/ml), glycerol (0.4% v/v), $MgCl_2$ (20 mM) and either oxalate (20 mM) for secreting conditions, or $CaCl_2$ (5 mM) for non-secreting conditions. Bright field images were taken every 5 min and fluorescence images were taken every 20 min for 2 h at 37°C with a Deltavision Spectris optical sectioning microscope (Applied Precision) using a 100x oil immersion objective (Olympus) with a numerical aperture of 1.40. The exposure time was set to 0.2 s, with a light intensity of 32% for bright field, 587 nm and 485 nm excitation lights. Following image acquisition, images were deconvolved using softWoRx 5.5 (standard "conservative" settings). Images were further processed with ImageJ-Fiji (National Institute of Health) using a binary mask for measuring cell growth. Red and green fluorescence was manually adjusted to discriminate T3SS-positive and T3SS-negative bacteria, respectively.

Fluorescence Microscopy—Quantification of Assembled T3SS Under Secreting and Non-secreting Conditions

ΔHOPEMTasd-based *Y. enterocolitica* AD4085 (EGFP-SctQ) and AD4306 (EGFP-SctD) cultures for microscopy (Kudryashev et al., 2013; Diepold et al., 2015) were inoculated from an overnight culture to an OD_{600} of 0.12. Cultures were incubated at 28°C for 1.5 h. After incubation, cultures were shifted to 37°C for 3 h. Next, 400 μl of culture was centrifuged (2,400 g, 2 min) and concentrated in 200 μl microscopy imaging buffer (100 mM HEPES pH 7.2, 100 mM NaCl, 5 mM ammonium sulfate, 20 mM sodium glutamate, 10 mM $MgCl_2$, 5 mM K_2SO_4, 0.5% (w/v) casamino acids) containing diaminopimelic acid (60 μg/ml) and $CaCl_2$ (5 mM) or EGTA (5 mM) according to the imaging conditions (non-secreting or secreting). To test for possible loss of T3SS during extended secretion, cultures were incubated under secreting or non-secreting conditions at 28°C for 1.5 h, and then shifted to 37°C for 3 h. For visualization, 2 μl of resuspended culture where mounted on a 1.5% (w/v) agar pad casted with the same buffer in a depression slide and visualized in a Deltavision Spectris Optical Sectioning Microscope (Applied Precision), equipped with a UApo N 100x/1.49 oil TIRF UIS2 objective (Olympus), using an Evolve EMCCD Camera (Photometrics). The sample was illuminated for 0.15 s with a 488 laser in a TIRF depth of 3440.0, except for the extended secretion assay, where the exposure time was 0.3 s under non-TIRF conditions. The micrographs where then deconvolved using softWoRx 5.5 (standard "conservative" settings) and further processed for presentation with ImageJ-Fiji. Cells were manually counted in several fields of view.

Needle Staining Protocol

MRS40-based *Y. enterocolitica* CH4006 ($SctF_{S5C}$) and a MRS40 wild-type control were inoculated from overnight cultures to an OD_{600} of 0.15 in secreting medium. Cultures were incubated at 28°C for 1.5 h and then shifted to 37°C for 2 h. At this point, 500 μl were transferred to a 2 ml tube and washed with minimal medium adjusted for secreting conditions. The cells were concentrated in 100 μl microscopy imaging buffer containing EGTA (5 mM) and CF-633 maleimide dye (Sigma-Aldrich, USA) (5 μM) for 5 min. The cells were then collected and washed with microscopy imaging buffer containing EGTA (5 mM) once or four times, as indicated. Images were acquired as z stacks of 11 images with a stacking of 0.15 μm. The micrographs where then deconvolved using softWoRx 5.5 (standard "conservative" settings) and further processed for presentation with ImageJ-Fiji.

Energy Charge Determination

Intracellular metabolites were extracted from the total cellular biomass of wildtype ΔHOPEMTasd cultures, used in this experiment for biosafety reasons, based on a sequential quenching-extraction approach. 3 ml culture aliquots were pipetted into 9 ml of 60% (v/v) cold methanol (−60°C). Cells were immediately pelleted by centrifugation (10 min, −10°C, 20,000 x g), and the supernatant was removed. Pellets were stored at −80°C until extracted. Intracellular metabolites were extracted by adding a volume equivalent to 300 µl per 3 ml of a sample at an OD_{600} of 1 of both extraction fluid {50% (v/v) methanol, 50% (v/v) TE buffer [10 mM TRIZMA (pH 7.0), 1 mM EDTA]; −20°C} and chloroform (−20°C) to each cell pellet. The resulting mixture was incubated at 4°C for 2 h on a shaking device (Eppendorf shaker) and centrifuged (10 min, −10°C, 20,000 x g). The upper phase of the two-phase system was filtered (0.22 µm, PTFE, 4 mm diameter, Phenomenex) and stored at −80°C until the polar metabolites were analyzed.

Quantification of nucleotides was performed using a LC-MS/MS. The chromatographic separation was performed on an Agilent Infinity II 1290 HPLC system using a SeQuant ZIC-HILIC column (150 × 2.1 mm; 3.5 µm, 100 Å, Merck, Germany) equipped with a 20 × 2.1 mm guard column of similar specificity (Merck, Germany) at a constant flow rate of 0.4 ml/min with mobile phase A being 20 mM ammonium acetate (Sigma-Aldrich, USA) adjusted to pH 9.2 with ammonium hydroxide (Honeywell, USA) and phase B being acetonitrile (Honeywell, USA).

The injection volume was 3 µl. The mobile phase profile consisted of the following steps and linear gradients: 0–1 min from 20% B to 25% B; 1–4 min from 25 to 35% B; 4–5 min from 35 to 80% B; 5–6 min constant at 80% B; 6–7 min from 80 to 20% B; 7–8 min constant at 20% B. An Agilent 6495 ion funnel mass spectrometer was used in negative mode with an electrospray ionization source and the following conditions: ESI spray voltage 3,500 V, sheath gas 350°C at 11 l/min, nebulizer pressure 20 psig and drying gas 225°C at 14 l/min. Compounds were identified based on their exact mass and retention time compared to standards. Extracted ion chromatograms of the [M-H]- forms were integrated using MassHunter software (Agilent, Santa Clara, CA, USA). Absolute concentrations were calculated based on an external calibration curve.

AUTHOR CONTRIBUTIONS

BM-D and AD conceived, designed experiments, and wrote the paper. BM-D, CH, SW, DC, NP, and AD performed the experiments. BM-D, CH, SW, NP, and AD analyzed the data.

ACKNOWLEDGMENTS

This work was supported by the Max Planck Society. Nucleotide analysis was performed by the Core Facility for Metabolomics and Small Molecules of the Max Planck Institute for Terrestrial Microbiology. We thank Kai Thormann, University of Gießen, for support with the visualization of needles.

REFERENCES

Akeda, Y., and Galán, J. E. (2005). Chaperone release and unfolding of substrates in type III secretion. *Nature* 437, 911–915. doi: 10.1038/nature03992

Armentrout, E. I., and Rietsch, A. (2016). The type III secretion translocation pore senses host cell contact. *PLOS Pathog.* 12:e1005530. doi: 10.1371/journal.ppat.1005530

Avican, K., Fahlgren, A., Huss, M., Heroven, A. K., Beckstette, M., Dersch, P., et al. (2015). Reprogramming of yersinia from virulent to persistent mode revealed by complex *in vivo* RNA-seq analysis. *PLoS Pathog.* 11:e1004600. doi: 10.1371/journal.ppat.1004600

Behnsen, J., Jellbauer, S., Wong, C. P., Edwards, R. A., George, M. D., Ouyang, W., et al. (2014). The cytokine IL-22 promotes pathogen colonization by suppressing related commensal bacteria. *Immunity* 40, 262–273. doi: 10.1016/j.immuni.2014.01.003

Böhme, K., Steinmann, R., Kortmann, J., Seekircher, S., Heroven, A. K., Berger, E., et al. (2012). Concerted actions of a thermo-labile regulator and a unique intergenic RNA thermosensor control Yersinia virulence. *PLoS Pathog.* 8:e1002518. doi: 10.1371/journal.ppat.1002518

Boland, A., Sory, M.-P., Iriarte, M., Kerbourch, C., Wattiau, P., and Cornelis, G. R. (1996). Status of YopM and YopN in the yersinia yop virulon: YopM of Y.enterocolitica is internalized inside the cytosol of PU5-1.8 macrophages by the YopB, D, N delivery apparatus. *EMBO J.* 15, 5191–5201. doi: 10.1002/j.1460-2075.1996.tb00904.x

Brubaker, R. R. (2005). Influence of Na(+), dicarboxylic amino acids, and pH in modulating the low-calcium response of *Yersinia pestis*. *Infect. Immun.* 73, 4743–4752. doi: 10.1128/IAI.73.8.4743-4752.2005

Büttner, D. (2012). Protein export according to schedule: architecture, assembly, and regulation of type III secretion systems from plant- and animal-pathogenic bacteria. *Microbiol. Mol. Biol. Rev.* 76, 262–310. doi: 10.1128/MMBR.05017-11

Charpentier, X., and Oswald, E. (2004). Identification of the secretion and translocation domain of the enteropathogenic and enterohemorrhagic *Escherichia coli* effector Cif, using TEM-1 beta-lactamase as a new fluorescence-based reporter. *J. Bacteriol.* 186, 5486–5495. doi: 10.1128/JB.186.16.5486-5495.2004

Cisz, M., Lee, P. C., and Rietsch, A. (2008). ExoS controls the cell contact-mediated switch to effector secretion in *Pseudomonas aeruginosa*. *J. Bacteriol.* 190, 2726–2738. doi: 10.1128/JB.01553-07

Cornelis, G., Vanooteghem, J., and Sluiters, C. (1987). Transcription of the yop regulon from *Y. enterocolitica* requires trans acting pYV and chromosomal genes. *Microb. Pathog.* 2, 367–379. doi: 10.1016/0882-4010(87)90078-7

Cornelis, G. R. (2002). Yersinia type III secretion: send in the effectors. *J. Cell Biol.* 158, 401–408. doi: 10.1083/jcb.200205077

Cornelis, G. R. (2006). The type III secretion injectisome. *Nat. Rev. Microbiol.* 4, 811–825. doi: 10.1038/nrmicro1526

Cornelis, G. R., Biot, T., Lambert de Rouvroit, C., Michiels, T., Mulder, B., Sluiters, C., et al. (1989). The Yersinia yop regulon. *Mol. Microbiol.* 3, 1455–1459. doi: 10.1111/j.1365-2958.1989.tb00129.x

Davis, A. J., and Mecsas, J. (2006). Mutations in the Yersinia pseudotuberculosis type III secretion system needle protein, YscF, that specifically abrogate effector translocation into host cells. *J. Bacteriol.* 189, 83–97. doi: 10.1128/JB.01396-06

Deng, W., Marshall, N. C., Rowland, J. L., McCoy, J. M., Worrall, L. J., Santos, A. S., et al. (2017). Assembly, structure, function and regulation of type III secretion systems. *Nat. Rev. Microbiol.* 15, 323–337. doi: 10.1038/nrmicro.2017.20

Dewoody, R. S., Merritt, P. M., and Marketon, M. M. (2013). Regulation of the Yersinia type III secretion system: traffic control. *Front. Cell. Infect. Microbiol.* 3:4. doi: 10.3389/fcimb.2013.00004

Diard, M., Garcia, V., Maier, L., Remus-Emsermann, M. N. P., Regoes, R. R., Ackermann, M., et al. (2013). Stabilization of cooperative virulence by the expression of an avirulent phenotype. *Nature* 494, 353–356. doi: 10.1038/nature11913

Diepold, A., Amstutz, M., Abel, S., Sorg, I., Jenal, U., and Cornelis, G. R. (2010). Deciphering the assembly of the Yersinia type III secretion injectisome. *EMBO J.* 29, 1928–1940. doi: 10.1038/emboj.2010.84

Diepold, A., Kudryashev, M., Delalez, N. J., Berry, R. M., and Armitage, J. P. (2015). Composition, formation, and regulation of the cytosolic c-ring, a dynamic component of the type III secretion injectisome. *PLOS Biol.* 13:e1002039. doi: 10.1371/journal.pbio.1002039

Diepold, A., Sezgin, E., Huseyin, M., Mortimer, T., Eggeling, C., and Armitage, J. P. (2017). A dynamic and adaptive network of cytosolic interactions governs protein export by the T3SS injectisome. *Nat. Commun.* 8:15940. doi: 10.1038/ncomms15940

Diepold, A., and Wagner, S. (2014). Assembly of the bacterial type III secretion machinery. *FEMS Microbiol. Rev.* 38, 802–822. doi: 10.1111/1574-6976.12061

Diepold, A., Wiesand, U., and Cornelis, G. R. (2011). The assembly of the export apparatus (YscR,S,T,U,V) of the Yersinia type III secretion apparatus occurs independently of other structural components and involves the formation of an YscV oligomer. *Mol. Microbiol.* 82, 502–514. doi: 10.1111/j.1365-2958.2011.07830.x

Enninga, J., Mounier, J., Sansonetti, P., Tran Van Nhieu, G., and Van Nhieu, G. T. (2005). Secretion of type III effectors into host cells in real time. *Nat. Methods* 2, 959–965. doi: 10.1038/nmeth804

Enninga, J., and Rosenshine, I. (2009). Imaging the assembly, structure and activity of type III secretion systems. *Cell. Microbiol.* 11, 1462–1470. doi: 10.1111/j.1462-5822.2009.01360.x

Fowler, J. M., and Brubaker, R. R. (1994). Physiological basis of the low calcium response in *Yersinia pestis*. *Infect. Immun.* 62, 5234–5241.

Fowler, J. M., Wulff, C. R., Straley, S., and Brubaker, R. R. (2009). Growth of calcium-blind mutants of *Yersinia pestis* at 37 C in permissive Ca2+-deficient environments. *Microbiology* 155, 2509–2521. doi: 10.1099/mic.0.028852-0

Galán, J. E. (2009). Common themes in the design and function of bacterial effectors. *Cell Host Microbe* 5, 571–579. doi: 10.1016/j.chom.2009.04.008

Grosdent, N., Maridonneau-Parini, I., Sory, M.-P., and Cornelis, G. R. (2002). Role of yops and adhesins in resistance of yersinia enterocolitica to phagocytosis. *Infect. Immun.* 70, 4165–4176. doi: 10.1128/IAI.70.8.4165-4176.2002

Håkansson, S., Schesser, K., Persson, C., Galyov, E. E., Rosqvist, R., Hombl,é, F., et al. (1996). The YopB protein of Yersinia pseudotuberculosis is essential for the translocation of Yop effector proteins across the target cell plasma membrane and displays a contact-dependent membrane disrupting activity. *EMBO J.* 15, 5812–5823. doi: 10.1002/j.1460-2075.1996.tb00968.x

Heroven, A. K., and Dersch, P. (2014). Coregulation of host-adapted metabolism and virulence by pathogenic yersiniae. *Front. Cell. Infect. Microbiol.* 4:146. doi: 10.3389/fcimb.2014.00146

Hoe, N., and Goguen, J. D. (1993). Temperature sensing in *Yersinia pestis*: translation of the LcrF activator protein is thermally regulated. *J. Bacteriol.* 175, 7901–7909. doi: 10.1128/jb.175.24.7901-7909.1993

Hueck, C. J. (1998). Type III protein secretion systems in bacterial pathogens of animals and plants. *Microbiol. Mol. Biol. Rev.* 62, 379–433.

Kaniga, K., Delor, I., and Cornelis, G. R. (1991). A wide-host-range suicide vector for improving reverse genetics in Gram-negative bacteria: inactivation of the blaA gene of Yersinia enterocolitica. *Gene* 109, 137–141. doi: 10.1016/0378-1119(91)90599-7

Kenjale, R., Wilson, J., Zenk, S., Saurya, S., Picking, W. L., and Blocker, A. J. (2005). The needle component of the type III secreton of Shigella regulates the activity of the secretion apparatus. *J. Biol. Chem.* 280, 42929–42937. doi: 10.1074/jbc.M508377200

Knodler, L. A., Vallance, B. A., Celli, J., Winfree, S., Hansen, B., Montero, M., et al. (2010). Dissemination of invasive Salmonella via bacterial-induced extrusion of mucosal epithelia. *Proc. Natl. Acad. Sci. U.S.A.* 107, 17733–17738. doi: 10.1073/pnas.1006098107

Kudryashev, M., Diepold, A., Amstutz, M., Armitage, J. P., Stahlberg, H., and Cornelis, G. R. (2015). Yersinia enterocolitica type III secretion injectisomes form regularly spaced clusters, which incorporate new machines upon activation. *Mol. Microbiol.* 95, 875–884. doi: 10.1111/mmi.12908

Kudryashev, M., Stenta, M., Schmelz, S., Amstutz, M., Wiesand, U., Castaño-Díez, D., et al. (2013). In situ structural analysis of the Yersinia enterocolitica injectisome. *Elife* 2:e00792. doi: 10.7554/eLife.00792

Kuhlen, L., Abrusci, P., Johnson, S., Gault, J., Deme, J., Caesar, J., et al. (2018). Structure of the core of the type III secretion system export apparatus. *Nat. Struct. Mol. Biol.* 25, 583–590. doi: 10.1038/s41594-018-0086-9

Kupferberg, L. L., and Higuchi, K. (1958). Role of calcium ions in the stimulation of growth of virulent strains of Pasteurella pestis. *J. Bacteriol.* 76, 120–121.

Lambert de Rouvroit, C., Sluiters, C., and Cornelis, G. R. (1992). Role of the transcriptional activator, VirF, and temperature in the expression of the pYV plasmid genes of Yersinia enterocolitica. *Mol. Microbiol.* 6, 395–409. doi: 10.1111/j.1365-2958.1992.tb01483.x

Lara-Tejero, M., Kato, J., Wagner, S., Liu, X., and Galán, J. E. (2011). A sorting platform determines the order of protein secretion in bacterial type III systems. *Science* 331, 1188–1191. doi: 10.1126/science.1201476

Marketon, M. M., DePaolo, R. W., DeBord, K. L., Jabri, B., and Schneewind, O. (2005). Plague bacteria target immune cells during infection. *Science* 309, 1739–1741. doi: 10.1126/science.1114580

Mehigh, R. J., Sample, A. K., and Brubaker, R. R. (1989). Expression of the low calcium response in *Yersinia pestis*. *Microb. Pathog.* 6, 203–217. doi: 10.1016/0882-4010(89)90070-3

Mills, E., Baruch, K., Charpentier, X., Kobi, S., and Rosenshine, I. (2008). Real-time analysis of effector translocation by the type III secretion system of enteropathogenic *Escherichia coli*. *Cell Host Microbe* 3, 104–113. doi: 10.1016/j.chom.2007.11.007

Mueller, C. A., Broz, P., Müller, S. A., Ringler, P., Erne-Brand, F., Sorg, I., et al. (2005). The V-antigen of Yersinia forms a distinct structure at the tip of injectisome needles. *Science* 310, 674–676. doi: 10.1126/science.1118476

Müller, A. J., Hoffmann, C., Galle, M., Van Den Broeke, A., Heikenwalder, M., Falter, L., et al. (2009). The, *S. typhimurium* effector sope induces caspase-1 activation in stromal cells to initiate gut inflammation. *Cell Host Microbe* 6, 125–136. doi: 10.1016/j.chom.2009.07.007

Nauth, T., Huschka, F., Schweizer, M., Bosse, J. B., Diepold, A., Failla, A. V., et al. (2018). Visualization of translocons in Yersinia type III protein secretion machines during host cell infection. *PLOS Pathog.* 14:e1007527. doi: 10.1371/journal.ppat.1007527

Navarro, L., Alto, N. M., and Dixon, J. E. (2005). Functions of the Yersinia effector proteins in inhibiting host immune responses. *Curr. Opin. Microbiol.* 8, 21–27. doi: 10.1016/j.mib.2004.12.014

Park, D., Lara-Tejero, M., Waxham, M. N., Li, W., Hu, B., Galán, J. E., et al. (2018). Visualization of the type III secretion mediated Salmonella-host cell interface using cryo-electron tomography. *Elife* 7:e39514. doi: 10.7554/eLife.39514

Pha, K. (2016). *Yersinia* type III effectors perturb host innate immune responses. *World, J. Biol. Chem.* 7:1. doi: 10.4331/wjbc.v7.i1.1

Philip, N. H., Zwack, E. E., and Brodsky, I. E. (2016). Activation and evasion of inflammasomes by yersinia. *Curr. Top. Microbiol. Immunol.* 397, 69–90. doi: 10.1007/978-3-319-41171-2_4

Portaliou, A. G., Tsolis, K. C., Loos, M. S., Zorzini, V., and Economou, A. (2016). Type III secretion: building and operating a remarkable nanomachine. *Trends Biochem. Sci.* 41, 175–189 doi: 10.1016/j.tibs.2015.09.005

Ramos-Morales, F. (2012). Impact of *Salmonella enterica* type III secretion system effectors on the eukaryotic host cell. *ISRN Cell Biol.* 2012, 1–36. doi: 10.5402/2012/787934

Rietsch, A., and Mekalanos, J. J. (2006). Metabolic regulation of type III secretion gene expression in *Pseudomonas aeruginosa*. *Mol. Microbiol.* 59, 807–820. doi: 10.1111/j.1365-2958.2005.04990.x

Roehrich, A. D., Guillossou, E., Blocker, A. J., and Martinez-Argudo, I. (2013). Shigella IpaD has a dual role: signal transduction from the type III secretion system needle tip and intracellular secretion regulation. *Mol. Microbiol.* 87, 690–706. doi: 10.1111/mmi.12124

Rundell, E. A., McKeithen-Mead, S. A., and Kazmierczak, B. I. (2016). Rampant cheating by pathogens? *PLOS Pathog.* 12:e1005792. doi: 10.1371/journal.ppat.1005792

Sánchez-Romero, M. A., and Casadesús, J. (2018). Contribution of SPI-1 bistability to *Salmonella enterica* cooperative virulence: insights from single cell analysis. *Sci. Rep.* 8:14875. doi: 10.1038/s41598-018-33137-z

Schlumberger, M. C., Müller, A., Ehrbar, K., Winnen, B., Duss, I., Stecher, B., et al. (2005). Real-time imaging of type III secretion: salmonella SipA injection into host cells. *Proc. Natl. Acad. Sci. U.S.A.* 102, 12548–12553. doi: 10.1073/pnas.0503407102

Shaulov, L., Gershberg, J., Deng, W., Finlay, B. B., and Sal-Man, N. (2017). The ruler protein escp of the enteropathogenic *Escherichia coli* type III secretion system is involved in calcium sensing and secretion hierarchy regulation by interacting with the gatekeeper protein SepL. *MBio* 8:e01733–e01716. doi: 10.1128/mBio.01733-16

Skurnik, M., Bölin, I., Heikkinen, H., Piha, S., and Wolf-Watz, H. (1984). Virulence plasmid-associated autoagglutination in Yersinia spp. *J. Bacteriol.* 158, 1033–1036.

Sory, M.-P., Boland, A., Lambermont, I., and Cornelis, G. R. (1995). Identification of the YopE and YopH domains required for secretion and internalization into the cytosol of macrophages, using the cyaA gene fusion approach. *Proc. Natl. Acad. Sci. U.S.A.* 92, 11998–12002. doi: 10.1073/pnas.92.26.11998

Stecher, B., Robbiani, R., Walker, A. W., Westendorf, A. M., Barthel, M., Kremer, M., et al. (2007). *Salmonella enterica* serovar typhimurium exploits inflammation to compete with the intestinal microbiota. *PLoS Biol.* 5, 2177–2189. doi: 10.1371/journal.pbio.0050244

Sturm, A., Heinemann, M., Arnoldini, M., Benecke, A., Ackermann, M., Benz, M., et al. (2011). The cost of virulence: retarded growth of Salmonella Typhimurium cells expressing type III secretion system 1. *PLoS Pathog.* 7:e1002143. doi: 10.1371/journal.ppat.1002143

Torruellas, J., Jackson, M. W., Pennock, J. W., and Plano, G. V. (2005). The *Yersinia pestis* type III secretion needle plays a role in the regulation of Yop secretion. *Mol. Microbiol.* 57, 1719–1733. doi: 10.1111/j.1365-2958.2005.04790.x

Veenendaal, A. K. J., Hodgkinson, J., Schwarzer, L., Stabat, D., Zenk, S., and Blocker, A. J. (2007). The type III secretion system needle tip complex mediates host cell sensing and translocon insertion. *Mol. Microbiol.* 63, 1719–1730. doi: 10.1111/j.1365-2958.2007.05620.x

Wang, H., Avican, K., Fahlgren, A., Erttmann, S. F., Nuss, A. M., Dersch, P., et al. (2016). Increased plasmid copy number is essential for Yersinia T3SS function and virulence. *Science* 353, 492–495. doi: 10.1126/science.aaf7501

Weigel, W. A., and Dersch, P. (2018). Phenotypic heterogeneity: a bacterial virulence strategy. *Microbes Infect.* 20, 570–577. doi: 10.1016/j.micinf.2018.01.008

Wiley, D. J., Rosqvist, R., and Schesser, K. (2007). Induction of the yersinia type 3 secretion system as an all-or-none phenomenon. *J. Mol. Biol.* 373, 27–37. doi: 10.1016/j.jmb.2007.07.077

Wilharm, G., and Heider, C. (2014). Interrelationship between type three secretion system and metabolism in pathogenic bacteria. *Front. Cell. Infect. Microbiol.* 4:150. doi: 10.3389/fcimb.2014.00150

Yother, J., and Goguen, J. D. (1985). Isolation and characterization of Ca2+-blind mutants of *Yersinia pestis*. *J. Bacteriol.* 164, 704–711.

4

The *Campylobacter jejuni* Type VI Secretion System Enhances the Oxidative Stress Response and Host Colonization

*Janie Liaw[1], Geunhye Hong[1], Cadi Davies[1], Abdi Elmi[1], Filip Sima[2], Alexandros Stratakos[2], Lavinia Stef[3], Ioan Pet[3], Abderrahman Hachani[1,4], Nicolae Corcionivoschi[2,3], Brendan W. Wren[1], Ozan Gundogdu[1] and Nick Dorrell[1]**

[1] Faculty of Infectious and Tropical Diseases, London School of Hygiene & Tropical Medicine, London, United Kingdom, [2] Bacteriology Branch, Veterinary Sciences Division, Agri-Food and Biosciences Institute, Belfast, United Kingdom, [3] Bioengineering of Animal Science Resources, Banat University of Agricultural Sciences and Veterinary Medicine – King Michael the I of Romania, Timisoara, Romania, [4] The Peter Doherty Institute for Infection and Immunity, Department of Microbiology and Immunology, University of Melbourne, Melbourne, VIC, Australia

***Correspondence:**
Nick Dorrell
nick.dorrell@lshtm.ac.uk

The role of the Type VI secretion system (T6SS) in *Campylobacter jejuni* is poorly understood despite an increasing prevalence of the T6SS in recent *C. jejuni* isolates in humans and chickens. The T6SS is a contractile secretion machinery capable of delivering effectors that can play a role in host colonization and niche establishment. During host colonization, *C. jejuni* is exposed to oxidative stress in the host gastrointestinal tract, and in other bacteria the T6SS has been linked with the oxidative stress response. In this study, comparisons of whole genome sequences of a novel human isolate 488 with previously sequenced strains revealed a single highly conserved T6SS cluster shared between strains isolated from humans and chickens. The presence of a functional T6SS in the 488 wild-type strain is indicated by expression of T6SS genes and secretion of the effector TssD. Increased expression of oxidative stress response genes *katA*, *sodB*, and *ahpC*, and increased oxidative stress resistance in 488 wild-type strain suggest T6SS is associated with oxidative stress response. The role of the T6SS in interactions with host cells is explored using *in vitro* and *in vivo* models, and the presence of the T6SS is shown to increase *C. jejuni* cytotoxicity in the *Galleria mellonella* infection model. In biologically relevant models, the T6SS enhances *C. jejuni* interactions with and invasion of chicken primary intestinal cells and enhances the ability of *C. jejuni* to colonize chickens. This study demonstrates that the *C. jejuni* T6SS provides defense against oxidative stress and enhances host colonization, and highlights the importance of the T6SS during *in vivo* survival of T6SS-positive *C. jejuni* strains.

Keywords: campylobacter, type 6 secretion system, oxidative stress, chicken colonization, catalase, superoxide dismutase

INTRODUCTION

Campylobacter jejuni, a Gram-negative microaerophilic bacteria, is the leading cause of bacterial foodborne gastroenteritis worldwide. *C. jejuni* infection in humans can lead to diarrhea, vomiting, abdominal pain, fever, with symptoms generally appearing 2–5 days following exposure to an infectious dose as low as 500–900 bacteria (Robinson, 1981; Kaakoush et al., 2015). Disease presentation can vary depending on geographical region, with infections in low- and middle-income countries typically presenting with watery, non-inflammatory diarrhea whilst infections in high income countries display more severe disease, presenting with bloody inflammatory diarrhea (Coker et al., 2002). Campylobacteriosis is generally self-limiting, however, around 1 in 1,000 cases can develop severe auto-immune complications such as Guillain-Barré syndrome or Miller Fisher syndrome (Ang et al., 2001).

Campylobacter jejuni is most commonly transmitted through the handling and consumption of raw or undercooked poultry, but can also be spread through unpasteurized milk, contaminated water and cross contamination with other foods (Young et al., 2007; Kaakoush et al., 2015). *C. jejuni* colonizes chickens and other avian species and an estimated 70% of raw chicken sold in supermarkets in the United Kingdom will be contaminated with *C. jejuni* (Kaakoush et al., 2015). *C. jejuni* was previously regarded as a harmless commensal in the digestive tract of chickens, but recent studies indicate that colonization by *C. jejuni* is not asymptomatic, resulting in weight loss and slow growth of the infected poultry (Hermans et al., 2012; Wigley, 2015). The spread of *C. jejuni* through chicken flocks in farms can have a vast economic impact on the poultry industry and an increased spread of *C. jejuni* in chickens can subsequently affect the rates of infection in humans (Newell and Fearnley, 2003; Skarp et al., 2016).

During host colonization and infection, *C. jejuni* is exposed to conditions in the host gastrointestinal tract that present as physical and chemical stresses, including oxidative stress (Kim et al., 2015; Flint et al., 2016). Oxidative stress involves the generation of reactive oxygen species (ROS) that cause damage to nucleic acids, membranes and proteins of bacteria. In order to survive in this hostile environment, *C. jejuni* must defend against oxidative stress with enzymes that degrade ROS, such as SodB (superoxide dismutase), KatA (catalase), and AhpC (hydroperoxide reductase) (Kim et al., 2015). Regulation of the *C. jejuni* oxidative stress response is controlled by multiple regulatory mechanisms involving PerR, Fur and CosR to respond to fluctuating levels of ROS. Two MarR-type transcriptional regulators, RrpA and RrpB, also play a role in oxidative stress response regulation (Gundogdu et al., 2015).

The Type VI Secretion System (T6SS) is a contact-dependent secretion machinery capable of delivering effector proteins to both prokaryotic and eukaryotic cells. First identified in *Vibrio cholerae* and *Pseudomonas aeruginosa*, the T6SS has since been found to be present in 25% of Gram-negative bacterial species (Mougous et al., 2006; Pukatzki et al., 2006). The structure of the T6SS resembles an inverted bacteriophage tail with homologous components. The T6SS consists of 13 core components (TssA-TssM) and accessory proteins such as the T6SS-associated gene (Tag) proteins (see **Table 1**). A functioning T6SS complex requires essential components such as the baseplate (TssEFGK), a membrane-anchoring structure (TssJLM), a contractile sheath (TssBC) wrapped around a needle-like tube (TssD) and a puncture tip (TssI) further sharpened by a spike (TagD) (Cianfanelli et al., 2016). Composed of interlocking TssB and TssC components, the contractile sheath

TABLE 1 | Components of the bacterial Type VI Secretion System.

TSS system	Orthologs	Putative function/location
TssA	VasJ/ImpA	Docks to membrane complex, recruits baseplate complex, initiates/coordinates polymerization of TssD with sheath
TssB	VipA/ImpB	Contractile sheath
TssC	VipB/ImpC	Contractile sheath
TssD	Hcp	Secreted tube, effector
TssE	HsiF	Baseplate
TssF	VasA/ImpG	Baseplate
TssG	VasB/ImpH	Baseplate
TssH	ClpV/VasG	AAA+ATPase, sheath recycling
TssI	VgrG	Expelled spike, effector
TssJ	VasD/Lip/SciN	Membrane complex
TssK	VasE/ImpJ	Baseplate
TssL	IcmH/DotU/VasF	Membrane complex
TssM	IcmF/VasK	Membrane complex
TagD	PAAR	Tip of expelled spike

is responsible for producing enough energy to force the TssD needle-like structure through the inner membrane out into the extracellular space and puncture a host membrane to deliver effector proteins (Cianfanelli et al., 2016; Salih et al., 2018). The extended contractile sheath is broken down and the components recycled by the TssH ATPase for further sheath assembly (Kapitein et al., 2013).

Delivery of effector proteins by the T6SS to target cells can exert a number of effects including colonization and niche establishment (Kapitein and Mogk, 2014; Ma et al., 2014; Drebes Dorr and Blokesch, 2018). T6SS effectors can target and eliminate bacterial and fungal competitors and also affect eukaryotic host cells (Murdoch et al., 2011; Trunk et al., 2018). To prevent self-intoxication by effector proteins, bacteria with the T6SS possess immunity proteins to neutralize the effects of the toxins (Kirchberger et al., 2017; Ringel et al., 2017; Fitzsimons et al., 2018). In competition with prokaryotic targets, T6SS can act either defensively or offensively; for example, the T6SS of *V. cholerae* and *Serratia marcescens* are offensive, apparently firing constantly and indiscriminately into the surrounding space, whilst the defensive T6SS of *P. aeruginosa* reacts only when fired upon in a "tit-for-tat" response (Gerc et al., 2015). T6SS effectors can subvert host cell processes by manipulating the host cytoskeleton, hindering host defense mechanisms, modulating the host inflammatory response and modifying host membrane structure (Hachani et al., 2016).

The T6SS can also defend against the production of ROS through secretion of effectors. For example, the T6SS-4 of *Yersinia pseudotuberculosis* secretes the effector YezP, which is able to bind to and sequester zinc ions and protect the bacteria from the effects of oxidative stress (Wang et al., 2015). The T6SS-4 of *Burkholderia thailandensis* also secretes effectors TseM for the uptake of manganese ions and TseZ for the uptake of zinc ions to mitigate the effects of oxidative stress. Similarly, enterohemorrhagic *Escherichia coli* secretes a T6SS effector, KatN, which facilitates survival of the bacteria in macrophages through decreasing the level of intracellular ROS (Wan et al., 2017).

Studies examining the prevalence of the T6SS in *C. jejuni* in Asia and Europe found a large variation in prevalence between regions. Harrison et al. (2014) observed in 2014 that up to 70% of isolates from chickens and humans in Vietnam were positive for the T6SS, whilst approximately only 3% of similar isolates from the United Kingdom were T6SS-positive. A further study in 2015 examining chicken isolates in Spain found a prevalence of 14%, whilst another study found that 28.8% of chicken isolates in Northern Ireland were T6SS-positive (Corcionivoschi et al., 2015; Ugarte-Ruiz et al., 2015). Other *Campylobacter* species can also carry the T6SS; the same study in Northern Ireland observed that 56.1% of *C. coli* found in retail chickens were T6SS-positive (Corcionivoschi et al., 2015). However, the large variation in prevalence may be due to differences in sample sizes, sample sources and in detection methods. Recent data suggests that the T6SS is becoming increasingly prevalent in *C. jejuni* strains, with indications that T6SS-positive strains are becoming more prevalent than T6SS-negative strains infecting chickens in farms, on raw poultry in supermarkets and even in hospital patients in the United Kingdom (Carmel Kelly, Agri-Food and Biosciences Institute, Personal Communication). A recent study in 2018 examining the presence of *C. jejuni* in wild birds of Finland observed that 49% of western jackdaw isolates and 72% of mallard duck isolates were T6SS-positive (Kovanen et al., 2018). This emphasizes the need to understand the role of the T6SS in *C. jejuni* and to develop intervention strategies to combat the rise of T6SS-positive *C. jejuni* strains (Sima et al., 2018).

In contrast to *V. cholerae* and *P. aeruginosa*, the role of the T6SS in *C. jejuni* is poorly understood. To date, only one *C. jejuni* T6SS cluster expressing a single TssD has been identified, compared to *P. aeruginosa* and *Yersinia pseudotuberculosis* which both possess multiple T6SS clusters exhibiting different functions (Lertpiriyapong et al., 2012). The structure of the *C. jejuni* T6SS is yet to be solved and TssD is thus far the only effector protein identified to be secreted by the *C. jejuni* T6SS (Lertpiriyapong et al., 2012; Bleumink-Pluym et al., 2013). Previous studies have demonstrated the *C. jejuni* T6SS may be important in host cell adherence and invasion, colonization, survival in bile salts and contact-dependent cytotoxicity toward red blood cells (Lertpiriyapong et al., 2012; Bleumink-Pluym et al., 2013). A recent study examined the structure of the TssD effector in *C. jejuni* and found that TssD is cytotoxic toward HepG2 human liver carcinoma cells (Noreen et al., 2018). However, whether the T6SS plays a role in the survival and infection of *C. jejuni* in poultry, a primary reservoir in humans is still unknown.

In this study, we investigated the role of the *C. jejuni* T6SS through whole genome sequencing of a T6SS-positive 488 wild-type strain (a recent human isolate from Brazil). We also sequenced the T6SS-positive 43431 wild-type strain (a human isolate from Canada) (Penner et al., 1983). We constructed defined isogenic mutants for genes encoding the contractile sheath components TssBC and needle structure TssD in the 488 wild-type strain and performed *in vitro* and *in vivo* characterization experiments in biologically relevant models. Our findings indicate that a functional T6SS is present in the *C. jejuni* 488 wild-type strain and the presence of the T6SS is important in defending against oxidative stress and enhancing *in vivo* survival, potentially thereby allowing strains harboring the T6SS to colonize and dominate in specific niches within a host.

RESULTS

Bioinformatic Analysis of T6SS Gene Clusters in *C. jejuni* 488 and Other T6SS-Positive Wild-Type Strains Reveals Synteny

Whole genome sequencing of *C. jejuni* 488 wild-type strain (a recent human isolate from Brazil) and *C. jejuni* wild-type strain 43431 (a human isolate from Canada) (Penner et al., 1983) was performed. *C. jejuni* wild-type strain RC039 (a chicken isolate from Northern Ireland) was previously sequenced (Corcionivoschi et al., 2015). The presence of a single T6SS cluster was observed in all three strains. All T6SS core components were identified, however, the TssH (ClpV) ATPase responsible for disassembly of the contracted sheath components is absent from the T6SS cluster of all *C. jejuni* strains sequenced thus far. The genome coordinates of the T6SS cluster in the *C. jejuni* 488 strain is listed in **Supplementary Table S1**. Comparisons of the 488, 43431, and RC039 genome sequences with previously published sequences for other T6SS-positive *C. jejuni* strains (Lertpiriyapong et al., 2012; Bleumink-Pluym et al., 2013) revealed a T6SS cluster that is highly conserved, sharing synteny between strains and also with other *Campylobacter* species isolated from humans and chickens (**Figure 1**). The 414 strain, isolated from wild bank voles in the United Kingdom, has a different gene arrangement in the T6SS cluster, but the same core components are still present.

T6SS Genes *tssB*, *tssC tssD* Are Expressed in the 488 Wild-Type Strain

Composed of interlocking TssB and TssC proteins, the contractile sheath is responsible for producing enough energy to force the TssD needle-like structure through the inner membrane out into the extracellular space and across host membranes (Cianfanelli et al., 2016). To investigate whether the *C. jejuni* 488 wild-type strain has a functional T6SS, the expression of the contractile sheath genes *tssB* and *tssC* as well as the *tssD* gene was investigated using RT-PCR. *tssB*, *tssC tssD* were all found to be expressed when the 488 wild-type strain is grown both in broth culture for 16 h and on blood agar for 24 h, indicating that the *C. jejuni* T6SS contractile sheath is produced under different growth conditions (**Figure 2**).

C. jejuni 488 Wild-Type Strain Has a Functional T6SS That Secretes TssD

Previous studies have used the secretion of TssD as evidence that the T6SS is functional in *C. jejuni* (Lertpiriyapong et al., 2012; Bleumink-Pluym et al., 2013). In order to determine whether the T6SS in the 488 wild-type strain is functional,

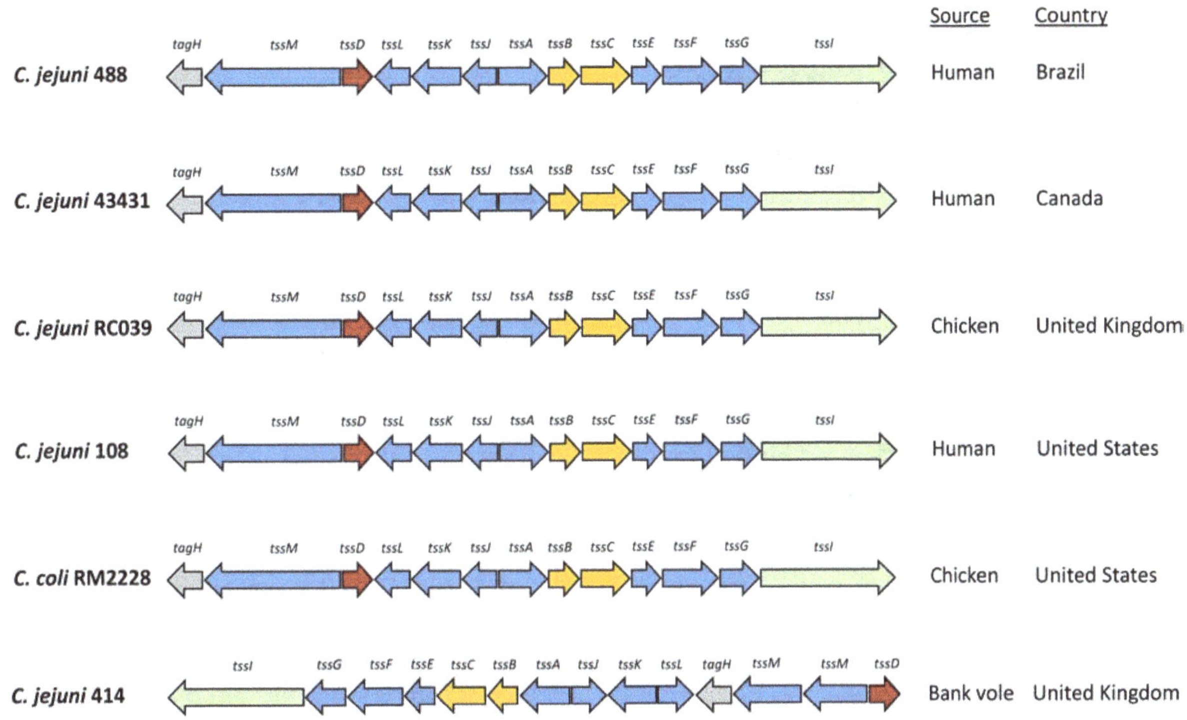

FIGURE 1 | Type VI secretion system gene clusters of *C. jejuni* strains. The *C. jejuni* 488 and 43431 wild-type strains were sequenced using whole genome sequencing in this study. The genome sequence of *C. jejuni* RC039 was published by Corcionivoschi et al. (2015). The genome sequences for *C. jejuni* 108 and *C. coli* RM2228 was published by Bleumink-Pluym et al. (2013). The genome sequence for *C. jejuni* 414 was published by Lertpiriyapong et al. (2012).

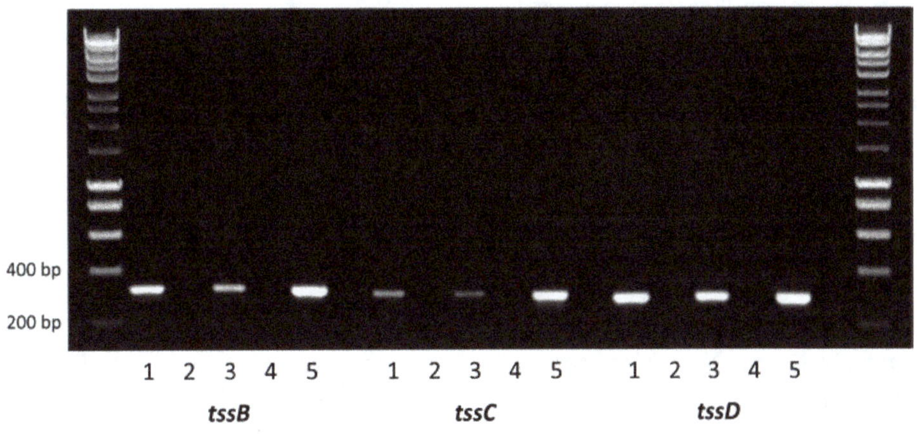

FIGURE 2 | Reverse transcription PCR analysis of T6SS gene expression in the 488 wild-type strain. RNA was isolated from 488 wild-type strain. Plate cultures were grown on blood agar plates and incubated for 24 h under microaerobic conditions. Broth cultures were grown in Brucella broth for 16 h at 37°C with shaking at 75 rpm under microaerobic conditions. Extracted RNA was converted to cDNA. RT-PCR was performed using *tssB*, *tssC*, and *tssD* primers. The first and last lanes are the molecular weight marker (HyperLadder 1 kb, Bioline, United Kingdom). Lane 1: 488 cDNA (plate culture); Lane 2: negative control (488 cDNA from plate culture synthesized without reverse transcriptase); Lane 3: 488 cDNA (broth culture); Lane 4: negative control (488 cDNA from broth culture synthesized without reverse transcriptase); and Lane 5: positive control (488 gDNA). Expected sizes are 316 bp (*tssB*), 300 bp (*tssC*), and 287 bp (*tssD*).

Western blotting was performed using a TssD antibody to detect the secretion of TssD. TssD is an approximately 18 kD protein that makes up the needle-like structure of the T6SS and has been shown in other bacteria to be important in the secretion of effector proteins (Cianfanelli et al., 2016). TssD is present in the whole cell lysate (**Figure 3A**) and also secreted into the supernatant of the 488 wild-type strain (**Figure 3B**), indicating that this strain has a functional T6SS. TssD is absent from both whole cell lysate and supernatant from the 488 *tssD* mutant.

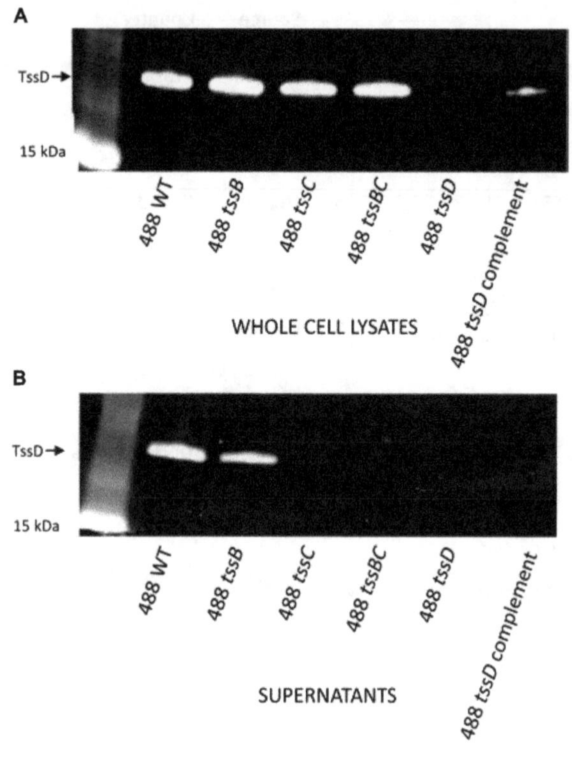

FIGURE 3 | Detection of TssD in *C. jejuni* whole cell lysates and supernatants. **(A)** Detection of TssD in *C. jejuni* whole cell lysates. Whole cell lysate samples were prepared from 16 h cultures of *C. jejuni* 488 wild-type strain, 488 *tssB* mutant, 488 *tssC* mutant, 488 *tssBC* double mutant, 488 *tssD* mutant, and 488 *tssD* complement grown in Brucella broth. 13 μg of samples were loaded onto SDS-PAGE. Western blotting was performed using a TssD antibody, with a recombinant TssD protein used as a positive control. **(B)** Detection of TssD in *C. jejuni* supernatants. Bacterial supernatant samples were prepared from 16 h cultures of *C. jejuni* 488 wild-type strain, 488 *tssB* mutant, 488 *tssC* mutant and 488 *tssBC* double mutant grown in Brucella broth. Supernatant samples were concentrated via TCA precipitation and 30 μg of samples were loaded onto SDS-PAGE. Western blotting was performed using a *C. jejuni* TssD antibody. *C. jejuni* TssD has an estimated molecular weight of 18 kDa.

Inactivation of Individual Contractile Sheath Components Does Not Abolish *C. jejuni* T6SS Function

488 *tssB* and *tssC* single mutants were constructed to investigate whether knocking out a contractile sheath component would result in a non-functional T6SS. Inactivation of either *tssB* or *tssC* reduces but does not completely abolish secretion of TssD (**Figure 3B**), indicating that the absence of one of the contractile sheath components does not result in a completely non-functional T6SS in *C. jejuni*. A 488 *tssBC* double mutant was also constructed to test the hypothesis that function of the *C. jejuni* T6SS is only abolished in the absence of both contractile sheath components. As hypothesized, TssD was present in the whole cell lysate but absent from the supernatant of the 488 *tssBC* double mutant, thereby demonstrating that the *C. jejuni* T6SS is not functional when the entire contractile sheath structure is missing.

T6SS in *C. jejuni* Is Associated With the Oxidative Stress Response

The T6SS has previously been linked with the oxidative stress response in *Y. pseudotuberculosis*, *B. thailandensis*, and enterohemorrhagic *E. coli* (Wang et al., 2015; Si et al., 2017; Wan et al., 2017). To investigate whether the *C. jejuni* T6SS is also associated with the oxidative stress response, the 488 wild-type strain, 488 *tssD* mutant and 81–176 wild-type strain were exposed to hydrogen peroxide (H_2O_2). Following 30 min exposure to 50 mM H_2O_2, the 488 wild-type strain exhibited significantly greater resistance to oxidative stress killing compared to the 488 *tssD* mutant and the 81-176 wild-type strain (**Figure 4A**). In order to investigate whether the increased susceptibility of the 488 *tssD* mutant to H_2O_2 is specific and not due to a potential membrane defect due to improper assembly of the T6SS in the bacterial membrane, antimicrobial susceptibility testing for the 488 wild-type strain, 488 tssD mutant and 488 tssD complement were performed. Disk diffusion assays were performed using ampicillin, amoxycillin/clavulanic acid, tetracycline and polymyxin B. A broth microdilution assay was performed using vancomycin. No differences in antimicrobial susceptibility were observed (**Supplementary Table S2**).

katA, *sodB*, and *ahpC* encode proteins involved directly in the breakdown of ROS. Expression of *katA*, *sodB*, and *ahpC* was investigated in the 488 wild-type strain and 488 *tssD* mutant using qRT-PCR. Expression of all three genes were significantly reduced in the 488 *tssD* mutant compared to the 488 wild-type strain. This data combined with the increased ability of the 488 wild-type strain to survive the effects of oxidative stress suggest that the T6SS is associated with the oxidative stress response in *C. jejuni* (**Figure 4B**).

T6SS Increases *C. jejuni* Cytotoxicity in the *Galleria mellonella* Model of Infection

The larvae of *G. mellonella* (Greater wax moth) are an established model to study the pathogenesis of *C. jejuni* (Senior et al., 2011). In order to investigate whether the presence of a T6SS in *C. jejuni* enhances bacterial cytotoxicity, *G. mellonella* larvae were injected with *C. jejuni* strains and larvae survival examined over a duration of 5 days. Only the T6SS-positive 488 wild-type strain was cytotoxic to *G. mellonella* larvae after 24 h post-injection (**Figure 5**). The T6SS-negative 81–176 wild-type strain also exhibited some cytotoxicity, but at a lower level compared to the 488 wild-type strain after 48 and 72 h. After 96 and 120 h, cytotoxicity of the 488 *tssD* mutant was also observed but at a significantly lower level than the 488 wild-type strain.

T6SS Enhances Both *C. jejuni* Interactions With and Invasion of Chicken Primary Intestinal Cells

Recent studies suggest that the prevalence of T6SS-positive *C. jejuni* strains is on the rise in high-income countries and there are indications that T6SS-positive strains are now prevalent over T6SS-negative strains infecting chickens in farms, on raw chicken in supermarkets and in hospital patients (Ugarte-Ruiz et al., 2015; Sima et al., 2018). To investigate whether the presence of the

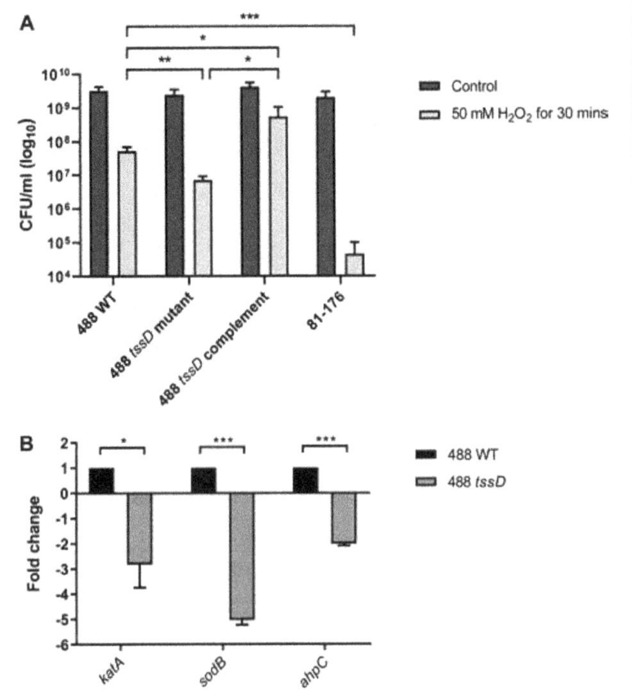

FIGURE 4 | Type VI secretion system of *C. jejuni* is involved in the oxidative stress response. **(A)** Survival of 488 wild-type strain, 488 *tssD* mutant, 488 *tssD* complement, and 81–176 wild-type strain following exposure to oxidative stress. The strains were exposed to 50 mM H_2O_2 for 30 min, then serial dilutions were performed and CFUs/ml counted. Asterisks denote a statistically significant difference ($^*p \leq 0.05$, $^{**}p \leq 0.01$, $^{***}p \leq 0.001$). **(B)** qRT-PCR analysis comparing expression of *katA*, *sodB*, and *ahpC* in the 488 wild-type strain and 488 *tssD* mutant. qRT-PCR analysis was performed using *katA*, *sodB*, and *ahpC* primers. Data was analyzed by the comparative CT method with *gyrA* housekeeping gene as the internal control. The relative expression of *katA*, *sodB*, and *ahpC* are shown. Asterisks denote a statistically significant difference ($^*p \leq 0.05$, $^{***}p \leq 0.001$).

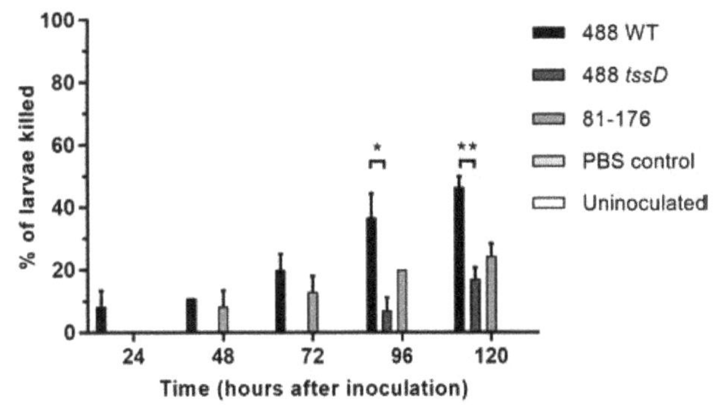

FIGURE 5 | Infection of *Galleria mellonella* larvae with the 488 wild-type strain, 488 *tssD* mutant or 81–176 wild-type strain. Ten *G. mellonella* larvae were injected per bacterial strain with a syringe in the right foremost leg. Controls injected with PBS only were included along with uninoculated controls. Larvae were incubated at 37°C with counts of dead larvae recorded every 24 h over a period of 5 days. Asterisks denote a statistically significant difference ($^*p \leq 0.05$, $^{**}p \leq 0.01$).

T6SS plays a role in the ability of *C. jejuni* to infect chickens, an *in vitro* model was used to examine the potential of *C. jejuni* to adhere to and invade chicken primary intestinal cells. The 488 wild-type strain exhibited significantly higher levels of adherence and invasion than the 488 *tssD* mutant. The T6SS-negative 81–176 wild-type strain also exhibited lower levels of adherence and invasion than the 488 wild-type strain, however, these differences were not significant (**Figure 6**).

T6SS Enhances the Ability of *C. jejuni* to Infect Chickens

To further investigate whether the presence of the T6SS plays a role in the ability of *C. jejuni* to infect chickens, chicken infection studies were performed. An identical pattern was observed after *in vivo* infection of 15-day old Ross 308 broiler chickens, where at 3 days post-infection the numbers of the 488 wild-type strain detected in the caeca were significantly higher than the numbers of the 488 *tssD* mutant or 81–176 wild-type strain (**Figure 7**). These results indicate that the presence of the T6SS is important in enhancing the ability of *C. jejuni* to colonize chickens.

DISCUSSION

The *C. jejuni* T6SS is a functional secretory mechanism that appears distinct from the well-elucidated *P. aeruginosa* and *V. cholerae* T6SS model systems. Whole genome sequencing of a novel 488 strain and the T6SS-positive 43431 strain revealed a single T6SS cluster containing one copy of the *tssD* gene that encodes the needle-like tube of the T6SS, but the absence of *tssH* which encodes the ATPase that breaks down and recycles the TssBC contractile sheath. This is in contrast to the T6SS model systems of *P. aeruginosa* and *V. cholerae* where multiple T6SS clusters are present with differing functions. The absence of a *tssH* ortholog had previously been observed in other *C. jejuni* strains in other studies (Lertpiriyapong et al., 2012; Bleumink-Pluym et al., 2013). *Burkholderia* species, *Helicobacter hepaticus*, *Francisella tularensis*, and *Salmonella enterica* also appear to lack a TssH component. Despite the absence of TssH, the presence of a functional T6SS in all these organisms including *C. jejuni* suggests there may be alternate mechanisms for contractile sheath recycling. In *V. cholerae* a study demonstrated that whilst TssH is not essential, it is important in increasing the efficiency of the T6SS in inter-bacterial competition assays (Bachmann et al., 2015).

Comparison of the *C. jejuni* strains sequenced in this study with previously published sequences of other *C. jejuni* strains as well as other *Campylobacter* species revealed a T6SS cluster that is very closely conserved with all core genes present in the same arrangement. *C. jejuni* 488 (human isolate from Brazil), 43431 (human isolate from Canada), 108 (human isolate from the United States), RC039 (chicken isolate from the United Kingdom), and even *C. coli* RM2228 (chicken isolate from the United States) all share the same conserved T6SS cluster. Only *C. jejuni* 414 had a different gene arrangement in the T6SS cluster. 414 is an environmental strain, isolated from a wild bank vole in the United Kingdom (Williams et al., 2010). It is possible that agricultural intensification practices which readily facilitate

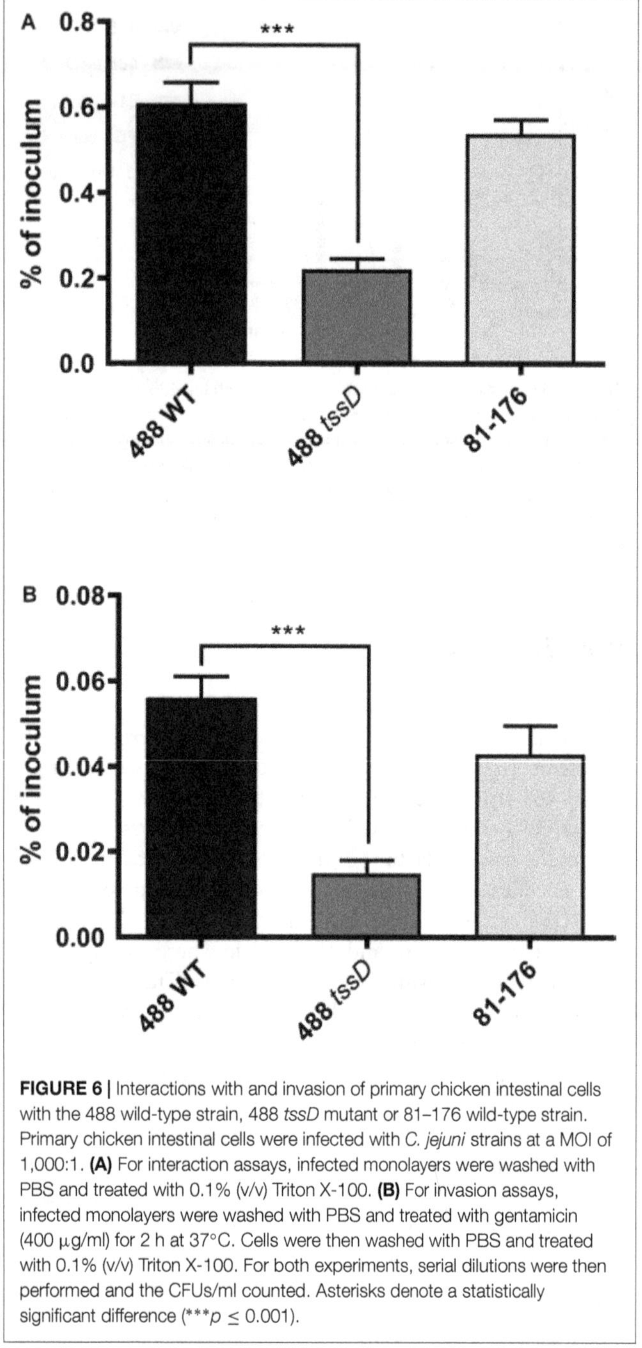

FIGURE 6 | Interactions with and invasion of primary chicken intestinal cells with the 488 wild-type strain, 488 *tssD* mutant or 81–176 wild-type strain. Primary chicken intestinal cells were infected with *C. jejuni* strains at a MOI of 1,000:1. **(A)** For interaction assays, infected monolayers were washed with PBS and treated with 0.1% (v/v) Triton X-100. **(B)** For invasion assays, infected monolayers were washed with PBS and treated with gentamicin (400 μg/ml) for 2 h at 37°C. Cells were then washed with PBS and treated with 0.1% (v/v) Triton X-100. For both experiments, serial dilutions were then performed and the CFUs/ml counted. Asterisks denote a statistically significant difference (***$p \leq 0.001$).

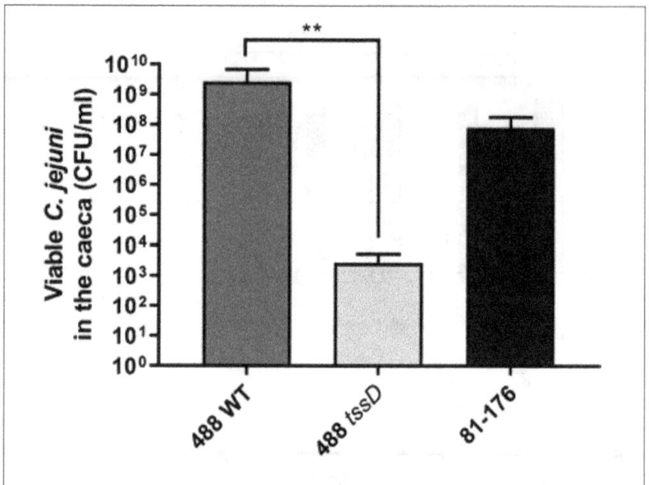

FIGURE 7 | Infection of broiler chickens with the 488 wild-type strain, 488 *tssD* mutant or 81–176 wild-type strain. Ten 15-day old Ross 308 broiler chickens were inoculated with approximately 1×10^8 CFU/ml of either the 488 wild-type strain, the 488 *tssD* mutant or the 81–176 wild-type strain. Chickens were euthanized 3 days post-infection. Caecum contents were plated and counts of viable *C. jejuni* in the samples performed. Asterisks denote a statistically significant difference (**$p \leq 0.01$).

passing of strains between chickens and humans could lead to these strains to share more of a conserved T6SS compared to the 414 environmental strain.

Further investigations indicated that the novel 488 strain has a functional T6SS capable of secreting the TssD effector, corroborating previous studies which have shown TssD to be secreted from 43431 and 108 strains (Lertpiriyapong et al., 2012; Bleumink-Pluym et al., 2013). However, the contractile sheath components TssBC and their function had not previously been studied in *C. jejuni*. In other bacteria, an intact contractile sheath structure is important for a fully functioning T6SS as removal of either TssB/VipA or TssC/VipB from the contractile sheaths described in *V. cholerae* result in a defective T6SS unable to secrete effectors (Basler et al., 2012; Kudryashev et al., 2015; Brackmann et al., 2018). In this study we have shown that both contractile sheath genes are expressed when the 488 strain is cultured in broth and on solid plates. Isogenic 488 *tssB* and *tssC* mutants were constructed and shown to still be able to secrete TssD at a reduced level compared to the wild-type strain. The observation that the *C. jejuni* T6SS does not require both TssB and TssC components to be present for the T6SS to be able to secrete TssD is unusual and differs from previous observations of the T6SS in *V. cholerae*. This suggests that in *C. jejuni*, as long as either TssB or TssC is present, the T6SS remains capable of secreting TssD at a reduced level. However, this does not suggest that the contractile sheath components in *C. jejuni* may differ from those in the T6SS model systems of *P. aeruginosa* and *V. cholerae*, rather that the contractile sheath components may be interchangeable or be able to compensate for the absence of the other component via a yet unknown process.

The importance of the T6SS in countering the effects of oxidative stress has previously been shown in *Y. pseudotuberculosis*, *B. thailandensis*, and enterohemorrhagic *E. coli* (Wang et al., 2015; Si et al., 2017; Wan et al., 2017). In this study, we show that the *C. jejuni* T6SS also appears to play a role, with the genes that encode KatA, SodB, and AhpC that are involved directly in the breakdown of ROS all expressed at significantly higher levels in the 488 wild-type strain compared to the 488 *tssD* mutant. The 488 wild-type strain with an intact T6SS is also more resistant to the effects of oxidative stress compared to the 488 *tssD* mutant. We speculate that TssD positively regulates the expression of genes involved in the breakdown of ROS, and in turn this results in greater resistance to oxidative stress in strains harboring an intact T6SS cluster.

A MarR family transcriptional regulator TctR was recently shown to regulate the T6SS-2 gene cluster in *B. pseudomallei* (Losada et al., 2018). Previous studies have also shown that the MarR family transcriptional regulators RrpA and RrpB are important in regulating both oxidative and aerobic stress responses in *C. jejuni* and therefore play a role in enhancing bacterial survival both in the hosts and in the environment (Gundogdu et al., 2011, 2015, 2016). As our results indicate that the *C. jejuni* T6SS is also associated with the oxidative stress response, it is tempting to speculate that the RrpA and RrpB regulators may in some way be linked to the T6SS. Further studies will be required to investigate this hypothetical link.

Based on our data we propose that presence of the T6SS cluster in *C. jejuni* strains also confers a competitive advantage to these strains within a host. The T6SS-positive 488 wild-type strain is more cytotoxic in the *G. mellonella* model than the T6SS-negative 81–176 wild-type strain and the 488 *tssD* mutant. This suggests that the presence of a T6SS increases the cytotoxicity of *C. jejuni* in the *G. mellonella* model of infection and secreted T6SS effectors may also be important in causing cytotoxicity to other organisms. The 81–176 strain was selected as a negative control in this study due to the absence of the T6SS in this strain. Despite lacking the T6SS, 81–176 is a hypervirulent strain capable of causing severe disease and harbors two plasmids, pTet and pVir, that play a role in increased virulence (Black et al., 1988; Bacon et al., 2000). Therefore, any differences observed between 488 and 81–176 could potentially be due to a diversity of virulence factors in these two strains rather than the presence or absence of the T6SS.

This study is the first to examine the role of T6SS of *C. jejuni* in a biologically relevant model. Lertpiriyapong et al. (2012) utilized a murine model and found that a T6SS-positive strain to be more interactive with and invasive in RAW 264.7 macrophage cells and have a higher colonization potential in IL-10-deficient mice. However, it has previously been shown that *C. jejuni* does not colonize mice in the same manner as in chickens, as *C. jejuni* colonizes mice at a significantly slower rate than chickens and some strains such as 81–176 do not appear to colonize mice at all (Wilson et al., 2010). The *C. jejuni* 488 wild-type strain exhibits higher levels of adherence to and invasion of chicken cells and is also able to infect chickens at a much higher rate that the *tssD* mutant. The results indicate that the ability of *C. jejuni* to infect chickens is enhanced by the presence of the T6SS and the T6SS may be important as a colonization factor in the natural host of *C. jejuni*. The increased ability of *C. jejuni* strains with the T6SS to infect and colonize chickens is a particular concern for the agricultural and food industries tasked with reducing *C. jejuni* load in both live chickens on farms and on raw chicken meat in the supermarket (Sima et al., 2018). From a public health perspective, the rise of T6SS in *C. jejuni* is also problematic as there are indications that strains with the T6SS may cause more severe disease in humans (Harrison et al., 2014).

In summary, in this study we confirmed the presence of a single T6SS cluster among several *C. jejuni* strains and confirmed that the functional T6SS is capable of secreting the TssD effector. Our results indicated that the *C. jejuni* T6SS is involved in the oxidative stress response. Using *in vitro* and *in vivo* models we demonstrated the increased ability of T6SS-positive *C. jejuni* to colonize the natural avian host. Our findings highlight the importance of further understanding the function of the T6SS present in an expanding population of *C. jejuni*, the potential importance of the T6SS in colonization and niche establishment in different hosts and the potential for T6SS-positive *C. jejuni* strains to cause more severe disease in both chickens and humans.

MATERIALS AND METHODS

Bacterial Strains and Growth Conditions

Campylobacter jejuni strains used in this study are listed in **Supplementary Table S3**. *C. jejuni* strains were grown at 37°C under microaerobic conditions (85% N_2, 15% CO_2 5% O_2) in a variable atmosphere chamber (Don Whitley Scientific, United Kingdom). Unless otherwise stated, *C. jejuni* were grown either on Columbia agar with 7% (v/v) horse blood (TCS Biosciences, United Kingdom) with the addition of Skirrow *Campylobacter* selective supplement or in Brucella broth (BD Diagnostics, United Kingdom). *E. coli* strains listed in **Supplementary Table S4** were grown on lysogeny broth (LB) agar plates or in LB broth at 37°C. The appropriate antibiotics were added as required at concentrations of 50 μg/ml kanamycin, 100 μg/ml ampicillin or 10 μg/ml chloramphenicol for *C. jejuni* growth, with the concentration of chloramphenicol for *E. coli* growth increased to 50 μg/ml. All reagents were obtained from Oxoid (United Kingdom) unless otherwise stated.

Whole Genome Sequencing

Genome sequencing of the *C. jejuni* 488 and 43431 (Poly et al., 2004) wild-type strains was performed as previously described by Ugarte-Ruiz et al. (2014). Briefly, sequencing was performed using the Illumina MiSeq 2 × 301 bp paired-end sequencing. To analyze the data quality, FastQC was used (Simon, 2010) followed by read trimming using Trimmomatic (v0.32) (leading' and "trailing" setting of 3, a "sliding window" setting of 4:20 and a "minlength" of 36 nucleotides) (Bolger et al., 2014). Reads were mapped using BWA-MEM (v0.7.7-r441) against the genome sequence of *C. jejuni* NCTC 11168 (AL111168) (Li and Durbin, 2009). Assembly on unmapped regions was performed using Velvet Optimizer (v2.2.5) using n50 optimization (Zerbino and Birney, 2008; Gladman and Seemann, 2012). Contigs were ordered against *C. jejuni* NCTC 11168 (AL111168) strains using ABACAS (v1.3.1) (Assefa et al., 2009). Genome annotation was performed using Prokka (Seemann, 2014). Genomes were visualized using Artemis and ACT software (Carver et al., 2012). T6SS ORFs were identified using BLAST (Altschul et al., 1990; Gish and States, 1993). The 488 and 43431 genome sequences were uploaded to the EBI ENA database (Accession number PRJEB31331).

Reverse Transcription PCR (RT-PCR) and Quantitative Real-Time PCR (qRT-PCR) Analyses

Total RNA was isolated using PureLink RNA Mini Kit (Thermo Fisher Scientific) from *C. jejuni* cultures grown for 16 h at

37°C with shaking at 75 rpm under microaerobic conditions in Brucella broth. TURBO DNA-free kit (Thermo Fisher Scientific) was used to remove DNA contamination and RNA was converted to cDNA using the SuperScript III First-Strand Synthesis System (Thermo Fisher Scientific). Reverse transcription PCR (RT-PCR) was performed according to the manufacturer's instructions with primers listed in **Supplementary Table S5**. Quantitative real-time PCR (qRT-PCR) was performed using primers listed in **Supplementary Table S5**, with SYBR Green Master Mix (Applied Biosystems, United Kingdom) on the ABI 7500 Real-Time PCR System machine (Applied Biosystems). qRT-PCR data was analyzed by the comparative C_T method with *gyrA* housekeeping gene as an internal control (Ritz et al., 2002; Schmittgen and Livak, 2008).

Construction of *tssB*, *tssC*, *tssD* Mutants and *tssBC* Double Mutant

Campylobacter jejuni mutants were constructed as previously described (Gundogdu et al., 2011). Briefly, the appropriate gene specific primers (see **Supplementary Table S5**) were used to amplify the gene of interest from *C. jejuni* genomic DNA. PCR products were cloned into a pGEM-T Easy vector (Promega, United Kingdom) and transformed into *E. coli* XL2-Blue if the unique restriction site was *Bam*HI or *Bgl*II. *E. coli* SCS110 were used if the restriction site was *Bcl*I. If none of these sites were present, inverse PCR mutagenesis was used to introduce a *Bgl*II site (Gundogdu et al., 2015). Plasmid DNA was digested with *Bam*HI, *Bcl*I, or *Bgl*II, a kanamycin or chloramphenicol resistance cassette was inserted and the resulting construct transformed into *E. coli*. Successful constructs were transformed into *C. jejuni* by electroporation and positive clones were confirmed by PCR and Sanger sequencing. For construction of a *C. jejuni tssBC* double mutant, the plasmid DNA construct used for the *C. jejuni tssC* mutant was transformed into *C. jejuni tssB* mutant by electroporation.

Preparation of Whole Cell Lysates and Supernatants for Protein Secretion Assays

Campylobacter jejuni strains from 24 h plate cultures were inoculated to OD_{600} 0.1 in Brucella broth and incubated at 37°C with shaking at 75 rpm under microaerobic conditions until late log phase. The broth cultures were centrifuged at 4,000 rpm at 4°C for 30 min to separate the pellet and the supernatant.

To prepare a whole cell lysate sample, a pellet was re-suspended in PBS and sonicated for 10 min on high setting using a Bioruptor (Diagenode, Belgium). Sonicated samples were centrifuged at 13,000 rpm for 5 min and the resulting supernatant was added to 2X Laemmli sample buffer (Sigma-Aldrich, United Kingdom) then boiled at 95°C for 10 min, followed by centrifugation at 13,000 rpm for 5 min. To prepare a supernatant sample, supernatant was filtered through a 0.2 μm-pore-size filter (Millipore, United Kingdom) to remove remaining cells and the titrate was concentrated using an Amicon Ultra-15 centrifugal filter (10 kDa) (Millipore). Trichloroacetic acid (TCA) precipitation with acetone washes was performed to further concentrate the samples as described previously (Link and LaBaer, 2011). Following acetone washes, the pellet was re-suspended in 2X Laemmli sample buffer and boiled at 95°C for 10 min, followed by centrifugation at 13,000 rpm for 5 min.

SDS-PAGE and Western Blot Analysis

BCA assay was performed to determine protein concentration in samples. 13 μg of whole cell lysate samples and 30 μg of supernatant samples were loaded along with Pageruler Plus Pre-stained Protein Ladder (Thermo Fisher Scientific, United Kingdom) onto NuPAGE Bis-Tris gel (12%) (Thermo Fisher Scientific) with MOPS running buffer (Thermo Fisher Scientific). Membrane transfer was performed using the iBlot 2 Dry Blotting System (Thermo Fisher Scientific). The membrane was blocked with 2% (w/v) milk overnight at 4°C, incubated with the TssD antibody in phosphate buffered saline with 0.1% (v/v) Tween-20 (PBS-T) for 1 h at room temperature, washed with PBS-T then incubated with the secondary goat anti-rabbit antibody in PBS-T for 1 h at room temperature. The membrane was washed twice with PBS-T, once with PBS scanned using the Odyssey Imaging System (LI-COR Biosciences, United Kingdom).

TssD Antibody Production

The polyclonal anti-TssD antibody was produced by Capra Science Antibodies AB (Sweden). The *tssD* gene cloned into an expression vector and recombinant TssD protein was isolated and purified. For production of the TssD antiserum, purified TssD was immunized into a rabbit. Two boosts with the antigen were performed, followed by the first bleed. A further boost with the antigen was performed followed by the second bleed; the process was repeated for a third bleed. Antiserum collected from the third bleed was affinity purified using a peptide-coupled column for the anti-TssD antibody.

Oxidative Stress Assay

Campylobacter jejuni from 24 h plate cultures were re-suspended in PBS, the OD_{600} was measured and the suspension adjusted with PBS to OD_{600} 1.0. Bacterial suspensions were exposed to 50 mM H_2O_2 for 30 min at 37°C stationary under microaerobic conditions. Serial dilutions were performed and dilutions plated onto blood agar plates. Plates were incubated at 37°C under microaerobic conditions and colonies counted after 48 h.

Antimicrobial Susceptibility Assays

The disk diffusion assays were performed with ampicillin (10 μg), amoxycillin/clavulanic acid (2:1, 30 μg), tetracycline (30 μg) or polymyxin B (300 units) disks (Oxoid) following the methodology published by the European Society of Clinical Microbiology (EUCAST) (EUCAST, 2019). Zones of growth inhibition were measured in millimeters and sensitivity (S) determined based on the EUCAST guidelines. Broth microdilution assays were performed with vancomycin (Sigma) and the minimum inhibitory concentration (MIC, μg/ml) was determined according to the methodology published by Wiegand et al. (2008).

Galleria mellonella Model of Infection

Galleria mellonella larvae were purchased from Livefoods Direct (United Kingdom). Bacterial cells harvested from 24 h plate cultures were re-suspended in PBS and OD_{600} adjusted to 0.1. Ten *G. mellonella* larvae per bacterial strain were injected with 10 μl bacterial suspension with a micro syringe (Hamilton, Switzerland) in the right foremost leg. Controls injected with PBS or not injected were also prepared. Larvae were incubated at 37°C, with counts of dead larvae recorded every 24 h for 5 days.

Chicken Cell Interaction and Invasion Assays

Isolation of chicken intestinal primary cells (Byrne et al., 2007) as well as interaction and invasion assays (Corcionivoschi et al., 2009) were performed as described previously. Briefly, biopsies from sections of small intestines from 6 to 12 week-old broiler chickens (Cobb 500) were placed in primary cell culture medium and primary cells were isolated. *C. jejuni* strains were grown for 24 h on Muller-Hinton agar under microaerobic conditions. Bacterial cells were washed and resuspended in tissue culture medium to an OD_{600} of 0.4, then added to chicken intestinal primary cells grown in tissue culture plates to yield a multiplicity of infection of 1000:1. Plates were centrifuged and incubated for 3 h at 37°C in a microaerophilic environment. For interaction assays, infected monolayers were washed with PBS and treated with 0.1% v/v Triton X-100. Serial dilutions were performed and the CFUs/ml were enumerated. For invasion assays, infected monolayers were washed with PBS and treated with gentamicin (400 μg/ml) for 2 h at 37°C. Cells were then washed with PBS and treated with 0.1% v/v Triton X-100. Serial dilutions were performed and the CFUs/ml were enumerated.

Chicken Infection Assay

Thirty male broiler chickens (Ross 308) were housed in isolation units on wood shaving bedding. The temperature in the isolation unit was kept between 22–25°C and thermostatically controlled. Broilers were fed *ad libitum* with a standard diet. *C. jejuni* strains were grown on Muller Hinton plates for 24 h under microaerobic conditions and resuspended in sterile distilled water. At 15 days old, ten broilers were inoculated with approximately 1×10^8 CFU/ml of either the 488 wild-type strain, the 488 *tssD* mutant or the 81–176 wild-type strain. The different batches of infected broilers were kept separated in sterile isolation units. After 3 days of infection, broilers were euthanized and *C. jejuni* was enumerated by analyzing the cecum content using the ISO17025 methodology for plate counting. All broilers were confirmed using cloacal swabs as being *Campylobacter* free at the time of infection. These experiments were performed in triplicate on three separate occasions.

Statistical Analysis

All experiments were performed with at least three biological replicates and three technical replicates, unless otherwise stated. Statistical analyses were performed using GraphPad Prism 7 (GraphPad Software, United States) and data were presented as mean ± SEM. Results were compared using unpaired *t*-test with $^*p \leq 0.05$, $^{**}p \leq 0.01$, $^{***}p \leq 0.001$.

ETHICS STATEMENT

The experiments were performed according to the legislation in place (Law 471/2002 and government ordinance 437/2002) and under the supervision of National Sanitary Veterinary Agency. The Ethics Committee of Banat University of Agricultural Sciences and Veterinary Medicine - King Michael I of Romania approved this work.

AUTHOR CONTRIBUTIONS

OG and ND conceived the study with input from AH and NC. JL, GH, CD, AE, FS, AS, and OG performed the experiments and contributed to this manuscript. JL, OG, and ND wrote the manuscript with significant input from LS, IP, NC, and BW.

FUNDING

The authors gratefully acknowledge the support of the Biotechnology and Biological Sciences Research Council Institute Strategic Programme BB/R012504/1 constituent project BBS/E/F/000PR10349. AH was supported by H2020-MSCA Global Fellowship grant 657766.

REFERENCES

Altschul, S. F., Gish, W., Miller, W., Myers, E. W., and Lipman, D. J. (1990). Basic local alignment search tool. *J. Mol. Biol.* 215, 403–410. doi: 10.1006/jmbi.1990.9999

Ang, C. W., De Klerk, M. A., Endtz, H. P., Jacobs, B. C., Laman, J. D., van der Meche, F. G., et al. (2001). Guillain-Barre syndrome- and miller fisher syndrome-associated campylobacter *jejuni* lipopolysaccharides induce anti-GM1 and anti-GQ1b antibodies in rabbits. *Infect. Immun.* 69, 2462–2469. doi: 10.1128/IAI.69.4.2462-2469.2001

Assefa, S., Keane, T. M., Otto, T. D., Newbold, C., and Berriman, M. (2009). ABACAS: algorithm-based automatic contiguation of assembled sequences. *Bioinformatics* 25, 1968–1969. doi: 10.1093/bioinformatics/btp347

Bachmann, V., Kostiuk, B., Unterweger, D., Diaz-Satizabal, L., Ogg, S., and Pukatzki, S. (2015). Bile salts modulate the mucin-activated type VI secretion system of pandemic *Vibrio cholerae*. *PLoS Negl. Trop. Dis.* 9:e0004031. doi: 10.1371/journal.pntd.0004031

Bacon, D. J., Alm, R. A., Burr, D. H., Hu, L., Kopecko, D. J., Ewing, C. P., et al. (2000). Involvement of a plasmid in virulence of *Campylobacter jejuni* 81-176. *Infect. Immun.* 68, 4384–4390. doi: 10.1128/iai.68.8.4384-4390.2000

Basler, M., Pilhofer, M., Henderson, G. P., Jensen, G. J., and Mekalanos, J. J. (2012). Type VI secretion requires a dynamic contractile phage tail-like structure. *Nature* 483, 182–186. doi: 10.1038/nature10846

Black, R. E., Levine, M. M., Clements, M. L., Hughes, T. P., and Blaser, M. J. (1988). Experimental *Campylobacter jejuni* infection in humans. *J. Infect. Dis.* 157, 472–479. doi: 10.1093/infdis/157.3.472

Bleumink-Pluym, N. M., van Alphen, L. B., Bouwman, L. I., Wosten, M. M., and van Putten, J. P. (2013). Identification of a functional type VI secretion system in

Campylobacter jejuni conferring capsule polysaccharide sensitive cytotoxicity. *PLoS Pathog.* 9:e1003393. doi: 10.1371/journal.ppat.1003393

Bolger, A. M., Lohse, M., and Usadel, B. (2014). Trimmomatic: a flexible trimmer for Illumina sequence data. *Bioinformatics* 30, 2114–2120. doi: 10.1093/bioinformatics/btu170

Brackmann, M., Wang, J., and Basler, M. (2018). Type VI secretion system sheath inter-subunit interactions modulate its contraction. *EMBO Rep.* 19, 225–233. doi: 10.15252/embr.201744416

Byrne, C. M., Clyne, M., and Bourke, B. (2007). *Campylobacter jejuni* adhere to and invade chicken intestinal epithelial cells in vitro. *Microbiology* 153(Pt 2), 561–569. doi: 10.1099/mic.0.2006/000711-710

Carver, T., Harris, S. R., Berriman, M., Parkhill, J., and McQuillan, J. A. (2012). Artemis: an integrated platform for visualization and analysis of high-throughput sequence-based experimental data. *Bioinformatics* 28, 464–469. doi: 10.1093/bioinformatics/btr703

Cianfanelli, F. R., Monlezun, L., and Coulthurst, S. J. (2016). Aim, load, fire: the type VI secretion system, a bacterial Nanoweapon. *Trends Microbiol.* 24, 51–62. doi: 10.1016/j.tim.2015.10.005

Coker, A. O., Isokpehi, R. D., Thomas, B. N., Amisu, K. O., and Obi, C. L. (2002). Human campylobacteriosis in developing countries. *Emerg. Infect. Dis.* 8, 237–244. doi: 10.3201/eid0803.010233

Corcionivoschi, N., Clyne, M., Lyons, A., Elmi, A., Gundogdu, O., Wren, B. W., et al. (2009). *Campylobacter jejuni* cocultured with epithelial cells reduces surface capsular polysaccharide expression. *Infect. Immun.* 77, 1959–1967. doi: 10.1128/IAI.01239-1238

Corcionivoschi, N., Gundogdu, O., Moran, L., Kelly, C., Scates, P., Stef, L., et al. (2015). Virulence characteristics of hcp (+) *Campylobacter jejuni* and Campylobacter coli isolates from retail chicken. *Gut Pathog.* 7:20. doi: 10.1186/s13099-015-0067-z

Drebes Dorr, N. C., and Blokesch, M. (2018). Bacterial type VI secretion system facilitates niche domination. *Proc. Natl. Acad. Sci. U.S.A.* 115, 8855–8857. doi: 10.1073/pnas.1812776115

EUCAST (2019). *Antimicrobial Susceptibility Testing: EUCAST Disk Diffusion Method.* Available at: http://www.eucast.org/ast_of_bacteria/disk_diffusion_methodology/ (accessed May 10, 2019).

Fitzsimons, T. C., Lewis, J. M., Wright, A., Kleifeld, O., Schittenhelm, R. B., Powell, D., et al. (2018). Identification of novel *Acinetobacter baumannii* Type VI secretion system antibacterial effector and immunity pairs. *Infect. Immun.* 86:e00297-18. doi: 10.1128/IAI.00297-218

Flint, A., Butcher, J., and Stintzi, A. (2016). Stress responses, adaptation, and virulence of bacterial pathogens during host gastrointestinal colonization. *Microbiol. Spectr.* 4:VMBF-0007-2015. doi: 10.1128/microbiolspec.VMBF-0007-2015

Gerc, A. J., Diepold, A., Trunk, K., Porter, M., Rickman, C., Armitage, J. P., et al. (2015). Visualization of the *Serratia* Type VI secretion system reveals unprovoked attacks and dynamic assembly. *Cell Rep.* 12, 2131–2142. doi: 10.1016/j.celrep.2015.08.053

Gish, W., and States, D. J. (1993). Identification of protein coding regions by database similarity search. *Nat. Genet.* 3, 266–272. doi: 10.1038/ng0393-266

Gladman, S., and Seemann, T. (2012). *VelvetOptimiser, v2.2.5.*

Gundogdu, O., da Silva, D. T., Mohammad, B., Elmi, A., Mills, D. C., Wren, B. W., et al. (2015). The *Campylobacter jejuni* MarR-like transcriptional regulators RrpA and RrpB both influence bacterial responses to oxidative and aerobic stresses. *Front. Microbiol.* 6:724. doi: 10.3389/fmicb.2015.00724

Gundogdu, O., da Silva, D. T., Mohammad, B., Elmi, A., Wren, B. W., van Vliet, A. H., et al. (2016). The *Campylobacter jejuni* oxidative stress regulator RrpB is associated with a genomic hypervariable region and altered oxidative stress resistance. *Front. Microbiol.* 7:2117. doi: 10.3389/fmicb.2016.02117

Gundogdu, O., Mills, D. C., Elmi, A., Martin, M. J., Wren, B. W., and Dorrell, N. (2011). The *Campylobacter jejuni* transcriptional regulator Cj1556 plays a role in the oxidative and aerobic stress response and is important for bacterial survival in vivo. *J. Bacteriol.* 193, 4238–4249. doi: 10.1128/JB.05189-5111

Hachani, A., Wood, T. E., and Filloux, A. (2016). Type VI secretion and anti-host effectors. *Curr. Opin. Microbiol.* 29, 81–93. doi: 10.1016/j.mib.2015.11.006

Harrison, J. W., Dung, T. T., Siddiqui, F., Korbrisate, S., Bukhari, H., Tra, M. P., et al. (2014). Identification of possible virulence marker from *Campylobacter jejuni* isolates. *Emerg. Infect. Dis.* 20, 1026–1029. doi: 10.3201/eid2006.130635

Hermans, D., Pasmans, F., Heyndrickx, M., Van Immerseel, F., Martel, A., Van Deun, K., et al. (2012). A tolerogenic mucosal immune response leads to persistent *Campylobacter jejuni* colonization in the chicken gut. *Crit. Rev. Microbiol.* 38, 17–29. doi: 10.3109/1040841X.2011.615298

Kaakoush, N. O., Castano-Rodriguez, N., Mitchell, H. M., and Man, S. M. (2015). Global epidemiology of *Campylobacter* infection. *Clin. Microbiol. Rev.* 28, 687–720. doi: 10.1128/CMR.00006-15

Kapitein, N., Bonemann, G., Pietrosiuk, A., Seyffer, F., Hausser, I., Locker, J. K., et al. (2013). ClpV recycles VipA/VipB tubules and prevents non-productive tubule formation to ensure efficient type VI protein secretion. *Mol. Microbiol.* 87, 1013–1028. doi: 10.1111/mmi.12147

Kapitein, N., and Mogk, A. (2014). Type VI secretion system helps find a niche. *Cell Host Microb.* 16, 5–6. doi: 10.1016/j.chom.2014.06.012

Kim, J. C., Oh, E., Kim, J., and Jeon, B. (2015). Regulation of oxidative stress resistance in *Campylobacter jejuni*, a microaerophilic foodborne pathogen. *Front. Microbiol.* 6:751. doi: 10.3389/fmicb.2015.00751

Kirchberger, P. C., Unterweger, D., Provenzano, D., Pukatzki, S., and Boucher, Y. (2017). Sequential displacement of Type VI secretion system effector genes leads to evolution of diverse immunity gene arrays in *Vibrio cholerae*. *Sci. Rep.* 7:45133. doi: 10.1038/srep45133

Kovanen, S., Rossi, M., Pohja-Mykra, M., Nieminen, T., Raunio-Saarnisto, M., Sauvala, M., et al. (2018). Population genetics and characterization of *Campylobacter jejuni* isolates in western jackdaws and game birds in Finland. *Appl. Environ. Microbiol.* 85:e02365-18. doi: 10.1128/AEM.02365-2318

Kudryashev, M., Wang, R. Y., Brackmann, M., Scherer, S., Maier, T., Baker, D., et al. (2015). Structure of the type VI secretion system contractile sheath. *Cell* 160, 952–962. doi: 10.1016/j.cell.2015.01.037

Lertpiriyapong, K., Gamazon, E. R., Feng, Y., Park, D. S., Pang, J., Botka, G., et al. (2012). *Campylobacter jejuni* type VI secretion system: roles in adaptation to deoxycholic acid, host cell adherence, invasion, and in vivo colonization. *PLoS One* 7:e42842. doi: 10.1371/journal.pone.0042842

Li, H., and Durbin, R. (2009). Fast and accurate short read alignment with burrows-wheeler transform. *Bioinformatics* 25, 1754–1760. doi: 10.1093/bioinformatics/btp324

Link, A. J., and LaBaer, J. (2011). Trichloroacetic acid (TCA) precipitation of proteins. *Cold Spring Harb. Protoc.* 2011, 993–994. doi: 10.1101/pdb.prot5651

Losada, L., Shea, A. A., and DeShazer, D. (2018). A MarR family transcriptional regulator and subinhibitory antibiotics regulate type VI secretion gene clusters in *Burkholderia pseudomallei*. *Microbiology* 164, 1196–1211. doi: 10.1099/mic.0.000697

Ma, L. S., Hachani, A., Lin, J. S., Filloux, A., and Lai, E. M. (2014). *Agrobacterium tumefaciens* deploys a superfamily of type VI secretion DNase effectors as weapons for interbacterial competition in planta. *Cell Host Microb.* 16, 94–104. doi: 10.1016/j.chom.2014.06.002

Mougous, J. D., Cuff, M. E., Raunser, S., Shen, A., Zhou, M., Gifford, C. A., et al. (2006). A virulence locus of *Pseudomonas aeruginosa* encodes a protein secretion apparatus. *Science* 312, 1526–1530. doi: 10.1126/science.1128393

Murdoch, S. L., Trunk, K., English, G., Fritsch, M. J., Pourkarimi, E., and Coulthurst, S. J. (2011). The opportunistic pathogen *Serratia marcescens* utilizes type VI secretion to target bacterial competitors. *J. Bacteriol.* 193, 6057–6069. doi: 10.1128/JB.05671-5611

Newell, D. G., and Fearnley, C. (2003). Sources of *Campylobacter* colonization in broiler chickens. *Appl. Environ. Microbiol.* 69, 4343–4351. doi: 10.1128/aem.69.8.4343-4351.2003

Noreen, Z., Jobichen, C., Abbasi, R., Seetharaman, J., Sivaraman, J., and Bokhari, H. (2018). Structural basis for the pathogenesis of *Campylobacter jejuni* Hcp1, a structural and effector protein of the Type VI Secretion System. *FEBS J.* 285, 4060–4070. doi: 10.1111/febs.14650

Penner, J. L., Hennessy, J. N., and Congi, R. V. (1983). Serotyping of *Campylobacter jejuni* and *Campylobacter coli* on the basis of thermostable antigens. *Eur. J. Clin. Microbiol.* 2, 378–383. doi: 10.1007/bf02019474

Poly, F., Threadgill, D., and Stintzi, A. (2004). Identification of *Campylobacter jejuni* ATCC 43431-specific genes by whole microbial genome comparisons. *J. Bacteriol.* 186, 4781–4795. doi: 10.1128/JB.186.14.4781-4795.2004

Pukatzki, S., Ma, A. T., Sturtevant, D., Krastins, B., Sarracino, D., Nelson, W. C., et al. (2006). Identification of a conserved bacterial protein secretion system in *Vibrio cholerae* using the *Dictyostelium* host model system. *Proc. Natl. Acad. Sci. U.S.A.* 103, 1528–1533. doi: 10.1073/pnas.0510322103

Ringel, P. D., Hu, D., and Basler, M. (2017). The role of Type VI secretion system effectors in target cell lysis and subsequent horizontal gene transfer. *Cell Rep.* 21, 3927–3940. doi: 10.1016/j.celrep.2017.12.020

Ritz, M., Garenaux, A., Berge, M., and Federighi, M. (2002). Determination of rpoA as the most suitable internal control to study stress response in *C. jejuni* by RT-qPCR and application to oxidative stress. *J. Microbiol. Methods* 76, 196–200. doi: 10.1016/j.mimet.2008.10.014

Robinson, D. A. (1981). Infective dose of *Campylobacter jejuni* in milk. *Br. Med. J.* 282:1584. doi: 10.1136/bmj.282.6276.1584

Salih, O., He, S., Planamente, S., Stach, L., MacDonald, J. T., Manoli, E., et al. (2018). Atomic structure of Type VI contractile sheath from *Pseudomonas aeruginosa*. *Structure* 26, 329–336.e3. doi: 10.1016/j.str.2017.12.005

Schmittgen, T. D., and Livak, K. J. (2008). Analyzing real-time PCR data by the comparative C(T) method. *Nat. Protoc.* 3, 1101–1108. doi: 10.1038/nprot.2008.73

Seemann, T. (2014). Prokka: rapid prokaryotic genome annotation. *Bioinformatics* 30, 2068–2069. doi: 10.1093/bioinformatics/btu153

Senior, N. J., Bagnall, M. C., Champion, O. L., Reynolds, S. E., La Ragione, R. M., Woodward, M. J., et al. (2011). Galleria mellonella as an infection model for *Campylobacter jejuni* virulence. *J. Med. Microbiol.* 60(Pt 5), 661–669. doi: 10.1099/jmm.0.026658-26650

Si, M., Wang, Y., Zhang, B., Zhao, C., Kang, Y., Bai, H., et al. (2017). The Type VI secretion system engages a Redox-regulated dual-functional heme transporter for zinc acquisition. *Cell Rep.* 20, 949–959. doi: 10.1016/j.celrep.2017.06.081

Sima, F., Stratakos, A. C., Ward, P., Linton, M., Kelly, C., Pinkerton, L., et al. (2018). A novel natural antimicrobial can reduce the *in vitro* and *in vivo* Pathogenicity of T6SS positive *Campylobacter jejuni* and *Campylobacter coli* chicken isolates. *Front. Microbiol.* 9:2139. doi: 10.3389/fmicb.2018.02139

Simon, A. (2010). *FastQC*. Available at: http://www.bioinformatics.babraham.ac.uk/projects/fastqc/, v0.11.2 (accessed March 5, 2018).

Skarp, C. P. A., Hanninen, M. L., and Rautelin, H. I. K. (2016). *Campylobacteriosis*: the role of poultry meat. *Clin. Microbiol. Infect.* 22, 103–109. doi: 10.1016/j.cmi.2015.11.019

Trunk, K., Peltier, J., Liu, Y. C., Dill, B. D., Walker, L., Gow, N. A. R., et al. (2018). The type VI secretion system deploys antifungal effectors against microbial competitors. *Nat. Microbiol.* 3, 920–931. doi: 10.1038/s41564-018-0191-x

Ugarte-Ruiz, M., Stabler, R. A., Dominguez, L., Porrero, M. C., Wren, B. W., Dorrell, N., et al. (2014). Prevalence of Type VI secretion system in spanish *Campylobacter jejuni* isolates. *Zoonoses Public Health* 62, 497–500. doi: 10.1111/zph.12176

Ugarte-Ruiz, M., Stabler, R. A., Dominguez, L., Porrero, M. C., Wren, B. W., Dorrell, N., et al. (2015). Prevalence of type VI secretion system in spanish *Campylobacter jejuni* isolates. *Zoonoses Public Health* 62, 497–500. doi: 10.1111/zph.12176

Wan, B., Zhang, Q., Ni, J., Li, S., Wen, D., Li, J., et al. (2017). Type VI secretion system contributes to Enterohemorrhagic *Escherichia coli* virulence by secreting catalase against host reactive oxygen species (ROS). *PLoS Pathog.* 13:e1006246. doi: 10.1371/journal.ppat.1006246

Wang, T., Si, M., Song, Y., Zhu, W., Gao, F., Wang, Y., et al. (2015). Type VI Secretion system transports Zn2+ to combat multiple stresses and host immunity. *PLoS Pathog.* 11:e1005020. doi: 10.1371/journal.ppat.1005020

Wiegand, I., Hilpert, K., and Hancock, R. E. (2008). Agar and broth dilution methods to determine the minimal inhibitory concentration (MIC) of antimicrobial substances. *Nat. Protoc.* 3, 163–175. doi: 10.1038/nprot.2007.521

Wigley, P. (2015). Blurred lines: pathogens, commensals, and the healthy Gut. *Front. Vet. Sci.* 2:40. doi: 10.3389/fvets.2015.00040

Williams, N. J., Jones, T. R., Leatherbarrow, H. J., Birtles, R. J., Lahuerta-Marin, A., Bennett, M., et al. (2010). Isolation of a novel *Campylobacter jejuni* clone associated with the bank vole, *Myodes glareolus*. *Appl. Environ. Microbiol.* 76, 7318–7321. doi: 10.1128/AEM.00511-510

Wilson, D. L., Rathinam, V. A. K., Qi, W. H., Wick, L. M., Landgraf, J., Bell, J. A., et al. (2010). Genetic diversity in *Campylobacter jejuni* is associated with differential colonization of broiler chickens and C57BL/6J IL10-deficient mice. *Microbiology* 156, 2046–2057. doi: 10.1099/mic.0.035717-35710

Young, K. T., Davis, L. M., and Dirita, V. J. (2007). *Campylobacter jejuni*: molecular biology and pathogenesis. *Nat. Rev. Microbiol.* 5, 665–679. doi: 10.1038/nrmicro1718

Zerbino, D. R., and Birney, E. (2008). Velvet: algorithms for de novo short read assembly using de Bruijn graphs. *Genome Res.* 18, 821–829. doi: 10.1101/gr.074492.107

5

A High-Throughput Interbacterial Competition Screen Identifies ClpAP in Enhancing Recipient Susceptibility to Type VI Secretion System-Mediated Attack by *Agrobacterium tumefaciens*

Hsiao-Han Lin[1,2], Manda Yu[1], Manoj Kumar Sriramoju[3], Shang-Te Danny Hsu[3], Chi-Te Liu[2,4] and Erh-Min Lai[1]**

[1] Institute of Plant and Microbial Biology, Academia Sinica, Taipei, Taiwan, [2] Institute of Biotechnology, National Taiwan University, Taipei, Taiwan, [3] Institute of Biological Chemistry, Academia Sinica, Taipei, Taiwan, [4] Agricultural Biotechnology Research Center, Academia Sinica, Taipei, Taiwan

***Correspondence:**
Chi-Te Liu
chiteliu@ntu.edu.tw
Erh-Min Lai
emlai@gate.sinica.edu.tw

The type VI secretion system (T6SS) is an effector delivery system used by Gram-negative bacteria to kill other bacteria or eukaryotic hosts to gain fitness. The plant pathogen *Agrobacterium tumefaciens* utilizes its T6SS to kill other bacteria, such as *Escherichia coli*. We observed that the *A. tumefaciens* T6SS-dependent killing outcome differs when using different T6SS-lacking, K-12 *E. coli* strains as a recipient cell. Thus, we hypothesized that the *A. tumefaciens* T6SS killing outcome not only relies on the T6SS activity of the attacker cells but also depends on the recipient cells. Here, we developed a high-throughput interbacterial competition platform to test the hypothesis by screening for mutants with reduced killing outcomes caused by *A. tumefaciens* strain C58. Among the 3,909 strains in the *E. coli* Keio library screened, 16 mutants with less susceptibility to *A. tumefaciens* C58 T6SS-dependent killing were identified, and four of them were validated by complementation test. Among the four, the *clpP* encoding ClpP protease, which is universal and highly conserved in both prokaryotes and eukaryotic organelles, was selected for further characterizations. We demonstrated that ClpP is responsible for enhancing susceptibility to the T6SS killing. Because ClpP protease depends on other adapter proteins such as ClpA and ClpX for substrate recognition, further mutant studies followed by complementation tests were carried out to reveal that ClpP-associated AAA$^+$ ATPase ClpA, but not ClpX, is involved in enhancing susceptibility to *A. tumefaciens* T6SS killing. Moreover, functional and biochemical studies of various ClpP amino acid substitution variants provided evidence that ClpA–ClpP interaction is critical in enhancing susceptibility to the T6SS killing. This study highlights the importance of recipient factors in determining the outcome of the T6SS killing and shows the universal ClpP protease as a novel recipient factor hijacked by the T6SS of *A. tumefaciens*.

Keywords: type VI secretion system, antibacterial activity, recipient cells, ClpP, ClpA, *Agrobacterium tumefaciens*, *Escherichia coli*

INTRODUCTION

Bacteria have evolved broad strategies in secreting antibiotics or protein toxins to antagonize other bacteria and gain fitness to fight for limited nutrients and space. Among them, the Gram-negative bacteria use a variety of protein secretion systems such as type I secretion system (T1SS) (García-Bayona et al., 2017, 2019), type IV secretion system (T4SS) (Souza et al., 2015; Bayer-Santos et al., 2019), contact-dependent inhibition (CDI; belongs to type V secretion system) (Aoki et al., 2005, 2010), and type VI secretion system (T6SS) (LeRoux et al., 2012; Basler et al., 2013) as antibacterial weapons. Bacteria that produce and deliver protein toxins, the effectors, through secretion systems to kill other bacteria are attacker cells, and the attacked cells are the recipient cells (Costa et al., 2015; Filloux and Sagfors, 2015). Attacker cells also produce cognate immunity proteins to neutralize effectors to prevent self-intoxication (Alteri and Mobley, 2016; Lien and Lai, 2017). A recipient cell is intoxicated if it does not have cognate immunity protein to neutralize the toxicity of its effector.

In the CDI system, non-immunity proteins in the recipient cell also participate in the bacterial competition outcome (Aoki et al., 2008, 2010; Diner et al., 2012; Willett et al., 2015; Jones et al., 2017). For example, the CDI effector CdiA-CT^{EC93} utilizes recipient's outer membrane protein BamA and the inner membrane protein AcrB to enter the recipient cell (Aoki et al., 2008). BamA belongs to the BAM complex that functions in outer membrane β-barrel proteins (OMPs) biogenesis. AcrB is an inner membrane protein that belongs to the multidrug efflux pump TolC complex. Another example is the necessity of the recipient *O*-acetylserine sulfhydrylase A (CysK) to the CDI effector CdiA-CT^{EC536} (Diner et al., 2012). In the recipient cell, CdiA-CT^{EC536} binds to CysK to increase its thermostability and its tRNase activity (Johnson et al., 2016). Interestingly, this CysK.CdiA-CT^{EC536} complex mimics the CysK.CysE complex, which is typically formed during *de novo* cysteine biogenesis, with a higher binding affinity (Johnson et al., 2016; Jones et al., 2017). Other examples are the recipient elongation factor Tu (EF-Tu) in activating the toxicity of CdiA-CT^{EC869} and CdiA-CT^{NC101} (Jones et al., 2017; Michalska et al., 2017), and the involvement of recipient PtsG in CdiA-CT^{3006} and CdiA-CT^{NC101} entry (Willett et al., 2015). To summarize, a variety of the non-immunity proteins in the recipient cells affect the CDI antagonizing outcome. As the bacterial secretion systems that serve as an antibacterial weapon share some universal characters, the above phenomenon raised a question of whether non-immunity proteins of the recipient cells also affect the bacterial antagonizing outcome in other secretion systems.

Recently, examples about the involvement of the recipient non-immunity proteins in T6SS competition outcome emerged. The first description is the involvement of the EF-Tu protein of the recipient cell for Tse6 effector-mediated killing by *Pseudomonas aeruginosa* (Whitney et al., 2015). Although recipient's EF-Tu was initially proposed to grant access of Tse6 into the recipient cytoplasm (Whitney et al., 2015), a further study demonstrated that Tse6 could penetrate the double bilayer of the EF-Tu-free liposome and exert its toxicity inside it (Quentin et al., 2018). The role of the recipient EF-Tu involved in an interbacterial competition of Tse6 remains elusive. A T6SS study in *Serratia marcescens* demonstrated that the recipient protein DsbA plays a role in activating *S. marcescens* T6SS effectors Ssp2 and Ssp4, but not Rhs2 (Mariano et al., 2018). The *S. marcescens* T6SS kills its Ssp2-sensitive siblings only when the recipient cells harbor *dsbA* homologs ($dsbA1^+$ $dsbA2^+$). The same results were also observed using Ssp4-sensitive recipient cells, but not Rhs2-sensitive strain as a recipient cell. The above findings highlight the necessity of a recipient factor to facilitate the T6SS attack. However, a systematic screening of the recipient factors that can either promote or reduce the susceptibility of the T6SS attack is still lacking.

This study aimed to explore the recipient genetic factors that affect the T6SS killing outcome using the well-characterized T6SS-possessing plant pathogen *Agrobacterium tumefaciens*, a causative agent of crown gall disease in many different plants. The *A. tumefaciens* strain C58 harbors three effector proteins: type VI DNase effector 1 (Tde1), Tde2, and putative type VI amidase effector (Tae). The Tde proteins are the main contributor to *A. tumefaciens* T6SS-dependent interbacterial competition (Ma et al., 2014). Using the T6SS-lacking *Escherichia coli* K12 strain as a model recipient cell, we report here a high-throughput, population level, interbacterial competition screening platform for identifying the recipient genetic factors that contribute to *A. tumefaciens* C58 T6SS's killing outcome. Among the 3,909 *E. coli* Keio mutants screened, we confirmed that at least six of them play a role in enhancing susceptibility to *A. tumefaciens* T6SS attack by an interbacterial competition assay and by complementation *in trans*. One of the confirmed genes, *caseinolytic protease P* (*clpP*), was highlighted in this study owing to its prominent phenotype. A functional ClpP complex consists of a tetradodecameric ClpP and its associated AAA$^+$ ATPase substrate-recognizing partner ClpA or ClpX (Olivares et al., 2015). Further mutant studies showed that *clpA*, but not *clpX*, is involved in the outcome of *A. tumefaciens* T6SS killing. Our data also suggest that the ClpAP complex formation mediates the outcome of T6SS killing. This work not only provides a new screening platform for elucidating factors that are involved in the interbacterial competition but also strengthens the importance of recipient genetic factors in the outcome of the T6SS antibacterial activity.

MATERIALS AND METHODS

Bacterial Strains, Plasmids, and Growth Conditions

The complete information about the strains and plasmids used in this study is described in **Table 1**. The *E. coli* Keio mutants (Baba et al., 2006) and the BW25113 wild type were obtained from the Keio collection from NBRP (NIG, Japan) and used as the recipient cells unless otherwise indicated. *A. tumefaciens* C58 wild type and the *tssL* mutants (Δ*tssL*) were used as the attacker cells. *A. tumefaciens* was grown at 25°C in 523 medium, and *E. coli* was grown in lysogeny broth (LB) medium at 37°C unless indicated. The plasmids were maintained in 20 μg/ml of kanamycin (Km),

TABLE 1 | Bacterial strains and plasmids.

Strain/plasmid	Relevant characteristics	Source/references
Agrobacterium tumefaciens		
C58 (EML530)	Wild-type virulence strain containing pTiC58 and pAtC58	Eugene Nester
C58:Δ*atu4333* (EML1073)	*atu4333* (*tssL*) in-frame deletion mutant of C58 background	(Ma et al., 2012)
Escherichia coli		
DH10B	Host for DNA cloning	Invitrogen
BW25113	Wild-type strain of the Keio Collection. *rrnB* DE*lacZ*4787 *HsdR*514 DE(*araBAD*)567 DE(*rhaBAD*)568 *rph*-1.	(Baba et al., 2006)
Keio collection	Systematic single-gene knockout mutants of *E. coli* BW25113	(Baba et al., 2006)
JW0427	BW25113 *clpP:kan*	(Baba et al., 2006)
JW0866	BW25113 *clpA:kan*	(Baba et al., 2006)
JW0428	BW25113 *clpX:kan*	(Baba et al., 2006)
EML5395	DH10B harboring pNptII	This study
EML5393	BW25113 wild-type harboring pNptII	This study
BL21(DE3)	Host for protein expression	(Studier and Moffatt, 1986)
Plasmids		
pTrc200HA	Sp^R, pTrc200 harboring C-terminal influenza hemagglutinin (HA) epitope, P*trc*, lacI^q, pVS1 origin	Laboratory collection
pRL662	Gm^R, a non-transferable broad-host range vector derived from pBBR1MCS2	(Vergunst et al., 2000)
pET22b(+)	Ap^R, *E. coli* overexpression vector harboring C-terminal 6xHis epitope	Novagen
pRL-*rpsL*	Gm^R, pRL662 expressing BW25113 *rpsL* gene	This study
pRL-*galk*	Gm^R, pRL662 expressing BW25113 *galK* gene	This study
pRL-*nupG*	Gm^R, pRL662 expressing BW25113 *nupG* gene	This study
pRL-*rpsL*^{Str}	Gm^R, pRL662 expressing DH10B *rpsL*^{Str} gene	This study
pNptII	Km^R, Gm^R, pRL662 expressing *nptII* gene	This study
pClpP-HA	Sp^R, pTrc200HA expressing ClpP-HA fusion protein	This study
pClpA-HA	Sp^R, pTrc200HA expressing ClpA-HA fusion protein	This study
pClpP$_{S111A}$-HA	Sp^R, pTrc200HA expressing ClpP-HA fusion protein with S111A substitution	This study
pClpP$_{H136A}$-HA	Sp^R, pTrc200HA expressing ClpP-HA fusion protein with H136A substitution	This study
pClpP$_{D185A}$-HA	Sp^R, pTrc200HA expressing ClpP-HA fusion protein with D185A substitution	This study
pClpP$_{R26A}$-HA	Sp^R, pTrc200HA expressing ClpP-HA fusion protein with R26A substitution	This study
pClpP$_{D32A}$-HA	Sp^R, pTrc200HA expressing ClpP-HA fusion protein with D32A substitution	This study
pClpX-ΔN-ter	Plasmid used for purifying ClpX-ΔN	Robert T. Sauer
pGFP-ssrA	Plasmid used for purifying GFP-ssrA	Robert T. Sauer
pClpP-tev-His	Ap^R, pET22b(+) expressing ClpP-tev-His, in which ClpP protein is fused with a TEV protease cleavage site and a His-tag in its C-terminal	Robert T. Sauer
pClpP$_{S111A}$-tev-His	Ap^R, pET22b(+) expressing ClpP-tev-His with ClpP S111A substitution	This study
pClpP$_{H136A}$-tev-His	Ap^R, pET22b(+) expressing ClpP-tev-His with ClpP H136A substitution	This study
pClpP$_{D185A}$-tev-His	Ap^R, pET22b(+) expressing ClpP-tev-His with ClpP D185A substitution	This study

100 μg/ml of spectinomycin (Sp), and 20 μg/ml of gentamycin for *E. coli.*

Plasmid Construction

All plasmids (**Table 1**) were confirmed by sequencing unless otherwise indicated. The complete list of primers used in this study is in **Table 2**. Plasmid pNptII was created by ligating the *Xho*I/*Bam*HI-digested *nptII* PCR product into the same restriction sites of pRL662. The plasmid was transformed into DH10B, and the resulting strain was designated as EML5395. The pRL-*rpsL*, pRL-*galK*, pRL-*nupG*, and pRL-*rpsL*^{Str} were created by ligating the *Xho*I/*Xba*I-digested PCR product into the same restriction sites of pRL662. The plasmid was transformed into DH10B, and the resulting strain was designated as EML5389, EML5390, EML5391, and EML5392. Plasmids pClpP-HA and pClpA-HA were created by ligating *Sac*I/*Pst*I-digested PCR products (*clpP* and *clpA* from BW25113 wild type without the stop codon, respectively) into pTrc200HA. The pClpP$_{S111A}$-HA was created by amplifying fragments using pTRC99C-F plus ClpP-S111A-rv and pTRC99C-R plus ClpP-S111A-fw as primers. The two fragments were then merged and amplified by PCR-Splicing by Overlapping Extension (SOEing) (Heckman and Pease, 2007). The resulting full-length *clpP*-containing fragment was digested by *Sac*I/*Pst*I and then ligated into pTrc200HA. All other pClpP-HA plasmids with a mutated form of ClpP were created similarly. The plasmid constructs ClpX (ClpX-ΔN-ter), wild-type ClpP-tev-His, and green fluorescent protein (GFP)-ssrA were a kind gift from Dr. Robert T. Sauer (MIT, Cambridge, United States). Site-directed mutagenesis was performed to generate the ClpP variants. All plasmids of pClpP-tev-His with a

TABLE 2 | Primer information.

Primer	Sequence (5′–3′)[a]	Plasmids
T7	TAATACGACTCACTATAGGG	pET22b(+)
T7T	GCTAGTTATTGCTCAGCGG	
pTRC99C-F	TTGCGCCGACATCATAAC	pTrc200HA
pTRC99C-R	CTGCGTTCTGATTTAATCTG	
rpsL-fw	AAAAACTCGAGGCAAAAGCTAAAACCAGGA	(1) pRL-*rpsL*
rpsL-rv	AAAAATCTAGACTTACTTAACGGAGAACCA	(2) pRL-rpsL^{Str}
galK-fw	AAAAACTCGAGCAGTCAGCGATATCCATT	pRL-galk
galK-rv	AAAAATCTAGAGCAAAGTTAACAGTCGGT	
nupG-fw	AAAAACTCGAGTCAAACACTCATCCGCAT	pRL-nupG
nupG-rv	AAAAATCTAGACCCGTTTTTCTTTGCGTAA	
NptII-fw-*Xho*I	AAAAACTCGAGAGACTGGGCGGTTTTATGGA	pNptII
NptII-rv-*Hin*dIII	AAAAAAAGCTTCTCTAGCGAACCCCAGAGTC	
ClpP-*Sac*I-fw	AAAAAGAGCTCATGTCATACAGCGGCGAACGAGATAAC	pClpP-HA
ClpP-*Pst*I-rv	AAAAACTGCAGATTACGATGGGTCAGAATCGAATCGAC	
ClpA-*Sac*I-fw	AAAAAGAGCTCATGCTCAATCAAGAACTGGAACTCAGTTT	pClpA-HA
ClpA-*Pst*I-rv	AAAAACTGCAGATGCGCTGCTTCCGCCTTGTGCTTT	
ClpP-S111A-fw	TGTATGGGCCAGGCGGCC**GCG**ATGGGCGCTTTCTTGCTG	(1) pClpP$_{S111A}$-HA
ClpP-S111A-rv	CAGCAAGAAAGCGCCCAT**CGC**GGCCGCCTGGCCCATACA	(2) pClpP$_{S111A}$-tev-His
ClpP-H136A-fw	AATTCGCGCGTGATGATT**GCC**CAACCGTTGGGCGGCTAC	(1) pClpP$_{H136A}$-HA
ClpP-H136A-rv	GTAGCCGCCCAACGGTTG**GGC**AATCATCACGCGCGAATT	(2) pClpP$_{H136A}$-tev-His
ClpP-D185A-fw	GAACGTGATACCGAGCGC**GCT**CGCTTCCTTTCCGCCCCT	(1) pClpP$_{D185A}$-HA
ClpP-D185A-rv	AGGGGCGGAAAGGAAGCG**AGC**GCGCTCGGTATCACGTTC	(2) pClpP$_{D185A}$-tev-His
ClpP-R26A-fw	GTCATTGAACAGACCTCA**GCC**GGTGAGCGCTCTTTTGAT	pClpP$_{R26A}$-HA
ClpP-R26A-rv	ATCAAAAGAGCGCTCACC**GGC**TGAGGTCTGTTCAATGAC	
ClpP-D32A-fw	CGCGGTGAGCGCTCTTTT**GCT**ATCTATTCTCGTCTACTT	pClpP$_{D32A}$-HA
ClpP-D32A-rv	AAGTAGACGAGAATAGAT**AGC**AAAAGAGCGCTCACCGCG	

[a]*Restriction enzyme sites are underlined, and mutated sequences are indicated in bold type.*

mutated *clpP* gene was constructed similar to that of pClpP$_{S111A}$-HA mentioned above with the differences below: Primer T7 was used instead of pTRC99C-F, and primer T7T was used instead of pTRC99C-R, and the restriction sites used were *Xba*I/*Xho*I.

Interbacterial Competition Assay

The optical densities of the cultured *A. tumefaciens* and *E. coli* were measured and adjusted to OD_{600} equals to 3.0 in 0.9% NaCl (w/v). The recipient *E. coli* cells were then further diluted to OD_{600} equals to 0.3 or 0.1, depending on the need of the assay. Afterward, the attacker and the recipient cultures were mixed in equal volume to make the attacker: recipient ratio 10:1 or 30:1, respectively. Ten microliters of the mixed bacterial culture was then spotted onto *Agrobacterium* Kill-triggering medium (AK medium, 3 g of K_2HPO_4, 1 g of NaH_2PO_4, 1 g of NH_4Cl, 0.15 g of KCl, and 9.76 g of MES, pH 5.5), solidified by 2% (w/v) agar, and then air-dried to enable contact-dependent competition. The competition plates were cultured at 25°C for 16 h. After the competition, bacteria were recovered using a loop and resuspended into 500 μl of 0.9% NaCl. The recovered bacterial suspension was then serially diluted and plated onto LB supplemented with spectinomycin to select recipient *E. coli* cells. After overnight culture at 37°C, the recovered colony formation unit (cfu) was counted and recorded. The T6SS-dependent susceptibility index (SI) was defined as the logarithm of the recovered *E. coli* cfu co-cultured with Δ*tssL* subtracted by that co-cultured with wild-type *A. tumefaciens*.

The High-Throughput Interbacterial Competition Platform

Pipetting steps of the screening platform were performed by the pipetting robot EzMate401 (Arise Biotech, Taiwan) unless otherwise specified. Fifty microliters of the cultured attacker *A. tumefaciens* was pelleted using 8,000 × *g* for 10 min at 15°C. After the medium was removed, the pellet was washed twice using 0.9% NaCl (w/v) and then adjusted to OD_{600} equals to 3.0. The OD_{600}-adjusted attacker cells were then dispensed as 300 μl into each well of a 2.2-ml Deepwell microplate (Basic Life, Taiwan). Each well was then added with 10 μl of the cultured recipient *E. coli* mutants and mixed well to make the attacker:target at 30:1 (v/v). After being mixed, the bacterial mixture was then added onto the competition plate. The competition plate was made by 25 ml of the AK medium with 2% (w/v) agarose solidified in a 96-well lid. The competition plate was then cultured at 25°C for 16 h before recovery. The recovery was performed by stamping a 96-well plate replicator to the competition spots followed by suspending the bacterial cells to a 96-well plate containing 200 μl of 0.9% NaCl in each well. After being mixed, 10 μl of the recovered bacterial suspension was spotted onto LB agar supplemented with kanamycin made in a 96-well lid, cultured at 37°C overnight, and then was observed. In the first screening, only *A. tumefaciens* C58 wild type was used as the attacker. In the second screening, both wild type and Δ*tssL* were used as the attackers. For the groups co-cultured with *A. tumefaciens* C58 wild type, the recovery suspension was either undiluted or diluted to 5 and 25 times before being spotted onto LB agar with kanamycin plate. For the groups co-cultured with *A. tumefaciens* C58 Δ*tssL*, the recovery suspensions were either undiluted or diluted to 10 and 100 times before spotted onto LB agar with kanamycin plate. At each stage, the *E. coli* mutants that formed multiple colonies were identified as the candidates.

Protein Production and Purification

Escherichia coli BL21(DE3) was used as a host to produce all proteins of interests. Cells were cultured in LB medium supplemented with appropriate antibiotics in 1-L flask. When OD_{600} reached 0.6, the bacterial culture was cooled to 16°C, and IPTG was added (final concentration of 0.5 mM) for the overexpression of the protein. The cells were further allowed to grow for 16 h, followed by centrifugation to pellet them and then resuspended in lysis buffer (50 mM of Tris, pH 8.0, 300 mM of NaCl, 1% Triton X-100, 10 mM of beta-mercaptoethanol, 1 mM of DTT, and 10% glycerol). The cells were lysed by sonication at 4°C (amplitude 10 for 5 s, followed by 15-s breaks; total sonication time was 6 min) (PRO Scientific, United States). The lysates were centrifuged at 20,000 rpm for 30 min at 4°C. The supernatants were collected and loaded onto Ni-NTA column (GE Healthcare, United States) equilibrated with wash buffer (50 mM of Tris, pH 8.0, and 300 mM of NaCl) and eluted by 6 ml of wash buffer containing 250 mM of imidazole. The eluted fractions of the protein were further subjected to size-exclusion chromatography (SEC) by Superdex 200, 16/60 column (GE Life Sciences, United States) in buffer containing 50 mM of Tris, pH 7.5, 100 mM of KCl, 25 mM of $MgCl_2$, 1 mM of DTT, and 10% glycerol. The protein purity was confirmed on 12% sodium dodecyl sulfate–polyacrylamide gel electrophoresis (SDS-PAGE). The samples were flash-frozen and stored in −80°C until further use.

Protein Degradation Assay

Green fluorescent protein (GFP) fluorescence based-degradation assays were carried out in Protein Degradation (PD) buffer (25 mM of HEPES, pH 7.5, 100 mM of KCl, 25 mM of $MgCl_2$, 1 mM of DTT, and 10% glycerol) containing 3 μM of GFP-ssrA as substrate and ATP regeneration system (16 mM of creatine phosphatase and 0.32 mg/ml of creatine kinase) as described previously (Sriramoju et al., 2018). In brief, 0.1 μM of $ClpX_6$ and 0.3 μM of $ClpP_{14}$ or its variants were mixed at 30°C and allowed to stand for 2 min. The protein degradation reaction was started by addition of ATP to a final concentration of 5 mM. The changes in the fluorescence were measured at 511 nm with an excitation wavelength at 467 nm in a 96-well format using Infinite M1000 PRO plate reader (Tecan, Switzerland).

Sodium Dodecyl Sulfate–Polyacrylamide Gel Electrophoresis and Western Blot Analysis

The Δ*clpP*:kan *E. coli* strains harboring appropriate plasmid were grown as the same procedure indicated in the *Interbacterial Competition Assay*. Cells were adjusted to OD_{600} of 5.0, collected at 5,000 × *g* for 5 min, and directly resuspended in 1 × SDS sample buffer. The samples were incubated at 96°C for 10 min and then analyzed by SDS-PAGE. Protein samples separated by SDS-PAGE were transferred to an Immobilon-P membrane (Merck Millipore, United States). The monoclonal anti-HA was used at a dilution of 1:10,000 (Yao-Hong Biotech Inc., Taiwan), and the goat–anti-rabbit conjugated to horseradish peroxidase secondary antibody was used at a dilution of 1:10,000 (GeneTex, Taiwan). The Western Lightning ECL Pro (PerkinElmer Life Sciences, United States) was used for color development and visualized by BioSpectrum 600 Imaging System (UVP, United States).

Statistical Analysis and Figure Production

Statistical analyses and figure production were performed using the R program (version 3.5.1) (R Core Team, 2018) and RStudio (version 1.1.456) (RStudio Team, 2015). R packages plyr (version 1.8.4) (Wickham, 2011) and multcompView (version 0.1-7) (Graves et al., 2015) were used for statistical analyses. Figures were produced using the R packages ggplot2 (version 3.0.0) (Wickham, 2016), Hmisc (version 4.1-1) (Harrell et al., 2018), and ggpubr (version 0.2) (Kassambara, 2018). Student's *t*-test, one-way analysis of variance (one-way ANOVA), and Tukey's honestly significant difference test (Tukey HSD test), in which significant difference threshold set as 0.05, were used in all cases.

RESULTS

The *Agrobacterium tumefaciens* T6SS Killing Outcome Differs Between Different *Escherichia coli* Strains

Using an optimized competition condition (AK medium agar that contains basic minerals at pH 5.5), we noticed that when co-cultured with wild-type *A. tumefaciens* C58, the recovered colony-forming unit (cfu) of *E. coli* BW25113 was always lower than that of DH10B (**Figure 1A**). Meanwhile, the recovered cfu of both *E. coli* strains was the same when co-cultured with Δ*tssL A. tumefaciens* C58 (hereafter referred to Δ*tssL*), a T6SS secretion-deficient mutant (**Figure 1A**). For more intuitive readout, we introduced T6SS-dependent SI, which reflects the strength of the T6SS killing. The SI was defined as the logarithm of the recovered *E. coli* cfu co-cultured with Δ*tssL* subtracted by that co-cultured with wild type. The mean SI between *A. tumefaciens* and BW25113 was significantly higher than that of between *A. tumefaciens* and DH10B with a *P*-value of 0.02 ($T \leq t$, two-tailed, **Figure 1B**). This result suggests that some genetic factors of BW25113 may enhance the *A. tumefaciens* C58 killing outcome in a T6SS-dependent manner.

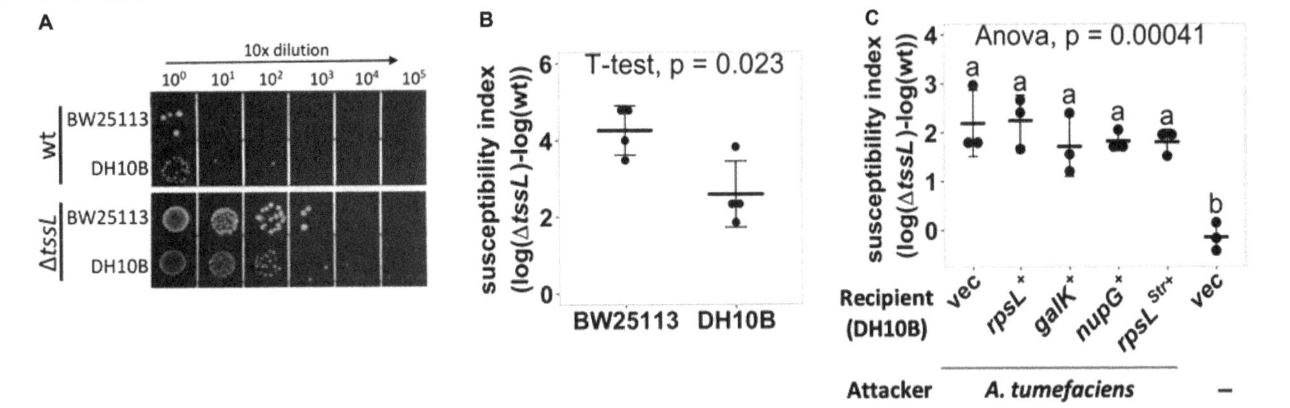

FIGURE 1 | *Agrobacterium tumefaciens* type VI secretion system (T6SS)-dependent antibacterial activity against *Escherichia coli* strains. **(A,B)** *A. tumefaciens* T6SS antibacterial activity against *E. coli* strains DH10B and BW25113. *A. tumefaciens* was co-cultured at a ratio of 30:1 with *E. coli* DH10B or BW25113, both *E. coli* strains harboring vector pRL662, on *Agrobacterium* Kill (AK) agar medium for 16 h. The bacterial mixtures were serially diluted and spotted **(A)** or quantified by counting cfu **(B)** on gentamicin-containing lysogeny broth (LB) agar plates to selectively recover *E. coli*. **(C)** *E. coli* DH10B was complemented by either vector only (vec) or derivative expressing *rpsL*, *galK*, *nupG*, or *rpsL*^{Str} *in trans* before being subjected to *A. tumefaciens* T6SS-dependent antibacterial activity assay as described in **(B)**. Susceptibility index (SI) was defined as the subtraction difference of the recovery log(cfu) of that attacked by Δ*tssL* to that attacked by wild-type *A. tumefaciens* C58. Data are mean ± SD of three independent experiments calculated by *t*-test with $P < 0.05$ for statistical significance **(B)** or single-factor analysis of variance (ANOVA) and Tukey honestly significant difference (HSD), in which two groups with significant differences are indicated with different letters (a and b) **(C)**.

We tested whether the genes that are functional in BW25113 but not in DH10B could be the cause of the higher SI in BW25113. The *galK* and *nupG* genes are functional in BW25113 but are pseudogenes in DH10B. The *rpsL* has a mutation in DH10B (*rpsL*^{Str}), which renders the strain resistant to streptomycin, but not in BW25113. The *rpsL*, *galK*, or *nupG* gene from BW25113 was cloned into pRL662 and expressed by constitutive *lacZ* promoter in DH10B as a recipient for a T6SS interbacterial competition assay (**Figure 1C**). The DH10B expressing the *rpsL*^{Str} (overexpressing *rpsL*^{Str}) was also included. The DH10B harboring empty vector (vec) served as a negative control. A group without attacker was also included to monitor whether the decrease in cfu after the competition solely comes from co-culture with *A. tumefaciens* attacker. The SIs were not significantly different between DH10B and any of the complemented groups, and each had an SI mean of about 2 (**Figure 1C**). The above approach was not able to identify the genetic factors that contributed to the enhanced resistance in DH10B, which may imply that precise control of transgene expression or multiple complementation would be required. Therefore, we developed a high-throughput screening method to identify the individual genes that contribute to the enhanced susceptibility of BW25113.

Establishment of a High-Throughput Interbacterial Competition Platform to Identify Recipient *Escherichia coli* Mutants With Less Susceptibility to *Agrobacterium tumefaciens* C58 T6SS Killing

We decided to screen the BW25113 single-gene mutant library (Keio collection from NBRP [NIG, Japan]: *E. coli*) for strains with less susceptibility to *A. tumefaciens* T6SS-mediated killing. An interbacterial competition assay starts from mixing the attacker and the recipient cells, followed by counting the recovered recipient *E. coli* on selective media (**Figure 2A**). This protocol only allowed screening of 10 mutants per day, which was not efficient enough for screening 3,909 strains of the Keio library.

Therefore, we developed a high-throughput interbacterial competition platform that enables 96 population-level, interbacterial competition simultaneously (**Figure 2B**). The recipient Keio *E. coli* strains were cultured in the 96-well, and the attacker *A. tumefaciens* was cultured in a flask. After the culture, the attacker was adjusted to OD_{600} equals to 3.0 and then dispensed to a 2.2-ml deep-well plate. The recipient cells were added into the attacker-containing plates in a volume ratio of 30 to 1. Ten microliters of the attacker-recipient mixtures were dropped on the competition surface made by agar solidified on a 96-well lid. A microplate replicator was used to stamp on the competition spots to recover the bacterial cells of each competition group. The recovered bacteria were suspended in the saline buffer (0.9% NaCl), mixed, and then spotted on the recipient-selection surface made by agar solidified on a microplate lid. The competition condition was set at the strength that enables *A. tumefaciens* to kill almost all BW25113 wild-type recipients so that only a few or no cells would survive. This setup made recognizing the resistant mutants simple – the ones with the multiple colonies are the candidates (**Figure 2B**).

All the 3,909 strains in the Keio were screened using *A. tumefaciens* C58 wild type as the attacker. In each screening, at least two wild type *E. coli* BW25113 replicates were incorporated and screened in parallel as parental controls. The Keio mutants that formed colonies in this stage were selected, and 196 strains showed enhanced resistant to *A. tumefaciens* C58 attack. The 196 strains were subjected to second screening using both wild

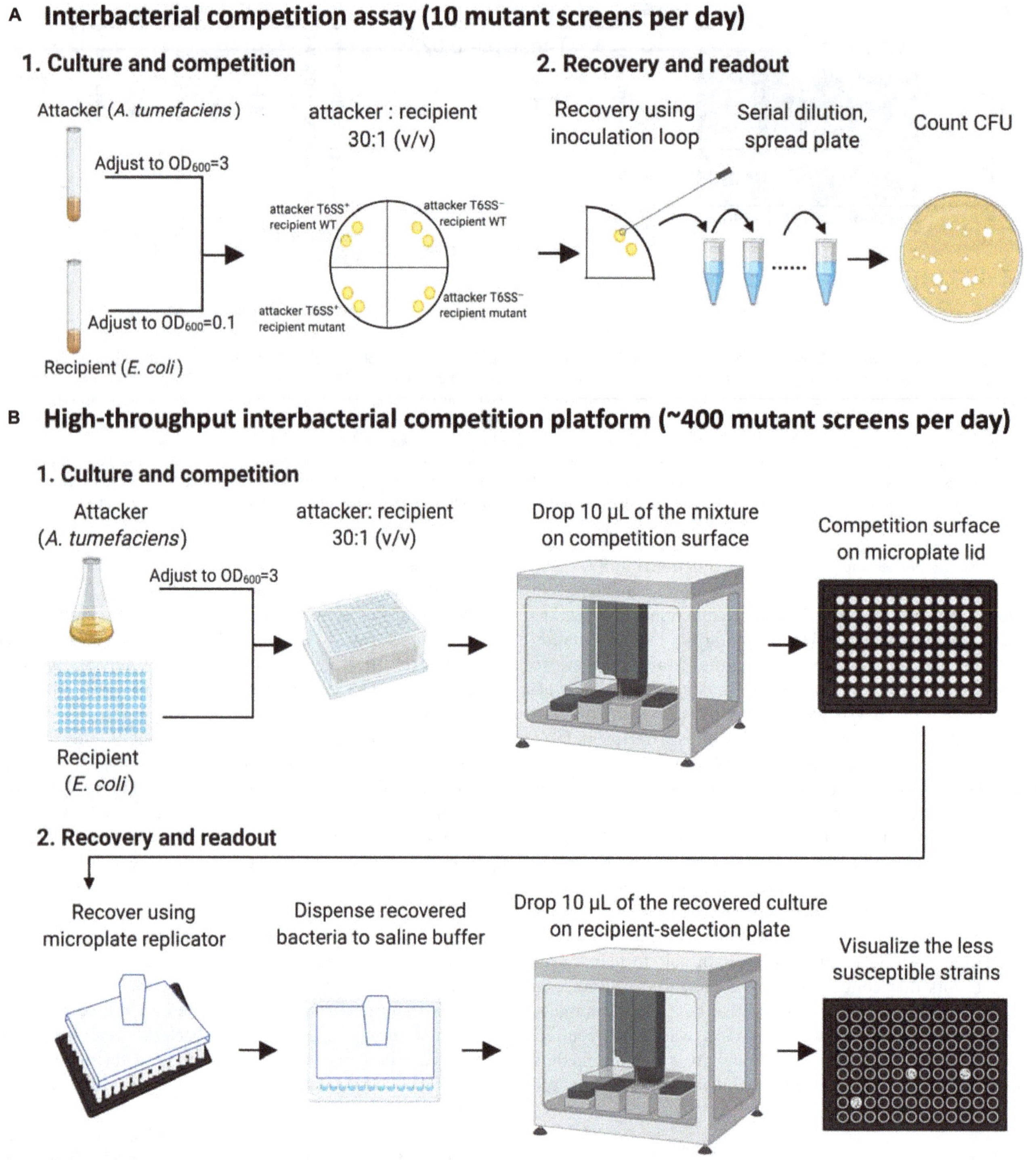

FIGURE 2 | The high-throughput interbacterial competition platform. **(A)** Interbacterial competition assay. Cultured attacker *Agrobacterium tumefaciens* and recipient *Escherichia coli* were mixed and then spotted on the *Agrobacterium* Kill (AK) agar medium to allow interbacterial competition for 16 h at 25°C followed by recovery of mixed cultures, serially diluted, and then spread onto lysogeny broth (LB) plate supplemented with appropriate antibiotics to select for recipient cells.
(B) High-throughput interbacterial competition screening platform. Recipient cells were grown and mixed with attacker *A. tumefaciens* in a 96-well plate. The bacterial mixture was dropped onto the AK agar medium competition surface using an automated pipetting system. The competition surface was made on a microplate lid. Recovery was performed using microplate replicator. The candidates are the strains that show multiple colonies grown after recovery as opposed to wild-type controls and most strains with no or few colonies. This high-throughput *A. tumefaciens* type VI secretion system (T6SS) killing platform enables ~400 mutant screens per day. This figure was created with BioRender (https://biorender.com/).

type and Δ*tssL* as the attackers. At this stage, we incorporated a grading system: Grade I mutants were at least 25 times less susceptible to C58 T6SS-dependent killing, whereas grade II mutants were at least 10 times less susceptible. Six grade I mutants and 10 grade II mutants were identified.

Confirmation of the *Escherichia coli* Mutants With Less Susceptibility to *Agrobacterium tumefaciens* C58 Type VI Secretion System Killing

The enhanced resistance of the six grade I mutants were further verified by an interbacterial competition assay and by complementation tests. For complementation, wild-type genes from BW25113 were cloned into plasmid pTrc200HA plasmid and expressed by *trc* promoter. Five out of six showed lower susceptibility to *A. tumefaciens* T6SS attack than that of BW25113 wild type (**Table 3** and **Supplementary Figure S1**). These are *clpP*, *gltA*, *ydhS*, *ydaE*, and *cbpA* mutants. The *yeaX* mutant, on the other hand, did not differ when compared with the wild type. The *cbpA* mutant showed a milder phenotype and could not be complemented *in trans* under the condition tested (**Table 3** and **Supplementary Figure S1**). As *cbpA* is the first gene in its operon, the failure in complementation could be due to the requirement of other gene(s) in the operon. Nevertheless, the verification performed above showed that the high-throughput interbacterial competition platform was reliable in identifying the recipient genetic factors that participate in T6SS killing.

The ClpP Protein Plays a Role in Enhancing Susceptibility to *Agrobacterium tumefaciens* Type VI Secretion System Killing

Because known recipient cell factors affecting antibacterial activity are often conserved components, we selected Δ*clpP*:kan (labeled as Δ*clpP*) for further studies. ClpP is a highly conserved, housekeeping AAA$^+$ serine protease that exists in prokaryotes, plastids, and mitochondria (Alexopoulos et al., 2012; Bhandari et al., 2018; Mahmoud and Chien, 2018). We performed a quantitative interbacterial competition assay using *A. tumefaciens* as the attacker and the BW25113 wild type, Δ*clpP*, or complemented strain *clpP*$^+$ as the recipient cells (**Figure 3A**). The initial cfu of the *E. coli* at 0 h was about 10^6 in all groups (one-way ANOVA with $P = 0.88$), indicating that any *E. coli* cfu difference at 16 h was not due to initial bacteria titer difference. The cfu among different recipient *E. coli* strains was not significantly different at 16 h when using *A. tumefaciens* Δ*tssL* (one-way ANOVA with $P = 0.67$), indicating that co-culture with T6SS-deficient strain will not cause recipient titer to differ. On the other hand, the recovered cfu of Δ*clpP* was about 10^4, whereas it was about 5×10^2 in BW25113 wild type and in *clpP*$^+$ after 16-h competition using wild-type *A. tumefaciens* (**Figure 3A**). The mean SI of the BW25113 wild type to *A. tumefaciens* C58 is significantly higher than that of Δ*clpP* (one-way ANOVA with $P = 0.02$, **Figure 3B**). The less susceptible phenotype of the Δ*clpP* can be fully complemented *in trans* (*clpP*$^+$) ($P = 0.96$ compared with BW25113 wild type). These results confirmed that *clpP* contributes to enhancing susceptibility to T6SS antibacterial activity of *A. tumefaciens* C58.

Effects of ClpP Catalytic Variants in Enhancing *Agrobacterium tumefaciens* Type VI Secretion System Antibacterial Activity and Protease Activity

A functional ClpP complex consists of a tetradodecameric ClpP ($ClpP_{14}$) and its associated AAA$^+$ ATPase substrate-recognizing partner ClpA or ClpX, both in a hexameric form (Olivares et al., 2015). The protease catalytic triad of the *E. coli* ClpP is composed of S111, H136, and D185 (counted from the Met1) (Maurizi et al., 1990; Wang et al., 1997). We tested whether the ClpP protease is essential in enhancing *E. coli* susceptibility to *A. tumefaciens* C58 T6SS attack. *E. coli* Δ*clpP* complemented with pTrc200HA expressing either wild-type or catalytic variants ClpP S111A, H136A, and D185A was used as a recipient strain. All ClpP variants contain a C-terminal HA tag. Two of the catalytic variants, S111A$^+$ and H136A$^+$, failed to complement, whereas surprisingly, the third catalytic variant, D185A$^+$, can fully complement the phenotype (**Figure 4A**). The difference of ClpP catalytic variants to complement Δ*clpP* was not due to their protein-expression level as determined by Western blot (**Figure 4B**). The protein migration of the $ClpP_{S111A}$ and $ClpP_{H136A}$ was slower than that of the $ClpP_{wt}$ and $ClpP_{D185A}$

TABLE 3 | *Escherichia coli* strains that showed reduced susceptibility to *Agrobacterium tumefaciens* T6SS attack.

No.	Resource (JW ID)	Disrupted gene	Gene products affected by kanamycin cassette insertion[a]	Reduced susceptibility[b]	Trans complementation[c]
1	JS0427	*clpP*	ClpAXP, ClpXP, ClpAP	O	O
2	JW0710	*gltA*	citrate synthase	O	O
3	JW1658	*ydhS*	FAD/NAD(P) binding domain-containing protein YdhS	O	O
4	JW1346	*ydaE*	Rac prophage; zinc-binding protein	O	Δ
5	JW0985	*cbpA*	Curved DNA-binding protein	O	X
6	JW1792	*yeaX*	Carnitine monooxygenase	X	n.d.

n.d., not determined. [a]*Gene products information was obtained from the EcoCyc database (Keseler et al., 2016).* [b]*Mutant strains with reduced susceptibility index (SI) and showed significant difference under $P < 0.05$ was labeled as O; those with no significant difference to that of wild type were labeled in X.* [c]*Plasmid-born gene that can fully complement the disrupted gene is labeled in O, partially complemented is labeled in Δ, and cannot be complemented is labeled in X.*

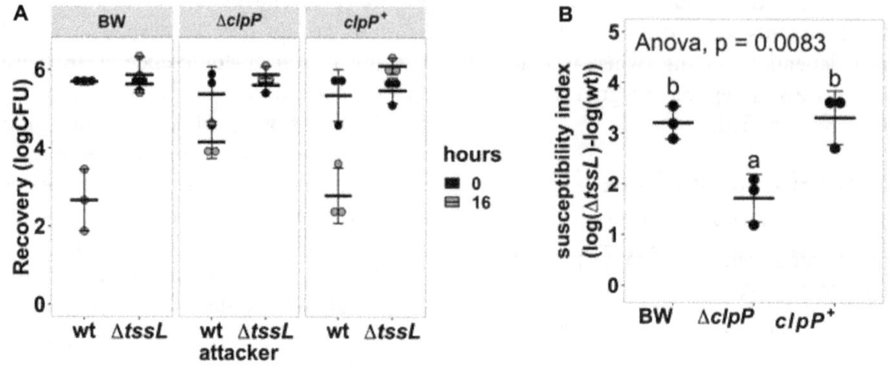

FIGURE 3 | *Agrobacterium tumefaciens* susceptibility to type VI secretion system (T6SS)-dependent antibacterial activity was reduced in *Escherichia coli clpP:kan* and can be fully complemented *in trans*. **(A)** Recovery of surviving *E. coli* cells at 0 h and 16 h after being co-cultured with either *A. tumefaciens* wild type C58 (wt) or Δ*tssL* at a ratio of 30:1. **(B)** The susceptibility index (SI) of *E. coli* BW25113 wild type (BW), Δ*clpP*, and Δ*clpP* complemented with *clpP* expressed on plasmid (*clpP*+) was calculated from the recovery rate shown in **(A)**. Statistical analysis involved single-factor analysis of variance (ANOVA) and Tukey honestly significant difference (HSD). Data are mean ± SD of three independent experiments, and two groups with significant differences are indicated with different letters (a and b) ($P < 0.05$ for statistical significance).

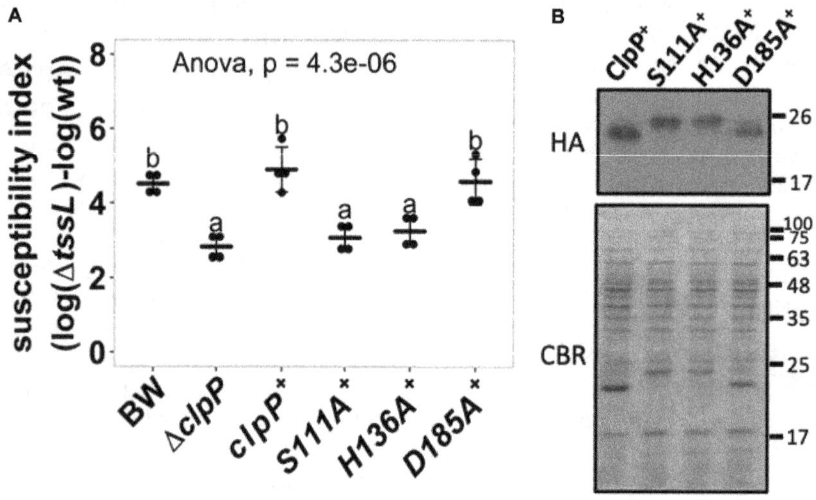

FIGURE 4 | Effects of ClpP protease catalytic variants in enhancing *Agrobacterium tumefaciens* type VI secretion system (T6SS) antibacterial activity. **(A)** The susceptibility index calculated from *A. tumefaciens* interbacterial activity assay against *Escherichia coli*. The *A. tumefaciens* C58 wild-type or Δ*tssL* were co-cultured at a ratio of 10:1 with *E. coli* BW25113 wild type (BW), Δ*clpP*, and Δ*clpP* complemented with *clpP* and its variants expressed on plasmid. The complemented *clpP* strains were either wild type (clpP+) or catalytic variants $ClpP_{S111A}$ (S111A+), $ClpP_{H136A}$ (H136A+), and $ClpP_{D185A}$ (D185A+), with C-terminus HA-tag. The susceptibility index (SI) of each *E. coli* was calculated from the logarithm recovery rate of the Δ*tssL* co-cultured group minus that of the wild-type co-cultured group. Data are mean ± SD of four biological replicates from two independent experiments. Statistical analysis involved single-factor analysis of variance (ANOVA) and Tukey honestly significant difference (HSD) with $P < 0.05$ for statistical significance. Two groups with significant differences are indicated with different letters (a and b). **(B)** The ClpP protein levels of the Δ*clpP* complemented strains used in **(A)**. The ClpP-expressing *E. coli* strains were cultured at the same condition used in interbacterial competition assay. Instead of co-culture with *A. tumefaciens*, protein samples were collected, normalized, and subjected to Western blot analysis of ClpP:HA and its variants. Representative result of three independent experiments is shown.

owing to their inability to remove the N-terminal propeptide (1–14 amino acids) as in $ClpP_{wt}$ and $ClpP_{D185A}$ (Maurizi et al., 1990; Bewley et al., 2006).

As $ClpP_{D185A}$ was able to complement the phenotype, we further investigated the ClpP protease activity of the above ClpP variants by a widely adopted ClpP protein degradation assay using GFP-ssrA as the model substrate. Loss of GFP fluorescence is used as a reporter to monitor substrate degradation by ClpXP as a function of time (Weber-Ban et al., 1999; Sriramoju et al., 2018). The results showed that over time, wild-type ClpP effectively degraded GFP-ssrA with a half-life of about 30 min (**Figure 5A**). Meanwhile, less than a 10% decrease of the GFP-ssrA signal was observed in GFP-ssrA only and wild type without ATP groups, both served as negative controls. The decreasing rates of the GFP-ssrA fluorescence of $ClpP_{S111A}$, $ClpP_{H136A}$, and $ClpP_{D185A}$ were significantly slower than those of $ClpP_{WT}$ and showed no significant difference among the three variants at the end of the test (**Figures 5A,B**). Although $ClpP_{D185A}$ showed no

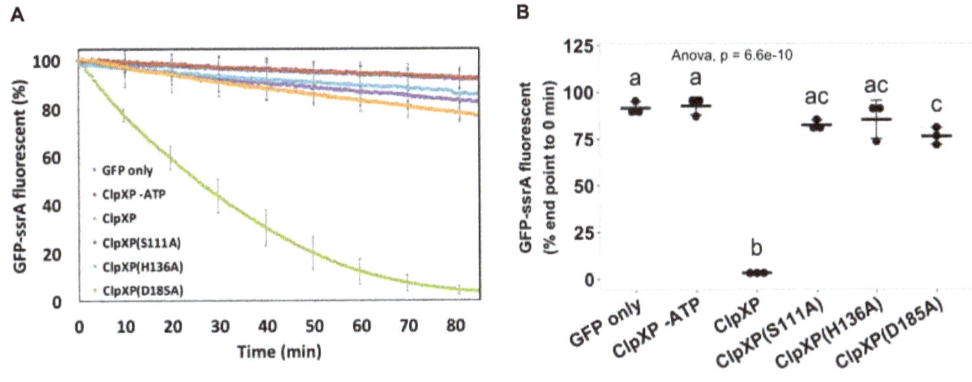

FIGURE 5 | Protease activity assay of the ClpP and its catalytic variants. The wild-type ClpP and its catalytic variants were each pre-assembled with ClpX followed by providing its substrate, the ssrA-tagged green fluorescent protein (GFP). The GFP fluorescent signals were monitored **(A)** over time, and **(B)** statistical analysis was measured at the end of the assay. Statistical analysis involved single-factor analysis of variance (ANOVA) and Tukey honestly significant difference (HSD) with $P < 0.05$ for statistical significance. Two groups with significant differences are indicated with different letters (a and b). Data are mean ± SD of three biological replicates from one representative result of at least two independent experiments.

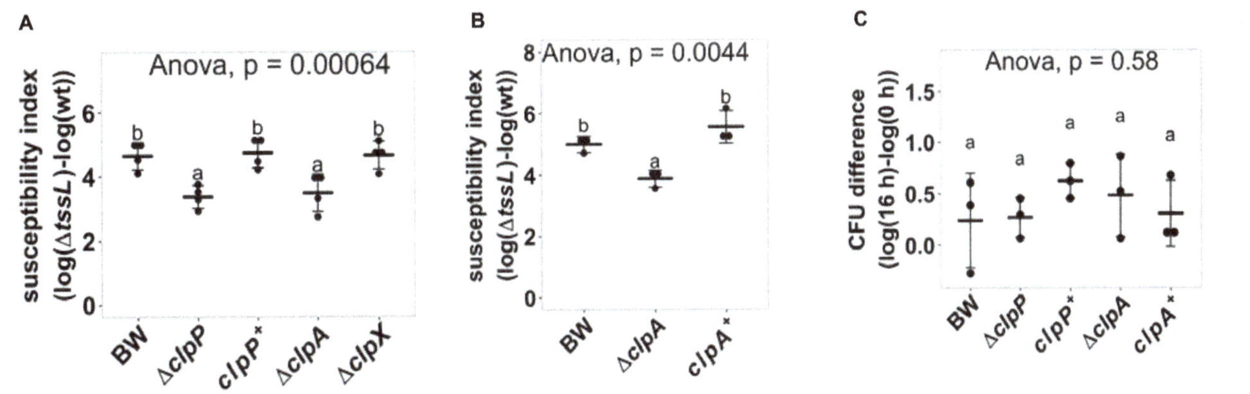

FIGURE 6 | ClpP associated AAA+ ATPase ClpA but not ClpX is involved in enhancing *Agrobacterium tumefaciens* type VI secretion system (T6SS) antibacterial activity. **(A)** *A. tumefaciens* T6SS antibacterial activity against *Escherichia coli* Δ*clpP* and its complement strain, Δ*clpA* and Δ*clpX*. The *A. tumefaciens* and the *E. coli* were co-cultured at a ratio of 10:1 on *Agrobacterium* Kill (AK) agar medium for 16 h. Afterward, the recovery of *E. coli* strains was quantified, and the susceptibility index was calculated by subtracting the difference of the recovered log(cfu) of that attacked by Δ*tssL* to that by wild-type *A. tumefaciens* C58. **(B)** *A. tumefaciens* T6SS antibacterial activity assay and the susceptibility index were performed as described in **(A)** using *E. coli* wild type (BW), Δ*clpA*, and Δ*clpA* complemented with *clpA* expressed on plasmid (*clpA*$^+$). **(C)** Growth of *E. coli* when co-culturing with the Δ*tssL A. tumefaciens*. Data in **(A–C)** are mean ± SD of at least three independent experiments. Statistical analysis involved single-factor analysis of variance (ANOVA) and Tukey honestly significant difference (HSD) with $P < 0.05$ for statistical significance. Two groups with significant differences are indicated with different letters (a and b).

statistically difference in GFP-ssrA degradation compared with ClpP$_{S111A}$ and ClpP$_{H136A}$ at the final time point, it showed significantly lower GFP-ssrA signal to that of the negative control groups (**Figure 5B**).

The ClpP-Associated AAA$^+$ ATPase ClpA but Not ClpX Is Involved in Enhancing Susceptibility to *Agrobacterium tumefaciens* Type VI Secretion System Activity

ClpP is a protein protease dependent on other adapter proteins such as ClpA and ClpX for substrate recognition (Maurizi, 1991; Gottesman et al., 1998). Therefore, we next determined whether the resistant phenotype of Δ*clpP* is mediated by ClpA or ClpX through the interbacterial competition assay of the deletion mutants Δ*clpA*:kan (hereafter referred to as Δ*clpA*) and Δ*clpX*:kan (hereafter referred to as Δ*clpX*) as recipients. SI demonstrates that Δ*clpA* was less susceptible to *A. tumefaciens* T6SS killing than BW25113 wild-type ($P = 0.02$), whereas Δ*clpX* was similar to BW25113 wild type ($P = 1.00$) (**Figure 6A**). The decreased *A. tumefaciens* T6SS killing phenotype of Δ*clpA* was fully complemented *in trans* (**Figure 6B**). No difference could be detected among the growth of the BW25113 wild-type, Δ*clpA*, Δ*clpP*, and their respective complemented strains when co-cultured with Δ*tssL* ($P = 0.58$) (**Figure 6C**). Therefore, the killing outcome is caused by *Agrobacterium* T6SS-mediated interbacterial competition rather than the growth rate of the different recipient strains under the competition condition. This suggested that ClpA could be the adapter that interacts with

ClpP leading to the enhanced susceptibility to T6SS attack in BW25113 wild type. In this case, the interaction between ClpA and ClpP should be required for enhancing *A. tumefaciens* T6SS killing. The interaction between ClpA and ClpP is well studied, and it has been demonstrated that the R26A and D32A variants of ClpP lose their ability to bind to ClpA by 50 and 100%, respectively (Bewley et al., 2006). Therefore, we complemented $ClpP_{R26A}$ and $ClpP_{D32A}$ in Δ*clpP* to determine whether the two variants could restore the susceptibility. The $R26A^{+}$ was able to complement (P = 0.96, compared to $ClpP^{+}$), whereas $D32A^{+}$ failed to complement and showed no statistical difference in SI than that of Δ*clpP* ($P < 10^{-4}$) (**Figure 7**). These results suggest that the phenotype observed in Δ*clpP* and in Δ*clpA* could be associated with ClpA–ClpP interaction. Because the retained N-terminal propeptide does not prevent ClpP–ClpA binding (Maurizi et al., 1990), the inability of unprocessed $ClpP_{S111A}$ and $ClpP_{H136A}$ in enhanced susceptibility is independent of ClpP–ClpA complex formation.

DISCUSSION

This study provides evidence that the genetic factors of the recipient cells play an important role in affecting the outcome of the T6SS antibacterial activity. The high throughput interbacterial competition platform developed in this study proved to be an effective method in identifying recipient factors that affect the outcome of *A. tumefaciens* T6SS antibacterial activity. Further exploration led to the confirmation of at least six genes (*clpP*, *clpA*, *gltA*, *ydhS*, *ydaE*, and *cbpA*) encoding known or putative cytoplasmic proteins (Keseler et al., 2016), whereas CbpA resides both in the cytoplasm and in the nucleoid (Orfanoudaki and Economou, 2014). None of these gene products were localized to the inner membrane, periplasm, outer membrane, or extracellular milieu. This result implies that the process affecting the outcome of *A. tumefaciens* T6SS killing to *E. coli* occurs in the cytoplasm, presumably after the injection of the T6SS puncturing apparatus. Previous studies have mainly focused on how attacker T6SS is regulated and sensed (Filloux and Sagfors, 2015; Alteri and Mobley, 2016; Hood et al., 2017). This study provides a new insight that recipient cell genes can also affect the T6SS killing outcome and that it could take place after the injection of the T6SS apparatus into the recipient cytoplasm.

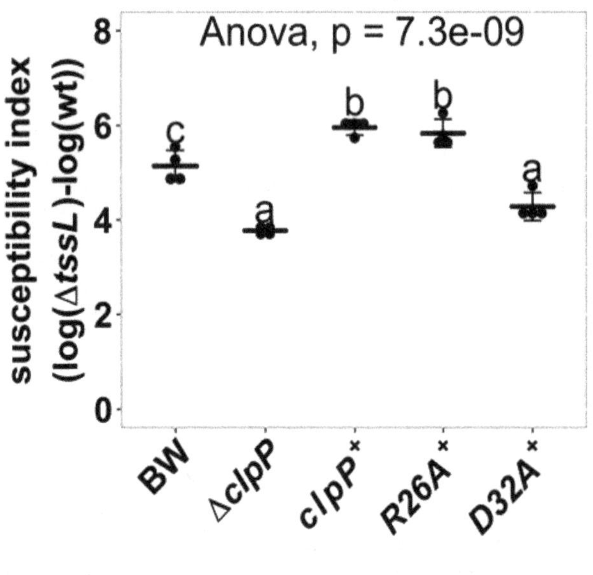

FIGURE 7 | Effects of ClpP variants impaired with ClpA-binding ability in enhancing *Agrobacterium tumefaciens* type VI secretion system (T6SS) antibacterial activity. Interbacterial competition assay between *A. tumefaciens* and *Escherichia coli* wild type, Δ*clpP*, and Δ*clpP* complement strains expressing wild-type ClpP (*clpP*$^{+}$), ClpAP complex formation mutants $ClpP_{R26A}$ ($R26A^{+}$), and $ClpP_{D32A}$ ($D32A^{+}$). The ClpAP complex forming ability is half than that of wild-type ClpP in $ClpP_{R26A}$ and is completely lost in $ClpP_{D32A}$ (Bewley et al., 2006). The T6SS killing data are mean $\pm$ SD of four biological replicates from two independent experiments. Statistical analysis involved single-factor analysis of variance (ANOVA) and Tukey honestly significant difference (HSD) with $P < 0.05$ for statistical significance. Two groups with significant differences are indicated with different letters (a and b).

Our data showed that ClpA but not ClpX, together with ClpP, contributes to the susceptibility of the recipient *E. coli* to *A. tumefaciens* T6SS killing. The *clpX* transcript level drops and fades 15 min after the onset of carbon starvation (Li et al., 2000), which is the condition used for our interbacterial competition. Thus, ClpX is probably not available to form the ClpXP complex during *Agrobacterium* T6SS attacks. The Δ*clpA* was indeed identified in the first screening but was accidentally misplaced and did not enter the second screening process. Therefore, Δ*clpA* did not appear in our final candidate list until we obtained the correct strain for confirmation. The results that the three catalytic variants $ClpP_{S111A}$, $ClpP_{H136A}$, and $ClpP_{D185A}$ did not significantly differ in their ability to degrade GFP-ssrA substrate suggested that the protease activity may not be the leading cause in enhancing *A. tumefaciens* T6SS attack. On the other hand, unlike $ClpP_{S111A}$ and $ClpP_{H136A}$, which do not exhibit significant protease activity as compared with that of the negative controls, $ClpP_{D185A}$ may possess weak protease activity, as the GFP-ssrA fluorescence level is significantly lower than that of the negative controls at the final time point. Thus, the involvement of the ClpP protease activity cannot be completely ruled out as the weak protease activity of $ClpP_{D185A}$ may be sufficient to exhibit its function in enhancing *A. tumefaciens* T6SS attack. Of note, the ClpP protease activity monitored by the *in vitro* protease activity assay using either ClpX or ClpA as a protein unfoldase showed a highly similar pattern among 24 ClpP variants (Bewley et al., 2006). As this GFP-ssrA degradation assay is an *in vitro* system and that it is difficult to monitor the ClpP protease activity of the recipient under competition condition, the role of ClpP protease remains elusive.

Our data also suggest that ClpAP complex is required in enhancing recipient susceptibility during *A. tumefaciens* T6SS killing on the basis of the results that ClpP variant that loses its ability to form a complex with ClpA did not complement the phenotype whereas those with ClpA binding ability do. This implies that the ClpA–ClpP complex, rather than ClpP alone, is the cause of the enhanced susceptibility to T6SS attack. As ClpP allosterically activates the polypeptide translocation activity of ClpA (Miller et al., 2013), the necessity of the ClpAP complex may depend on the unfoldase activity of ClpA. The detailed mechanism on how recipient ClpAP is involved in T6SS susceptibility enhancement awaits further investigations. One promising future direction would be identifying the potential ClpA substrates and their effects on increasing susceptibility of T6SS attack.

Hijacking a highly conserved and essential molecule of the recipient cell to improve attacker fitness is not uncommon. The examples are CdiA-CT^{EC93} hijacking essential proteins BamA and AcrB, CdiA-CT^{EC536} hijacking the recipient CysK, and Ssp2 and Ssp4 hijacking recipient DsbA (Aoki et al., 2008; Diner et al., 2012; Mariano et al., 2018). The ClpP protease, on the other hand, is highly conserved in both prokaryotes and eukaryotic organelles like plastid and mitochondria (Culp and Wright, 2016; Moreno et al., 2017). The ClpP protease cooperates with different AAA$^+$ ATPases in different organisms. It works with ClpA and ClpX in Gram-negative bacteria; with ClpC and ClpE in Gram-positive bacteria; with ClpC1, ClpC2, and ClpD in the chloroplast; and with ClpX in human mitochondria. In all these cases, the ClpP protease seems to play a central role in protein homeostasis. Dysfunction of the system can lead to severe developmental defects, a reduction in the pathogenicity, or lethality (Cole et al., 2015; Nishimura and Van Wijk, 2015; Bhandari et al., 2018). The current result suggests that the ClpP protease system could be another target hijacked by the T6SS attacker to improve its competitive advantage.

To our knowledge, the involvement of the ClpAP complex in enhancing the recipient's susceptibility to *A. tumefaciens* T6SS activity has not been described in the contact-dependent competitor elimination systems in Gram-negative bacteria like T1SS, T4SS, CDI, and T6SS. It would be of interest to uncover how and what *A. tumefaciens* factors hijack this universal and highly conserved ClpP and its associated AAA$^+$ ATPase substrate recognizing partner. The current finding provides additional evidence to support that T6SS can manipulate the essential and highly conserved molecules of recipient cells to achieve better inhibition of the performance (Russell et al., 2014). Elucidating the underlying molecular mechanisms of ClpAP and other recipient factors would be the next direction to understand further how genetic factors can affect the recipient susceptibility to the T6SS attacks.

AUTHOR CONTRIBUTIONS

H-HL, MY, and E-ML conceived and designed the experiments. H-HL performed most of the experiments. MS contributed to the protease activity assay. MS and S-TH provided the materials and tools for the protease activity assay. S-TH, C-TL, and E-ML supervised the execution of the experiments. H-HL and E-ML, with contributions from MY, MS, S-TH, and C-TL wrote the manuscript. All authors read and approved the final manuscript.

FUNDING

The funding for this project was provided by the Ministry of Science and Technology of Taiwan (MOST) (Grant Nos. 104-2311-B-001-025-MY3 to E-ML; 107-2628-M-001-005-MY3 to S-TH; and 107-2811-M-001-1574 to MS) and Academia Sinica Investigator Award to E-ML (Grant No. AS-IA-107-L01).

ACKNOWLEDGMENTS

We thank National BioResource Project (NIG, Japan): *E. coli* for providing the Keio collection. We also thank Lai lab members for discussion and suggestions. We acknowledge the staffs in the Plant Cell Biology Core Laboratory and the DNA Sequencing Core Laboratory at the Institute of Plant and Microbial Biology, and Biophysics Facility at the Institute of Biological Chemistry, Academia Sinica, Taiwan, and Chia Lee for technical support.

REFERENCES

Alexopoulos, J. A., Guarné, A., and Ortega, J. (2012). ClpP: a structurally dynamic protease regulated by AAA+ proteins. *J. Struct. Biol.* 179, 202–210. doi: 10.1016/j.jsb.2012.05.003

Alteri, C. J., and Mobley, H. L. T. (2016). The versatile type VI secretion system. *Microbiol. Spectr.* 4:26.

Aoki, S. K., Diner, E. J., De Roodenbeke, C. T. K., Burgess, B. R., Poole, S. J., Braaten, B. A., et al. (2010). A widespread family of polymorphic contact-dependent toxin delivery systems in bacteria. *Nature* 468, 439–442. doi: 10.1038/nature09490

Aoki, S. K., Malinverni, J. C., Jacoby, K., Thomas, B., Pamma, R., Trinh, B. N., et al. (2008). Contact-dependent growth inhibition requires the essential outer membrane protein BamA (YaeT) as the receptor and the inner membrane transport protein AcrB. *Mol. Microbiol.* 70, 323–340. doi: 10.1111/j.1365-2958.2008.06404.x

Aoki, S. K., Pamma, R., Hernday, A. D., Bickham, J. E., Braaten, B. A., and Low, D. A. (2005). Contact-dependent inhibition of growth in *Escherichia coli*. *Science* 309, 1245–1248. doi: 10.1126/science.1115109

Baba, T., Ara, T., Hasegawa, M., Takai, Y., Okumura, Y., Baba, M., et al. (2006). Construction of *Escherichia coli* K-12 in-frame, single-gene knockout mutants: the Keio collection. *Mol. Syst. Biol.* 2:2006.0008.

Basler, M., Ho, B. T., and Mekalanos, J. J. (2013). Tit-for-tat: type VI secretion system counterattack during bacterial cell-cell interactions. *Cell* 152, 884–894. doi: 10.1016/j.cell.2013.01.042

Bayer-Santos, E., Cenens, W., Matsuyama, B. Y., Di Sessa, G., Mininel, I. D. V., and Farah, C. S. (2019). The opportunistic pathogen *Stenotrophomonas maltophilia* utilizes a type IV secretion system for interbacterial killing. *PLoS Pathog.* 15:e1007651. doi: 10.1371/journal.ppat.1007651

Bewley, M. C., Graziano, V., Griffin, K., and Flanagan, J. M. (2006). The asymmetry in the mature amino-terminus of ClpP facilitates a local symmetry match in ClpAP and ClpXP complexes. *J. Struct. Biol.* 153, 113–128. doi: 10.1016/j.jsb.2005.09.011

Bhandari, V., Wong, K. S., Zhou, J. L., Mabanglo, M. F., Batey, R. A., and Houry, W. A. (2018). The role of ClpP protease in bacterial pathogenesis and human diseases. *ACS Chem. Biol.* 13, 1413–1425. doi: 10.1021/acschembio.8b00124

Cole, A., Wang, Z., Coyaud, E., Voisin, V., Gronda, M., Jitkova, Y., et al. (2015). Inhibition of the mitochondrial protease ClpP as a therapeutic strategy for human acute myeloid leukemia. *Cancer Cell* 27, 864–876. doi: 10.1016/j.ccell.2015.05.004

Costa, T. R. D., Felisberto-Rodrigues, C., Meir, A., Prevost, M. S., Redzej, A., Trokter, M., et al. (2015). Secretion systems in Gram-negative bacteria: structural and mechanistic insights. *Nat. Rev. Microb.* 13, 343–359. doi: 10.1038/nrmicro3456

Culp, E., and Wright, G. D. (2016). Bacterial proteases, untapped antimicrobial drug targets. *J. Antibiot.* 70, 366–377. doi: 10.1038/ja.2016.138

Diner, E. J., Beck, C. M., Webb, J. S., Low, D. A., and Hayes, C. S. (2012). Identification of a target cell permissive factor required for contact-dependent growth inhibition (CDI). *Genes Dev.* 26, 515–525. doi: 10.1101/gad.182345.111

Filloux, A., and Sagfors, A. (2015). "3 - News and views on protein secretion systems," in *The Comprehensive Sourcebook of Bacterial Protein Toxins (Fourth Edition)*, eds J. Alouf, D. Ladant, and M. R. Popoff, (Boston: Academic Press), 77–108. doi: 10.1016/b978-0-12-800188-2.00003-3

García-Bayona, L., Gozzi, K., and Laub, M. T. (2019). Mechanisms of resistance to the contact-dependent bacteriocin CdzC/D in *Caulobacter crescentus*. *J. Bacteriol.* 201:e538-18. doi: 10.1128/JB.00538-18

García-Bayona, L., Guo, M. S., and Laub, M. T. (2017). Contact-dependent killing by *Caulobacter crescentus* via cell surface-associated, glycine zipper proteins. *eLife* 6:e24869. doi: 10.7554/eLife.24869

Gottesman, S., Roche, E., Zhou, Y., and Sauer, R. T. (1998). The ClpXP and ClpAP proteases degrade proteins with carboxy-terminal peptide tails added by the SsrA-tagging system. *Genes Dev.* 12, 1338–1347. doi: 10.1101/gad.12.9.1338

Graves, S., Piepho, H.-P., Selzer, L., and Dorai-Raj, S. (2015). "multcompView: visualizations of paired comparisons," in *R package version 0.1-7*.

Harrell, F. E. Jr., Dupont, C., and Others, M. (2018). *Hmisc: Harrell Miscellaneous*. Vienna: R Foundation for Statistical Computing.

Heckman, K. L., and Pease, L. R. (2007). Gene splicing and mutagenesis by PCR-driven overlap extension. *Nat. Protoc.* 2, 924–932. doi: 10.1038/nprot.2007.132

Hood, R. D., Peterson, S. B., and Mougous, J. D. (2017). From striking out to striking gold: discovering that type VI secretion targets bacteria. *Cell Host Microbe* 21, 286–289. doi: 10.1016/j.chom.2017.02.001

Johnson, P. M., Beck, C. M., Morse, R. P., Garza-Sánchez, F., Low, D. A., Hayes, C. S., et al. (2016). Unraveling the essential role of CysK in CDI toxin activation. *Proc. Natl. Acad. Sci. U.S.A.* 113, 9792–9797. doi: 10.1073/pnas.1607112113

Jones, A. M., Garza-Sánchez, F., So, J., Hayes, C. S., and Low, D. A. (2017). Activation of contact-dependent antibacterial tRNase toxins by translation elongation factors. *Proc. Natl. Acad. Sci. U.S.A.* 114, E1951–E1957. doi: 10.1073/pnas.1619273114

Kassambara, A. (2018). *ggpubr: 'ggplot2' Based Publication Ready Plots*. New York, NY: Springer.

Keseler, I. M., Mackie, A., Santos-Zavaleta, A., Billington, R., Bonavides-Martínez, C., Caspi, R., et al. (2016). The EcoCyc database: reflecting new knowledge about *Escherichia coli* K-12. *Nucleic Acids Res.* 45, D543–D550. doi: 10.1093/nar/gkw1003

LeRoux, M., De Leon, J. A., Kuwada, N. J., Russell, A. B., Pinto-Santini, D., Hood, R. D., et al. (2012). Quantitative single-cell characterization of bacterial interactions reveals type VI secretion is a double-edged sword. *Proc. Natl. Acad. Sci. U.S.A.* 109, 19804–19809. doi: 10.1073/pnas.1213963109

Li, C., Tao, Y. P., and Simon, L. D. (2000). Expression of different-size transcripts from the *clpP-clpX* operon of *Escherichia coli* during carbon deprivation. *J. Bacteriol.* 182, 6630–6637. doi: 10.1128/jb.182.23.6630-6637.2000

Lien, Y.-W., and Lai, E.-M. (2017). Type VI secretion effectors: methodologies and biology. *Front. Cell Infect. Microbiol.* 7:254. doi: 10.3389/fcimb.2017.00254

Ma, L.-S., Hachani, A., Lin, J.-S., Filloux, A., and Lai, E.-M. (2014). *Agrobacterium tumefaciens* deploys a superfamily of type VI secretion dnase effectors as weapons for interbacterial competition in planta. *Cell Host Microbe* 16, 94–104. doi: 10.1016/j.chom.2014.06.002

Ma, L.-S., Narberhaus, F., and Lai, E.-M. (2012). IcmF family protein TssM exhibits ATPase activity and energizes type VI secretion. *J. Biol. Chem.* 287, 15610–15621. doi: 10.1074/jbc.M111.301630

Mahmoud, S. A., and Chien, P. (2018). Regulated proteolysis in bacteria. *Annu. Rev. Biochem.* 87, 677–696. doi: 10.1146/annurev-biochem-062917-012848

Mariano, G., Monlezun, L., and Coulthurst, S. J. (2018). Dual role for DsbA in attacking and targeted bacterial cells during type VI secretion system-mediated competition. *Cell Rep.* 22, 774–785. doi: 10.1016/j.celrep.2017.12.075

Maurizi, M. R. (1991). ATP-promoted interaction between Clp A and Clp P in activation of Clp protease from *Escherichia coli*. *Biochem. Soc. Trans.* 19, 719–723. doi: 10.1042/bst0190719

Maurizi, M. R., Clark, W. P., Kim, S. H., and Gottesman, S. (1990). Clp P represents a unique family of serine proteases. *J. Biol. Chem.* 265, 12546–12552.

Michalska, K., Gucinski, G. C., Garza-Sánchez, F., Johnson, P. M., Stols, L. M., Eschenfeldt, W. H., et al. (2017). Structure of a novel antibacterial toxin that exploits elongation factor Tu to cleave specific transfer RNAs. *Nucleic Acids Res.* 45, 10306–10320. doi: 10.1093/nar/gkx700

Miller, J. M., Lin, J., Li, T., and Lucius, A. L. (2013). E. coli ClpA catalyzed polypeptide translocation is allosterically controlled by the protease ClpP. *J. Mol. Biol.* 425, 2795–2812. doi: 10.1016/j.jmb.2013.04.019

Moreno, J. C., Tiller, N., Diez, M., Karcher, D., Tillich, M., Schöttler, M. A., et al. (2017). Generation and characterization of a collection of knock-down lines for the chloroplast Clp protease complex in tobacco. *J. Exp. Bot.* 68, 2199–2218. doi: 10.1093/jxb/erx066

Nishimura, K., and Van Wijk, K. J. (2015). Organization, function and substrates of the essential Clp protease system in plastids. *Biochim. Biophys. Acta* 1847, 915–930. doi: 10.1016/j.bbabio.2014.11.012

Olivares, A. O., Baker, T. A., and Sauer, R. T. (2015). Mechanistic insights into bacterial AAA+ proteases and protein-remodelling machines. *Nat. Rev. Microbiol.* 14, 33–44. doi: 10.1038/nrmicro.2015.4

Orfanoudaki, G., and Economou, A. (2014). Proteome-wide subcellular topologies of *E. coli* polypeptides database (STEPdb). *Mol. Cell. Proteomics* 13, 3674–3687. doi: 10.1074/mcp.O114.041137

Quentin, D., Ahmad, S., Shanthamoorthy, P., Mougous, J. D., Whitney, J. C., and Raunser, S. (2018). Mechanism of loading and translocation of type VI secretion system effector Tse6. *Nat. Microbiol.* 3, 1142–1152. doi: 10.1038/s41564-018-0238-z

R Core Team, (2018). *R: A Language and Environment for Statistical Computing*. Vienna: R Foundation for Statistical Computing.

RStudio Team, (2015). *RStudio: Integrated Development for R*. Boston, MA: RStudio, Inc.

Russell, A. B., Peterson, S. B., and Mougous, J. D. (2014). Type VI secretion system effectors: poisons with a purpose. *Nat. Rev. Microbiol.* 12, 137–148. doi: 10.1038/nrmicro3185

Souza, D. P., Oka, G. U., Alvarez-Martinez, C. E., Bisson-Filho, A. W., Dunger, G., Hobeika, L., et al. (2015). Bacterial killing via a type IV secretion system. *Nat. Commun.* 6:6453. doi: 10.1038/ncomms7453

Sriramoju, M. K., Chen, Y., Lee, Y.-T. C., and Hsu, S.-T. D. (2018). Topologically knotted deubiquitinases exhibit unprecedented mechanostability to withstand the proteolysis by an AAA+ protease. *Sci. Rep.* 8:7076. doi: 10.1038/s41598-018-25470-0

Studier, F. W., and Moffatt, B. A. (1986). Use of bacteriophage T7 RNA polymerase to direct selective high-level expression of cloned genes. *J. Mol. Biol.* 189, 113–130. doi: 10.1016/0022-2836(86)90385-2

Vergunst, A. C., Schrammeijer, B., Den Dulk-Ras, A., De Vlaam, C. M. T., Regensburg-Tuïnk, T. J. G., and Hooykaas, P. J. (2000). VirB/D4-dependent protein translocation from *Agrobacterium* into plant cells. *Science* 290, 979–982. doi: 10.1126/science.290.5493.979

Wang, J., Hartling, J. A., and Flanagan, J. M. (1997). The structure of ClpP at 2.3 Å resolution suggests a model for ATP-dependent proteolysis. *Cell* 91, 447–456. doi: 10.1016/s0092-8674(00)80431-6

Weber-Ban, E. U., Reid, B. G., Miranker, A. D., and Horwich, A. L. (1999). Global unfolding of a substrate protein by the Hsp100 chaperone ClpA. *Nature* 401, 90–93. doi: 10.1038/43481

Whitney, J. C., Quentin, D., Sawai, S., Leroux, M., Harding, B. N., Ledvina, H. E., et al. (2015). An interbacterial NAD(P)+ glycohydrolase toxin requires elongation factor Tu for delivery to target cells. *Cell* 163, 607–619. doi: 10.1016/j.cell.2015.09.027

Wickham, H. (2011). The split-apply-combine strategy for data analysis. *J. Stat. Softw.* 40:29.

Wickham, H. (2016). *ggplot2: Elegant Graphics for Data Analysis*. New York, NY: Springer-Verlag.

Willett, J. L. E., Gucinski, G. C., Fatherree, J. P., Low, D. A., and Hayes, C. S. (2015). Contact-dependent growth inhibition toxins exploit multiple independent cell-entry pathways. *Proc. Natl. Acad. Sci. U.S.A.* 112, 11341–11346. doi: 10.1073/pnas.1512124112

6

Interaction of *Bacteroides fragilis* Toxin with Outer Membrane Vesicles Reveals New Mechanism of Its Secretion and Delivery

Natalya B. Zakharzhevskaya[1*], *Vladimir B. Tsvetkov*[1,2,3*], *Anna A. Vanyushkina*[1], *Anna M. Varizhuk*[1], *Daria V. Rakitina*[1], *Victor V. Podgorsky*[1], *Innokentii E. Vishnyakov*[4,5], *Daria D. Kharlampieva*[1], *Valentin A. Manuvera*[1], *Fedor V. Lisitsyn*[6], *Elena A. Gushina*[6], *Vassili N. Lazarev*[1,7] and *Vadim M. Govorun*[1,7,8]

[1] Federal Research and Clinical Centre of Physical-Chemical Medicine Federal Medical Biological Agency, Moscow, Russia, [2] Department of Polyelectrolytes and Surface-Active Polymers, Topchiev Institute of Petrochemical Synthesis, Moscow, Russia, [3] Department of Molecular Virology, FSBI Research Institute of Influenza, Ministry of Health of the Russian Federation, Saint Petersburg, Russia, [4] Lab of Genome Structural Organization, Institute of Cytology, Russian Academy of Sciences, Saint Petersburg, Russia, [5] Institute of Nanobiotechnologies, Peter the Great St. Petersburg Polytechnic University, Saint Petersburg, Russia, [6] N.F. Gamalei Federal Research Centre for Epidemiology and Microbiology, Ministry of Health Russian Federation, Moscow, Russia, [7] Lab of Systems Biology, Moscow Institute of Physics and Technology, Dolgoprudny, Russia, [8] Department of Proteomics, Shemyakin-Ovchinnikov Institute of Bioorganic Chemistry of the Russian Academy of Sciences, Moscow, Russia

***Correspondence:**
Natalya B. Zakharzhevskaya
natazaha@gmail.com
Vladimir B. Tsvetkov
v.b.tsvetkov@gmail.com

The only recognized virulence factor of enterotoxigenic *Bacteroides fragilis* (ETBF) that accompanies bloodstream infections is the zinc-dependent non-lethal metalloprotease *B. fragilis* toxin (BFT). The isolated toxin stimulates intestinal secretion, resulting in epithelial damage and necrosis. Numerous publications have focused on the interrelation of BFT with intestinal inflammation and colorectal neoplasia, but nothing is known about the mechanism of its secretion and delivery to host cells. However, recent studies of gram-negative bacteria have shown that outer membrane vesicles (OMVs) could be an essential mechanism for the spread of a large number of virulence factors. Here, we show for the first time that BFT is not a freely secreted protease but is associated with OMVs. Our findings indicate that only outer surface-exposed BFT causes epithelial cell contact disruption. According to our *in silico* models confirmed by Trp quenching assay and NMR, BFT has special interactions with outer membrane components such as phospholipids and is secreted during vesicle formation. Moreover, the strong cooperation of BFT with polysaccharides is similar to the behavior of lectins. Understanding the molecular mechanisms of BFT secretion provides new perspectives for investigating intestinal inflammation pathogenesis and its prevention.

Keywords: toxin delivery, lipid protein interactions, shot gun lipidomics, Electron microscopy, fluorescence quenching, NMR

INTRODUCTION

Of the numerous microbial species that inhabit the gastrointestinal tract of mammals, Bacteroidetes is the most abundant gram-negative bacterial phylum (Ley et al., 2008). The anaerobe *Bacteroides fragilis* is a common colonic symbiont with an affinity for mucosal colonization, although it makes up only 1 to 2% of the cultured fecal flora (Huang et al., 2011). There are two molecular subtypes, non-toxigenic *B. fragilis* (NTBF) and enterotoxigenic *B. fragilis* (ETBF). ETBF is an intestinal bacterium that has been associated with inflammatory bowel disease and colorectal cancer in humans (Prindiville et al., 2000; Toprak et al., 2006). The only well-studied virulence factor specific to ETBF is the secreted metalloprotease *B. fragilis* toxin (BFT) (Moncrief et al., 1995; Franco et al., 1997). BFT can affect zonula adherens and tight junctions in the intestinal epithelium by cleaving E-cadherin (Wu et al., 1998), resulting in rearrangements of the actin cytoskeleton of epithelial cells. BFT is synthesized as a 44.4-kDa precursor (pBFT), which is then processed into a 21-kDa mature BFT (mBFT) that is secreted into the supernatant of cultured cells (Kling et al., 1997). Three toxin isoforms have been described, BFT1, BFT2, and BFT3, with isoform BFT2 being the most common (Scotto d'Abusco et al., 2000). Although BFT is a secreted protease, nothing is known about the mechanisms of its secretion and transport to host cells. Gram-negative bacteria have evolved mechanisms to deliver virulence factors to the host (Koster et al., 2000). Well-studied examples include type III secretion systems (Galán et al., 2014), type IV secretion systems (Wallden et al., 2010), and type VI secretion systems, which are required for virulence factor transport to host cells (Hachani et al., 2016). Genomic studies of *B. fragilis* have not shown evidence of type III, IV, autotransporter, or two-partner secretion systems (Wilson et al., 2015). However, *B. fragilis* was shown to possess genes for Hly type I secretion systems, which are similar to the hemolysin type I secretion system HlyDb of *Escherichia coli* (Wang et al., 1991). Type VI secretion systems (T6SS) were recently discovered in a few Bacteroidetes strains, thereby extending the presence of these systems beyond Proteobacteria. Comprehensive analysis of all sequenced human gut Bacteroidales strains has shown that more than half contain T6SS loci (Coyne et al., 2016). T6SS as a multiprotein complex is specially organized into three distinct genetic architectures (GA) where GA1 and GA2 loci are present on conserved integrative conjugative elements (ICE) and are transferred and shared among diverse human gut Bacteroidales species. But GA3 loci are not contained on conserved ICE and are confined to *B. fragilis*. Thorough research has showed that GA3 loci of *B. fragilis* could be a source of numerous novel effector and immunity proteins (Chatzidaki-Livanis et al., 2016). But there is no evidence that T6SS may be used for *B. fragilis* toxin secretion.

Rather than secrete virulence factors into the surrounding milieu, where they could be degraded by host proteases, many gram-negative pathogens utilize outer membrane vesicles (OMVs) as a mechanism of delivering active proteins and other moieties into host cells (Kulp and Kuehn, 2010). Toxin delivery mediated by OMVs is recognized as a potent virulence mechanism for many pathogens (Ellis and Kuehn, 2010). It is now well known that both non-pathogenic and pathogenic gram-negative bacteria constitutively release OMVs (Kuehn and Kesty, 2005). OMVs are spherical proteoliposomes that have an average diameter ranging from 20 to 150 nm and that are enriched with outer membrane proteins, phospholipids, polysaccharides, and numerous proteins of a wide molecular mass range (Mashburn-Warren et al., 2008). Many periplasm-located virulence factors are enriched in OMVs, including Shiga toxin produced by *E. coli* and Cag toxin produced by *Helicobacter pylori* (Ismail et al., 2003; Kesty and Kuehn, 2004). The large number of enzyme-containing OMVs produced by *B. fragilis* suggests that OMV transport may be an important export pathway (Patrick et al., 1996; Cerdeño-Tárraga et al., 2005). Intracellular, periplasmic and outer membrane-bound proteases have been identified in *B. fragilis* (Elhenawy et al., 2014). Moreover, *B. fragilis* OMVs which contain surface located polysaccharide A have been shown to play an anti-inflammatory role by acting on regulatory T (Treg) cells (Shen et al., 2012). Many hydrolytic enzymes, which are generally considered pathogenic factors, may be bound to the membrane and/or secreted (Gibson and Macfarlane, 1988). Toxins secreted by enterotoxigenic *E. coli* and *V. cholerae* have been found to associate with LPS on the outer surface of OMVs (Horstman and Kuehn, 2002; Chatterjee and Chaudhuri, 2011), in a manner similar to lectins. Lectins are usually characterized by weak interactions between carbohydrates and proteins through hydrogen and coordinate bonds (Richards et al., 1979). Because the *B. fragilis* genome does not encode for known secretion system genes involved in BFT secretion and transport, we reasoned that BFT might be delivered to host cells by OMVs. Consequently, the toxin is incorporated in vesicle membranes during membrane formation due to interactions with outer membrane components, such as lipids and LPS. In the present study, we demonstrate that BFT is associated with OMV membranes through hydrophobic and electrostatic interactions and forms hydrogen and coordinate bonds with membrane components, similar to the behavior of lectins.

RESULTS

OMV Production by NTBF and ETBF and BFT2 Detection in Association with OMVs

To analyze the surface structure of both NTBF and ETBF strains, we examined the bacteria by TEM, which revealed the formation of OMVs on the cell surface (**Figure 1A**). It was observed that both strains (ETBF and NTBF) of *B. fragilis* produce vesicles (**Figures 1A,B** for ETBF and Supplementary Figures 2A,B for NTBF) with sizes ranging from 20 to 100 nm (**Figure 1C**). To avoid contamination with bacteria, small volume of OMV containing solution were cultivated on blood agar plates under anaerobic conditions for 2 days. *B. fragilis* colonies were not observed on blood agar plates.

After isolation of OMV containing fraction from 250 ml cultured cells, we measured the total protein concentration of the ETBF and NTBF OMV preparations, which was ~40–60 μg in 50 μl. For toxin detection, we analyzed 40 μg ETBF and NTBF OMV preparations by western blot using polyclonal antibodies (anti-BFT2) specific to mBFT2 and pBFT2. As a result, we observed the association of mBFT2 with ETBF vesicles (**Figure 1D**). OMV-depleted medium was also used for toxin detection. Briefly, 100 ml OMV-free medium was lyophilized under reduced pressure by a rotary evaporator and analyzed by western blot with polyclonal antibodies (anti-BFT2). We did not detect any visible amount of free toxin. pBFT2 was not detected in the OMV fraction or in OMV-depleted medium. The cells fractions were also examined for toxin existence by

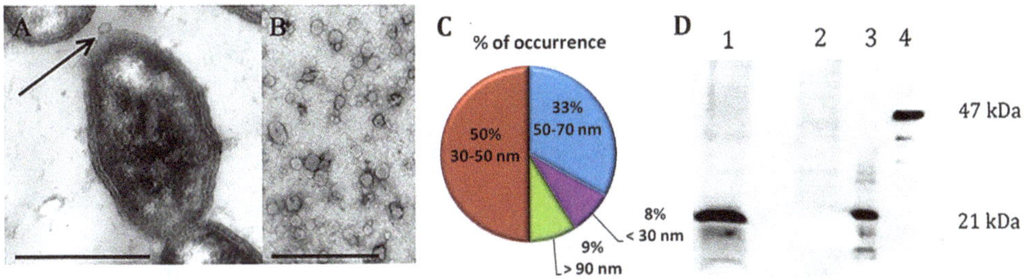

FIGURE 1 | *B. fragilis* produces outer membrane vesicles (OMV), containing BFT. TEM of thin section of ETBF cells during vesicle production **(A)** and isolated ETBF OMVs **(B)**, at magnification: x 10,000. Scale bars represent 1 μm for **(A)** and 300 nm for **(B)**. **(C)** OMV size distribution diagram determined from measurements of about 1000 OMVs from 10 samples **(D)**–5 μg of extracted OMV proteins of each strain (ETBF–1; NTBF–2) were run on 10% SDS-PAGE followed by western blot with antibody against BFT2. 100 ng of each recombinant forms of the toxin were also added (3–mBFT2 and 4–pBFT2).

western blot using polyclonal antibodies (anti-BFT2) specific to mBFT2 and pBFT2. As a result we detected major part of the pBFT2 in membrane fraction and small amount of pBFT2 in periplasm fraction of ETBF cells (Supplementary Figures 1A,B). We examined cells fractions by Q-TOF analysis (Supplementary Information 1).

To confirm the localization of the toxin in the bacterial membrane and in the OMV preparation, we performed immunoelectron microscopic analyses of thin sections using gold nanoparticles coupled with anti-BFT2 antibodies. We detected gold particles coupled with anti-BFT2 antibodies on the membrane and in the periplasm of ETBF (**Figures 2A,C, indicated by arrow**), which confirmed the previous results obtained by western blot analysis. There was no labeling of the same structure in NTBF cells (**Figure 2H** and Supplementary Figure 2A). We observed several labels located in the cytoplasm of bacterial cells, potentially indicating toxin formation (**Figures 2B–D**). Dynamics of OMV formation and release from the bacterial cell surface were monitored (**Figure 2B, indicated by arrow**). Importantly, we observed label predominantly located on the outer membrane (**Figure 2D, indicated by arrow**). ETBF and NTBF OMV samples were negatively stained and labeled with anti-BFT2 antibodies coupled with gold particles. We also examined freely isolated OMVs preparation for toxin localization by immunogold staining. We observed that the label was located on the surface of the ETBF OMV, indicating that the toxin was associated with the outer membrane (**Figures 2E–G**). There was no labeling of the same structure in NTBF OMVs (**Figure 2I** and Supplementary Figure 2B).

Shot-Gun Lipidomics of the *B. fragilis* Outer Membrane

To detect the components of the *B. fragilis* membrane, which the toxin could potentially interact with, shot-gun mass spectrometric analysis of the isolated membrane lipids and LPS extracts was performed. In the fragmentation spectra of membrane lipids, we primarily detected characteristic ions of polar groups of phospholipids, variable fatty acid residues capable of forming different diacylglycerol esters, cycles, and other compounds with water loss. The full list of the identified ions is shown in Supplementary information 2 (Table 1). As expected, the most represented ions in the spectrum belonged to the classes of phosphatidylethanolamine (PE), phosphatidylcholine (PC), and diacylglycerol (DG) (**Figure 3**).

To determine the specific molecular structure of *B. fragilis* LPS, we performed comprehensive mass spectrometry analysis. We used the Tri-Reagent method to extract LPS from *B. fragilis* cell membranes (Elhenawy et al., 2014). To profile the extracted LPS, we used direct injection electrospray-time-of-flight mass spectrometry in negative ion mode as described in the **Materials and Methods** section. As a result, we identified 38 different LPS compounds in the *B. fragilis* LPS preparation [Supplementary information 2 (Table 2)]. Among the detected ions, we reliably identified lipid A-disaccharide-1-P, 3-deoxy-D-manno-octulosonyl-lipid IV(A), KDNalpha2-3Galbeta1-4Glcbeta-Cer[d18:1/24:1(15Z)] and numerous galactosylceramides and glucosylceramides (polysaccharide chains consisting of 4 to 8 carbohydrate units). The identified lipid A-disaccharide-1-P structure was the same as that previously described by Elhenawy et al. (Patrick et al., 1996). As expected, the most represented ions in the spectrum belonged to classes of cerebrosides that are normally produced by *B. fragilis* cells. The mass spectrometry metabolomic data have been deposited to UCSD Center for Computational Mass Spectrometry (MassIVE ID: MSV000080382).

Modeling and Docking of Phospholipids (PC and PE), lipid A, Polysaccharide Chain, and BFT2 (mBFT2, pBFT2)

Two phospholipids of the most abundant classes represented in *B. fragilis* membranes (PC and PE) according to our shot-gun lipidomics data and the main components of LPS [lipid A and polysaccharide chain (PSC)] were docked to pBFT2 and mBFT2 surfaces. Modeling of the pBFT2 and mBFT2 surfaces according to hydrophobic potential distribution, cavities, and potential donors and acceptors of hydrogen bond distribution is shown in Supplementary Figures 3, 4.

The conformations of mBFT2 complexes with PE, PC, lipid A, and PSC with best values of binding energies are shown

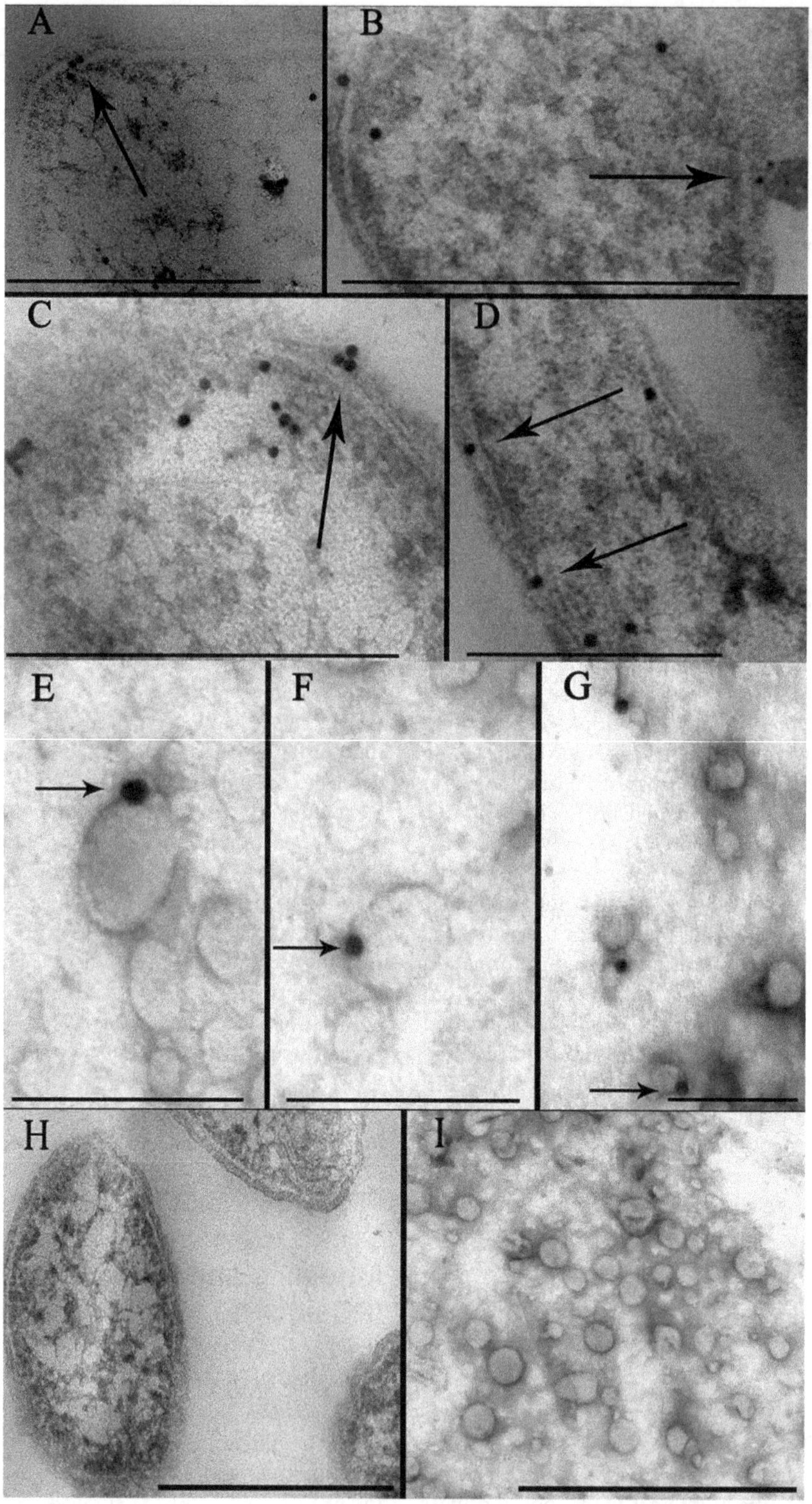

FIGURE 2 | Identification of toxin cell and OMV localization via immune-microscopy with antibodies against BFT. (A–D) Thin sections of ETBF cells analyzed by TEM contain some labels (black dots) coupled with antibodies against BFT fixed on periplasm and membrane (indicated by arrow). Several labels coupled with antibodies against BFT fixed on cytoplasm indicating probable toxin formation. Scale bars represent 300 nm for **(A)** and **(D)**, 500 nm for **(B)** and **(C)**. **(E–G)**—Negatively stained OMV preparations isolated from ETBF culture and coincubated with labels, (black dots indicated by arrow) coupled with antibodies against BFT were analyzed by TEM. Scale bars represent 100 nm for **(E,F)** and 150 nm for **(G)**. **(H)** Thin section of NTBF cells analyzed by TEM contains no fixed labels coupled with antibodies against BFT. **(I)** Negatively stained OMV preparations isolated from NTBF culture contain no fixed labels coupled with antibodies against BFT. Scale bars represent 600 nm for **(H)** and 400 nm for **(I)**.

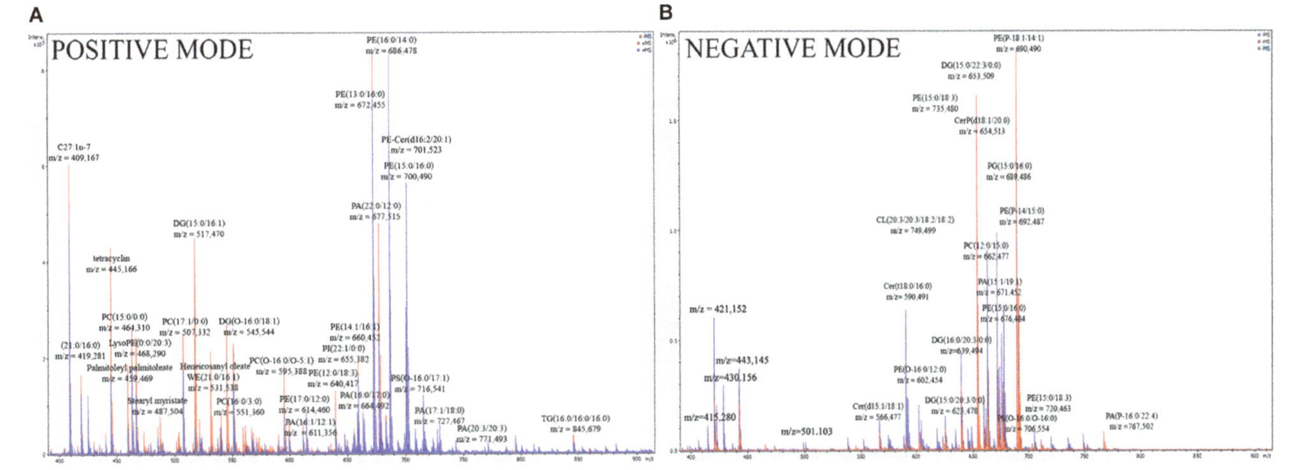

FIGURE 3 | Full mass spectra of *B. fragilis* lipids show the most represented lipids of *B. fragilis* membrane. (A) MS analysis of ETBF (colored in red) and NTBF (colored in blue) membrane in positive linear mode. **(B)** MS analysis of ETBF (colored in red) and NTBF (colored in blue) membrane in negative linear mode. *B. fragilis* cells membrane lipids were extracted by Folch method (see material and methods), dissolved in 200 μl ethanol and analyzed by quadruple time-of-flight tandem mass spectrometer. Mass spectrum of ETBF and NTBF in positive and negative linear mode showed the same cluster of peaks, indicating the most represented classes of lipids (PC, PE, DG, PA).

in **Figures 4, 5**. As is evident from Supplementary information 2 (Table 3), hydrophobic interactions as well as electrostatic make a significant contribution ($\Delta G_{non-polar}$) to the binding energy upon complex formation for both proteins (mBFT2 and pBFT2). The Coulomb contribution (ΔG_{el}) in the case of pBFT2 complex formation is insignificant (ΔG_{el} comparable to $\Delta G_{non-polar}$) compared with mBFT2 complex formation due to the latter's interaction with the zinc ion. Furthermore, the loss of conformational mobility during binding by the ligand as well as by the target leads to a decrease in entropy (TΔS) which reduces binding energy. Also note that electrostatic component of solvation energy (ΔG_{polar}) significantly decreases binding energy.

Lipids can form H-bonds with amino acid residues on pBFT2/mBFT2 groove surfaces (Supplementary Figures 5, 6, PC acts as an acceptor, and PE can be either a donor or an acceptor).

Importantly, the nitrogen group of PE tends to form donor-acceptor bonds with amino acids located in the mBFT2 cavity (**Figure 4A, indicated by arrow**). In contrast, hydrophobic contributions are greater in the case of pBFT2 probably due to the larger size of the pBFT2 surface groove compared to that of mBFT2.

Lipid A, as a main component of LPS, also forms H-bonds with amino acid residues on the mBFT2 groove surface (**Figure 5A**). The lipid A molecule contains two-fold the amount of fatty acid residues compared to PE and PC and therefore makes a significant hydrophobic contribution to mBFT2-lipid A complex formation [(Supplementary information 2 (Table 3)]. In accordance with Elhenawy et al., the lipid A molecule contains a phosphate group, but PSC may exist without the phosphate group in an aqueous medium (Elhenawy et al., 2014). PSC is composed of long chains of monosaccharide units bound together by glycosidic linkages, which form multiple H-bonds with mBFT2 amino acids (**Figure 5C**). These interactions may have a significant impact on polysaccharide chain-mBFT2 complex formation.

Importantly, non-ester phosphate oxygen atoms of PC/PE (**Figures 4B,D**), lipid A (**Figure 5B**), and PSC (**Figure 5D**) tend to form coordinate bonds with the zinc ion in the active center of mBFT2. Carbonyl oxygen atoms of PC/PE might also form such bonds with the zinc ion. According to our data, electrostatic contributions are higher for the lipid-mBFT2 complex than for the lipid-pBFT2 complex, indicating possible coordinate bond formation [$\Delta Gel_{\text{(PE+pBFT)}}$; $\Delta Gel_{\text{(PC+pBFT)}} < \Delta Gel_{\text{(PE+mBFT)}}$; $\Delta Gel_{\text{(PC+mBFT)}}$] [(Supplementary information 2 (Table 3)].

Trp Fluorescence Quenching Assay and 1H-NMR Spectroscopy of BFT-Lipid Complexes

In the above molecular modeling and docking experiments, we identified the most abundant classes of phospholipids of the *B. fragilis* membrane (PE and PC) and demonstrated their interaction with the mBFT2 and pBFT2 surfaces *in silico*. Next, the propensity of mBFT2 and pBFT2 to form complexes with PC was tested using 1H-NMR and Trp fluorescence quenching (**Figure 6**). Comparison of NMR spectra of PC alone and PC mixed with pBFT2/mBFT2 (**Figures 6A,B**) revealed changes in the chemical shifts and peak widths of the fatty acid signals (0—4 ppm), which indicated changes in PC conformation and mobility upon complex formation.

The Trp fluorescence quenching assay, a popular method for investigating lipid-protein interactions (Dua et al., 1995; Kraft et al., 2009), was chosen because BFT2 contains 4 Trp residues in its catalytic site. Proteinase K was used as a negative control, and BSA, which is known to bind lipids in the medium nanomolar range (Charbonneau and Tajmir-Riahi, 2010), was used as a positive control. Intrinsic protein fluorescence was monitored at the Trp/Tyr emission maximum upon excitation at 295 nm

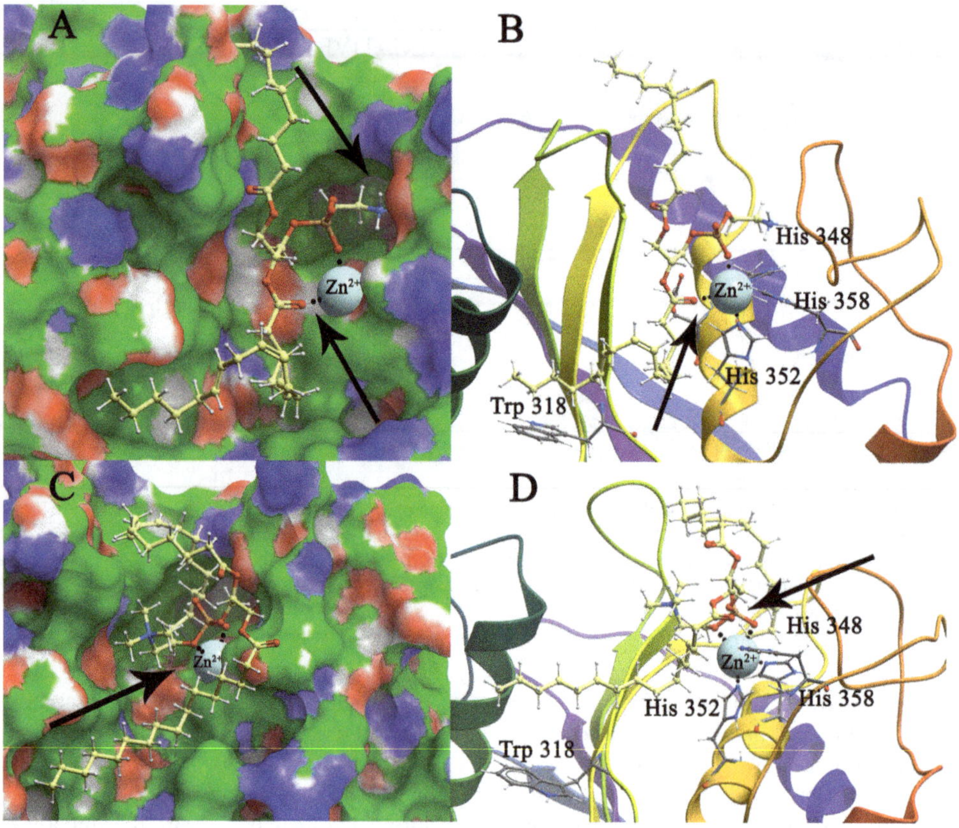

FIGURE 4 | Structure model of mBFT and best (according to the binding energy) ligands (A)—PC and **(C)**—PE location on the mBFT Conolly surface, painted depending on the values of the hydrophobic potential—green, donors—blue, acceptors—red, resulting docking via ICM. The atoms of the ligands are painted in the following colors: polar hydrogens—blue, nitrogen—dark blue, oxygen—red, phosphorus—orange, carbon—white. Zn ions are painted in blue. The non-polar hydrogens not shown. Black dot lines indicate hydrogen bonds. Oxygen of lipid phosphate group colored in red forming coordination bonds with zinc ion. Nitrogen group of PE forming donor-acceptor bounds with amino acids indicated by arrow. Detailed image of mBFT active center with PC **(B)** and PE **(D)**.

(Trp fluorescence, selectively, **Figures 6C,D**) or 280 nm (Trp and Tyr fluorescence, **Figures 6E,F**) in the presence of increasing concentrations of PC organized in liposomes by reverse-phase evaporation. The results suggest the formation of 1:1 protein-lipid complexes in a low ionic strength buffer and the formation of 3:1 mBFT2-lipid complexes in the standard PBS buffer. Importantly, the presence of larger aggregates with a different stoichiometry at high lipid concentrations cannot be excluded, as Trp fluorescence is likely only sensitive to initial saturation.

According to our docking models, non-ester phosphate oxygen atoms of the lipids tend to form coordinate bonds with the His-bound zinc ion in the active center of mBFT2. To test the model and the potential involvement of these coordinate bonds, we analyzed a BFT2 mutant with no His residues and, thus, no zinc ions in the active site. Both mutant forms (mBFT2-mut and pBFT2-mut) demonstrated enhanced affinity to PC, which may be attributed to their increased hydrophobicity, as the charged His residues had been replaced with polar but uncharged Tyr residues. The fact that mBFT2-mut bound with PC more efficiently than the wild-type protein argues against a major contribution by zinc to complex formation.

The Trp fluorescence quenching assay demonstrated that the most represented lipids of the *B. fragilis* cell membrane (PC and PE) form complexes with mBFT2, but to determine the lipid chemical groups capable of such interactions, NMR spectroscopy was performed. Similar to Trp fluorescence quenching assay results, constant values (K_d) calculated for PC-mBFT2 and PE-mBFT2 complexes had slight differences, confirming the specific nature of a protein-lipid interaction. Thus, PC was used as a model of protein-lipid complex formation. We used 5 μM of each form of BFT2 (pBFT2 and mBFT2) and 0.6 μM PC in a water solution to study complex formation. Common 1D proton (with WATERGATE water suppression) (**Figures 6A,B**) and 2D DOSY NMR spectra of PC, BFT2 forms and mixtures were obtained. L-α-phosphatidylcholine (P3556, Sigma Aldrich) was used as the model PC. We observed that PC formed a micelle suspension in the water solution. According to the diffusion NMR spectroscopy results, the micelles consisted of a rather large number of molecules (~10 molecules per micelle). This result corresponds to the literature on this topic (Mashburn-Warren et al., 2008). The diffusion coefficients of pBFT2 and mBFT2 in water solutions were D = −8.4 log(m^2/s) and D = −8.9

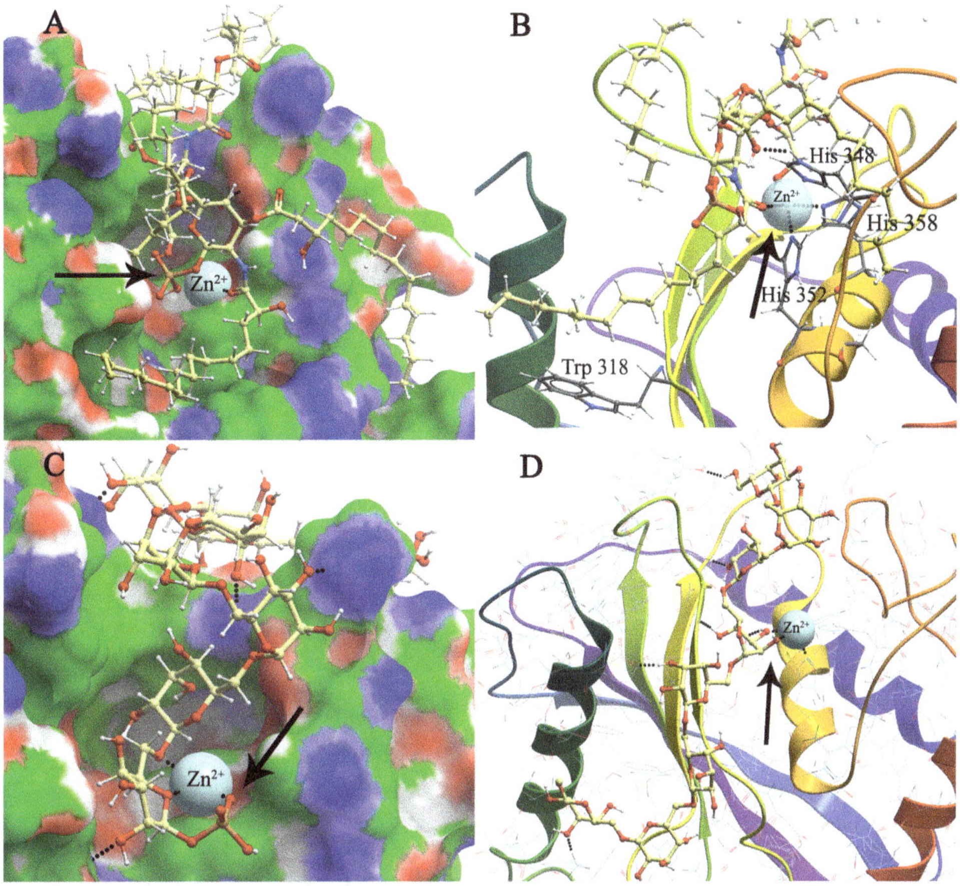

FIGURE 5 | Modeling and docking of protein-lipid A and polysaccharide chain association. Structure model of mBFT and best (according to the binding energy) ligand–lipid A **(A)** and polysaccharide chain **(C)** location on the mBFT Conolly surface, painted depending on the values of the hydrophobic potential—green, donors–blue, acceptors–red, resulting docking via ICM. Oxygen of lipid phosphate group colored in red forming coordination bonds with zinc ion (indicated by arrow). The atoms of the ligands are painted in the following colors: Polar hydrogens–blue, nitrogen–dark blue, oxygen–red, phosphorus–orange, carbon–white. Zn ions are painted in blue. The non-polar hydrogens not shown. Black dot lines indicate hydrogen bonds. Oxygen of lipid phosphate group colored in red forming coordination bonds with zinc ion. Detailed image of mBFT active center with lipid A **(B)** and polysaccharide chain **(D)**.

$\log(m^2/s)$, respectively. The diffusion coefficient for PC in the water solution was $D = -8.2 \log(m^2/s)$. The diffusion coefficients of PC and pBFT2 in the mixture were altered [$D = -9.1 \log(m^2/s)$ and $D = -8.6 \log(m^2/s)$, respectively] (**Figure 6A**) compared to the diffusion coefficients of each alone. The lipid molecules in the mixture were less mobile than in micelles in solution, and the protein molecules were also slightly less mobile in the mixture. In addition, the chemical shifts and peak widths of the fatty acid of PC in the mixture were slightly changed. Peak width changes in this case may be caused only by T_2 relaxation time, i.e., by PC mobility or conformation change. All these changes together may be explained by phospholipids-protein complex formation. Only one type of diffusion coefficient for PC and pBFT2 was present in the mixture, indicating that only one type of protein-phospholipid complex was present in the solution. The difference between the diffusion of free pBFT and pBFT2 in complex was not large. Consequently, complex formation probably causes only a protein conformation change. The results could be interpreted as the association of small lipid particles with the protein molecule core and PC shell. The results of NMR experiments with mBFT2 were similar to those described above (**Figure 6B**). mBFT2 also formed a complex in mixture with PC. However, the mBFT2 molecules were also partially self-aggregated, which was shown by 2D DOSY results. There were two fractions in the mBFT2 solution with diffusion coefficients $D = -8.9 \log (m^2/s)$ and $D = -9.3 \log (m^2/s)$. The mobility of the protein was also lower in the mixture with PC than individually, and PC in the mixture was less mobile as well. The diffusion coefficients of PC and mBFT2 in mixture were $D = -8.7 \log(m^2/s)$ and $D = -9 \log(m^2/s)$, respectively. The NMR data have been deposited to UCSD Center for Computational Mass Spectrometry (MassIVE ID: MSV000080385).

OMV-Associated BFT Is Biologically Active

E-cadherin is a 120-kDa type I transmembrane protein essential to the intercellular adhesion of adjacent epithelial cells, which are the primary known substrate for BFT protease activity (Remacle et al., 2014). Given that mBFT2 was associated with OMVs,

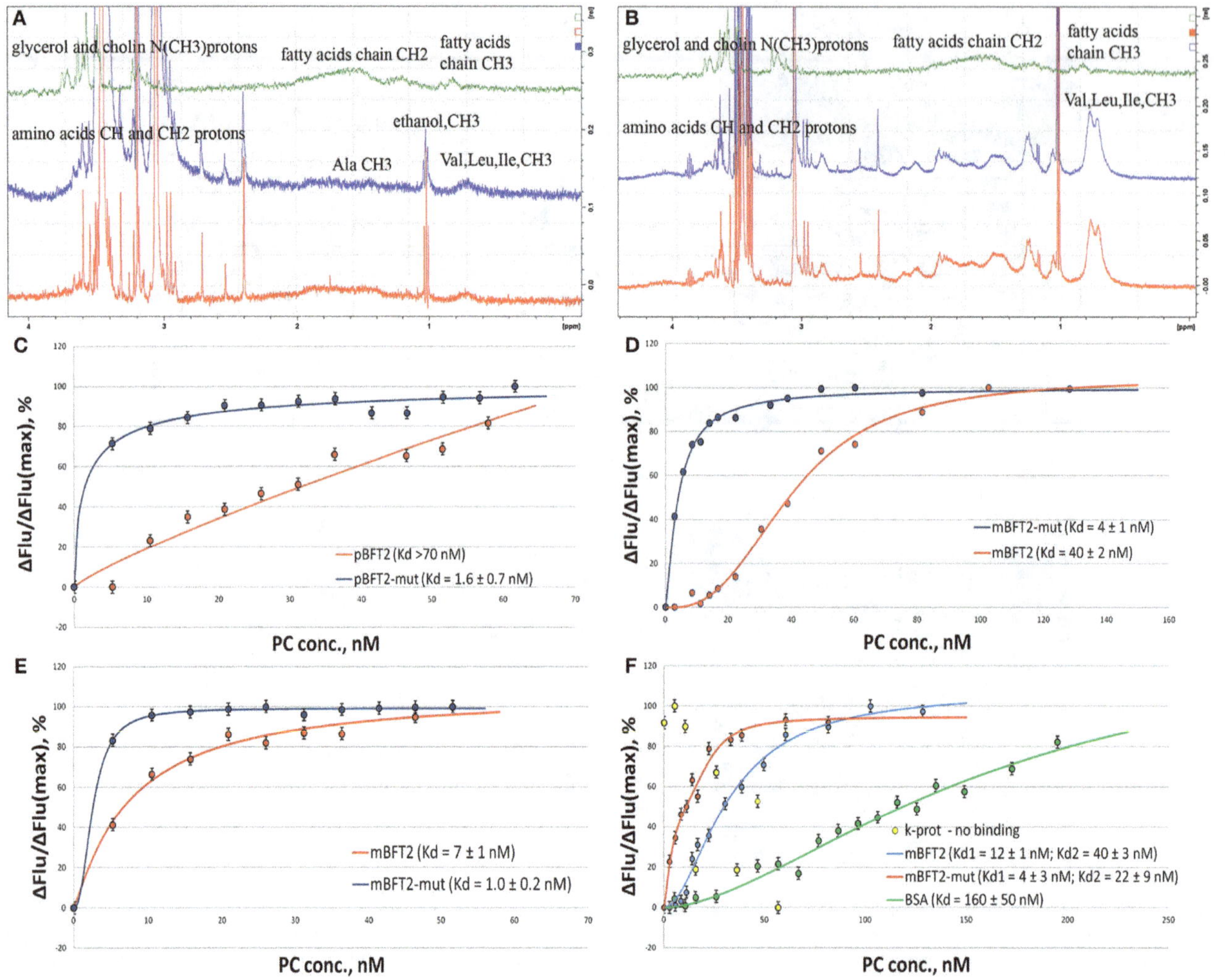

FIGURE 6 | 500 MHz 1D proton. NMR spectra of individual PC, pBFT2, and mBFT2 or their mixture **(A,B)** and fluorescence quenching assay**(C–F)**. **(A)** 500 MHz 1H-NMR spectra of PC (green), pBFT2 (blue), and their mixture (red), (0–4 ppm region). **(B)** 500 MHz 1H-NMR spectra of PC (green), mBFT2 (blue), and their mixture (red). **(C–F)** Trp fluorescence quenching. Conditions: The standard PBS buffer **(C–E)** or the low ionic strength buffer with Zn **(F)**; excitation at 295 **(C,D)** or 280 nm **(E,F)** 20°C. Protein concentration was 3 nM. Error bars indicate standard deviation for three measurements.

vesicle treatment should promote E-cadherin degradation in HT-29 cells. Using western blot analysis (**Figure 7B**), we observed time-dependent degradation of the 120-kDa subunit E-cadherin and its complete cleavage after 2 h of treatment with ETBF OMV in HT-29 cells. To confirm the effect of mBFT2-containing OMVs of ETBF on E-cadherin degradation, we used NTBF OMV at the same time points, and there was no effect.

The effect of toxins on E-cadherin could be dependent on mBFT2 OMV localization. BFT2 can be located inside the vesicles, in the vesicle membrane, or on the OMV surface. We produced two types of liposomes that were reverse-phase constructed with PC. In the first case, the toxin was encapsulated into the liposomes by a reverse-phase evaporation method, while in the second case, mBFT2 was added to the prepared liposomes. We verified the encapsulation of BFT2 into liposomes and analyzed whether unbound BFT2 was present in the medium by western blot (**Figure 7C**). We found that all of the added BFT2 was associated with liposomes, as we did not observe free BFT2 in the medium after centrifugation. Two types of liposomes with mBFT2 and pBFT2 were used for E-cadherin degradation experiments.

We observed complete E-cadherin degradation in HT-29 cells after 2 h of treatment with liposomes with added mBFT2 (**Figure 7A**). The same effect was shown using mBFT2 without liposomes. There was no E-cadherin cleavage when HT-29 cells were incubated with mBFT2 encapsulated into the liposomes. As expected, we did not observe any effect of pBFT2 on E-cadherin.

As described previously, OMVs can be used for virulence factor delivery to host cells. OMVs isolated from ETBF (**Figure 7D**) and NTBF (**Figure 7E**) were labeled with the lipophilic dye DiI, and two forms of the toxin [mBFT2 (**Figure 7F**) and pBFT2 (**Figure 7G**)] were independently added

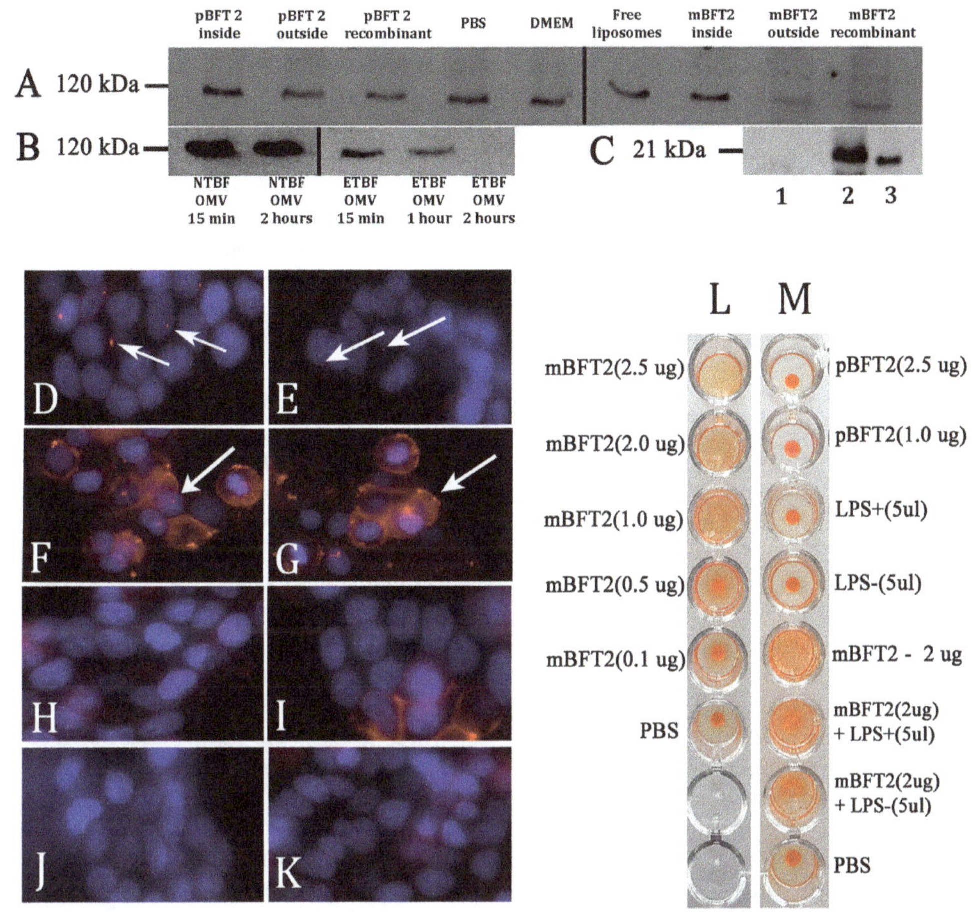

FIGURE 7 | Toxin containing liposomes and OMVs show proteolytic activity against HT-29 cell line E-cadherin and form complexes (A–K). Hemagglutination test **(L–M)** **(A)** Biological effects of the toxin to E-cadherin dependent of its localization. 12 nM pBFT2 and 14.2 nM mBFT2 encapsulated into liposome (pBFT2 inside and mBFT2 inside) or added to prepared liposomes—(pBFT2 outside and mBFT2 outside) were coincubated with HT-29 cells. Recombinant proteins were also coincubated with HT-29 cells (12 nM pBFT2–pBFT2 recombinant; 14.2 nM mBFT2–mBFT2 recombinant). PBS, DMEM and Free liposomes were used as negative controls. **(B)** Biological effect of the toxin containing OMVs to E-cadherin is time depended. 50 µg of total ETBF OMV proteins were coincubated with HT-29 cells for 15 min (ETBF OMV for 15 min), for 1 h (ETBF OMV for 1 h), for 2 h (ETBF OMV for 2 h). The same amounts of NTBF OMV proteins were coincubated with HT-29 cells for 15 min (NTBF OMV for 15 min) or for 2 h (NTBF OMV for 2 h). Extracted HT-29 cells proteins **(A,B)** were run on 10% SDS-PAGE followed by western blot with antibody against E-cadherin. **(C)** Toxin encapsulation and toxin-liposome association were examined by western blot. 14.2 nM mBFT2 with previously added prepared liposomes were dissolved in sterile culture media. After ultracentrifugation step supernatant was examined to unbound toxin—(lane 1), 14.2 nM mBFT2 encapsulated into the liposomes were treated with Proteinase K (20 ng/µl) and run on 10% SDS-PAGE followed by western blot with antibody against mBFT2–(lane 2). Recombinant protein—14.2 nM mBFT2—lane 3. **(D–K)** Complexes formation was examined by fluorescent microscopy. 3 µg OMVs, isolated from ETBF-**(D)** and NTBF-**(E)**; 12 nM pBFT2-**(F)** and 14.2 nM mBFT2-**(G)** were added to 100 µl prepared liposomes; 14.2 nM mBFT2-**(H)** and 12 nM pBFT2-**(I)** were encapsulated into the liposomes. **(J)**-10 µl VybrantDil were added to PBS and centrifuged at 100,000 g. **(K)**-100 µl liposomes. All samples **(D–I, K)** were labeled with VybrantDil (red) and coincubated with HT-29 cells for 1 h. Nuclei were stained with DAPI (blue). Arrows indicate protein-lipid complexes located on cells surfaces. **(L)**-Hemagglutination activity of mBFT2 depends on toxin concentration. **(M)**-Hemagglutination activity of mBFT2 and pBFT2 in a presence of LPS.

to the prepared liposomes and then incubated with HT-29 cells for 1 h. We also tested two forms of the toxin [mBFT2 (**Figure 7H**) and pBFT2 (**Figure 7I**)] encapsulated in liposomes for their ability to form complexes. As a control, we used free DiI-labeled liposomes that were also incubated with HT-29 cells for 1 h (**Figure 7J**). Moreover, to reduce possible false positive cell coloring, we dissolved 10 µl of stock DiI solution in PBS and centrifuged it at 100,000 × g; the resulting sediment dissolved in PBS was used for HT-29 cell labeling (**Figure 7K**). In agreement with our previous results, mBFT2 and pBFT2 added to the prepared liposomes formed complexes located on the cell surface (**Figure 7F,G, protein-lipid complexes indicated by arrows**). We observed ETBF OMVs and NTBF OMVs located on the cell surface, confirming that OMVs are used for protein delivery. Additionally, the relatively few NTBF OMVs located on the cell surface compared with ETBF OMVs may indicate that the toxin facilitates adherence between OMVs and cell membranes. We did not observe any labeled liposomes with encapsulated toxins on the cell surface, confirming the role of the toxin in complex formation.

Hemagglutination Test

Since pBFT2 and mBFT2 tend to form H-bonds and coordinate bonds with membrane components, including LPS, we examined the hemagglutination and lectin activity for both types of the toxin. First, increasing concentrations (0.1–2.5 μg) of mBFT2 were tested for the ability to induce hemagglutination. We detected erythrocyte hemagglutination with mBFT2 at concentrations of 2.5 and 2 μg (**Figures 7L,M**). pBFT2 did not demonstrate hemagglutination activity. We also identified inhibition of hemagglutination when mBFT2 was premixed with LPS isolated from ETBF and NTBF. LPS alone did not demonstrate hemagglutination activity (**Figure 7M**).

DISCUSSION

OMVs are considered to be one of the types of bacterial secretion system. Moreover, this secretion mechanism is well known in *B. fragilis* (Patrick et al., 1996; Elhenawy et al., 2014). Recently it has been described that *B. fragilis* contains T6SS, which is likely a source of numerous novel effector and immunity proteins (Coyne et al., 2016). But there is no evidence that this could be the mechanism for toxin secretion. In our study we hypotized that OMVs can be utilized for *B. fragilis* toxin secretion.

In our experiments, we demonstrated that both strains (ETBF and NTBF) of *B. fragilis* produce vesicles, and we detected mBFT2 in vesicles by western blot assay, suggesting that OMVs could be the mechanism of BFT secretion. As expected, microscopy assay results were in agreement with cells fractions and OMVs western blot results. We observed labeled antibodies against BFT2 in the periplasm, in membrane and in the vesicle membranes. Moreover, pBFT2 was detected primarily in membrane fraction but was not detected in OMVs suggesting possible toxin maturation in cells membrane. An NTBF cell fraction and OMVs isolated from NTBF culture were used as negative controls in all experiments.

The main visual biological effect of toxin exposure is that mBFT2 affects zonula adherens by cleaving E-cadherin. We used OMVs isolated from ETBF and NTBF to evaluate their biological activity against E-cadherin. As expected, we detected time-dependent E-cadherin degradation upon ETBF OMV treatment, but no degradation with NTBF OMV treatment, confirming that the toxin is active and associated with OMVs.

According to a recent publication, there is a special mechanism of OMV protein sorting. It was shown in *Campylobacter jejuni* that CDT toxin is not associated with membranes and is localized on the inner surface of the vesicles. This result was confirmed by OMV protease treatment, during which the toxin was not degraded because it was inside the vesicles (Lindmark et al., 2009). We used Proteinase K (20 ng/μl) treatment to determine possible toxin localization by western blot analysis and found that BFT2 was fully degraded within 10 min of Proteinase K treatment. These results indicate that the toxin is located on the OMV surface. To confirm surface-located toxin activity against E-cadherin, we prepared several types of liposomes with different localizations of the mBFT2. pBFT2 was used as a negative control because the immature toxin form does not contribute to E-cadherin degradation (Wu et al., 1998). In HT-29 cells treated with all liposome-toxin preparations, we observed E-cadherin degradation only when the toxin was added to the previously prepared liposomes, indicating that OMV-associated BFT2 is located on OMV surface. We observed toxin-liposome complexes labeled with the lipophilic dye DiI on the surface of HT-29 cells. Complex formation occurred only in the presence of toxin, which acted as an adhesive element. As expected, both types of OMV (isolated from ETBF and NTBF) were found on the HT-29 cell surface. Most likely, the ETBF and NTBF vesicle membranes contain adhesion proteins that facilitate OMV binding to the cell surface followed by internalization.

BFT could interact with a membrane protein receptor sensitive to depletion of membrane cholesterol (Wu et al., 2006). In this study, we hypothesized that BFTs interact with OMV membrane components, including phospholipids and LPS before binding with the potential receptor. First, we identified the *B. fragilis* membrane lipids and LPS using mass spectrometry. As expected, the most represented ions in the spectrum belonged to PE and PC classes, as they are prevalent lipid components of gram-negative bacteria membranes (Epand et al., 2007). Furthermore, we identified the lipid A and polysaccharide chain structures of *B. fragilis* LPS.

These results were further used for modeling and docking experiments. The mass spectrometric analysis results we obtained completely corresponded to data previously reported by Elhenawy et al. (2014). It should be noted that Elhenawy et al. previously characterized the same structure of lipid A and showed no difference between bacterial outer membrane and OMV lipid A structure. We identified that *B. fragilis* LPS consisted of a poly- and oligosaccharide region composed by monogalactosyl and -glucosyl units (up to 8 carbohydrate units in the chain) linked to lipid A-disaccharide.

We used the identified phospholipids, lipid A, and polysaccharide chain structures to model their interaction with mBFT2 and pBFT2. Polysaccharide chain and lipid A showed comparable binding energy values in docking with mBFT2. As expected, we observed the formation of multiple H-bonds between monosaccharide units of polysaccharide chain and amino acid residues of mBFT2, but an unusual effect was the coordinate bond formation between the oxygen of phosphate groups and zinc ion. This interaction is similar to the formation of non-covalent bonds in lectins, which have special binding sites for polysaccharides and form coordinate bonds with metal ions (Sharon, 1987; Abhilash et al., 2013). However, lectins are characterized by non-covalent interaction with sugars, not with lipids. The docking procedure for pBFT2 and LPS components was not performed because we did not expect the immature form of the protein to bind to LPS.

Despite the fact that mBFT2 is a soluble protease, we demonstrated, through the docking modeling that both mBFT2 and pBFT2 might hydrophobically interact with phospholipids. Carbonyl oxygen atoms of PC/PE (as it was shown for LPS components) formed coordinate bonds with the zinc ion located in the active center of mBFT2 after its processing. By diffusion NMR spectroscopy and Trp fluorescence quenching assays, we evaluated the formation of pBFT2-lipid and mBFT2-lipid complexes. NMR data indicated that the fatty acid residues participate directly in these interactions. The mutant protein mBFT2-mut, which does not contain a zinc ion in the active site, demonstrated enhanced affinity for PC, which argues against a major role for the coordinate bonds. We also observed enhanced affinity of the mutant form of pBFT2 for PC, which could result from the conformational alterations caused by the mutation or somewhat increased hydrophobicity.

High lipid-protein tropism was also shown in cell culture experiments. The formation of mBFT2-lipid complexes associated with the cell surface was demonstrated by microscopic assay. It was also shown that labeled vesicles were located on the cell surface. Our microscopy results confirmed previous experiments reported by Sears et al. where labeled recombinant toxin was also located on the cell surface (Wu et al., 2006).

Based on the obtained results, we propose a mechanism of toxin secretion (**Figure 8**). pBFT2 interacts with cellular membrane lipids and accumulates in the inner membrane. In periplasm possibly it undergoes processing via proteolytic cleavage by a *B. fragilis* cysteine protease, forming the active version of the toxin (mBFT2) (Herrou et al., 2016). Oxygen atoms of lipid phosphate groups located on the inner surface of the outer membrane bilayer interact with the active center of mBFT2, simultaneously forming coordinate bonds with the zinc ion. Thermal motion of the protein leads to a local stretching of the lipid, facilitating the cessation of hydrophobic interactions with its membrane pair. Fatty acid tails of lipids tend to occupy the free grooves in mBFT2, resulting in the promotion of mBFT2 outside the outer membrane. At this point, vesicle formation could occur, and the toxin incorporated into the OMV membrane will be delivered to the host cell. However, the proposed model of toxin promotion through the membrane does not exclude the possibility of potential secretion system involvement.

The protein could also be promoted to the OMV surface, forming new, stronger electrostatic and hydrogen bonds with LPS components and disrupting previous focal and hydrophobic bonds between the lipid and protein. Further protein motion becomes impossible due to significant hydrogen bond formation between the LPS carbohydrate moiety and the toxin. The same protein-carbohydrate communication was demonstrated previously in numerous studies for lectins (Soult et al., 2014). Lectins and carbohydrates are linked by a number of relatively weak interactions that ensure specificity. The interactions between one cell surface with carbohydrates and another with lectins resemble the action of Velcro in that each interaction is relatively weak but the composite is strong. Today, the adhesins and toxins produced by *Vibrio cholerae*, *Shigella dysenteriae*, and *Bordetella pertussis* are the most significant microbial lectins (Sandros et al., 1994). To confirm the potential lectin activity of mBFT2, we tested the ability of the toxin to induce hemagglutination. Here, we show for the first time that mBFT2 has hemagglutination activity. However, lectin activity was determined by the ability of LPS to inhibit hemagglutination. We premixed mBFT2 with LPS isolated from ETBF and NTBF and demonstrated alteration of the hemagglutination activity of mBFT2. Erythrocytes tended to form pellets when LPS had been mixed with mBFT2. Of note, pBFT2 did not display hemagglutination activity. We suggest that pBFT2 does not have the ability to induce hemagglutination but acquires this property during processing. Two forms of the toxin that have different hemagglutination properties might also exhibit different interaction with lipids. Thus, we demonstrated that mBFT2 has strong lectin activity that could be necessary for its biological functions.

We believe that the strong lectin-like protein-membrane association identified here could be used in two potential mechanisms of toxin-host cell interaction. Toxin-lipid or toxin-LPS association leading to the local toxin concentration increasing on the surface of target cells may increase contact of the toxin with a corresponding substrate or receptor. Moreover, toxin associated with vesicles could be taken up via endocytosis by eukaryotic cells or undergo a membrane flip-flop mechanism and persist in the intracellular environment.

MATERIALS AND METHODS

Bacterial Strains and Growth Conditions

Enteropathogenic *B. fragilis* BOB25 (Nikitina et al., 2015) and non-toxigenic *B. fragilis* 323-J-86 (clinical isolates kindly provided from the Federal Research and Clinical Centre of Physical-Chemical Medicine Federal Medical Biological Agency, Moscow, Russia) were grown on blood agar plates containing either 5% defibrinated horse blood or brain heart infusion broth supplemented with hemin (5 g/ml) under anaerobic conditions.

Cell Line Medium and Culture Conditions

Human colonic epithelial cells (HT-29) obtained from the American Type Culture Collection (ATCC Number HTB-38) were seeded in 25 cm^2 flasks at 37°C under 5% CO_2 in DMEM (Life Technologies, USA) containing 10% fetal bovine serum (FBS, Life Technologies, USA) and 2 mM GlutaMax (Life Technologies, USA).

Recombinant Proteins and Antibodies

Immature and mature forms of recombinant toxins (mBFT2, pBFT2) were prepared as described previously (Kharlampieva et al., 2015). The mutant forms of BFT (mBFT2-mut, pBFT2-mut) were obtained by site-directed mutagenesis, where zinc-chelating histidine residues were mutated to tyrosine residues (H348Y, H352Y, and H358Y). Detailed information about how the mutant forms of the toxin have been described previously (Kharlampieva et al., 2015).

For BFT2-specific antibody preparation, 100 μg recombinant pBFT2 in 1x PBS was injected to rabbits four times at intervals of 3–4 weeks. Fourteen days after the final injection, 15 ml blood was collected. Immunoglobulin fraction separation from the serum was performed with protein A-sepharose.

OMV Purification

Overnight-cultured *B. fragilis* (ETBF and NTBF) strains were centrifuged at 4500 × g at 4°C. To remove residual cells, the supernatant was filtered using a 0.45-μm pore membrane (Millex GV; Millipore). The filtrate was subjected to ultracentrifugation

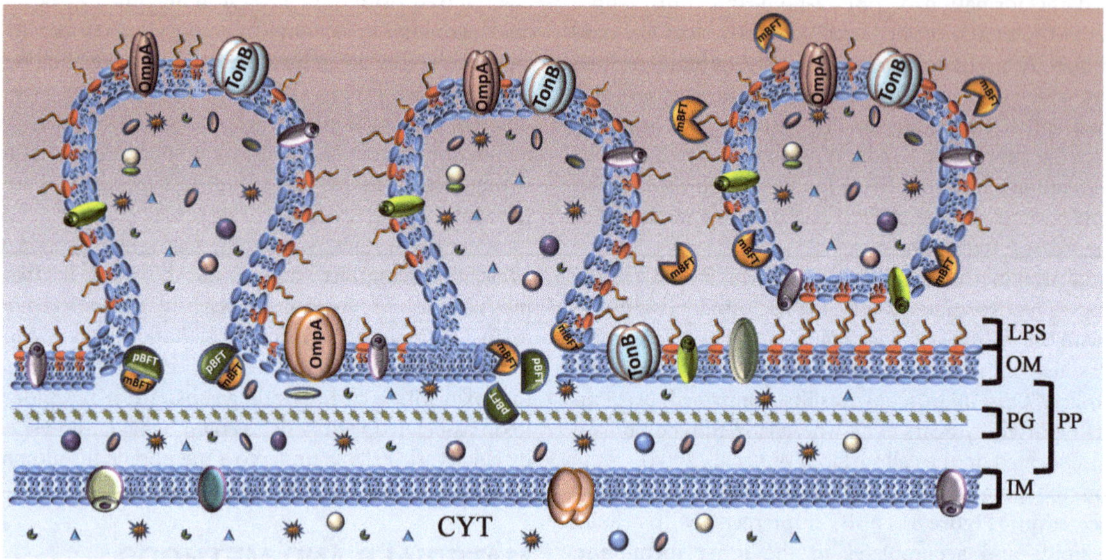

FIGURE 8 | Model of toxin capture during vesicle formation. Toxin is shown as complex of two subunits. Part of the toxin that will be processed (pBFT) and degraded is colored in dark green. Active part of the toxin (mBFT) colored in orange. OM, outer membrane; LPS, lipopolysaccharide; PG, peptidoglycan; PP, periplasm; IM, inner membrane; CYT, cytoplasma. At the beginning of vesicle formation, the major part of the toxin is not processed and could be found in membrane. During vesicle formation toxin could be processed by *B. fragilis* cysteine protease. Free grooves, located on the protein surface, formed during toxin processing interact with fatty acid residues of outer membrane lipids by hydrophobic interaction. Toxin promoted to the OMV surface where it interact with LPS. Incorporated or tightly binding toxin delivered to the target cell by OMVs.

at 100,000 × g for 2 h (Optima L-90K ultracentrifuge; Beckman Coulter). The supernatant was discarded, and the pellet was washed with sterile PBS and filtered through a 0.2-μm pore polyvinylidene difluoride (PVDF) membrane (Millex GV; Millipore). The ultracentrifugation step was repeated. The vesicle pellet was resuspended in 150 mM NaCl (pH 6.5). Protein concentration was quantified using a 2D-quant kit (GE Healthcare Life Sciences).

Cell Fractionation

Cell fractionation was performed as described by Lindmark et al. (2009). Precipitated proteins from cell fractions were collected by centrifugation at 12,000 × g, washed with acetone, dried and dissolved in Laemmli sample buffer. Protein concentration was quantified using a 2D-quant kit (GE Healthcare Life Sciences). In total, 40–60 μg each extract sample was used for SDS-PAGE and western blot assay.

Cells Fractions LC-MS/MS Analysis

Detail information about **SDS PAGE** and **In-gel trypsin digestion** of cell fractions proteins can be found in Supplemental information 2. LC-MS/MS analysis of tryptic peptides was carried out using Ultimate-3000 HPLC system (Thermo Scientific) coupled to a maXis qTOF after HDC-cell upgrade (Bruker) with a nano-electrospray source. Chromatographic separation of peptides was performed on a C-18 reversed phase column (Zorbax 300SB-C18, 150 mm x 75 um, particle diameter 3.5 um, Agilent). Gradient parameters were as follows: 5–35% acetonitrile in aqueous 0.1% (v/v) formic acid, duration 120 min, column flow 0.3 ul/min. Positive MS and MS/MS spectra were aquired using AutoMS/MS mode (capillary voltage 1700, curtain gas flow 4 l/min, curtain gas temperature 170 C, spectra rate 10 Hz, 4 precursors, m/z range 50–2200, active exclusion after 2 spectra, release after 0.5 min). Detail information about **Search Database Creation** and **Proteins and Peptides Identification** can be found in Supplemental information 2.

SDS-PAGE and Western Blot Analysis

The isolated OMVs and different cellular extracts were mixed with Laemmli sample buffer (1:1) containing CHAPS and separated by SDS-PAGE. A total of 40 μg each (NTBF and ETBF) OMV sample and 40–60 μg periplasmic, cytoplasmic, and membrane fractions were used for SDS-PAGE and subsequent western blot analysis. We used BFT2-specific antibodies and horseradish peroxidase-linked anti-rabbit IgG (from sheep, dilution 1:10,000, GE Healthcare, USA). The membranes were processed with ECL Plus western blot detection reagents (GE Healthcare, USA) according to the manufacturer's guidelines. The signals were detected on a ChemiDoc MP (BioRad, USA).

Electron Microscopy and Immunogold Labeling

Ultrathin sections of ETBF and NTBF cells were prepared as previously described (Farquhar, 1956). A volume of 5 μl of each OMV samples was negatively stained with 2% (wt/vol) uranyl acetate for 3 min and examined using a Zeiss Libra 120 electron microscope (Zeiss, Germany).

For immunogold labeling, cells were fixed by the addition of formaldehyde and glutaraldehyde to final concentrations of 4 and 0.1–0.2%, respectively, dehydrated with ethanol in increasing concentrations (70, 96%) and embedded in LR-White resin (Polyscience, INC, USA). To visualize the distribution of the BFT protein in *B. fragilis* cells, BFT2-specific antibodies diluted 1:50 in PBS (1×) and conjugates of protein A with 15 nm colloid gold particles (Aurion, The Netherlands) were used. OMVs were adsorbed onto carbon-coated nickel grids for 2 min and coincubated with labels, coupled with antibodies against BFT, and then negatively stained. Immunogold labeled samples were examined using a Zeiss Libra 120 electron microscope (Zeiss, Germany).

Lipid Extraction

For lipid extraction, 1 ml liquid culture (ETBF and NTBF) was used. Samples were incubated at –77°C for 15 min, then at room temperature for 3 min and centrifuged at 10,000 × g for 20 min. The resulting cell pellets were used for lipid extraction by a modified Folch protocol (Folch et al., 1957). LPS was isolated using the Tri-Reagent method described by Yi and Hackett (2000).

Shot-Gun Lipidomics

Identification of extracted membrane lipids and LPS was performed using a quadrupole time-of-flight tandem mass spectrometer (Q-TOF Maxis, Bruker Daltonics, Germany) with an updated collision cell for electrospray ionization source. Metabolite identification was confirmed by the fragmentation of the detected parent ions. External phospholipid standards (choline, phosphatidylcholine, phosphatidylserine, phosphatidylethanolamine, phosphatidylglycerol, phosphatidic acid, and tetracycline; Sigma Aldrich) were used to optimize the MS/MS-acquisition conditions. We used the following databases for lipid identification: LIPID MAPS database (LIPID MAPS Lipidomics Gateway, a free resource sponsored by the National Institute of General Medical Sciences, USA; http://www.lipidmaps.org), Byrdwell G. Resources for Lipid Analysis in the twenty-first Century (http://www.byrdwell.com), Metlin (Scrips Center for Mass Spectrometry, USA; https://masspec.scripps.edu) and Galactosylceramides and Glucosylceramides (Cerebrosides) (http://www.lipidhome.co.uk/).

Modeling and Docking

No BFT2 crystal structures have been reported thus far, so the atom coordinates for creating 3D models of this protein were taken from the XRD-based structure of its homolog BFT3 (PDB: 3p24 http://www.rcsb.org/pdb/explore/explore.do?structureId=3p24) by substituting several amino acid residues (see Supplemental information 2). The 3D models of the targets (PE, PC, Lipid A, and polysaccharide chain of LPS) were created with the Molsoft ICM version 3.8-3 application (Wesson and Eisenberg, 1992; Abagyan et al., 1994; Totrov and Abagyan, 2001a,b). Detailed information about the modeling and docking procedure can be found in Supplemental information 2.

Trp Fluorescence Quenching Assay

Intrinsic fluorescence of the Trp and Tyr residues was measured after the addition of different amounts of vesicles constructed from PC to 3 nM mBFT, pBFT2, mBFT2, pBFT-mut, mBFT-mut, Proteinase K, or BSA solutions in the standard PBS buffer (Merck) or a low ionic strength buffer (1 nM $ZnSO_4$ in 1:50 diluted PBS). Each protein solution was mixed gently after the addition of the PC vesicles and stored at room temperature for 1–2 min prior to measurements. Fluorescence emission spectra were registered at 20°C using a Chirascan spectrometer (Applied Photophysics) equipped with a thermostatically controlled cuvette holder with slit widths of 4 and 6 nm upon excitation at 280 or 295 nm. Light scattering by liposomes was taken into account. The quenching curves were fitted with equation (1)

$$Y = \frac{Y_{\max} \times X^n}{X^n + K_d^n} \tag{1}$$

where Y is fluorescence quenching and n is the Hill coefficient ($n = 1 \pm 0.3$ unless otherwise specified).

Fitting was performed using DataFit 9 software.

NMR Analysis of Protein-Lipid Complexes

The samples for NMR spectroscopy [500 μg mBFT2, 500 μg phosphatidylcholine (Sigma Aldrich, USA)] were dissolved in water (100 μl D_2O was added to each sample for the lock signal stabilization) and phosphate buffer (pH 7.4). All spectra were obtained on a Bruker Advance III 500 MHz NMR spectrometer (Bruker, USA) equipped with a Prodigy TCI cryogenic triple-channel probe. The sample temperature was kept at 300 K during the experiments. 2D DOSY (the stimulated echo pulse sequence with bipolar gradient pulses was used) and common 1D proton spectra were measured for the study of protein-lipid complex formation (Chou et al., 2004; Balayssac et al., 2009). The water peak in all experiments was suppressed by WATERGATE pulse sequence with five pairs of symmetric gradients (125 ms delay for binomial water suppression and 200 ms delay for gradient recovery). The NMR data processing and analysis were performed using Bruker TopSpin v.3.2 NMR.

Preparation of Liposomes by Reverse-Phase (REV) Evaporation

To prepare liposomes, 30 μl phosphatidylcholine or phosphatidylethanolamine in chloroform solution (100 mg/ml) and 300 μl PBS with 1 ml diethyl ether were added to a 50 ml round-bottom flask with a long extension neck, and the solvent was removed under reduced pressure by a rotary evaporator. Prepared liposomes were dissolved in 200 μl PBS.

Cell Culture Experiments

To examine the biological activity of BFT2-containing OMVs, HT-29 cells were co-incubated for 2 h with 40–60 μg total OMV proteins isolated from ETBF and NTBF. After co-incubation, cells were washed with 1x PBS buffer several times and mixed with 50 μl 1x Laemmli sample buffer containing CHAPS. To detect E-cadherin cleavage, western blot analysis with E-cadherin monoclonal mouse antibody (dilution 1:1000, Invitrogen, USA) and horseradish peroxidase-linked anti-mouse IgG (from sheep, dilution 1:10,000, GE Healthcare, USA) was performed. The membranes were processed with ECL Plus western blot detection reagents (GE Healthcare, USA) according to the manufacturer's guidelines. The signals were detected on a ChemiDoc MP (BioRad, USA).

To determine mBFT2 localization (on the outer or inner surface of the OMV membrane) essential for biological activity against E-cadherin, two different types of liposomes were obtained by reverse-phase evaporation. For encapsulated toxin preparation, 14.2 ng mBFT2 and 12 nM pBFT2 were encapsulated into 30 μl (100 mg/ml) liposomes by reverse-phase evaporation method, described earlier ("Material and Methods"—"Preparation of liposomes by reverse-phase (REV) evaporation"). Proteolysis of unencapsulated mBFT2 was performed using Proteinase K (20 ng/μl) treatment. Toxin encapsulation was verified by western blot with BFT-specific antibodies. For the toxin added to the prepared liposomes, 14.2 ng mBFT2 and 12 nM pBFT2 were added to 30 μl previously prepared liposomes (100 mg/ml), and the mBFT2-liposome mix was purified by one ultracentrifugation step at 100,000 × g for 1 h. The amount of unbound mBFT2 in the medium was determined by western blot with BFT2-specific antibodies. Both types of liposomes were co-incubated with HT-29 cells for 1 h. After incubation, cells were washed several times with 1 × PBS and mixed with 50 μl 1x Laemmli sample buffer containing CHAPS. To detect E-cadherin cleavage, western blot analysis with anti E-cadherin antibody was performed.

For visual assessment of protein-lipid complexes (mBFT2/pBFT2-liposomes) and OMV fixed on the cell surface, fluorescence microscopy was performed. Briefly, isolated OMVs of NTBF and ETBF (40 μg each) and 50 μl prepared liposomes (100 mg/ml) were separately labeled with Vybrant DiI in a 30 min incubation and purified again by one step of ultracentrifugation at 100,000 × g for 1 h. Labeled OMVs, liposomes alone, prepared liposomes with added mBFT2 or pBFT2 and encapsulated toxin preparations were co-incubated with HT-29 cells for 1 h. The cells were then washed ~three times, incubated with DAPI for nuclei labeling and observed with a Nikon Eclipse E800 microscope (Nikon, Japan) or an Olympus Live Cell Imaging System (Olympus IX51, Japan).

Hemagglutination Assay

A hemagglutination assay was performed using red blood cells (RBCs) from humans. Blood was provided by volunteer donors (Lewis $O^{\alpha-\beta+}$). Written informed consent from participants was obtained and approved by the ethical committee of the Federal Research and Clinical Centre of Physical-Chemical Medicine Federal Medical Biological Agency, Moscow, Russia (approval number 1a/2016). Heparinized whole human blood erythrocytes were washed three times by centrifugation at 200 × g and resuspended to 1.5% packed cell volume in 1× PBS. mBFT2 in increasing concentrations (0.1–2.5 μg), 5 μl LPS (isolated from 20 ml ETBF and 20 ml NTBF) and pBFT (2.5 and 1 μg) were independently mixed with the erythrocyte suspension in a round-bottomed 96-well dish and agitated by hand. Separately, mBFT2 (2 μg) was premixed with ETBF LPS or NTBF LPS, and then prepared solutions were mixed with the erythrocyte suspension in a round-bottomed 96-well dish and agitated by hand. A positive result was recorded if hemagglutination occurred within 10 min.

AUTHOR CONTRIBUTIONS

NZ, VT, AAV, AMV, and VP designed and performed experiments, analyzed data, and wrote the paper; DR, IV designed and performed experiments, FL, EG, DK, VM, and VL performed experiments; VG supervised the project.

FUNDING

This research was supported by RSF grant 14-24-00159 and RSF 14-25-00013.

ACKNOWLEDGMENTS

We thank Prof. Galina E. Pozmogova from Federal Research and Clinical Centre of Physical-Chemical Medicine of the Federal Medical Biological Agency for the critical review of the manuscript, Prof. Maria A. Lagarkova from Federal Research and Clinical Centre of Physical-Chemical Medicine of the Federal Medical Biological Agency for cell culture cultivation, Nina V. Seina, Ekaterina V. Surko, and Eskender Osmanov for TEM preparations.

REFERENCES

Abagyan, R., Totrov, M., and Kuznetsov, D. (1994). ICM, a new method for protein modeling and design: applications to docking and structure prediction from the distorted native conformation. *J. Comput. Chem.* 15, 488–506. doi: 10.1002/jcc.540150503

Abhilash, J., Dileep, K. V., Palanimuthu, M., Geethanandan, K., Sadasivan, C., and Haridas, M. (2013). Metal ions in sugar binding, sugar specificity and structural stability of Spatholobus parviflorus seed lectin. *J. Mol. Model.* 19, 3271–3278. doi: 10.1007/s00894-013-1854-4

Balayssac, S., Delsuc, M. A., Gilard, V., Prigent, Y., and Malet-Martino, M. (2009). Two-dimensional DOSY experiment with excitation sculpting water suppression for the analysis of natural and biological media. *J. Magn. Reson.* 196, 78–83. doi: 10.1016/j.jmr.2008.09.022

Cerdeño-Tárraga, A. M., Patrick, S., Crossman, L. C., Blakely, G., Abratt, V., Lennard, N., et al. (2005). Extensive DNA inversions in the *B. fragilis* genome control variable gene expression. *Science* 307, 1463–1465. doi: 10.1126/science.1107008

Charbonneau, D. M., and Tajmir-Riahi, H. A. (2010). Study on the interaction of cationic lipids with bovine serum albumin. *J. Phys. Chem. B* 114, 1148–1155. doi: 10.1021/jp910077h

Chatterjee, D., and Chaudhuri, K. (2011). Association of cholera toxin with *Vibrio cholerae* outer membrane vesicles which are internalized by human intestinal epithelial cells. *FEBS Lett.* 585, 1357–1362. doi: 10.1016/j.febslet.2011.04.017

Chatzidaki-Livanis, M., Geva-Zatorsky, N., and Comstock, L. E. (2016). *Bacteroides fragilis* type VI secretion systems use novel effector and immunity proteins to antagonize human gut Bacteroidales species. *Proc. Natl. Acad. Sci. U.S.A.* 113, 3627–3632. doi: 10.1073/pnas.1522510113

Chou, J. J., Baber, J. L., and Bax, A. (2004). Characterization of phospholipid mixed micelles by translational diffusion. *J. Biomol. NMR* 29, 299–308. doi: 10.1023/B:JNMR.0000032560.43738.6a

Coyne, M. J., Roelofs, K. G., and Comstock, L. E. (2016). Type VI secretion systems of human gut Bacteroidales segregate into three genetic architectures, two of which are contained on mobile genetic elements. *BMC Genomics* 17:58. doi: 10.1186/s12864-016-2377-z

Dua, R., Wu, S. K., and Cho, W. (1995). A structure-function study of bovine pancreatic phospholipase A2 using polymerized mixed liposomes. *J. Biol. Chem.* 270, 263–268. doi: 10.1074/jbc.270.1.263

Elhenawy, W., Debelyy, M. O., and Feldman, M. F. (2014). Preferential packing of acidic glycosidases and proteases into Bacteroides outer membrane vesicles. *MBio* 5, e00909–e00914. doi: 10.1128/mBio.00909-14

Ellis, T. N., and Kuehn, M. J. (2010). Virulence and immunomodulatory roles of bacterial outer membrane vesicles. *Microbiol. Mol. Biol. Rev.* 74, 81–94. doi: 10.1128/MMBR.00031-09

Epand, R. F., Savage, P. B., and Epand, R. M. (2007). Bacterial lipid composition and the antimicrobial efficacy of cationic steroid compounds (Ceragenins). *Biochim. Biophys. Acta* 1768, 2500–2509. doi: 10.1016/j.bbamem.2007.05.023

Farquhar, M. G. (1956). Preparation of ultrathin tissue sections for electron microscopy review and compilation of procedures. *Lab. Invest.* 5, 317–337.

Folch, J., Lees, M., and Sloane Stanley, G. H. (1957). A simple method for the isolation and purification of total lipides from animal tissues. *J. Biol. Chem.* 226, 497–509.

Franco, A. A., Mundy, L. M., Trucksis, M., Wu, S., Kaper, J. B., and Sears, C. L. (1997). Cloning and characterization of the *Bacteroides fragilis* metalloprotease toxin gene. *Infect. Immun.* 65, 1007–1013.

Galán, J. E., Lara-Tejero, M., Marlovits, T. C., and Wagner, S. (2014). Bacterial type III secretion systems: specialized nanomachines for protein delivery into target cells. *Annu. Rev. Microbiol.* 68, 415–438. doi: 10.1146/annurev-micro-092412-155725

Gibson, S. A., and Macfarlane, G. T. (1988). Characterization of proteases formed by *Bacteroides fragilis*. *J. Gen. Microbiol.* 134, 2231–2240. doi: 10.1099/00221287-134-8-2231

Hachani, A., Wood, T. E., and Filloux, A. (2016). Type VI secretion and anti-host effectors. *Curr. Opin. Microbiol.* 29, 81–93. doi: 10.1016/j.mib.2015.11.006

Herrou, J., Choi, V. M., Bubeck Wardenburg, J., and Crosson, S. (2016). Activation mechanism of the *Bacteroides fragilis* cysteine peptidase, fragipain. *Biochemistry* 55, 4077–4084. doi: 10.1021/acs.biochem.6b00546

Horstman, A. L., and Kuehn, M. J. (2002). Bacterial surface association of heat-labile enterotoxin through lipopolysaccharide after secretion via the general secretory pathway. *J. Biol. Chem.* 277, 32538–32545. doi: 10.1074/jbc.M203740200

Huang, J. Y., Lee, S. M., and Mazmanian, S. K. (2011). The human commensal *Bacteroides fragilis* binds intestinal mucin. *Anaerobe* 17, 137–141. doi: 10.1016/j.anaerobe.2011.05.017

Ismail, S., Hampton, M. B., and Keenan, J. I. (2003). *Helicobacter pylori* outer membrane vesicles modulate proliferation and interleukin-8 production by gastric epithelial cells. *Infect. Immun.* 71, 5670–5675. doi: 10.1128/IAI.71.10.5670-5675.2003

Kesty, N. C., and Kuehn, M. J. (2004). Incorporation of heterologous outer membrane and periplasmic proteins into *Escherichia coli* outer membrane vesicles. *J. Biol. Chem.* 279, 2069–2076. doi: 10.1074/jbc.M307628200

Kharlampieva, D., Manuvera, V., Podgorny, O., Grafskaia, E., Kovalchuk, S., Pobeguts, O., et al. (2015). Recombinant fragilysin isoforms cause E-cadherin cleavage of intact cells and do not cleave isolated E-cadherin. *Microb. Pathog.* 83–84, 47–56. doi: 10.1016/j.micpath.2015.05.003

Kling, J. J., Wright, R. L., Moncrief, J. S., and Wilkins, T. D. (1997). Cloning and characterization of the gene for the metalloprotease enterotoxin of *Bacteroides fragilis*. *FEMS Microbiol. Lett.* 146, 279–284. doi: 10.1111/j.1574-6968.1997.tb10205.x

Koster, M., Bitter, W., and Tommassen, J. (2000). Protein secretion mechanisms in Gram-negative bacteria. *Int. J. Med. Microbiol.* 290, 325–331. doi: 10.1016/S1438-4221(00)80033-8

Kraft, C. A., Garrido, J. L., Leiva-Vega, L., and Romero, G. (2009). Quantitative analysis of protein-lipid interactions using tryptophan fluorescence. *Sci. Signal.* 2:pl4. doi: 10.1126/scisignal.299pl4

Kuehn, M. J., and Kesty, N. C. (2005). Bacterial outer membrane vesicles and the host-pathogen interaction. *Genes Dev.* 19, 2645–2655. doi: 10.1101/gad.1299905

Kulp, A., and Kuehn, M. J. (2010). Biological functions and biogenesis of secreted bacterial outer membrane vesicles. *Annu. Rev. Microbiol.* 64, 163–184. doi: 10.1146/annurev.micro.091208.073413

Ley, R. E., Hamady, M., Lozupone, C., Turnbaugh, P. J., Ramey, R. R., Bircher, J. S., et al. (2008). Evolution of mammals and their gut microbes. *Science* 320, 1647–1651. doi: 10.1126/science.1155725

Lindmark, B., Rompikuntal, P. K., Vaitkevicius, K., Song, T., Mizunoe, Y., Uhlin, B. E., et al. (2009). Outer membrane vesicle-mediated release of cytolethal distending toxin (CDT) from *Campylobacter jejuni*. *BMC Microbiol.* 9:220. doi: 10.1186/1471-2180-9-220

Mashburn-Warren, L., McLean, R. J., and Whiteley, M. (2008). Gram-negative outer membrane vesicles: beyond the cell surface. *Geobiology* 6, 214–219. doi: 10.1111/j.1472-4669.2008.00157.x

Moncrief, J. S., Obiso, R. Jr., Barroso, L. A., Kling, J. J., Wright, R. L., Van Tassell, R. L., et al. (1995). The enterotoxin of *Bacteroides fragilis* is a metalloprotease. *Infect. Immun.* 63, 175–181.

Nikitina, A. S., Kharlampieva, D. D., Babenko, V. V., Shirokov, D. A., Vakhitova, M. T., Manolov, A. I., et al. (2015). Complete genome sequence of an enterotoxigenic *Bacteroides fragilis* clinical isolate. *Genome Announc.* 3:e00450-15. doi: 10.1128/genomeA.00450-15

Patrick, S., McKenna, J. P., O'Hagan, S., and Dermott, E. (1996). A comparison of the haemagglutinating and enzymic activities of *Bacteroides fragilis* whole cells and outer membrane vesicles. *Microb. Pathog.* 20, 191–202. doi: 10.1006/mpat.1996.0018

Prindiville, T. P., Sheikh, R. A., Cohen, S. H., Tang, Y. J., Cantrell, M. C., Silva, J., et al. (2000). *Bacteroides fragilis* enterotoxin gene sequences in patients with inflammatory bowel disease. *Emerging Infect. Dis.* 6, 171–174. doi: 10.3201/eid0602.000210

Remacle, A. G., Shiryaev, S. A., and Strongin, A. Y. (2014). Distinct interactions with cellular E-cadherin of the two virulent metalloproteinases encoded by a *Bacteroides fragilis* pathogenicity island. *PLoS ONE* 9:e113896. doi: 10.1371/journal.pone.0113896

Richards, R. L., Moss, J., Alving, C. R., Fishman, P. H., and Brady, R. O. (1979). Choleragen (cholera toxin): a bacterial lectin. *Proc. Natl. Acad. Sci. U.S.A.* 76, 1673–1676. doi: 10.1073/pnas.76.4.1673

Sandros, J., Rozdzinski, E., Zheng, J., Cowburn, D., and Tuomanen, E. (1994). Lectin domains in the toxin of *Bordetella pertussis*: selectin mimicry linked to microbial pathogenesis. *Glycoconj. J.* 11, 501–506. doi: 10.1007/BF00731300

Scotto d'Abusco, A. S., Del Grosso, M., Censini, S., Covacci, A., and Pantosti, A. (2000). The alleles of the bft gene are distributed differently among enterotoxigenic *Bacteroides fragilis* strains from human sources and can be present in double copies. *J. Clin. Microbiol.* 38, 607–612.

Sharon, N. (1987). Bacterial lectins, cell-cell recognition and infectious disease. *FEBS Lett.* 217, 145–157. doi: 10.1016/0014-5793(87)80654-3

Shen, Y., Giardino Torchia, M. L., Lawson, G. W., Karp, C. L., Ashwell, J. D., and Mazmanian, S. K. (2012). Outer membrane vesicles of a human commensal mediate immune regulation and disease protection. *Cell Host Microbe* 12, 509–520. doi: 10.1016/j.chom.2012.08.004

Soult, M. C., Dobrydneva, Y., Wahab, K. H., Britt, L. D., and Sullivan, C. J. (2014). Outer membrane vesicles alter inflammation and coagulation mediators. *J. Surg. Res.* 192, 134–142. doi: 10.1016/j.jss.2014.05.007

Toprak, N. U., Yagci, A., Gulluoglu, B. M., Akin, M. L., Demirkalem, P., Celenk, T., et al. (2006). A possible role of *Bacteroides fragilis* enterotoxin in the aetiology of colorectal cancer. *Clin. Microbiol. Infect.* 12, 782–786. doi: 10.1111/j.1469-0691.2006.01494.x

Totrov, M., and Abagyan, R. (2001a). "Protein-Ligand docking as an energy optimization problem," in *Drug-Receptor Thermodynamics: Introduction and Applications*, ed R. B. Raffa (John Wiley & Sons), 603–624.

Totrov, M., and Abagyan, R. (2001b). Rapid boundary element solvation electrostatics calculations in folding simulations: successful folding of a 23-residue peptide. *Biopolymers* 60, 124–133. doi: 10.1002/1097-0282(2001)60:2<124::AID-BIP1008>3.0.CO;2-S

Wallden, K., Rivera-Calzada, A., and Waksman, G. (2010). Type IV secretion systems: versatility and diversity in function. *Cell. Microbiol.* 12, 1203–1212. doi: 10.1111/j.1462-5822.2010.01499.x

Wang, R. C., Seror, S. J., Blight, M., Pratt, J. M., Broome-Smith, J. K., and Holland, I. B. (1991). Analysis of the membrane organization of an *Escherichia coli* protein translocator, HlyB, a member of a large family of prokaryote and eukaryote surface transport proteins. *J. Mol. Biol.* 217, 441–454. doi: 10.1016/0022-2836(91)90748-U

Wesson, L., and Eisenberg, D. (1992). Atomic solvation parameters applied to molecular dynamics of proteins in solution. *Protein Sci.* 1, 227–235. doi: 10.1002/pro.5560010204

Wilson, M. M., Anderson, D. E., and Bernstein, H. D. (2015). Analysis of the outer membrane proteome and secretome of *Bacteroides fragilis* reveals a multiplicity of secretion mechanisms. *PLoS ONE* 10:e0117732. doi: 10.1371/journal.pone.0117732

Wu, S., Lim, K. C., Huang, J., Saidi, R. F., and Sears, C. L. (1998). *Bacteroides fragilis* enterotoxin cleaves the zonula adherens protein, E-cadherin. *Proc. Natl. Acad. Sci. U.S.A.* 95, 14979–14984. doi: 10.1073/pnas.95.25.14979

Wu, S., Shin, J., Zhang, G., Cohen, M., Franco, A., and Sears, C. L. (2006). The *Bacteroides fragilis* toxin binds to a specific intestinal epithelial cell receptor. *Infect. Immun.* 74, 5382–5390. doi: 10.1128/IAI.00060-06

Yi, E. C., and Hackett, M. (2000). Rapid isolation method for lipopolysaccharide and lipid A from gram-negative bacteria. *Analyst* 125, 651–656. doi: 10.1039/b000368i

7

Versatility of the BID Domain: Conserved Function as Type-IV-Secretion-Signal and Secondarily Evolved Effector Functions within *Bartonella*-Infected Host Cells

*Alexander Wagner, Colin Tittes and Christoph Dehio**

Biozentrum, University of Basel, Basel, Switzerland

Correspondence:
Christoph Dehio
christoph.dehio@unibas.ch

Bartonella spp. are facultative intracellular pathogens that infect a wide range of mammalian hosts including humans. In order to subvert cellular functions and the innate immune response of their hosts, these pathogens utilize a VirB/VirD4 type-IV-secretion (T4S) system to translocate *Bartonella* effector proteins (Beps) into host cells. Crucial for this process is the Bep intracellular delivery (BID) domain that together with a C-terminal stretch of positively charged residues constitutes a bipartite T4S signal. This function in T4S is evolutionarily conserved with BID domains present in bacterial toxins and relaxases. Strikingly, some BID domains of Beps have evolved secondary functions to modulate host cell and innate immune pathways in favor of *Bartonella* infection. For instance, BID domains mediate F-actin-dependent bacterial internalization, inhibition of apoptosis, or modulate cell migration. Recently, crystal structures of three BID domains from different Beps have been solved, revealing a conserved fold formed by a four-helix bundle topped with a hook. While the conserved BID domain fold might preserve its genuine role in T4S, the highly variable surfaces characteristic for BID domains may facilitate secondary functions. In this review, we summarize our current knowledge on evolutionary and structural traits as well as functional aspects of the BID domain with regard to T4S and pathogenesis.

Keywords: Type-IV-secretion, VirB/VirD4, Bartonella, α-proteobacteria, Bartonella effector proteins, relaxases, BID domain, pathogenesis

INTRODUCTION

Type-IV-secretion (T4S) systems are multiprotein complexes embedded in the cell envelope of Gram-negative and Gram-positive bacteria and some archaea (Berge et al., 2017). They represent versatile nanomachines that fulfill diverse functions including (1) contact-dependent transfer of DNA (conjugation), (2) contact-dependent transfer of bacterial effector proteins into eukaryotic host cells, (3) contact-dependent toxin delivery into bacterial cells, (4) secretion of DNA into the extracellular milieu, and (5) uptake of DNA from the environment (Waksman, 2019). T4S systems can be, based on their architectural complexity, categorized into two classes: T4AS (12 subunits) and T4BS (>25 subunits) systems (Waksman, 2019). Based on the paradigmatic *Agrobacterium tumefaciens* VirB/VirD4 T4AS system, the subunits are named VirB1–11 and VirD4 (Li and Christie, 2018). VirB2–11 are essential for the assembly of the T4S system machinery and substrate translocation. The membrane-bound ATPase VirD4—also known as the T4S coupling protein (T4CP)—is crucial for the recognition of T4S substrates prior to translocation.

The majority of T4S substrates possess a non-cleavable T4S signal at their C-termini consisting of only a few positively charged or hydrophobic residues (Christie et al., 2014). However, some T4S signals form a larger structural scaffold, as for instance, the globular TSA domain of conjugative relaxase TraI encoded by plasmid R1 (Redzej et al., 2013). Another example constitutes the approximately 100-aa-long BID (Bep intracellular delivery) domain that together with a short positively charged C-terminal tail forms a bipartite T4S signal proposed to interact with the T4CP (Schulein et al., 2005; Stanger et al., 2017). The BID domain is present in α-proteobacterial toxins, relaxases, and Beps (*Bartonella* effector proteins) (**Figure 1A**), the latter representing numerous host cell-targeted effectors of pathogenic *Bartonella* species (Wagner and Dehio, 2019). The vast majority of BID domain-containing T4S substrates are genetically linked to a T4S system that resembles the canonical *A. tumefaciens* VirB/VirD4 T4S system (**Figure 1B**). VirD4-T4CPs associated with BID domain-containing T4S substrates form a monophyletic group among T4CP subtypes, indicating a coevolutionary trajectory to maintain interaction of this sublineage with BID domains (Schulein et al., 2005). Multiple studies with the model pathogen *Bartonella henselae* (*Bhe*) showed that Beps are translocated *via* a VirB/VirD4 T4S system into various host cell types to modulate diverse cellular and innate immune functions allowing *Bartonella* to spread and establish long-lasting hemotrophic infections in its mammalian host (Schulein et al., 2005; Schmid et al., 2006; Truttmann et al., 2011a; Okujava et al., 2014).

Beps are multi-domain proteins. A majority of Beps possess an N-terminal FIC (Filamentation induced by cAMP) domain that confers posttranslational modifications, a central connecting OB (oligonucleotide binding) fold, and a C-terminal BID domain (Engel et al., 2011; Harms et al., 2017b). A previous genome analysis revealed that 70% of all Beps and the interbacterial toxin VbhT (present on conjugative plasmid pVbh encoding the Vbh (VirB homologous) T4S system in certain *Bartonella* spp.) display the canonical FIC-OB-BID architecture (Engel et al., 2011). Furthermore, all Bep repertoires present in the *Bartonella* genus harbor Beps with a derived domain composition, which likely evolved from a single primordial FIC-OB-BID ancestor *via* repeated gene duplication and diversification events. The diversification of Bep repertoires occurred independently in three distinct *Bartonella* lineages, resulting in Bep197–234 in *B. ancashensis* of lineage 1 (L-1), Bep1–10 in lineage 3 (L-3), and BepA-I in the most species-rich lineage 4 (L-4) (Harms et al., 2017). Instead of a FIC domain, the derived Beps possess tandem-repeated tyrosine phosphorylation (pY) motifs that are phosphorylated by endogenous host cell kinases, and/or additional BID domains (Wagner and Dehio, 2019). While the original function as T4S signal is preserved among C-terminal BID domains, some BID domains have secondarily evolved effector functions within host cells. These functions include inhibition of apoptosis, bacterial uptake *via* rearrangement of the F-actin cytoskeleton, and modulation of cell migration of infected host cells (Truttmann et al., 2011a; Pulliainen et al., 2012; Okujava et al., 2014).

In this review, we will focus on the evolution and classification of BID domains based on their presence in different T4S substrates. We will furthermore discuss structural and functional aspects of the BID domain with regard to T4S and the subversion of host cell function.

CLASSIFICATION AND STRUCTURAL FEATURES OF BID DOMAINS

Classification of BID Domains

BID domains display high sequence variability. Their classification is mainly based on their position within the multi-domain relaxases and Beps (**Figure 1A**; Stanger et al., 2017). C-terminal BID domains that serve as part of the T4S signal are designated as tBIDx and nonterminal BID domains as BIDx, with "x" representing a number indicating whether this BID domain is the first, second, third, or fourth BID domain counted from the N-terminus (**Figure 1A**). In the Beps, tBIDs have been further subclassified into ancestral tBIDs found in the canonical FIC-OB-BID architecture and derived tBIDs of pY- and multi-BID domain-containing Beps (Stanger et al., 2017).

A recent study reported the presence of BID domains fused to toxin domains (PezT and Zeta) of toxin/antitoxin modules (Harms et al., 2017a). These PezT/Zeta-BID proteins are encoded by conjugative plasmids that are prevalent in various α-proteobacterial genera such as *Agrobacterium*, *Chelativorans*, *Ochrobactrum*, and *Sinorhizobium*. Although it is not clear whether these PezT/Zeta-BID proteins are translocated through a T4S system, their genetic conservation to a *virB/virD4*-like T4S system locus suggests that these proteins are *bona fide* T4S substrates (**Figure 1B**; Harms et al., 2017a; Wagner and Dehio, 2019). Therefore, we extend the classification of BID domains by introducing tBIDα for those present in toxins found in various α-proteobacterial species. In a phylogenetic tree, tBIDα domains form a monophyletic group similar to tBID2 domains of α-proteobacterial relaxases, tBID1 domains of *Bartonella* TraA-relaxases/VbhTs, and the ancient and derived tBID domains found in Beps, confirming that the tBIDα domains form a new class of BID domains (**Figure 1C**, left). Interestingly, tBIDα domains are more closely related to the tBID domains of Beps than to tBID2 domains of α-proteobacterial relaxases, even though PezT/Zeta-BID proteins are encoded adjacent to the latter (**Figure 1B**). Thus, tBIDα domains are likely not the result of gene duplication and reshuffling events of relaxase tBID1/2 domains as proposed for the tBID1 domain of VbhT that is virtually identical to the tBID1 domains of *Bartonella* TraA relaxases (Harms et al., 2017a).

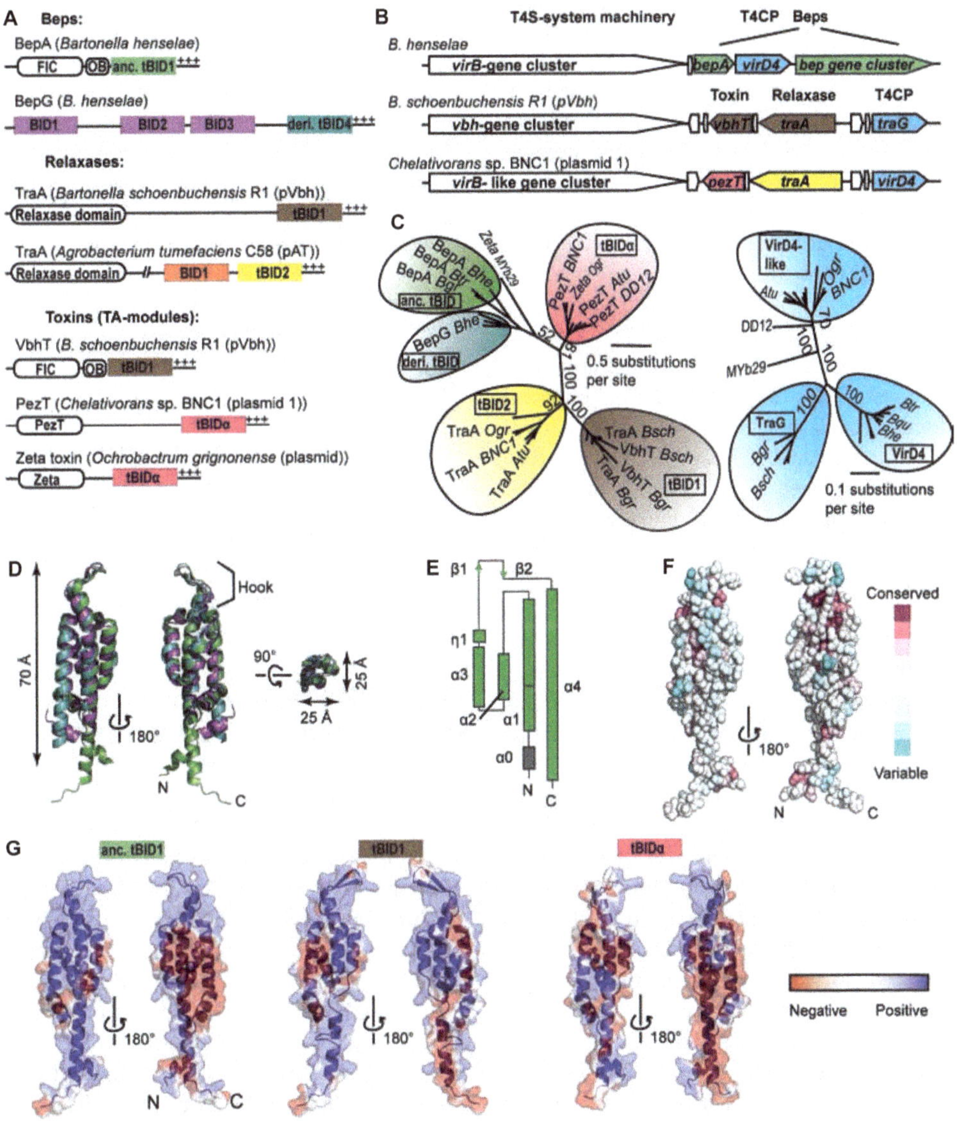

FIGURE 1 | Classification and structural features of BID domains. **(A)** Domain architecture of BID domain-containing type-IV-secretion (T4S) substrates found within α-proteobacteria. N-terminal, catalytic domains (FIC, relaxase domain, PezT, Zeta) and the OB (oligonucleotide binding) fold are displayed as white rectangles, respectively. BIDx and tBIDx domains are colored based on the subclass. +++, positively charged tail; anc., ancestral; deri., derived. **(B)** Synteny of representative BID domain-containing T4S substrate genes and adjacent *virB/virD4-like* T4S-system locus and genes involved in plasmid conjugation (the latter two are represented in white). The color code of BID domain-encoding genes is the same as of the respective BID domains displayed in **(A)**. Homologs of T4S coupling protein (T4CP) are depicted in blue. **(C)** Simplified neighbor-joining distance-based tree representations of the multiple sequence alignment of (left) terminal BIDs [tBIDs, color code as in **(A)**] and (right) the soluble domains of VirD4-like T4CPs that are associated with the tBIDs. Highlighted are representative proteins (per subfamily) encoded by: *B. grahamii* (*Bgr*), *B. tribocorum* (*Btr*), *B. henselae* (*Bhe*), *B. schoenbuchensis pVbh* (*Bsch*), *Agrobacterium tumefaciens* C58 pAT (*Atu*), *Chelativorans* sp. BNC1 plasmid 1 (BNC1), *Ochrobactrum grignonense* plasmid (*Ogr*), *Ochrobactrum sp.* MYb29 (MYb29), and *Shinella sp.* DD12 (DD12). **(D)** The similarity and compact nature of the BID fold is highlighted through superposition of the three solved BID domains: *Bro*Bep6_tBID1 (green; PDB: 4YK1), *Bcl*Bep9_tBID1 (cyan; PDB: 4YK2), and *Bhe*BepE_BID1 (purple; PDB: 4YK3). **(E)** Topology representation of *Bro*Bep6_tBID1. **(D,E)** are redrawn from Stanger et al. (2017) to adapt the color code to the remaining figure. **(F)** Residue conservation is rather low among BID domains of Beps. Depicted is the overall conservation score of BID domains mapped on the surface representation of *Bro*Bep6_tBID1. The color code is based on the ConSurf color scale (Ashkenazy et al., 2016). **(G)** Electrostatic potential mapped on the surfaces of experimentally determined (anc. tBID1 of *Bro*Bep6) and modeled (tBID1 of VbhT from *Bsch* and tBIDα from PezT from BNC1) tBID domains. Protein backbones are depicted as cartoon representation. The color code highlighting the electrostatic potential ranges from red (negative) to blue (positive).

The coevolutionary trajectory of tBID domains with their cognate T4CP is evident for tBID1 domains (TraA/VbhT) and TraG and for ancestral/derived tBIDs (Beps) with VirD4 (**Figure 1C**). In contrast, tBID2 (α-proteobacterial relaxases)- and tBIDα (PezT/Zeta-BID)-containing proteins supposedly interact with the same VirD4-like T4CP (**Figure 1C**, right), although these tBID domains are as distantly related to each other as tBID1 domains and ancestral/derived tBID domains (**Figure 1C**, left). It is worth mentioning that translocation of tBID-containing substrates through heterologous VirB/VirD4 T4S systems has been experimentally proven in multiple instances (e.g., Schulein et al., 2005; Harms et al., 2017a). For instance, the tBID2 domain of α-proteobacterial relaxase TraA (encoded on *Atu* pAT) fused to Cre-recombinase (Cre) translocates through the *Bhe* VirB/VirD4 T4S system with similar efficiency as Cre-tBID-fusions of different *Bhe*-Beps (Schulein et al., 2005). We therefore believe that coevolution of tBID domains with their BID-associated VirD4-T4CPs has not yet led to the establishment of discrete specificities in recognition – despite the remarkable sequence variability of BID domains.

Structural Features of BID Domains

Recently, the crystal structures of BID domains representative for three different classes have been solved, including an ancestral tBID1 domain of *B. rochalimae* Bep6, a derived tBID1 domain of *B. clarridgeiae* Bep9, and a derived BID1 domain of *Bhe*-BepE (Stanger et al., 2017). All three BID domains are folded to a rigid, antiparallel four-helix bundle topped with a hook that accommodates a position opposite to both termini (**Figures 1D,E**). The shape of the three BID domains is elongated with a length of approximately 70 Å and a diameter of 25 Å, suggesting that this conserved fold might be crucial for the primary secretion signal function of the BID domain in T4S (Stanger et al., 2017). It is tempting to speculate that the hook might play a role in the interaction with the T4CP and/or other components of the VirB/VirD4 T4S machinery. Helix-1 (α1) and helix-4 (α4) can either be straight or kinked (**Figure 1D**). This conformational variability of BID domains at their extremities might be the result of different domain compositions in the remaining part of the protein and/or facilitate novel interactions with host target proteins. Interestingly, the T4S activity of a Cre-tBID1-fusion lacking α1 was reduced to 30% compared to full-length Cre-tBID1, suggesting an important role of α1 in translocation (Schulein et al., 2005).

While the hydrophobic core of BID domains is conserved, their surfaces are highly variable. The plasticity of BID domains is highlighted by the fact that BID domains of relaxases and Beps display on average 14% similarity (Stanger et al., 2017). Sequence similarity is also rather low within the various BID domain classes (**Figure 1F**), with the highest degree of similarity observed within tBID1 domains of *Bartonella* TraA and VbhT, respectively. In general, tBIDx subclasses display a higher degree of conservation than BIDx classes, which might be due to a relieved selection pressure of BIDx domains to interact with the T4CP. Although the surface composition among BID domains is poorly conserved, their surface charge distribution seems to be rather consistent, displaying two highly positively charged areas separated by a negatively charged patch (Stanger et al., 2017). This mainly positive charge distribution suggests that BID domains likely interact with a negatively charged surface on the interaction partner. Furthermore, slight differences in the charge distribution between BID domain classes and even among closely related BID domain orthologs can be observed (**Figure 1G**), suggesting subtle functional differences with respect to T4S efficiency (tBIDx) and effector function (BIDx/tBIDx).

Summarizing, we believe that the conserved rigid fold of the BID domain facilitates its role as T4S signal, whereas the highly variable surface might enable the evolution of secondary functions within host cells.

BID DOMAIN-MEDIATED HOST CELL MODULATIONS

The remarkable degree of host adaptation of pathogenic *Bartonella* spp. to their mammalian hosts has been attributed to a large extent to the VirB/VirD4 T4S system and its translocated Beps (Siamer and Dehio, 2015; Dehio and Tsolis, 2017; Wagner and Dehio, 2019). Most of the Bep-mediated host cell modulations are BID domain dependent and include apoptosis inhibition, F-actin rearrangements, and host cell migration. BID domain-mediated phenotypes are best understood on the molecular and cellular level for human pathogenic *Bhe* and *B. quintana* (*Bqu*). Both species belong to L-4 and thus their Beps are designated with a letter code (BepA, BepB, and so on, **Figure 2A**).

BepA-tBID1 Mediates Apoptosis Inhibition in a Host-Specific Manner

Bhe and *Bqu* enhance the proliferation of human endothelial cells (ECs) by inhibiting apoptosis (Kirby and Nekorchuk, 2002; Schmid et al., 2006; Pulliainen et al., 2012). The antiapoptotic activity was assigned to the ancestral tBID1 domain of *Bhe*-BepA and *Bqu*-BepA.2, respectively (**Figure 2B**). *Bhe*-BepA-tBID1 physically interacts with the catalytic subunit C2 of human adenylyl cyclase isoform 7 (AC7) to potentiate cAMP production (Pulliainen et al., 2012). AC7 is a plasma membrane-bound enzyme, which requires activation and association of its two catalytic subunits C1 and C2 to convert ATP into cAMP (Sadana and Dessauer, 2009). *Bhe*-BepA-tBID1 potentiates the cAMP-triggering effect of GTP-bound $G\alpha_S$ in a physiological context and in a pharmacological context together with the plant-derived drug forskolin, which intercalates C1 and C2 into a catalytically active form (Pulliainen et al., 2012). Thus, it is plausible to assume that *Bhe*-BepA-tBID1 allosterically enhances C1 and C2 subunit association in order to elevate cAMP production. The molecular restraints of the *Bhe*-BepA-tBID1 interaction with C2 (AC7) are currently unknown. However, a *Bhe*-BepA construct consisting only of helix-4 of the ancestral tBID1 domain and the adjacent C-terminal stretch did not inhibit apoptosis, suggesting that helix-4 alone is not sufficient for the antiapoptotic activity mediated by *Bhe*-BepA-BID (Schmid et al., 2006).

Interestingly, neither the BepA paralogs BepB or BepC of *Bhe* nor the BepA ortholog from the rat-associated *B. tribocorum* (*Btr*) displayed antiapoptotic activity (Schmid et al., 2006). The latter is in line with previous observations that only L-4 species associated with significant clinical manifestations in humans (e.g., *Bhe* and *Bqu*) possess antiapoptotic activity toward human ECs (Kirby and Nekorchuk, 2002).

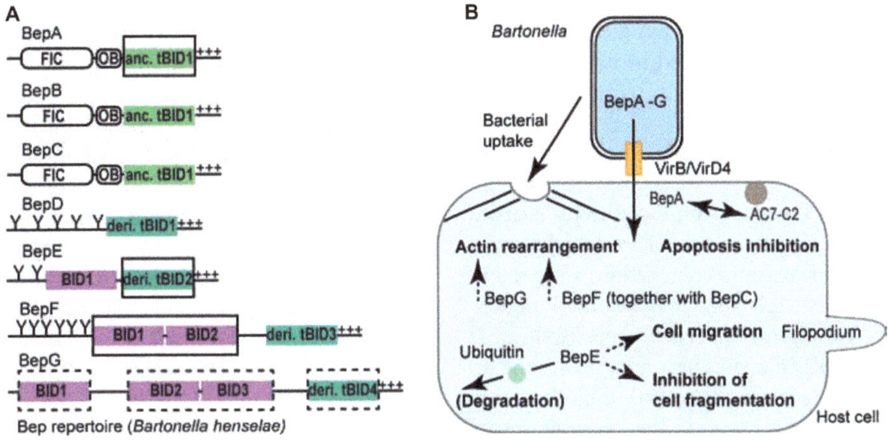

FIGURE 2 | BID domain-mediated host cell modulations. **(A)** Representative Bep repertoire of the model organism *Bartonella henselae* highlighting various classes of BID domains. BID domains with experimentally proven or suspected host-modulating function are highlighted with a full or dashed rectangle, respectively. OB, Oligonucleotide binding fold; Y, Tyrosine phosphorylation motif; +++, positively charged tail; anc., ancestral; deri., derived. **(B)** Schematic representation of BID-mediated host cell modulations. Following the VirB/VirD4 T4S system-mediated translocation into host cells, distinct BID domains [highlighted in **(A)**] alter host cell signaling processes allowing *Bartonella* to survive and propagate within the mammalian host. Host cells can counteract Bep-mediated functions by degrading the effectors following ubiquitination of their BID domains as shown for the BID domains of *Bqu*-BepE. Confirmed BID-target interactions are displayed with a continuous arrow, whereas dashed arrows indicate BID-mediated host cell modulations for which the target protein(s) are currently unknown. AC7-C2, catalytic subunit C2 of human adenylyl cyclase isoform 7 (AC7).

Multi-BID Domain-Containing Effectors BepG and BepF Trigger Invasome Formation

Bhe cells are internalized into ECs either individually *via* endocytosis or as bacterial aggregates in the course of the formation of a unique cellular structure, the invasome (Dehio et al., 1997). Invasome formation is a multistep process, that, following bacterial accumulation at the EC surface, involves F-actin rearrangements and stress fiber formation underneath the engulfed bacterial aggregate (Dehio et al., 1997). Furthermore, in contrast to the T4S system-independent endocytic uptake of *Bhe* into ECs, invasome formation is strictly VirB/VirD4 dependent (Schmid et al., 2004) and is redundantly triggered by either BepG or through the combined action of BepC and BepF (**Figure 2B**; Rhomberg et al., 2009; Truttmann et al., 2011b).

BepG of *Bhe* consists solely of four BID domains that are connected *via* short linker sequences. Hence, BepG likely promotes invasome formation *via* at least one of these four BID domains through interaction with yet unknown host target protein(s) (Rhomberg et al., 2009). Similarly, invasome formation mediated by BepF (together with BepC) is triggered by its two nonterminal BID domains BID1 and BID2, but not by its derived tBID3 domain (Truttmann et al., 2011a). Interestingly, BID2 and tBID3 are more similar to each other than to BID1. The overall low sequence conservation of these three BID domains allows no conclusion on why BID1 and BID2 contribute to invasome formation, but tBID3 is negligible in this process. We speculate that, besides certain, non-conserved residues at the surface of BID domains, also the relative position of BID domains within multi-domain architectures may be critical for effector function.

BepE-BID Domains Antagonize Cell Fragmentation and Promote Host Cell Migration

Bartonella spp. supposedly infect dendritic cells at the dermal site of inoculation and exploit these migratory cells as Trojan horses in order to reach the bloodstream, where bacteria infect, replicate, and persist within erythrocytes (Scherer et al., 1993; Schulein et al., 2001; Okujava et al., 2014; Vieira-Damiani et al., 2016). *In vivo* dissemination into the bloodstream is VirB/VirD4 dependent and relies on the function of BepE (**Figure 2B**; Okujava et al., 2014). *Bhe*-BepE is a pY-containing Bep that contains two BID domains (**Figure 2A**). Although *Bhe*-BepE interacts *via* its pY motifs with several host cell signaling proteins (Selbach et al., 2009), the dissemination of the bacteria into the bloodstream is exclusively dependent on the BID domains. *In vitro*, the derived tBID2 domain of *Bhe*-BepE interferes with a deleterious cell fragmentation phenotype triggered by other Beps (Okujava et al., 2014). Inhibition of the cell fragmentation phenotype is not only restricted to *Bhe*-BepE but appears to be a conserved function among BepE homologs including *Bqu*-BepE and *Btr*-BepE (Okujava et al., 2014).

Besides the cytoprotective effect against other Beps, translocated *Bhe*-BepE promotes the migratory capability of dendritic cells (Okujava et al., 2014). It needs to be determined whether this effect is mediated by the BID domains of BepE or by its pY motifs. However, it is conceivable that the promotion of cell migration is BID dependent, as BID domains of *Bhe*-BepE are sufficient to enable *Bartonella* cells to reach the bloodstream *in vivo* (Okujava et al., 2014).

A recent study showed that the tandemly repeated BID domains of *Bqu*-BepE but not of *Bhe*-BepE become ubiquitinated within host cells followed by proteasomal degradation (Wang et al., 2018). Whether or not this ubiquitination plays a role in effector function of *Bqu*-BepE needs to be addressed in future research.

CONCLUDING REMARKS

The BID domain constitutes together with a positively charged C-terminal tail a T4S-signal that is crucial for the interbacterial transfer of relaxases (alongside plasmid conjugation) and protein toxins by various α-proteobacteria and for the interkingdom transfer of effectors by pathogenic *Bartonella* spp. Besides its genuine role in T4S, several BID domains have adopted secondary functions within host cells such as apoptosis inhibition and F-actin rearrangements. On the basis of the recently solved BID domain structures, their conserved fold may play a crucial role in T4S, whereas the plasticity of the surfaces seems to have facilitated novel interaction areas with host target proteins (Stanger et al., 2017). Future structure/function-related studies should aim to systematically determine key residues of BID domain interactions with the T4CP and/or other T4S system components and with host target proteins. Regarding the latter, comparative analyses of BID domain-host protein interactions evolved in specific *Bartonella*-mammal pairs will enable us to address the role of Beps in host adaptation.

Independent studies showed that T4S substrates are translocated to the recipient cytosol in an unfolded state (Amyot et al., 2013; Trokter and Waksman, 2018). Due to its structural similarity with the intramolecular chaperone IpaD of type-III-secretion systems, the BID domain might similarly act as an unfoldase to prime toxins, relaxases, and Beps for translocation (Stanger et al., 2017). Future work may address the question if BID domains indeed function as chaperones prior to and after T4S. Furthermore, using multidisciplinary approaches such as X-ray crystallography and cryo-electron tomography, future efforts could pave the way for elucidating long-lasting questions regarding the T4S pathway(s) of relaxases and effectors by using BID domain-containing T4S substrates.

AUTHOR CONTRIBUTIONS

AW and CT designed the figures. AW, CT, and CD wrote the manuscript.

FUNDING

This work was supported by grant 31003A_173119 to CD from the Swiss National Science Foundation (SNSF, www.snf.ch).

REFERENCES

Amyot, W. M., Dejesus, D., and Isberg, R. R. (2013). Poison domains block transit of translocated substrates via the *Legionella pneumophila* Icm/Dot system. *Infect. Immun.* 81, 3239–3252. doi: 10.1128/iai.00552-13

Ashkenazy, H., Abadi, S., Martz, E., Chay, O., Mayrose, I., Pupko, T., et al. (2016). ConSurf 2016: an improved methodology to estimate and visualize evolutionary conservation in macromolecules. *Nucleic Acids Res.* 44, W344–W350. doi: 10.1093/nar/gkw408

Berge, C., Waksman, G., and Terradot, L. (2017). Structural and molecular biology of type IV secretion systems. *Curr. Top. Microbiol. Immunol.* 413, 31–60. doi: 10.1007/978-3-319-75241-9_2

Christie, P. J., Whitaker, N., and Gonzalez-Rivera, C. (2014). Mechanism and structure of the bacterial type IV secretion systems. *Biochim. Biophys. Acta* 1843, 1578–1591. doi: 10.1016/j.bbamcr.2013.12.019

Dehio, C., Meyer, M., Berger, J., Schwarz, H., and Lanz, C. (1997). Interaction of *Bartonella henselae* with endothelial cells results in bacterial aggregation on the cell surface and the subsequent engulfment and internalisation of the bacterial aggregate by a unique structure, the invasome. *J. Cell Sci.* 110, 2141–2154.

Dehio, C., and Tsolis, R. M. (2017). Type IV effector secretion and subversion of host functions by *Bartonella* and *Brucella* species. *Curr. Top. Microbiol. Immunol.* 413, 269–295. doi: 10.1007/978-3-319-75241-9_11

Engel, P., Salzburger, W., Liesch, M., Chang, C. C., Maruyama, S., Lanz, C., et al. (2011). Parallel evolution of a type IV secretion system in radiating lineages of the host-restricted bacterial pathogen *Bartonella*. *PLoS Genet.* 7:e1001296. doi: 10.1371/journal.pgen.1001296

Harms, A., Liesch, M., Korner, J., Quebatte, M., Engel, P., and Dehio, C. (2017). A bacterial toxin-antitoxin module is the origin of inter-bacterial and inter-kingdom effectors of *Bartonella*. *PLoS Genet.* 13:e1007077. doi: 10.1371/journal.pgen.1007077

Harms, A., Segers, F. H., Quebatte, M., Mistl, C., Manfredi, P., Korner, J., et al. (2017). Evolutionary dynamics of pathoadaptation revealed by three independent acquisitions of the VirB/D4 type IV secretion system in *Bartonella*. *Genome Biol. Evol.* 9, 761–776. doi: 10.1093/gbe/evx042

Kirby, J. E., and Nekorchuk, D. M. (2002). *Bartonella*-associated endothelial proliferation depends on inhibition of apoptosis. *Proc. Natl. Acad. Sci. USA* 99, 4656–4661. doi: 10.1073/pnas.072292699

Li, Y. G., and Christie, P. J. (2018). The agrobacterium VirB/VirD4 T4SS: mechanism and architecture defined through in vivo mutagenesis and chimeric systems. *Curr. Top. Microbiol. Immunol.* 418, 233–260. doi: 10.1007/82_2018_94

Okujava, R., Guye, P., Lu, Y. Y., Mistl, C., Polus, F., Vayssier-Taussat, M., et al. (2014). A translocated effector required for *Bartonella* dissemination from derma to blood safeguards migratory host cells from damage by co-translocated effectors. *PLoS Pathog.* 10:e1004187. doi: 10.1371/journal.ppat.1004187

Pulliainen, A. T., Pieles, K., Brand, C. S., Hauert, B., Bohm, A., Quebatte, M., et al. (2012). Bacterial effector binds host cell adenylyl cyclase to potentiate Galphas-dependent cAMP production. *Proc. Natl. Acad. Sci. USA* 109, 9581–9586. doi: 10.1073/pnas.1117651109

Redzej, A., Ilangovan, A., Lang, S., Gruber, C. J., Topf, M., Zangger, K., et al. (2013). Structure of a translocation signal domain mediating conjugative transfer by type IV secretion systems. *Mol. Microbiol.* 89, 324–333. doi: 10.1111/mmi.12275

Rhomberg, T. A., Truttmann, M. C., Guye, P., Ellner, Y., and Dehio, C. (2009). A translocated protein of *Bartonella henselae* interferes with endocytic uptake of individual bacteria and triggers uptake of large bacterial aggregates via the invasome. *Cell. Microbiol.* 11, 927–945. doi: 10.1111/j.1462-5822.2009.01302.x

Sadana, R., and Dessauer, C. W. (2009). Physiological roles for G protein-regulated adenylyl cyclase isoforms: insights from knockout and overexpression studies. *Neurosignals* 17, 5–22. doi: 10.1159/000166277

Scherer, D. C., Deburon-Connors, I., and Minnick, M. F. (1993). Characterization of *Bartonella bacilliformis* flagella and effect of antiflagellin antibodies on invasion of human erythrocytes. *Infect. Immun.* 61, 4962–4971.

Schmid, M. C., Scheidegger, F., Dehio, M., Balmelle-Devaux, N., Schulein, R., Guye, P., et al. (2006). A translocated bacterial protein protects vascular endothelial cells from apoptosis. *PLoS Pathog.* 2:e115. doi: 10.1371/journal.ppat.0020115

Schmid, M. C., Schulein, R., Dehio, M., Denecker, G., Carena, I., and Dehio, C. (2004). The VirB type IV secretion system of *Bartonella henselae* mediates invasion, proinflammatory activation and antiapoptotic protection of endothelial cells. *Mol. Microbiol.* 52, 81–92. doi: 10.1111/j.1365-2958.2003.03964.x

Schulein, R., Guye, P., Rhomberg, T. A., Schmid, M. C., Schroder, G., Vergunst, A. C., et al. (2005). A bipartite signal mediates the transfer of type IV secretion substrates of *Bartonella henselae* into human cells. *Proc. Natl. Acad. Sci. USA* 102, 856–861. doi: 10.1073/pnas.0406796102

Schulein, R., Seubert, A., Gille, C., Lanz, C., Hansmann, Y., Piemont, Y., et al. (2001). Invasion and persistent intracellular colonization of erythrocytes. A unique parasitic strategy of the emerging pathogen *Bartonella*. *J. Exp. Med.* 193, 1077–1086. doi: 10.1084/jem.193.9.1077

Selbach, M., Paul, F. E., Brandt, S., Guye, P., Daumke, O., Backert, S., et al. (2009). Host cell interactome of tyrosine-phosphorylated bacterial proteins. *Cell Host Microbe* 5, 397–403. doi: 10.1016/j.chom.2009.03.004

Siamer, S., and Dehio, C. (2015). New insights into the role of *Bartonella* effector proteins in pathogenesis. *Curr. Opin. Microbiol.* 23, 80–85. doi: 10.1016/j.mib.2014.11.007

Stanger, F. V., De Beer, T. A. P., Dranow, D. M., Schirmer, T., Phan, I., and Dehio, C. (2017). The BID domain of type IV secretion substrates forms a conserved four-helix bundle topped with a hook. *Structure* 25, 203–211. doi: 10.1016/j.str.2016.10.010

Trokter, M., and Waksman, G. (2018). Translocation through the conjugative type 4 secretion system requires unfolding of its protein substrate. *J. Bacteriol.* 200:e00615-17. doi: 10.1128/jb.00615-17

Truttmann, M. C., Guye, P., and Dehio, C. (2011). BID-F1 and BID-F2 domains of *Bartonella henselae* effector protein BepF trigger together with BepC the formation of invasome structures. *PLoS One* 6:e25106. doi: 10.1371/journal.pone.0025106

Truttmann, M. C., Rhomberg, T. A., and Dehio, C. (2011). Combined action of the type IV secretion effector proteins BepC and BepF promotes invasome formation of *Bartonella henselae* on endothelial and epithelial cells. *Cell. Microbiol.* 13, 284–299. doi: 10.1111/j.1462-5822.2010.01535.x

Vieira-Damiani, G., Ericson, M. E., Da Silva, M. N., Gupta, K., Soares, T. B., De Almeida, A. R., et al. (2016). *Bartonella henselae* initial infection of mature human erythrocytes observed in real time using bacterial endogenous fluorescence. *J. Trop. Dis. Public Health* 4:207. doi: 10.4172/2329-891x.1000207

Wagner, A., and Dehio, C. (2019). Role of distinct type-IV-secretion systems and secreted effector sets in host adaptation by pathogenic *Bartonella* species. *Cell. Microbiol.* 21:e13004. doi: 10.1111/cmi.13004

Waksman, G. (2019). From conjugation to T4S systems in Gram-negative bacteria: a mechanistic biology perspective. *EMBO Rep.* 20:e47012. doi: 10.15252/embr.201847012

Wang, C., Fu, J., Wang, M., Cai, Y., Hua, X., Du, Y., et al. (2018). *Bartonella quintana* type IV secretion effector BepE-induced selective autophagy by conjugation with K63 polyubiquitin chain. *Cell. Microbiol.* 21:e12984. doi: 10.1111/cmi.12984

8

Two-Partner Secretion: Combining Efficiency and Simplicity in the Secretion of Large Proteins for Bacteria-Host and Bacteria-Bacteria Interactions

Jeremy Guérin[1], Sarah Bigot[2], Robert Schneider[3], Susan K. Buchanan[1] and Françoise Jacob-Dubuisson[4]*

[1] Laboratory of Molecular Biology, National Institute of Diabetes and Digestive and Kidney Diseases, National Institutes of Health, Bethesda, MD, USA, [2] Molecular Microbiology and Structural Biochemistry, Centre National de La Recherche Scientifique UMR 5086–Université Lyon 1, Institute of Biology and Chemistry of Proteins, Lyon, France, [3] NMR and Molecular Interactions, Université de Lille, Centre National de La Recherche Scientifique, UMR 8576–Unité de Glycobiologie Structurale et Fonctionnelle, Lille, France, [4] Université de Lille, Centre National de La Recherche Scientifique, Institut National de La Santé et de La Recherche Médicale, CHU Lille, Institut Pasteur de Lille, U1019–UMR 8204–Centre d'Infection et d'Immunité de Lille, Lille, France

Correspondence:
Françoise Jacob-Dubuisson
francoise.jacob@ibl.cnrs.fr

Initially identified in pathogenic Gram-negative bacteria, the two-partner secretion (TPS) pathway, also known as Type Vb secretion, mediates the translocation across the outer membrane of large effector proteins involved in interactions between these pathogens and their hosts. More recently, distinct TPS systems have been shown to secrete toxic effector domains that participate in inter-bacterial competition or cooperation. The effects of these systems are based on kin vs. non-kin molecular recognition mediated by specific immunity proteins. With these new toxin-antitoxin systems, the range of TPS effector functions has thus been extended from cytolysis, adhesion, and iron acquisition, to genome maintenance, inter-bacterial killing and inter-bacterial signaling. Basically, a TPS system is made up of two proteins, the secreted TpsA effector protein and its TpsB partner transporter, with possible additional factors such as immunity proteins for protection against cognate toxic effectors. Structural studies have indicated that TpsA proteins mainly form elongated β helices that may be followed by specific functional domains. TpsB proteins belong to the Omp85 superfamily. Open questions remain on the mechanism of protein secretion in the absence of ATP or an electrochemical gradient across the outer membrane. The remarkable dynamics of the TpsB transporters and the progressive folding of their TpsA partners at the bacterial surface in the course of translocation are thought to be key elements driving the secretion process.

Keywords: type V secretion, two-partner secretion, Omp85 transporter, gram-negative bacteria, outer membrane, contact-dependent growth inhibition

INTRODUCTION: AN OVERVIEW OF TYPE V SECRETION

Two-Partner secretion (TPS) represents a branch of so-called type V secretion. Widespread in Gram-negative bacteria, type V secretion encompasses several subtypes, identified a–e, that share several general features (**Figure 1**). The cores of type V systems are composed of one or two proteins. The effector ("passenger") proteins or domains are transported exclusively across the outer membrane, following Sec-dependent export to the periplasm. In subtypes Va, Vc, Vd, and Ve, the passenger domain is fused to the membrane domain. The latter is necessary and was once thought to be sufficient for secretion of the passenger domain, hence the generic name of "autotransporters" (Pohlner et al., 1987; Leyton et al., 2012). In subtype Vb (i.e., the TPS pathway), in contrast, the passenger protein generically called "TpsA" is separate from its cognate "TpsB" transporter. In the case of TPS systems, thus, a TpsB transporter can have more than one effector, but this does not generally seem to be the case.

The passenger proteins or domains secreted by the type V pathway are generally long and form fibrous structures, often β helices. They frequently contain repeated sequences determining repetitive folds that appear to be specific to the secretion subtype (see below). The transporter components form transmembrane β-barrel pores. In the available X-ray structures, the β barrels are plugged after secretion by one α helix for type Va and Vb systems, three α helices for type Vc systems and an extended polypeptide segment for type Ve systems (Oomen et al., 2004; Meng et al., 2006; Barnard et al., 2007; Clantin et al., 2007; van den Berg, 2010; Fairman et al., 2012; Shahid et al., 2012). No hydrolysable energy source or electrochemical gradient powers type V translocation, and the processes of secretion and folding are thought to be coupled. In line with the latter feature, general properties of the passenger domains include their slow intrinsic folding rate, paucity in Cys residues, high solubility and low propensity to aggregate prior to folding (Junker et al., 2006; Hartmann et al., 2009; Junker and Clark, 2010). Last but not least, a defining feature of the type V pathway is that protein secretion in all subtypes depends on transporters of the Omp85 superfamily (Webb et al., 2012; Heinz and Lithgow, 2014).

In classical autotransporters (ATs; type Va), the passenger domains are mainly adhesins, proteases, or esterases. The same polypeptide contains in succession the passenger domain and the 12-stranded, transmembrane β-barrel domain (**Figure 1**). Proteolytic processing between the two domains frequently occurs for classical ATs. The prototypical fold of the passenger domain is a β helix, but other structures also occur (Emsley et al., 1996; Otto et al., 2005; van den Berg, 2010). ATs have been the focus of most studies on type V secretion, and they were thoroughly reviewed in several recent articles (Leyton et al., 2012; Grijpstra et al., 2013; van Ulsen et al., 2014).

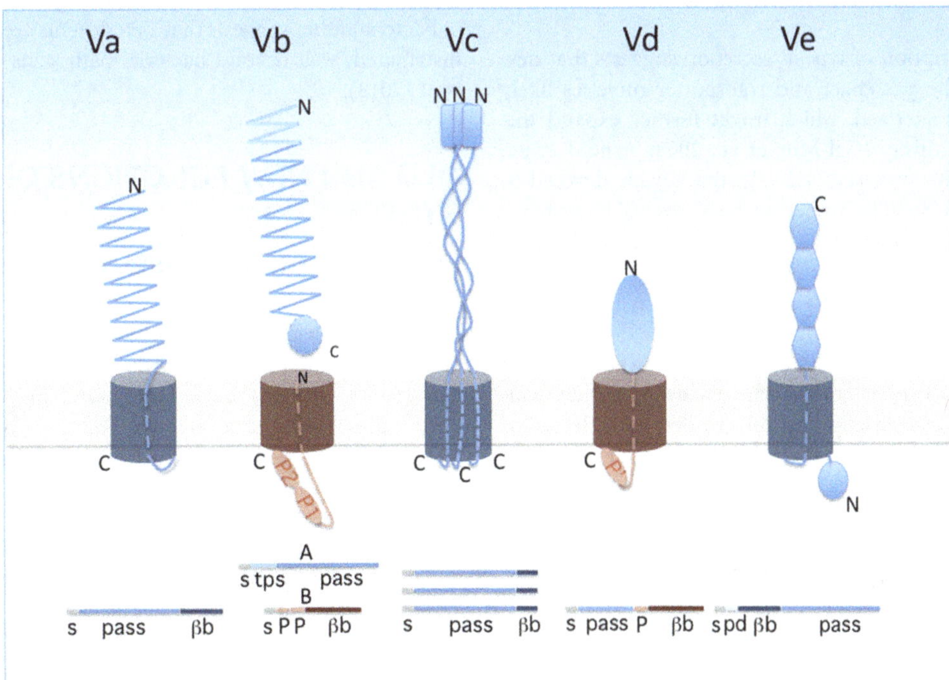

FIGURE 1 | Type V secretion subtypes. The proteins involved in each system are represented in their final form, i.e., after completion of secretion. A linear representation is shown underneath the schematics. The two types of β barrels are colored in dark blue (12-stranded barrel) and dark red (16-stranded barrel). The orientation of each protein is indicated by its N and C termini (denoted N and C). The POTRA domains (small ovals) are denoted P1, P2, and P' (the latter being a POTRA-like domain in PlpD). s, signal peptide; pass, passenger domain; βb, β-barrel domain; tps, TPS domain of TpsA proteins; pd, periplasmic domain of type Ve proteins.

Trimeric ATs (type Vc) are adhesins that may contribute to biofilm formation of pathogenic bacteria and have no known enzymatic activity (Hoiczyk et al., 2000; Cotter et al., 2005; Kim et al., 2006; Linke et al., 2006; Bentancor et al., 2012). They are homotrimers whose passenger domains assemble into long, rather rigid stalks with a "head," and harbor domains rich in β structure interspersed with helical coiled coils (reviewed in Fan et al., 2016). Each monomer contributes its four C-terminal β strands to the pore-forming transmembrane β barrel (Leo et al., 2012).

Type Ve proteins are intimins and invasins (Tsai et al., 2010; Leo et al., 2015b; Heinz et al., 2016). In these proteins, the 12-stranded transmembrane β barrel precedes the passenger domain, making them "reverse ATs" (Tsai et al., 2010; Fairman et al., 2012; Oberhettinger et al., 2012). Their modular passenger domains are composed of IgG-like and lectin-like domains. These proteins appear to also have periplasmic extensions involved in dimerization (Leo et al., 2015a).

The little studied type Vd proteins, of which PlpD of *P. aeruginosa* is the prototype, are hybrids between AT and TPS systems. Homologs of PlpD are restricted to specific lineages of Proteobacteria, Fusobacteria, Bacteroidetes, and Chlorobi, suggesting that they may have been acquired by horizontal transfer (Salacha et al., 2010). The passenger protein carries the four sequence blocks typical of patatin-like proteins (PLP) (da Mata Madeira et al., 2016) and has lipolytic activity. It is released into the milieu from the precursor by proteolytic cleavage. The transporter domain, which remains in the outer membrane after maturation of the precursor, is related to TpsB proteins (Salacha et al., 2010).

This short description of type V secretion suggests that new arrangements of the passenger and transporter moieties likely remain to be characterized, which might further expand this broad secretion pathway (Gal-Mor et al., 2008; Arnold et al., 2010; Jacob-Dubuisson et al., 2013). In this review devoted to type Vb secretion, we will first describe the basics of TPS systems. We will then develop functional aspects of the systems involved in contact-dependent growth inhibition (CDI), which thus far appear to be confined to the TPS pathway and are not found in other subtypes of type V secretion. We will cover the structural and mechanistic aspects of the TPS pathway, and to do so we will compare with other Type V systems where relevant. Earlier work will only be mentioned briefly, and thus readers are referred to previous reviews for more details (Jacob-Dubuisson et al., 2013; van Ulsen et al., 2014; Fan et al., 2016).

TPS SYSTEMS: GENERALITIES

The term Two-Partner Secretion was initially coined to define a distinct secretion pathway exemplified by a handful of systems including ShlAB of *Serratia marcescens*, FhaBC of *Bordetella pertussis*, HpmAB of *Proteus mirabilis*, and HMW1ABC and HMW2ABC of non-typeable *Haemophilus influenzae* (Poole et al., 1988; Schiebel et al., 1989; Domenighini et al., 1990; Uphoff and Welch, 1990; Barenkamp and St Geme, 1994; Willems et al., 1994; Hertle et al., 1999; Jacob-Dubuisson et al., 2001). As implied by the name, the core of a TPS system consists of two proteins, the secretory passenger protein and its transporter across the outer membrane, generically called TpsA and TpsB partners, respectively. In most instances, the genes coding for a TPS system are part of the same operon, but other genetic arrangements have been found (Jacob-Dubuisson et al., 2013) (**Figure 2**). The degree of specificity of a TpsB transporter for its cognate partner varies between systems, and some TpsBs can secrete more than one TpsA (Julio and Cotter, 2005) or appear to be more promiscuous than others (van Ulsen et al., 2008; ur Rahman and van Ulsen, 2013).

The first TPS systems to be characterized were found to secrete cytolysins or adhesins in pathogenic bacteria (Jacob-Dubuisson et al., 2001, 2004). The list rapidly expanded to include other TPS systems with new or unknown functions in various bacterial genera (**Table 1**). Later, a whole new group of TPS systems were found to mediate inter-bacterial interactions involving molecular recognition of closely related bacteria and leading to collective—cooperative or competitive behaviors (Aoki et al., 2005, 2010; Willett et al., 2015b). These "contact-dependent growth inhibition" (CDI) systems will be described in more detail below. Insight into these new TPS functions has considerably boosted interest in the field.

Thus, more and more TPS systems have been characterized over the years, overwhelmingly in pathogens. Whether this reflects their actual distribution in Gram-negative bacteria is very much in doubt, as pathogenic bacteria are much more extensively studied than environmental bacteria. Actually, the discovery of CDI systems and of their roles in collective behaviors of bacteria rather suggests that TPS systems are likely to be widely distributed, well beyond bacterial pathogens (Jacob-Dubuisson et al., 2013).

OLD AND NEW FUNCTIONS OF TPS SYSTEMS

Functions of TPS Systems in Bacterial Pathogens

In pathogenic bacteria, TpsA cytolysins/hemolysins are probably rather common (**Table 1**). Orthologs of the prototypic ShlA and HpmA proteins have been found in various genera. In other cases the specific activities of the TpsA proteins have not necessarily been determined. In many instances, the TPS operons are up-regulated upon bacterial entry into the host, and experimental cellular and animal models of infection indicate their importance in host-pathogen interactions. Examples include the RscA protein of *Yersinia enterocolitica* that limits systemic dissemination (Nelson et al., 2001), and the TpsA proteins PfhB1 and B2 of *Pasteurella multocida* and PdtA of *P. aeruginosa* that were shown to contribute to virulence in models of mouse septicemia and *Caenorhabditis elegans* infection, respectively (Fuller et al., 2000; Faure et al., 2014).

Specific functions have nevertheless been ascribed to several TpsA proteins. Thus, some are involved in iron acquisition, including HxuA of *H. influenzae* (Fournier et al., 2011) and possibly HlpA in the root-colonizing bacterium *Pseudomonas*

TABLE 1 | Diverse functions of TpsA proteins.

Class	Organism	Function	Reference
CYTOLYSINS/HEMOLYSINS			
ShlA	*Serratia marcescens*	Cytolysin, hemolysin, pore forming toxin, autophagy induction	Braun et al., 1992; Hertle et al., 1999; Konninger et al., 1999
HpmA	*Proteus mirabilis*	Cytolysin, hemolysin	Uphoff and Welch, 1990; Zwihart and Welch, 1990
EthA	*Edwardsiella tarda*	Cytolysin, hemolysin, host cell adherence, internalization process in fish	Hirono et al., 1997; Strauss et al., 1997; Wang et al., 2010
HhdA	*Haemophilus ducreyi*	Hemolysin	Palmer and Munson, 1995
PhlA	*Photorhabdus luminescens*	Hemolysin	Brillard et al., 2002
ExlA	*Pseudomonas aeruginosa*	Exolysin, plasma membrane rupture of human cells, pore forming toxin	Elsen et al., 2014; Basso et al., 2017
PROTEASES			
LepA	*Pseudomonas aeruginosa*	Induction of inflammatory responses trough human protease-activated receptors (PARs)	Kida et al., 2008, 2011
IRON ACQUISITION			
HxuA	*Haemophilus influenzae*	Heme acquisition from hemopexin	Cope et al., 1994, 1995
ADHESINS			
FHA	*Bordetella pertussis*	Adhesion to epithelial cells, biofilm formation, immunomodulation	Locht et al., 1993; Anderson et al., 2012; Serra et al., 2012
HMW1/HMW2	*Haemophilus influenzae*	Adhesion to epithelial cells	St Geme and Yeo, 2009
EtpA	*Escherichia coli*	Intestinal colonization, adhesion to host cells by binding to the tip of flagella	Roy et al., 2009
EtpB transporter	*Escherichia coli*	Adhesion to epithelial cells	Fleckenstein et al., 2006
CdrA	*Pseudomonas aeruginosa*	Biofilm, binding to Psl exopolysaccharides	Borlee et al., 2010
Ap58 (EnfA) transporter	*Escherichia coli*	Adhesion and hemagglutination activities	Monteiro-Neto et al., 2003
CDI SYSTEMS			
CdiA	Enterobacteria species, *Pseudomonas aeruginosa*	Contact dependent growth inhibition, biofilm	Aoki et al., 2005; Ruhe et al., 2015; Mercy et al., 2016
BcpA	*Burkholderia* species	Contact dependent growth inhibition, autoaggregation, biofilm, kin recognition, contact-dependent signaling	Anderson et al., 2012, 2014; Garcia et al., 2013, 2016
HecA*	*Dickeya dadantii*	Adhesin, attachment and aggregation on leaves, killing of epidermal cells	Rojas et al., 2002
HrpA*	*Neisseria meningitidis*	Adhesin, binding to epithelial cells, intracellular escape, immune evasion, biofilm formation	Schmitt et al., 2007; Tala et al., 2008; Neil and Apicella, 2009
HxfA*, HxfB*	*Xylella fatidiosa*	Autoaggregation	Guilhabert and Kirkpatrick, 2005
XacFhaB*	*Xanthomonas axonopodis*	Adhesin, biofilm formation	Gottig et al., 2009
FhaB*	*Xanthomonas fuscans*	Vascular transmission to bean seeds	Darsonval et al., 2009
MchA*	*Moraxella catarrhalis*	Adhesin, binding to epithelial cells	Plamondon et al., 2007
MhaB*	*Moraxella catarrhalis*	Adhesin, binding to epithelial cells	Balder et al., 2007
AbFhaB*	*Acinetobacter baumannii*	Adhesin, binding to epithelial cells and fibronectin	Perez et al., 2016
UNKNOWN FUNCTION			
RscA	*Yersinia enterolitica*	Limitation of splenic dissemination	Nelson et al., 2001
LspA1/LspA2	*Haemophilus ducreyi*	Inhibition of phagocytosis	Dodd et al., 2014
OtpA	*Escherichia coli*	Unknown	Choi et al., 2007
PdtA	*Pseudomonas aeruginosa*	Virulence in nematode model	Faure et al., 2014
BpaA	*Burkholderia pseudomallei*	Unknown	Brown et al., 2004
HlpA	*Pseudomonas putida*	Seed and Root colonization	Molina et al., 2006
PfhB1, PfhB2	*Pasteurella multocida*	Virulence in septicemic mouse model	Fuller et al., 2000

**Predicted CDI system based on genetic analysis.*

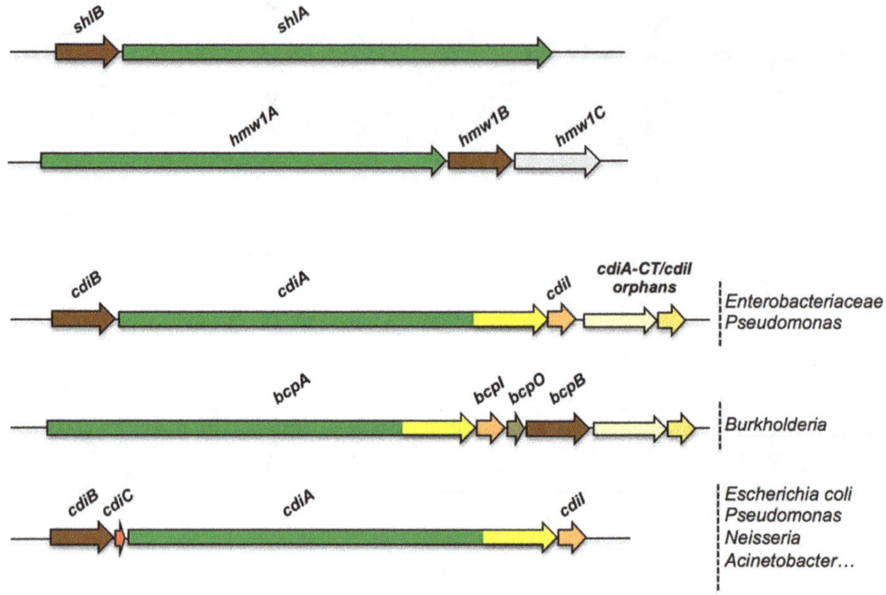

FIGURE 2 | Organization of TPS operons. Typical TPS operons are compared with operons coding for CDI systems found in various bacterial genera. Orphan variant *cdiA-CT/cdiI* cassettes are found downstream of some *cdi* operons that likely serve for homologous recombination with full-length *cdiA* genes, thus contributing to the polymorphism of the toxin moieties.

putida KT2440 (Molina et al., 2006). At the surface of the cell, HxuA interacts with hemopexin, a serum glycoprotein involved in heme recycling. This interaction causes release of the heme from hemopexin, making it available for import by the dedicated HxuC receptor (Fournier et al., 2011). In the case of enterotoxigenic *Escherichia coli* (ETEC), the TpsA protein EtpA is necessary for intestinal colonization. By binding to the tips of flagella, EtpA mediates bacterial adherence to intestinal cells (Roy et al., 2009). The TpsA proteins LspA1 and LspA2 of *H. ducreyi* are required for full virulence of this pathogen by inhibiting phagocytosis through the phosphorylation of the eukaryotic Src tyrosine kinase (Vakevainen et al., 2003; Ward et al., 2003; Dodd et al., 2014). In *P. aeruginosa*, the secreted TpsA protein LepA is a protease that activates the inflammatory response (Kida et al., 2008). Finally, the TpsB protein EtpB and its homolog EnfA, renamed Ap58, of enteroaggregative *E. coli* AEC O111H12 are involved in the adherence and hemagglutination activities of these isolates (Monteiro-Neto et al., 2003; Fleckenstein et al., 2006).

CDI Systems

First described in the *E. coli* EC93 strain isolated from rats, bacterial growth inhibition of neighboring cells was revealed to occur by direct interactions and to imply a specific TPS system which was renamed CDI (Aoki et al., 2005). Growth inhibition is mediated by toxic activities associated with the last ~300 C-terminal residues of the CdiA proteins, called CdiA-CT (**Figure 3A**). Upon cell contact, the surface-exposed CdiA binds the target cell, and its CdiA-CT is delivered, most likely after being cleaved off the rest of the protein, into the target bacterium. CDI^+ cells produce an immunity protein, CdiI, which protects them from fratricide by interacting with the cognate CdiA-CT and blocking its toxic activity. CDI systems are widespread among α, β, and γ Proteobacteria (Ruhe et al., 2013), but the genetic organization of those systems differs between species. Most of them share the classical *cdiBAI* locus found in *E. coli* EC93 (Aoki et al., 2005), but the *cdi* genes of *Burkholderia* species constitute a unique class with the distinct *bcp* (*Burkholderia* CDI proteins) nomenclature. This atypical *bcpAIB* gene organization can also comprise an accessory *bcpO* gene between *bcpI* and *bcpB* (Anderson et al., 2012) (**Figure 2**). Depending on the species, it codes for a predicted periplasmic lipoprotein or for a cytoplasmic protein of unknown function, which is necessary for the function of BcpA (Anderson et al., 2012). In addition, orphan variant *cdiA-CT/cdiI* cassettes are found downstream of the *cdi* operons in some species that likely serve for homologous recombination with full-length *cdiA* genes contributing to the variability of the CdiA-CT domain between CdiA proteins. Finally, several Proteobacteria contain a *cdiBCAI*-type operon, with *cdiC* encoding a protein predicted to belong to the toxin acyltransferase family (Ruhe et al., 2013; Ogier et al., 2016) (**Figure 2**). The function of the CdiC protein is unknown, but it might be involved in CdiBA biogenesis and/or post-translational modifications of CdiA.

Like TpsA proteins, CdiAs are composed of large regions rich in β structure, including the N-terminal TPS domain. They however differ from typical TpsA proteins in their C termini (**Figure 3A**). Sequence alignments have indicated that CdiA proteins share conserved C-proximal motifs of unknown function, such as (Q/E)LYN in *Burkholderia*, VENN in other bacteria or yet other motifs in some *Pseudomonas* (Aoki et al., 2005; Anderson et al., 2012; Mercy et al., 2016) (**Figure 3A**).

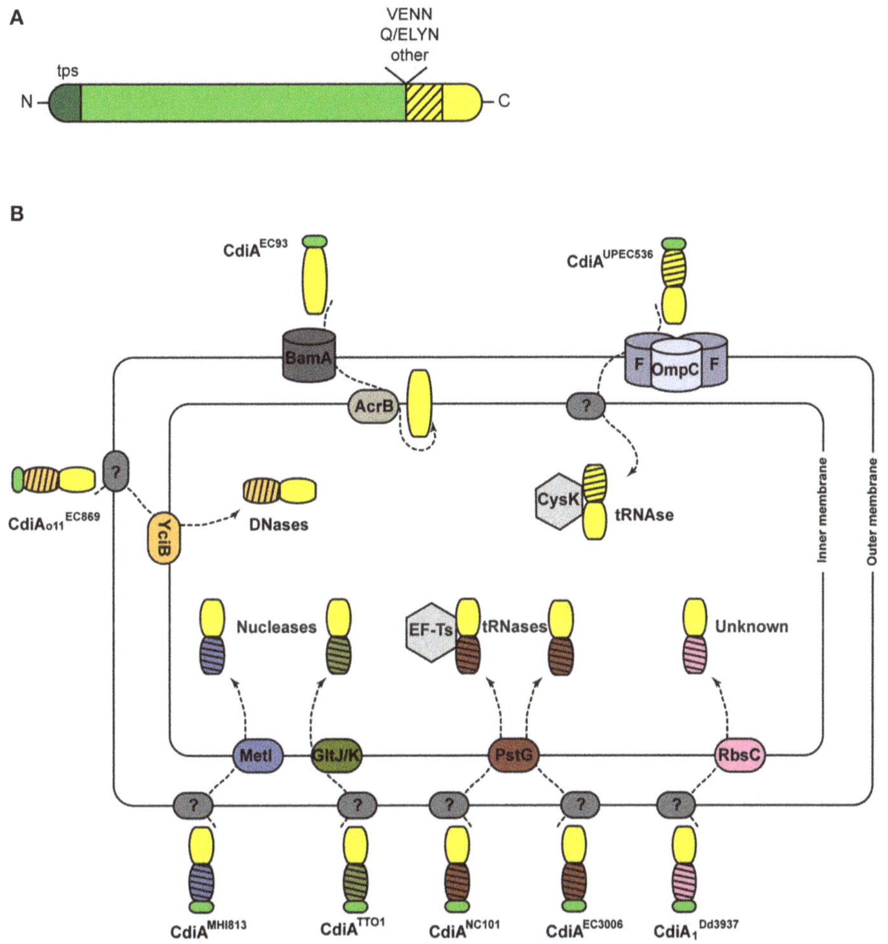

FIGURE 3 | CDI systems. (A) Linear representation of a typical CdiA protein. In addition to the TPS domain (in darker shade of green), found in all TpsA proteins and necessary for secretion, CdiA proteins also harbor specific sequence motifs such as VENN or (Q/E)LYN that separate the long central region from the CdiA-CT domain. The first part of the CT domain (hatched) is necessary for import into the target cell, while the second part carries the toxic activity of the protein. **(B)** Cell entry pathways of CdiA-CT. The pre-toxin motif that demarcates the variable CdiA-CT is represented in green. The receptors of CdiA-CT domains at the surface of the target bacteria remain unknown in most cases (indicated by ?). CdiA-CT^{EC93} of *E. coli* EC93 is predicted to be a pore-forming domain that inserts into the inner membrane. For the other CdiA-CT domains, their N-terminal domains (hatched) are colored according to the membrane proteins putatively involved in their entry into the cytoplasm. The tRNase activities of CdiA-CT^{UPEC536} and CdiA^{NC101} are activated by the cytoplasmic cysteine synthase A CysK and the translational elongation factor EF-Ts, respectively. The CdiA toxin of *E. coli* EC869 is a DNase, and *E. coli* NC101 and EC3006 produce tRNases. The CdiA-CT moieties of *E. coli* MHI813 and *Photorhabdus luminescens* TTO1 harbor conserved nuclease_NS2 and endonuclease_VII domains, respectively. The toxic activity of CdiA produced by *Dickeya dadantii* 3937 is unknown.

The VENN motif of CdiA^{UPEC536} was shown not to be required for toxin import in the target cell (Beck et al., 2014a). One hypothesis is that the conserved motifs might be involved in the proteolytic processing of the CdiA proteins to release their C-terminal domains, as for the bacterial intein-like (BIL) domain of CdiA of *P. syringae* (Amitai et al., 2003). Beyond the conserved motifs, the sequences diverge abruptly, and therefore the so-called "CdiA-CT" domains are highly variable. They have been identified as the toxic domains, carrying DNase, tRNase, or pore-forming activities (Aoki et al., 2010; Zhang et al., 2011; Ruhe et al., 2013; Webb et al., 2013).

The toxins need to reach the cytosol of target cells by crossing both bacterial membranes (**Figure 3B**). The study of their translocation pathways has revealed complex mechanisms that do not seem to be conserved among CDI systems. They have mostly been investigated in Enterobacteria, and a summary of these findings is depicted in **Figure 3B**. The CdiA proteins must bind outer membrane receptors before their CdiA-CT moieties are translocated into the target cells. Only two such receptors have been identified to date, BamA for CdiA^{EC93} and heterotrimeric osmoporins composed of OmpC and OmpF for CdiA^{UPEC536} (Aoki et al., 2008; Beck et al., 2016). The current model proposes that after recognition, proteolytic cleavage releases the CdiA-CT from the full CdiA protein through an unknown mechanism. The CdiA-CT is translocated into the periplasm, where it recognizes an inner membrane receptor. Import across the cytoplasmic membrane exploits specific membrane proteins, and the N-terminal part of the CdiA-CT domain plays a crucial role in this step (Willett et al., 2015a) (**Figure 3B**). Once inside the cell, the CdiA-CT domains deploy their toxic activity, which is dictated by their sequences and their folds (Zhang et al., 2011). Activation of nuclease activity generally depends on host factors. The O-acetylserine sulfhydrylase CysK and the elongation factor Ts (Ef-Ts) are required for the activities of CdiA-CT$^{\mathrm{UPEC536}}$ and CdiA$^{\mathrm{NC101}}$, respectively (Diner et al., 2012; Kaundal et al., 2016; Jones et al., 2017).

The observations that CDI systems mostly target closely related species and that CdiA proteins preferentially bind kin receptors, thus allowing interactions between self-bacteria, suggest a role for CDI systems beyond competition in collective behaviors of bacteria. This hypothesis has recently been confirmed in *Burkholderia,* which use CDI proteins to establish signaling between CDI^{+} neighbors and thus to affect gene expression in immune recipient bacteria (Garcia et al., 2016). This "contact-dependent signaling" (CDS) implies a functional CdiA-CT domain, but it is restricted to specific toxic domains. In line with signaling functions, some CDI systems help to retain genetic elements through a surveillance mechanism (Ruhe et al., 2016). This property is consistent with the fact that most *cdi* genes are typically found on genomic or pathogenicity islands (Klee et al., 2000; Dobrindt et al., 2002; Tuanyok et al., 2008; Tumapa et al., 2008; Siddaramappa et al., 2011; Willett et al., 2015b; Ruhe et al., 2016). The maintenance of genetic material by CDI is linked to toxin exchange between sibling cells and might serve to maintain the *cdi*-containing islands in a population.

Many TpsA adhesins have now been redefined as CdiA proteins (**Table 1**). Some of them contribute to the virulence of necrogenic bacterial phytopathogens, including *Dickeya dadantii* (Rojas et al., 2002), *Xylella fastidiosa* (Guilhabert and Kirkpatrick, 2005), and *Xanthomonas axonopodis* (Gottig et al., 2009), with activities ranging from adherence to biofilm formation to epidermal cell killing. Interestingly, some CdiA proteins appear to mediate biofilm formation, but in a CDI-independent manner (Garcia et al., 2013; Ruhe et al., 2015). Whether TpsA proteins might generally be multifunctional remains an open question, but this would be quite conceivable given their large sizes.

REGULATION OF *TPS* EXPRESSION

Although *tps* genes appear to be expressed during infection and no specific regulatory pathways have been ascribed to this regulation, several factors modulating TPS production have been characterized (**Table 2**). To date, the two-component system BvgAS is the best-studied regulatory pathway, controlling *fhaB* and *fhaC* gene expression of *B. pertussis* (Scarlato et al., 1991). Other signal transduction systems have been identified as regulators of *tps* operons in several bacterial species. Quite frequently, the mechanism of production is closely related to the function of the TpsA protein. Thus, a large number of TPS systems are produced upon iron limitation, such as HxuABC involved in iron acquisition (Wong and Lee, 1994; Cope et al., 1995), or cytolysins/hemolysins whose production in low-iron conditions might be a means for the bacteria to release iron from eukaryotic cells or erythrocytes. In *P. aeruginosa*, the intracellular level of cyclic diguanylate monophosphate (c-di-GMP) controls the *cdrAB* operon (Borlee et al., 2010) through the transcriptional regulator FleQ (Baraquet and Harwood, 2015). In addition, the PhoBR two-component system and PUMA3 cell-surface signaling, both activated upon phosphate starvation, positively control the production of the PdtAB system (Llamas et al., 2009; Faure et al., 2014). Finally, two CDI systems are regulated by the post-transcriptional regulator RsmA (Mercy et al., 2016).

ADDITIONS TO THE CORE: OTHER PROTEINS INVOLVED IN TPS SYSTEMS

A number of TPS systems comprise more than two partners (**Figure 2**). This is typically the case for the *cdiI, cdiO, cdiC* genes of CDI systems. In non-typeable *H. influenzae,* TPS systems are encoded by three-gene operons, *hmw1abc* and *hmw2abc* (Barenkamp and St Geme, 1994). *hmw1c* and *hmw2c* code for cytoplasmic glycosyltransferases. HMW1C covalently modifies Asn residues in repeated sequences of HMW1 with mono- and di-hexoses, which increases the stability of the adhesin against proteolytic degradation and antagonizes its release from the cell surface (Grass et al., 2003, 2010; Gross et al., 2008). Other TpsA proteins are also glycosylated (Fleckenstein et al., 2006), as are the passenger domains of a subset of proteins secreted by the type Va pathway (Benz and Schmidt, 2001; Moormann et al., 2002; Charbonneau et al., 2007; Charbonneau and Mourez, 2008; Côté et al., 2013). In addition to slowing down proteolytic degradation, these modifications appear to modify the properties of the adhesins and to modulate their secretion.

The hemopexin TpsA protein HxuA of *H. influenzae* is part of a three-gene operon, in which *hxuB* codes for the TpsB transporter and *hxuC* for a TonB-dependent transporter (Cope et al., 1995; Fournier et al., 2011). All three proteins are necessary to capture heme bound to hemopexin as an iron source. After binding hemopexin, HxuA would trigger heme release for its capture by HxuC (Zambolin et al., 2016).

Finally, some TpsA proteins undergo proteolytic maturation in the course of secretion, but the genes coding for their putative maturation proteases appear not to be part of the TPS-coding operons. Thus, the mature FHA adhesin of *B. pertussis* results from several proteolytic maturation steps (Coutte et al., 2001; Mazar and Cotter, 2006; Melvin et al., 2015). The protease involved in the release of the mature FHA protein from the cell surface is a subtilisin autotransporter called SphB1 (Coutte et al., 2001, 2003). Although no other substrates are known for SphB1, its gene does not belong to the locus encompassing *fhaB* and *fhaC*. Nevertheless, all three are regulated in a coordinated fashion, being part of the virulence regulon of *B. pertussis* (Antoine et al., 2000). In *P. aeruginosa*, the adhesin CdrA is a substrate of the periplasmic protease LapG whose activity is controlled by the intracellular level of c-di-GMP (Cooley et al., 2015; Rybtke et al., 2015). At low c-di-GMP level, LapG cleaves the periplasmic C-terminal tail of CdrA and releases this adhesin from the cell surface to prevent CdrA-dependent biofilm formation. Yet unidentified proteases are involved in the maturation of other TpsA proteins (Ward et al., 1998; Grass and St Geme, 2000; Schmitt et al., 2007).

TABLE 2 | Factors involved in the regulation of TPS operons.

tps genes	Organism	Regulation	Reference
hxuABC	*Haemophilus influenzae*	Iron-limitation, Fur regulator	Wong and Lee, 1994; Cope et al., 1995
ethBA	*Edwarsiella tarda*	Iron-limitation, Fur and EthR regulators, EsrAB two-component system	Hirono et al., 1997; Wang et al., 2009, 2010
phlBA	*Photorhabdus luminescens*	Iron-limitation	Brillard et al., 2002
shlBA	*Serratia marcescens*	Iron-limitation, RcsB regulator, RssAB two-component system	Poole and Braun, 1988; Lin et al., 2010; Di Venanzio et al., 2014
etpBAC	*Escherichia coli*	Iron-limitation	Haines et al., 2015
rscBAC	*Yersinia enterolitica*	RscR regulator	Nelson et al., 2001
cdrAB	*Pseudomonas aeruginosa*	c-di-GMP level, FleQ regulator	Borlee et al., 2010; Baraquet and Harwood, 2015
fhaB-fhaC	*Bordetella pertussis*	BvgAS two-component system	Scarlato et al., 1991
lspB-lspA2	*Haemophilus ducreyi*	CpxRA two component system, Fis protein	Labandeira-Rey et al., 2009, 2013
pdtB-pdtA	*Pseudomonas aeruginosa*	Phosphate limitation, PhoBR two-component system, PUMA3 system	Llamas et al., 2009; Faure et al., 2014
cdiBAI	*Pseudomonas aeruginosa*	RsmA regulator	Mercy et al., 2016

ANATOMY OF TPS SYSTEMS

TpsA Proteins

TpsA proteins are large exoproteins (~100–650 kDa) that progressively fold at the cell surface in the course of secretion across the outer membrane (see below). In spite of their different functions, all TpsA proteins harbor long stretches of imperfect repeats and are predicted to have high contents of β strand structure organized in fibrous, β-helix folds (Kajava and Steven, 2006a). First observed in pectate lyase (Yoder et al., 1993), the β-helix structure is a solenoid composed of long, parallel β sheets along the axis of the helix (Kajava et al., 2001; Kajava and Steven, 2006b). Its overall shape is provided by the stacking of coils, each of which is composed of three short β strands and forms a complete turn of the β helix. Each β strand interacts via hydrogen bonds with the closest β strands from previous and following coils, forming long parallel β sheets along the axis of the molecule. The interior of a β-helix protein is tightly packed with mostly hydrophobic residues, resulting in a very stable fold (Kajava and Steven, 2006a). Analysis of available structures has also highlighted structural elements that project out of the β-helical core and might carry out specific functions. The notion that the β helix serves as a scaffold to present functional loops or domains at a distance from the bacterial surface does not preclude the possibility that it also has specific functions of its own, such as mediating homotypic interactions that may contribute to biofilm formation (Menozzi et al., 1994; Ruhe et al., 2015).

The structural study of TpsA proteins is complicated by their large size and poor solubility. The fact that they must be secreted by their specific partners to acquire their native fold is a limiting factor for overexpression. Using X-ray crystallography, the majority of structures solved thus far are N-terminal TpsA fragments containing the "TPS" domain, or C-terminal fragments associated with toxin activities of CDI systems. One full-length TpsA structure has been solved, that of HxuA from *H. influenzae* (Zambolin et al., 2016).

All TpsA proteins share a conserved, ~250-residue TPS domain, a.k.a. the secretion domain, corresponding to the minimal region needed for secretion. Located at the N terminus of the mature protein, this essential region mediates molecular recognition of the TpsB transporter in the periplasm, while coupling secretion and folding at the surface of the cell (see below) (Schönherr et al., 1993; Uphoff and Welch, 1994; Renauld-Mongénie et al., 1996; Jacob-Dubuisson et al., 1997; Grass and St Geme, 2000; Clantin et al., 2004; Surana et al., 2004; Hodak et al., 2006; Yeo et al., 2007; Weaver et al., 2009). Two subfamilies of TPS domains have been identified on the basis of sequence alignments (Yeo et al., 2007; Jacob-Dubuisson et al., 2009) and appear distinctly in the phylogenetic tree of TPS domains (**Figure 4**) (Yeo et al., 2007; Jacob-Dubuisson et al., 2009). In addition, subgroups can be defined based on TpsA functions, probably reflecting specificities in the steps of recognition and secretion initiation for these different groups. Thus far, four structures containing TPS domains are available, two of the first family, Fha30 of *B. pertussis* (Clantin et al., 2004) and HpmA265 of *P. mirabilis* (Weaver et al., 2009), and two of the second family, Hmw1-PP (*H. influenza;* Yeo et al., 2007), and HxuA of *H. influenzae* (Baelen et al., 2013; Zambolin et al., 2016).

TpsA proteins form right-handed β helices with three parallel β sheets, referred to as PB1, PB2, and PB3 (**Figure 5A**). The N-terminal β strands cap the β-helix tip by protecting the hydrophobic core from the solvent. The interior of the first β-helix coil is stabilized by a cluster of conserved aromatic residues from β_4, β_5, and β_6 (the nomenclature used here for strand numbering is that proposed in Baelen et al., 2013) (**Figure 5A**) (Clantin et al., 2004). Thereafter, the coils become more regular to eventually display a triangular-shaped cross-section in the C-terminal moiety of the TPS domain (**Figure 5B**). TPS domains present structural elements protruding from the β-helical core. Thus, in the middle of the TPS domain, an anti-parallel β sheet forms a β-sandwich structure with the core of the β helix (**Figure 5B**). In Hmw1-PP, the β sheet is formed by three β strands, with an α helix replacing the fourth one. TpsA proteins

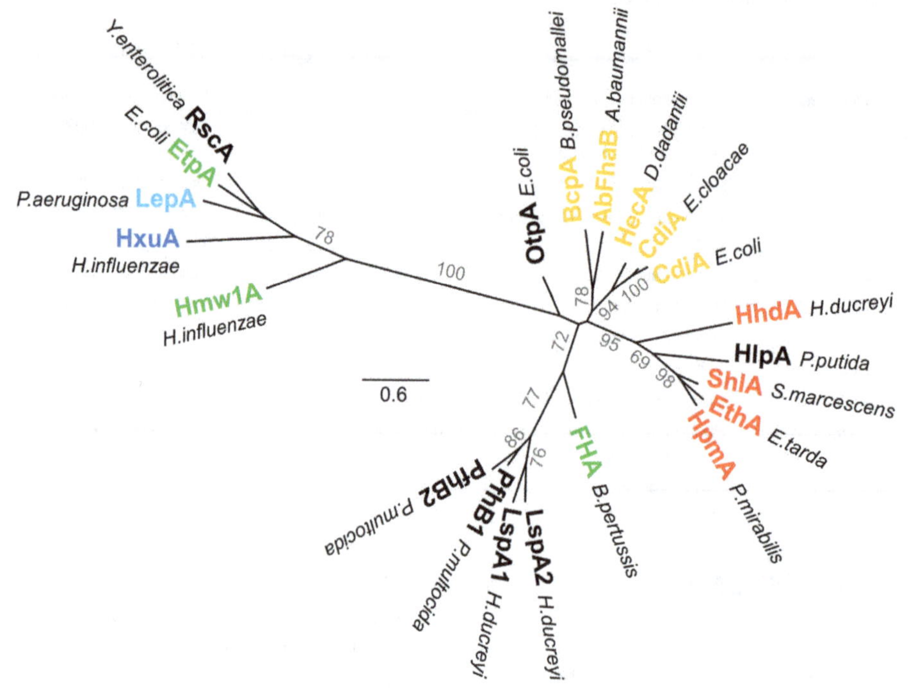

FIGURE 4 | Phylogenetic tree of TPS domains. Phylogenetic tree of TPS domains of TpsA proteins cited in this review. The tree shows the subdivision of TpsA proteins into two different families. The proteins also globally form clusters according to function (red for cytolysins/hemolysins, green for adhesins, orange for CDI systems, blue for proteases, dark blue for iron acquisition). The limits of the TPS domains included in the analysis were defined using both sequence similarities and secondary structure predictions, with available X-ray structures used as references. The amino acid sequences were aligned using Promals3D (Pei et al., 2008). PhyML implemented in Geneious v7.1.2 was used to generate an unrooted phylogenetic tree, where scale bars represent the number of substitutions per site, and bootstrap values above 50 (percentages of 1,000 replicates) are shown next to the branches.

also contain a highly conserved NPNG motif which forms a β turn between strands β_{10} in PB2 and β_{11} in PB3 and is crucial for folding and secretion (Jacob-Dubuisson et al., 1997; St Geme and Grass, 1998; Grass and St Geme, 2000; Hodak et al., 2006). Close to the N-terminus and only shared by Fha30 and HpmA265, a second anti-parallel β hairpin (denoted $\beta_{7/8}$*) that harbors a conserved motif, NPNL, is also important for secretion (Schönherr et al., 1993; Jacob-Dubuisson et al., 1997; Hodak et al., 2006). As this anti-parallel β hairpin is absent from the second family of TPS domains, it is not essential for TpsA proteins in general but probably reflects specific secretion and/or folding properties of the TPS domains in the first family (**Figure 4**).

Due to their large size, little is known about the structural organization of full-length TpsA proteins beyond their TPS domains. Electron microscopy has been used to describe the global shape of 500-Å-long FHA (Makhov et al., 1994; Kajava et al., 2001). Based on electron microscopy and X-ray data, the most likely model for full-length FHA is that of a straight, elongated β helix formed from long regions of tandem repeats. The adherence functions of the protein likely map to extended loops and extra-helical motifs along the mature helix. A non-repeat domain of unknown structure that follows the β helix is also important for function (Kajava et al., 2001; Melvin et al., 2015). Folding of this domain requires the non-secreted C-terminal portion of the FHA precursor that is processed to form the mature protein and controls its release (Noel et al., 2012; Melvin et al., 2015).

The structure of the relatively small TpsA protein HxuA (96.3 kDa, 120 Å long) is shown in **Figure 5B**. HxuA is a right-handed β helix whose N-terminal and C-terminal moieties have different orientations because of a kink in PB1. This twist in the middle of the β helix divides the protein in two segments: the N-terminal moiety with the TPS domain, and the C-terminal moiety associated with HxuA function (**Figures 5A,B**). The latter is highly asymmetric due to α helices and long loops, including the essential M loop, that protrude from the β-helical core. The last residues resolved in the structure form an amphipathic α helix whose hydrophobic face interacts with PB1 while the other is solvent-exposed (**Figure 5B**).

Analysis of the HxuA-hemopexin complex by transmission electron microscopy and X-ray crystallography has revealed that hemopexin interacts only with the C-terminal moiety of HxuA (Zambolin et al., 2016). The interaction with hemopexin induces a large-scale motion of the M loop (**Figure 5B**) which then forms polar interactions with residues in the heme-binding pocket of hemopexin that trigger heme release.

In the HxuA structure, the 66 C-terminal amino acids are not detected in the electron density map. Similar to that of HMW1, the C terminus of HxuA is expected to remain in the periplasm. This anchor domain harbors a disulfide bond, which creates

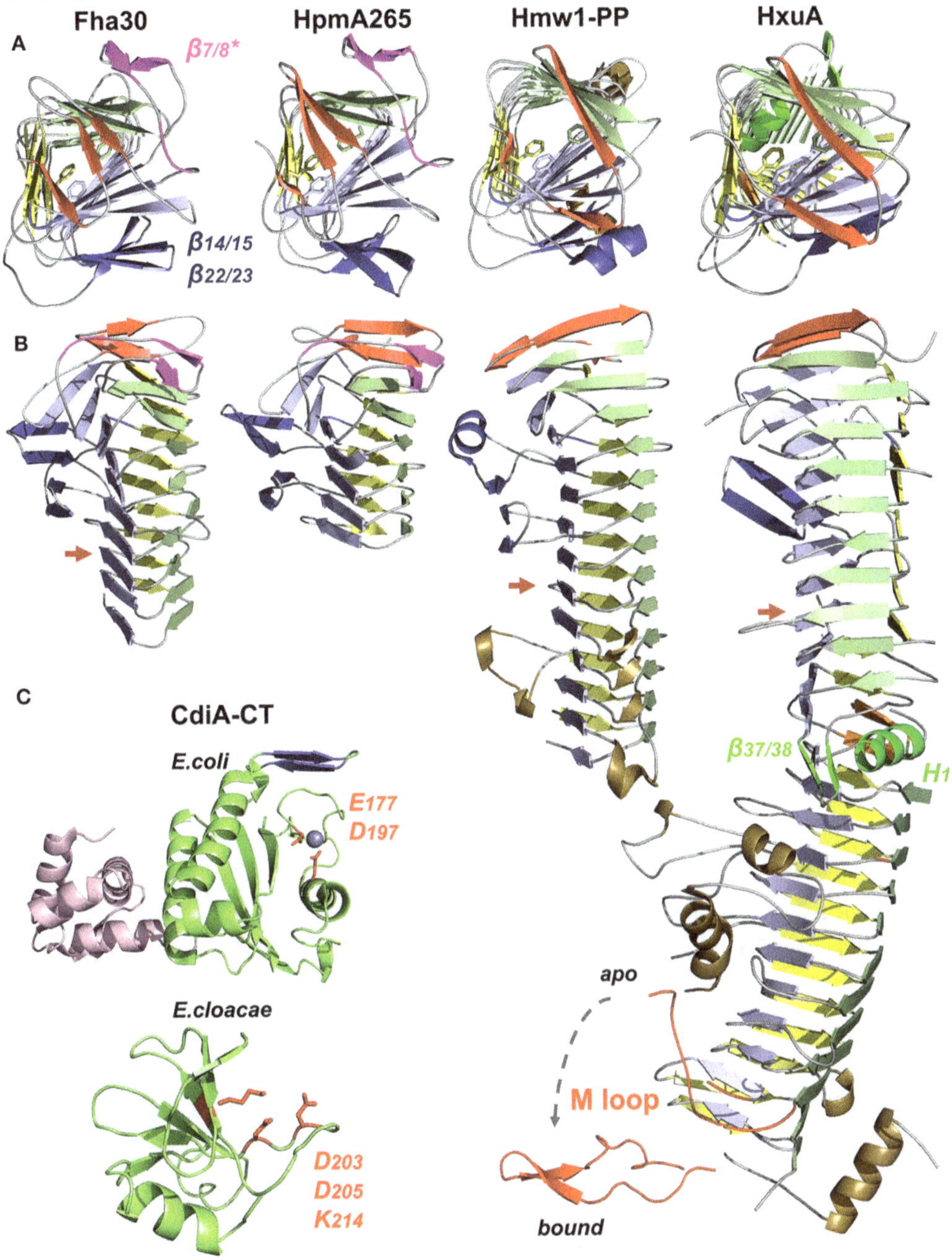

FIGURE 5 | X-ray structures of TpsA proteins. Cartoon representations of Fha30 (PDB entry 1rwr), HpmA265 (3fy3), Hmw1-PP (2odl), HxuA (4mr6 and 4rt6), CdiA-CT of *E. coli* EC869 (4g6u), and CdiA-CT of *E. cloacae* (4ntq). The parallel β sheets PB1, PB2, and PB3 are colored in light green, blue, and yellow, respectively. The first β strands corresponding to the N-terminal cap are represented in red. The NPNG motif and the extra-helical β-sheet $\beta_{14/15}$–$\beta_{22/23}$ conserved among TpsA proteins are in blue, and specific elements from the FHA subfamily (the NPNL motif and $\beta_{7/8}^{*}$) are in magenta. To harmonize the nomenclature between proteins, the numbers given to the structural elements may differ from those in the original publications. **(A)** Views from the N-terminal top of the β-helix axis. Residues of the aromatic cluster are shown in stick representation. **(B)** Side view of TpsA structures. Red arrows indicate the end of the TPS domain. Of note, β_{14} is replaced by an α helix in Hmw1-PP, and part of that β sheet is missing in full-length HxuA. In these two structures, the extra-helical elements in the C-terminal moiety are in brown. For HxuA, structural elements responsible for the twist in the middle of the β helix are highlighted in green (α helix H1 in PB1, and β hairpin β_{37}/β_{38}). The M loop (in red) is represented in two conformations, with and without hemopexin, denoted bound and apo, respectively. **(C)** Structures of the CdiA-CT domains of CdiA proteins. The nuclease domain is highlighted in green, with the side chains of the active site residues in red. For the CdiA-CT of *E. coli*, the active-site Zn^{2+} ion is shown as a sphere, and the N-terminal α-helical bundle is colored in pink. The β hairpin involved in forming β-sheet structure with the immunity protein is in blue. The structures of the toxins were solved in complex with their respective immunity proteins (not represented), arguing that the CdiA-CT moieties must be in inactive conformations.

a globular loop region that locks the TpsA C terminus in the pore of its TpsB partner (Buscher et al., 2006). Preventing HxuA release into the supernatant must be important to couple heme release and import. The presence or absence of this C-terminal anchor domain possibly reflects functional differences among TpsA proteins.

To date, no full structure has been reported of the very large CdiA proteins (180–650 kDa), but several structures of CdiA-CT domains have been obtained by producing the toxic domain in complex with its cognate CdiI immunity protein. For CdiA-CT of *E. coli* EC869, the structure starts ~80 residues after the VENN motif. The N-terminal and C-terminal domains of CdiA-CT form a 4-helix bundle and a central β sheet sandwiched between four α helices, respectively (**Figure 5C**). The second domain is structurally similar to type IIS restriction endonucleases, with a Zn^{2+} ion in the active site (Kachalova et al., 2008; Morse et al., 2012). Adjacent to the active site, a β hairpin interacts with the immunity protein by β augmentation, forming an anti-parallel β sheet (Morse et al., 2012). The structure of another CdiA-CT corresponding to the last 75 amino acids of the *E. cloacae* CdiA protein in interaction with its immunity protein shows a completely different fold, displaying structural homology with the nuclease domain of colicin E3. The toxin domain is folded into one α helix followed by a five-stranded anti-parallel β sheet and is expected to cleave 16S rRNA (**Figure 5C**) (Beck et al., 2014b). These two CdiA-CT moieties share no function, sequence or structural homologies, reflecting how bacteria use two-partner secretion and the modular organization of CdiA proteins to deliver various kinds of toxins into target cells.

TpsB Transporters

The second partner in a TPS system is the TpsB protein. These proteins belong to the ubiquitous Omp85 superfamily, whose best-known members are the essential BamA transporters that assemble proteins in the outer membrane of Gram-negative bacteria (reviewed in Bos et al., 2007; Knowles et al., 2009; Hagan et al., 2011; Ricci and Silhavy, 2012). All the X-ray structures of Omp85 transporters thus far available show that these transporters share major structural features (Clantin et al., 2007; Gruss et al., 2013; Noinaj et al., 2013; Albrecht et al., 2014; Ni et al., 2014; Maier et al., 2015; Bakelar et al., 2016; Gu et al., 2016; Han et al., 2016). For TpsB transporters, the only structure reported thus far is that of FhaC (Clantin et al., 2007; Maier et al., 2015) (**Figure 6A**).

The C-terminal moiety of FhaC forms a 16-stranded, anti-parallel β barrel in the outer membrane, which has been shown to serve as the pore for the translocation of its FHA partner across the outer membrane (Baud et al., 2014). The β barrel is preceded by two periplasmic Polypeptide Transport-Associated (POTRA) domains in tandem, called POTRA1 and POTRA2. The POTRA domain fold is βααββ, with an anti-parallel β sheet flanked by two α helices on one side of the sheet. POTRA domains have been proposed to mediate protein-protein interactions, probably by β augmentation (Kim et al., 2007). The POTRA domains of several TpsB proteins have been shown to recognize the TPS domains of their respective TpsA partners (Surana et al., 2004; Hodak et al., 2006; Delattre et al., 2011; ur Rahman et al., 2014; Garnett et al., 2015; Grass et al., 2015). A major binding site for the FHA TPS domain in FhaC is a hydrophobic groove formed by the edge of the β sheet and the flanking α helix of the barrel-proximal POTRA2 domain (Delattre et al., 2011). This site appears to be well suited to accommodate amphipathic polypeptide segments of FHA, which interacts with FhaC in an extended, not-yet folded conformation (Hodak et al., 2006).

The β barrel of FhaC is occluded by the N-terminal α helix, H1, which crosses the barrel pore with its N terminus at the cell surface and its C terminus in the periplasm. Although not required for activity, similar helices are predicted in most TpsB proteins (Guérin et al., 2014). This N-terminal α helix might facilitate biogenesis as well as stabilize the "resting" form of the transporter (see below). The α helix H1 is followed by a 30-residue periplasmic linker in an extended conformation that joins H1 to the N terminus of the membrane-distal POTRA1 domain (Maier et al., 2015). Unlike H1, which is dispensable, the linker is necessary for FhaC secretion activity (Guédin et al., 2000; Clantin et al., 2007). The X-ray structure of FhaC has revealed that the linker occupies the FHA binding site along POTRA2. One of its functions might thus be to regulate accessibility of the binding site in a competitive mechanism (Guérin et al., 2014; Maier et al., 2015).

The β barrel of FhaC is also partially occluded by a long extracellular loop, L6, a hallmark feature of Omp85 transporters (Moslavac et al., 2005; Arnold et al., 2010). The Arg of the highly conserved VRGY/F motif at the tip of L6 forms a salt bridge with the Asp of another conserved motif, F/GxDxG, located on the β strand β13 of the barrel (Maier et al., 2015). This interaction thus positions L6 within the β barrel in a similar manner in all available Omp85 structures (Gruss et al., 2013; Noinaj et al., 2013; Albrecht et al., 2014; Ni et al., 2014; Bakelar et al., 2016; Gu et al., 2016; Han et al., 2016). Like the barrel-proximal POTRA domain, L6 is essential for the activity of Omp85 proteins. The functions of these critical pieces of the machinery remain unclear (Delattre et al., 2010; Leonard-Rivera and Misra, 2012; Rigel et al., 2013).

PATHWAY OF TPSA PROTEINS ACROSS THE CELL ENVELOPE

The pathway of TpsA proteins from the cytoplasm to the cell surface has been reviewed in (Jacob-Dubuisson et al., 2004; van Ulsen et al., 2014). After an overview of current knowledge, we will spell out the unresolved questions on the transport mechanism.

Export across the Inner Membrane and the Periplasm

TpsA proteins are synthesized as preproteins, and their N-terminal signal peptide determines Sec-dependent export across the cytoplasmic membrane (Grass and St Geme, 2000; Chevalier et al., 2004). Some of them have an extended signal peptide that harbors a semi-conserved N-terminal extension (Jacob-Dubuisson et al., 2004; van Ulsen et al., 2014), which is also found in subsets of classical and trimeric AT proteins (Peterson et al., 2006; Desvaux et al., 2007; Szczesny and Lupas, 2008). Among

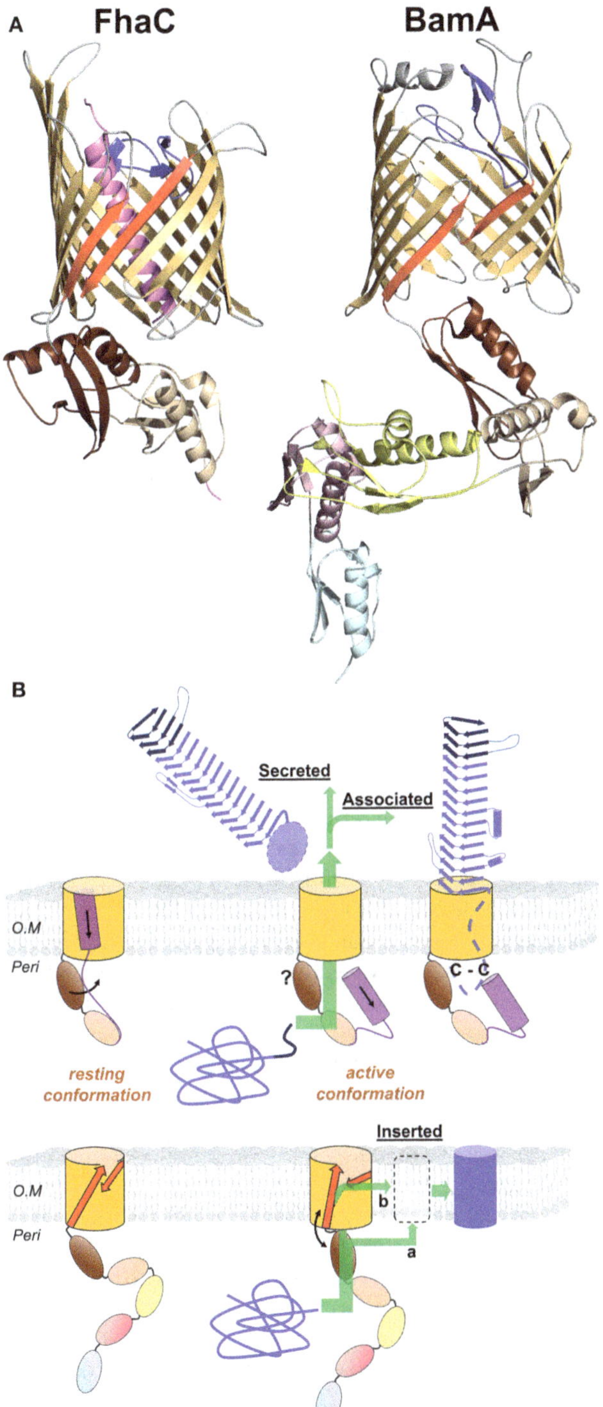

FIGURE 6 | Omp85 transporters: X-ray structures to mechanistic models. (A) Cartoon representations of FhaC from *B. pertussis* (PDB entry 4ql0) and BamA from *N. gonorrhoeae* (4k3b). The common structural features include the 16-strand barrel in gold, the L6 loop in blue and the last two POTRA domains in wheat and brown (POTRA1 and POTRA2 for FhaC). The β_1 and β_{16} strands are shown in red. Specific elements include the N-terminal α helix of FhaC in purple, and the POTRA3-2-1 domains of BamA in yellow, pink, and cyan, respectively. **(B)** Mechanistic models for TpsB transporters and BamA proteins (upper and lower diagrams, respectively). The substrates *(Continued)*

FIGURE 6 | Continued
are colored blue, unfolded in the periplasm and folded in their final locations. For FhaC, the motions of the N-terminal α helix H1 and of the POTRA2 domain are shown with black arrows (see text). The TPS domain (dark blue) interacts with the POTRA domains, and the TpsA protein is translocated through the barrel pore (green arrow). The location of the POTRA domains at this stage remains to be determined. Depending on the subfamily, the TpsA is secreted into the milieu or remains associated with its transporter by a small globular periplasmic domain harboring a disulfide bond (C-C). For BamA, the available structures indicate at least two conformations, one in which POTRA5 is away from the β barrel and β_1 and β_{16} are close to one another with H bonds formed between them, and another characterized by the occurrence of a lateral gate caused by the reorientation of β_1–β_8 and POTRA5. This gate might serve for progressive folding of the substrate through the formation of a hybrid barrel with BamA, before its release in the outer membrane (green arrow denoted b; BAM-budding model). Local destabilization of the bilayer close to the β_1–β_{16} junction might also facilitate direct insertion of the prefolded substrate in the membrane (green arrow denoted a; BAM-assisted model). The L6 loop and the rest of the BAM complex are not represented.

TPS systems, the function of these extended signal peptides has been investigated only in the case of the TpsA preprotein FhaB, which is the precursor of FHA in *B. pertussis*. This study has revealed that the extension optimizes biogenesis by slowing down export and delaying signal peptide cleavage (Chevalier et al., 2004). The role of the extension has also been studied for several AT proteins, as reviewed in (Desvaux et al., 2006; van Ulsen et al., 2014). It was shown in the case of EspP that, by prolonging the association of the AT with the inner membrane, the extended signal peptide might prevent non-productive folding of the passenger domain in the periplasm (Szabady et al., 2005).

Following Sec-dependent export, the TpsA proteins reach the periplasm, where they remain in extended conformations for their interactions with their TpsB transporters. How the not-yet-folded TpsA secretion intermediates are protected from degradation, misfolding, or aggregation in the periplasm has been investigated in very few systems. Chaperone requirement by TpsA proteins might depend on their size, the proteolytic activity in the periplasm of the host bacterium, and the rates at which they tend to aggregate or to misfold. The proteins that form long β solenoids are generally slow to fold and do not have a strong tendency to aggregate, two properties favorable to Type V secretion (Hodak et al., 2006; Junker et al., 2006; Junker and Clark, 2010).

The time window during which TpsA periplasmic intermediates retain secretion competence markedly depends on the system. For the OtpAB system of *E. coli* O157:H7, expression of the OtpB transporter could be triggered after that of its TpsA partner with no detrimental effect on secretion, demonstrating that export across the cytoplasmic membrane and secretion across the outer membrane need not be temporally coupled (Choi and Bernstein, 2009). In contrast, periplasmic intermediates of FHA appeared to rapidly become secretion-incompetent *in vivo* (Guédin et al., 1998). Similarly, when secretion was reconstituted *in vitro*, delaying the addition of FhaC-containing proteoliposomes to FHA-producing spheroplasts strongly impaired translocation into the vesicles (Fan et al., 2012).

While *bona fide* periplasmic intermediates are detectable for some TpsA proteins, including ShlA, OtpA and a few others (Schiebel et al., 1989; van Ulsen et al., 2008; Choi and Bernstein, 2009), in other TPS systems, in contrast, they appear to be quickly degraded. Thus, HMW1 and FhaB were proteolyzed by the protease-chaperone DegP if their secretion was impeded, probably to limit the development of envelope stress (St Geme and Grass, 1998; Baud et al., 2009). On the other hand, in the case of FHA, DegP was also shown to facilitate secretion (Baud et al., 2009, 2011). In particular, a specific form of DegP associated with the cytoplasmic membrane was found to bind non-native FHA fragments with strong affinity, indicating that it might be a "holding chaperone" (Baud et al., 2009, 2011). The involvement of DegP has been shown in type Va, Vc, and Ve systems, suggesting that it might be general in the type V pathway (Mogensen and Otzen, 2005; Grosskinsky et al., 2007; Oberhettinger et al., 2012).

Translocation across the Outer Membrane: Function of the TpsB Partner

Molecular recognition between the two partners is mediated by the TPS domain and the POTRA domains of the TpsA and TpsB proteins, respectively (Surana et al., 2004; Hodak et al., 2006; Delattre et al., 2011; Garnett et al., 2015). The TPS domain of the TpsA protein must be in an extended conformation for interaction with the POTRA domains of the TpsB transporter, as shown for the FHA/FhaC and HMW1/HMW1B pairs (Hodak et al., 2006; Grass et al., 2015). Surface plasmon resonance experiments with the FHA/FhaC pair have indicated interactions of micromolar affinity between the two proteins and suggested that association and dissociation occur very fast (Delattre et al., 2011). Similarly, NMR experiments on the LepAB system of *P. aeruginosa* have shown fast exchange between the bound and free forms, which also supports the idea that TpsA-TpsB interactions are dynamic (Garnett et al., 2015). While this may be expected from the fact that the partners must dissociate after secretion, this property is likely to have some bearing on the mechanisms of transport (see below). What constitutes the "secretion signal" of a TpsA protein is imperfectly defined but most likely involves a combination of conserved and non-conserved residues, as well as some extended amphipathic structure, likely for β augmentation of the POTRA β sheets (Hodak et al., 2006; Kim et al., 2007; Gatzeva-Topalova et al., 2010). Crystal structures of the soluble periplasmic domain of the Omp85 proteins BamA and TamA indicate that POTRA domains may generally interact with other proteins by β augmentation (Kim et al., 2007; Gruss et al., 2013).

Binding of the TPS domain to the POTRA domains is followed by the transport of the TpsA protein to the cell surface, most likely in an extended conformation, but a large gap persists in our understanding of the translocation step itself (**Figure 6B**). The path of translocation of FHA across the outer membrane has been investigated by *in vivo* cross-linking. This identified several regions of FhaC that interact with FHA: the surface of the POTRA domains, the inner lining of the β-barrel pore, and specific surface loops (Baud et al., 2014). Similarly, in particular two regions in the N-terminal and central parts of the TPS domain of FHA interact with FhaC. The interaction map reveals a funnel-like pathway, with the conformationally flexible TPS domain entering the channel in a non-exclusive manner and exiting along a specific four-stranded β sheet at the cell surface (Baud et al., 2014). Translocation initially appears to proceed in discrete steps, which is consistent with a repetitive, cyclic process (Baud et al., 2014).

Two models of translocation have been proposed. According to the first one, the TpsA protein forms a hairpin in the pore. Its TPS domain remains bound to the POTRA domains throughout the entire process, while the rest is progressively translocated and folds at the cell surface. In this scenario, the TPS domain is released at a late or final stage of translocation (Mazar and Cotter, 2006). In an alternative model, the TPS domain reaches the surface first and nucleates the folding of the rest of the protein (Hodak and Jacob-Dubuisson, 2007). Several pieces of evidence suggest that the latter mechanism is at play, notably the efficient secretion of N-terminal truncates of TpsA proteins (Jacob-Dubuisson et al., 2004), and the accessibility of the N-terminus of stalled FHA constructs at the cell surface (Guérin et al., 2014). In addition, the stable TPS fold and the observation that a TPS domain can initiate TpsA folding *in vitro* (Walker et al., 2004; Weaver et al., 2009) indicate that the TPS domain may have a similar role in initiating folding in two-partner secretion as that suggested for the stable C-terminal core of the passenger domain in autotransporter secretion (see below; Junker et al., 2006, 2009; Peterson et al., 2010; Renn et al., 2012; Besingi et al., 2013).

Irrespective of the model, the same basic questions arise: how is the TpsA protein pulled or pushed into the pore? What initiates the process and what drives it forward? Does the TpsB transporter cycle between different conformations in order to mediate the progressive transport of its substrate? It should be noted that no high-energy, hydrolyzable compounds such as ATP are available in the periplasm, and that the semi-permeable outer membrane cannot sustain an electrochemical gradient based on small ions, although a Donnan potential may exist (see below; Sen et al., 1988). The process should thus involve transitions between conformations separated by low energy barriers.

The dynamics of the FhaC transporter has been investigated using electron paramagnetic resonance (EPR), which provides information on the mobility of specific regions of the protein as well as the distances between them. These experiments revealed that FhaC exists in an equilibrium of several conformations. The first equilibrium concerns the N-terminal α helix H1 which spontaneously moves to the periplasm (Guérin et al., 2014). The movement of H1 breaks linker-POTRA interactions, thus allowing the TPS domain of the substrate protein to bind to the POTRA domains (**Figure 6B**). The equilibrium between the resting, closed conformation of FhaC and the open conformation of FhaC with H1 in the periplasm might thus be displaced by the binding of FHA (Guérin et al., 2014; Maier et al., 2015). Similarly, in the LepB transporter of *P. aeruginosa*, the linker may transiently interact with POTRA2 and be displaced by the substrate (Garnett et al., 2015).

The second equilibrium concerns the conserved loop L6 that is folded back inside the pore from the cell surface and interacts with the inner wall of the barrel (Guerin et al., 2015; Maier et al.,

2015). Although this loop, and in particular its VRGY hallmark motif, is essential for activity (Clantin et al., 2007; Delattre et al., 2010), its function remains obscure. It does not seem to have a direct role in substrate pulling (Baud et al., 2014) and appears relatively rigid in EPR experiments (Guerin et al., 2015). Notably, in BamA, attaching L6 to the barrel does not inhibit growth, so large-scale motion of L6 does not seem to be required for BamA function (Noinaj et al., 2014). Nevertheless, the position of L6 appears to change in the pore and to modulate channel opening (Guerin et al., 2015). Although these experiments have revealed that, overall, TpsB proteins are highly dynamic, they fall short of describing the full secretion cycle.

Secretion and folding are most likely coupled in the TPS pathway. This has long been proposed to explain how secretion could proceed in the absence of classical sources of energy. Thus, once a TpsA protein emerges at the cell surface and starts to fold into a β helix, the difference in free energy between the extended and the folded forms is thought to drive secretion (Jacob-Dubuisson et al., 2004). This model has been extensively probed for type Va AT proteins whose passenger domains also fold into long β solenoids. These β helices appear to unfold and fold in several steps, and many of them appear to have a stable core that initiates folding (Oliver et al., 2003; Renn and Clark, 2008). The passenger domain of a classical AT protein forms a hairpin in the pore in the course of secretion, and thus its C-terminal portion reaches the cell surface first (Bernstein, 2007; Junker et al., 2009; Zhai et al., 2011). In many cases the C-terminal region of the passenger has a greater thermostability than the rest of the protein, and this difference is thought to promote its vectorial folding, which may then drive secretion (Junker et al., 2006, 2009; Peterson et al., 2010; Renn et al., 2012; Besingi et al., 2013). The initiation of translocation, before passenger folding can occur, may then be linked to the energetically favorable folding and membrane insertion of the β barrel, with BamA lowering the kinetic barrier (Moon et al., 2013; Gessmann et al., 2014). Consistent with the hypothesis of folding-driven secretion, mutations that impair folding of the C-terminal passenger region or the β helix in general have been observed to reduce or abolish secretion (Peterson et al., 2010; Renn et al., 2012; Drobnak et al., 2015). However, it has been noted that the free energy typically associated with protein folding is orders of magnitude smaller than the energetic cost of protein transport across a membrane as it has been measured, for example, for translocation across the chloroplast envelope (Kang'ethe and Bernstein, 2013a). Nevertheless, the possibility of reconstituting type V secretion systems *in vitro* and obtaining translocation of TpsA proteins and AT passengers into liposomes demonstrates that, in these systems, protein translocation across a membrane is indeed possible without input of external energy (Norell et al., 2014). One solution that has been proposed to this apparent conundrum is a "Brownian ratchet"-type mechanism in which random thermal motion obtains directionality via an effectively irreversible step, here, the folding of the transport substrate on the extracellular side, which prevents backtracking of the protein chain (Peterson et al., 2010; Drobnak et al., 2015). Apart from the folding free energy, the required free energy for this process would be contributed by the mechanisms that keep secretion substrates unfolded in the periplasm, i.e., most likely chaperones (Baud et al., 2009; Jacob-Dubuisson et al., 2013). Such mechanisms have been described theoretically (Simon et al., 1992; Depperschmidt et al., 2013) and demonstrated experimentally e.g. for transport into the endoplasmatic reticulum (Matlack et al., 1999), suggesting that they may also be involved in bacterial type V secretion.

Still, it has been observed that, when engineered into an AT sequence, even a disordered domain that does not assume a stable structure could be secreted. This occurred even if the remaining passenger domain fragment was too short to fold (Kang'ethe and Bernstein, 2013b). A Brownian ratchet mechanism thus cannot be at play in this case. However, removal of negatively charged residues in the passenger was observed to inhibit secretion in this system. In this context, it is interesting to note that sizable Donnan potentials—with the periplasmic side negative—have been observed across the *E. coli* outer membrane and traced to the presence of negatively charged oligosaccharides (Sen et al., 1988). The observation that a disordered, negatively charged polypeptide can be secreted thus suggests that an electrochemical potential based on large, impermeable charged molecules may indeed be present across the bacterial OM and play a role in type V secretion. In addition, the process might also benefit from entropic effects due to the difference between the crowded periplasmic environment and the extracellular milieu (Fan et al., 2016); however, extracellular crowding agents have not been observed to affect AT secretion (Drobnak et al., 2015).

The same principles of differential stability between distinct regions of the secreted β helix and of vectorial folding observed in AT proteins likely apply to TPS systems as well, and therefore the region emerging first from the TpsB channel probably nucleates folding of the β helix at the cell surface. The conserved TPS domain is an obvious candidate for this function, and several data support the idea. Early studies have indicated that the TPS domain of ShlA was able to template the folding of the unfolded full-length protein to form the active toxin *in vitro* (Schiebel et al., 1989; Schönherr et al., 1993). Similar experiments with the TPS domain of HpmA have shown that cooperative β strand interactions mediate the folding of neighboring full-length proteins, a process called "template-assisted hemolysis" (Weaver et al., 2009). Two more recent pieces of work have addressed the unfolding properties of the TPS domains of FHA and HpmA, by using atomic force microscopy (Alsteens et al., 2013) or chemical denaturation (Wimmer et al., 2015), respectively. Both studies have shown that TPS domains unfold in several steps and harbor highly stable core subdomains. In the second case, the presence of the folded core subdomain allowed rapid folding of the rest of the TPS domain *in vitro*. It is tempting to speculate that these core regions of the TPS domain fold early in the course of secretion and nucleate folding of the rest by β augmentation concomitant with translocation, and that a Brownian ratchet-type of mechanism is at play in TPS secretion as well.

Translocation initiation in TPS systems cannot be linked to the free energy gained from β barrel folding and membrane insertion, as has been proposed for AT proteins (Moon et al., 2013), since the two processes are independent. Here, the specific but transient interactions observed between the TpsB transporter and the TPS domain of its substrate likely play a role (Delattre et al., 2011).

The possibility that the TpsB transporter assists in the initial folding of its partner has been suggested by recent observations in two different TPS systems. Thus, specific interactions were shown to occur between parts of the FHA TPS domain and specific surface β strands and loops of FhaC (Baud et al., 2014). The edge of this small surface-exposed β sheet of FhaC might guide the secretion of the TPS domain and template its initial folding at the cell surface by β augmentation (Baud et al., 2014). Interestingly, the corresponding loops of HMW1B appear to tether the HMW1 adhesin at the cell surface of *H. influenzae* (Grass et al., 2015). Thus, specific structural features at the extracellular surface of the TpsB transporter might be involved in the secretion of the cognate TpsA partner and possibly also retain its N terminus close to the cell surface.

What Can We Learn for the TPS Pathway from the Role of BamA in Type V Secretion?

TpsB transporters are Omp85 proteins specialized in the transport across the outer membrane of soluble protein substrates (Heinz and Lithgow, 2014). In parallel with the role of a specialized Omp85 transporter for type Vb secretion, there have been multiple demonstrations that another Omp85 transporter, BamA, and indeed the BAM complex, is involved in the folding and insertion of most outer membrane proteins, including classical ATs (type Va) (Jain and Goldberg, 2007; Ieva and Bernstein, 2009; Sauri et al., 2009; Ieva et al., 2011), trimeric ATs (Lehr et al., 2010) and type Ve intimins (Bodelón et al., 2009; Oberhettinger et al., 2012). Omp85 transporters thus form the mechanistic basis of type V secretion.

In spite of the many structures now available of BamA and the BAM complex (**Figure 6A**), our models for the molecular mechanisms of protein assembly in the outer membrane remain somewhat speculative (Hagan et al., 2011; Noinaj et al., 2015). Several studies have shown that BamA opens laterally between its first and last β strands in the outer membrane and that this opening is required for function (Noinaj et al., 2013, 2014; Albrecht et al., 2014; Iadanza et al., 2016). Another important feature common to all BamA structures is a decreased hydrophobic thickness where the first and last β strands meet, which causes a local thinning of the outer membrane (Noinaj et al., 2013, 2014). Two popular mechanistic models for BamA-mediated protein assembly are the BAM-assisted and BAM-budding models (**Figure 6B**). It should be noted that they have not been experimentally proven, and it is possible that different models apply to different classes of OMPs. The BAM-assisted model postulates that some OMPs can fold without help from accessory proteins and need only a locally destabilized outer membrane in which to insert the fully folded OMP. BamA locally disturbs the outer membrane where its first and last β strands meet, and it could serve as a folding catalyst by lowering the kinetic barrier to nascent OMP insertion (Burgess et al., 2008; Noinaj et al., 2013, 2015; Gessmann et al., 2014). The BAM-budding model takes into account the requirement for lateral opening of BamA and might explain how BAM helps to fold OMPs that do not spontaneously fold on their own. In this model, an unfolded OMP would be delivered to the BAM complex by periplasmic chaperones such as SurA and Skp. The nascent OMP would then be sequentially folded by pairing individual β strands with the first and last β strands of BamA separated by the lateral opening. In this model, β strands from the nascent OMP would be added to BamA, forming a hybrid BamA-OMP barrel, and eventually the new OMP would separate from BamA and move away laterally into the outer membrane (**Figure 6B**).

Classical AT proteins (type Va) are composed of both a β barrel moiety and a soluble passenger domain, and several pieces of work have indicated that the BAM complex is involved in both the insertion of the β barrel moiety into the membrane and the translocation of the passenger domain to the bacterial surface (Ieva et al., 2008; Ieva and Bernstein, 2009; Sauri et al., 2009). For the AT protein EspP, an assembly intermediate was detected in the periplasm whose topology resembled that of the assembled protein, with a segment preceding the barrel moiety embedded in a "proto-barrel" (Ieva et al., 2008). Interactions were detected between the BAM complex and both the barrel and the passenger domains of the AT substrate (Ieva and Bernstein, 2009). Formation of the β barrel domain thus appears to proceed to a certain extent in the periplasm, with a β hairpin that corresponds to a segment C-terminal of the passenger incorporated in its pore. According to these authors, the proto-barrel would then undergo a conformational change before translocation is initiated. The passenger domain would interact with the POTRA domains of BamA and progressively move through a channel, composed of BamA and/or the AT barrel (Pavlova et al., 2013). These observations are at odds with the model that the β barrel of the AT protein assembles progressively, hairpin by hairpin, in the outer membrane as suggested by the budding model, and they argue that the lateral opening of the BamA barrel might play another role in the assembly/secretion process of ATs.

What about TPS systems? TpsA proteins are soluble and have no transmembrane domain, and thus they represent "simpler" substrates than AT proteins. *In vitro* reconstitution of TPS secretion has shown that, while TpsB proteins are inserted into the OM by the BAM complex like most outer membrane proteins (Norell et al., 2014), they form autonomous secretion ports for their TpsA substrates (Fan et al., 2012). In other words, the translocation of a TpsA protein only requires its TpsB partner and does not proceed through a channel also involving BamA. A TpsB transporter thus mediates the translocation of its soluble TpsA substrate by itself.

The role of the POTRA domains in Omp85 transporters is likely to go beyond the recruitment of substrate proteins, as suggested by a point mutation in POTRA2 that affects the function of FhaC but not the binding of FHA (Delattre et al., 2011). This mutation changes a highly conserved Asp residue in the TpsB family that participates in periplasmic interactions between the POTRA2 domain, the linker and the barrel (Maier et al., 2015). The POTRA domains might thus contribute to addressing the TpsA protein to the pore of the TpsB transporter. Similar suggestions were made for the POTRA domains of HMW1B and LepB (Garnett et al., 2015; Grass et al., 2015).

Their role in shuttling the passenger to the barrel might explain why PlpD, the prototypic Vd protein, harbors a POTRA-like domain. Since the Patatin domains of the passenger are part of the same polypeptide as the TpsB-barrel-like transporter moiety, the POTRA-like domain is not necessary to recruit the substrate.

Both BamA and TpsB transporters most likely work in a cyclic manner and go through their "conformational cycle" several times in the course of secretion of their long substrates (**Figure 6B**). The conformational changes that they undergo remain to be described, but we propose that they involve concerted motions of the three conserved structural components essential for activity, i.e., the β barrel, the L6 loop and the barrel-proximal POTRA domain. A few observations support this hypothesis. It has been proposed that the L6 loop of BamA cycles between several conformations, and that its conformation is modulated by other Bam proteins via the POTRA5 domain (Rigel et al., 2013). A functional connection between the latter and L6 in BamA has also been found in a search for intragenic suppressors of a mutation that disrupts the L6-barrel interaction (Dwyer et al., 2013). Functional links between L6 and the barrel are clearly established. For instance, the FhaC channel becomes larger if the interaction between L6 and the wall of the barrel is disrupted (Guerin et al., 2015). Similarly, two conductance states have been recorded for the HMW1B transporter. The higher-conductance state is occasionally visited by the protein and likely corresponds to a more open channel (Duret et al., 2008).

Our current hypothesis for the mechanism of two-partner secretion is that the TpsB barrel cycles between narrow-channel and open-channel states. As seen with BamA, the conformational changes might induce a reorientation of β1 and POTRA2, with the formation of a lateral opening between the first and last strands of the β barrel. This lateral opening could be used to enlarge the β barrel with the insertion of amphipathic β hairpin(s) from periplasmic portions of the protein, thus hoisting a first portion of substrate bound to the POTRA domains toward the surface. After the substrate is released on the extracellular side of the outer membrane to initiate folding, possibly along a template provided by extracellular parts of the barrel, the inserted region switches back to the periplasm to repeat the cycle. We hypothesize also that L6 can stabilize these conformations by forming distinct interactions with specific regions of the β barrel in each of the two states. The TpsA protein might thus "hitch-hike" on spontaneous conformational changes of its transporter for translocation. Together with extracellular-only folding as required for a Brownian ratchet mechanism, and possibly a Donnan potential, our proposed mechanism accounts for the vectorial translocation of TpsA proteins across the bacterial OM.

CONCLUSION

TPS systems are widespread among Gram-negative bacteria, both pathogenic and environmental. They serve many different functions that participate in the interactions of the bacteria with their environment, be it the host cell or bacterial competitors. The diversity of type V systems deployed by bacteria is probably yet larger than we have come to realize, with hybrid systems made up of parts borrowed from a variety of protein domains. The mechanisms of transport of such diverse and sometimes extremely long domains remain poorly understood. Endeavors to decipher those mechanisms will undoubtedly illuminate the inner workings of Omp85 transporters.

AUTHOR CONTRIBUTIONS

All authors listed have made substantial, direct and intellectual contribution to the work, and approved it for publication.

ACKNOWLEDGMENTS

We thank Maarten Ghequire for help with the Geneious software and phylogenetic trees. JG and SKB are supported by the Intramural Research Program of the NIH, the National Institute of Diabetes and Digestive and Kidney Diseases (NIDDK). SB is supported by a FINOVI grant and CNRS. The work of FJ has been supported over the years by the ANR (grant ANR-10-BLAN-1306), INSERM, CNRS, and Région Nord Pas de Calais. RS gratefully acknowledges funding via a "Projets exploratoires premier soutien" (PEPS) grant from the CNRS and the University of Lille. We also acknowledge support from TGE RMN THC (FR-3050, France) and FRABio (Univ. Lille, CNRS, FR 3688).

REFERENCES

Albrecht, R., Schutz, M., Oberhettinger, P., Faulstich, M., Bermejo, I., Rudel, T., et al. (2014). Structure of BamA, an essential factor in outer membrane protein biogenesis. *Acta Crystallogr. D Biol. Crystallogr.* 70, 1779–1789. doi: 10.1107/S1399004714007482

Alsteens, D., Martinez, N., Jamin, M., and Jacob-Dubuisson, F. (2013). Sequential unfolding of beta helical protein by single-molecule atomic force microscopy. *PLoS ONE* 8:e73572. doi: 10.1371/journal.pone.0073572

Amitai, G., Belenkiy, O., Dassa, B., Shainskaya, A., and Pietrokovski, S. (2003). Distribution and function of new bacterial intein-like protein domains. *Mol. Microbiol.* 47, 61–73. doi: 10.1046/j.1365-2958.2003.03283.x

Anderson, M. S., Garcia, E. C., and Cotter, P. A. (2012). The *Burkholderia bcpAIOB* genes define unique classes of two-partner secretion and contact dependent growth inhibition systems. *PLoS Genet.* 8:e1002877. doi: 10.1371/journal.pgen.1002877

Anderson, M. S., Garcia, E. C., and Cotter, P. A. (2014). Kind discrimination and competitive exclusion mediated by contact-dependent growth inhibition systems shape biofilm community structure. *PLoS Pathog.* 10:e1004076. doi: 10.1371/journal.ppat.1004076

Antoine, R., Alonso, S., Raze, D., Coutte, L., Lesjean, S., Willery, E., et al. (2000). New virulence-activated and virulence-repressed genes identified by systematic gene inactivation and generation of transcriptional fusions in *Bordetella pertussis*. *J. Bacteriol.* 182, 5902–5905.

Aoki, S. K., Diner, E. J., de Roodenbeke, C. T., Burgess, B. R., Poole, S. J., Braaten, B. A., et al. (2010). A widespread family of polymorphic contact-dependent toxin delivery systems in bacteria. *Nature* 468, 439–442. doi: 10.1038/nature09490

Aoki, S. K., Malinverni, J. C., Jacoby, K., Thomas, B., Pamma, R., Trinh, B. N., et al. (2008). Contact-dependent growth inhibition requires the essential outer membrane protein BamA (YaeT) as the receptor and the inner membrane transport protein AcrB. *Mol. Microbiol.* 70, 323–340. doi: 10.1111/j.1365-2958.2008.06404.x

Aoki, S. K., Pamma, R., Hernday, A. D., Bickham, J. E., Braaten, B. A., and Low, D. A. (2005). Contact-dependent inhibition of growth in *Escherichia coli*. *Science* 309, 1245–1248. doi: 10.1126/science.1115109

Arnold, T., Zeth, K., and Linke, D. (2010). Omp85 from the thermophilic cyanobacterium *Thermosynechococcus elongatus* differs from proteobacterial Omp85 in structure and domain composition. *J. Biol. Chem.* 285, 18003–18015. doi: 10.1074/jbc.M110.112516

Baelen, S., Dewitte, F., Clantin, B., and Villeret, V. (2013). Structure of the secretion domain of HxuA from *Haemophilus influenzae*. *Acta Crystallogr. Sect. F Struct. Biol. Cryst. Commun.* 69, 1322–1327. doi: 10.1107/S174430911302962X

Bakelar, J., Buchanan, S. K., and Noinaj, N. (2016). The structure of the beta-barrel assembly machinery complex. *Science* 351, 180–186. doi: 10.1126/science.aad3460

Balder, R., Hassel, J., Lipski, S., and Lafontaine, E. R. (2007). *Moraxella catarrhalis* strain O35E expresses two filamentous hemagglutinin-like proteins that mediate adherence to human epithelial cells. *Infect. Immun.* 75, 2765–2775. doi: 10.1128/IAI.00079-07

Baraquet, C., and Harwood, C. S. (2015). FleQ DNA Binding consensus sequence revealed by studies of FleQ-dependent regulation of biofilm gene expression in *Pseudomonas aeruginosa*. *J. Bacteriol.* 198, 178–186. doi: 10.1128/JB.00539-15

Barenkamp, S. J., and St Geme, J. W. I. (1994). Genes encoding high-molecular-weight adhesion proteins of nontypeable *Haemophilus influenzae* are part of gene clusters. *Infect. Immun.* 62, 3320–3328.

Barnard, T. J., Dautin, N., Lukacik, P., Bernstein, H. D., and Buchanan, S. K. (2007). Autotransporter structure reveals intra-barrel cleavage followed by conformational changes. *Nat. Struct. Mol. Biol.* 14, 1214–1220. doi: 10.1002/0471140864.ps1709s47

Basso, P., Ragno, M., Elsen, S., Reboud, E., Golovkine, G., Bouillot, S., et al. (2017). *Pseudomonas aeruginosa* pore-forming exolysin and Type IV Pili Cooperate to induce host cell lysis. *MBio* 8, e02250–e02216. doi: 10.1128/mBio.02250-16

Baud, C., Guérin, J., Petit, E., Lesne, E., Dupre, E., Locht, C., et al. (2014). Translocation path of a substrate protein through its Omp85 transporter. *Nat. Commun.* 5:5271. doi: 10.1038/ncomms6271

Baud, C., Gutsche, I., Willery, E., de Paepe, D., Drobecq, H., Gilleron, M., et al. (2011). Membrane-associated DegP in *Bordetella* chaperones a repeat-rich secretory protein. *Mol. Microbiol.* 80, 1625–1636. doi: 10.1111/j.1365-2958.2011.07672.x

Baud, C., Hodak, H., Willery, E., Drobecq, H., Locht, C., Jamin, M., et al. (2009). Role of DegP for two-partner secretion in *Bordetella*. *Mol. Microbiol.* 74, 315–329. doi: 10.1111/j.1365-2958.2009.06860.x

Beck, C. M., Diner, E. J., Kim, J. J., Low, D. A., and Hayes, C. S. (2014a). The F pilus mediates a novel pathway of CDI toxin import. *Mol. Microbiol.* 93, 276–290. doi: 10.1111/mmi.12658

Beck, C. M., Morse, R. P., Cunningham, D. A., Iniguez, A., Low, D. A., Goulding, C. W., et al. (2014b). CdiA from *Enterobacter cloacae* delivers a toxic ribosomal RNase into target bacteria. *Structure* 22, 707–718. doi: 10.1016/j.str.2014.02.012

Beck, C. M., Willett, J. L., Cunningham, D. A., Kim, J. J., Low, D. A., and Hayes, C. S. (2016). CdiA effectors from uropathogenic *Escherichia coli* use heterotrimeric osmoporins as receptors to recognize target bacteria. *PLoS Pathog.* 12:e1005925. doi: 10.1371/journal.ppat.1005925

Bentancor, L. V., Camacho-Peiro, A., Bozkurt-Guzel, C., Pier, G. B., and Maira-Litran, T. (2012). Identification of Ata, a multifunctional trimeric autotransporter of *Acinetobacter baumannii*. *J. Bacteriol.* 194, 3950–3960. doi: 10.1128/JB.06769-11

Benz, I., and Schmidt, M. A. (2001). Glycosylation with heptose residues mediated by the *aah* gene product is essential for adherence of the AIDA-I adhesin. *Mol. Microbiol.* 40, 1403–1413.

Bernstein, H. D. (2007). Are bacterial 'autotransporters' really transporters? *Trends Microbiol.* 15, 441–447. doi: 10.1016/j.tim.2007.09.007

Besingi, R. N., Chaney, J. L., and Clark, P. L. (2013). An alternative outer membrane secretion mechanism for an autotransporter protein lacking a C-terminal stable core. *Mol. Microbiol.* 90, 1028–1045. doi: 10.1111/mmi.12414

Bodelón, G., Marín, E., and Fernandez, L. A. (2009). Role of periplasmic chaperones and BamA (YaeT/Omp85) in folding and secretion of intimin from enteropathogenic *Escherichia coli* strains. *J. Bacteriol.* 191, 5169–5179. doi: 10.1128/JB.00458-09

Borlee, B. R., Goldman, A. D., Murakami, K., Samudrala, R., Wozniak, D. J., and Parsek, M. R. (2010). *Pseudomonas aeruginosa* uses a cyclic-di-GMP-regulated adhesin to reinforce the biofilm extracellular matrix. *Mol. Microbiol.* 75, 827–842. doi: 10.1111/j.1365-2958.2009.06991.x

Bos, M. P., Robert, V., and Tommassen, J. (2007). Biogenesis of the gram-negative bacterial outer membrane. *Annu. Rev. Microbiol.* 61, 191–214. doi: 10.1146/annurev.micro.61.080706.093245

Braun, V., Hobbie, S., and Ondraczek, R. (1992). *Serratia marcescens* forms a new type of cytolysin. *FEMS Microbiol. Lett.* 100, 299–306.

Brillard, J., Duchaud, E., Boemare, N., Kunst, F., and Givaudan, A. (2002). The PhlA hemolysin from the entomopathogenic bacterium *Photorhabdus luminescens* belongs to the two-partner secretion family of hemolysins. *J. Bacteriol.* 184, 3871–3878.

Brown, N. F., Logue, C. A., Boddey, J. A., Scott, R., Hirst, R. G., and Beacham, I. R. (2004). Identification of a novel two-partner secretion system from *Burkholderia pseudomallei*. *Mol. Genet. Genomics* 272, 204–215. doi: 10.1007/s00438-004-1039-z

Burgess, N. K., Dao, T. P., Stanley, A. M., and Fleming, K. G. (2008). Beta-barrel proteins that reside in the *Escherichia coli* outer membrane *in vivo* demonstrate varied folding behavior *in vitro*. *J. Biol. Chem.* 283, 26748–26758. doi: 10.1074/jbc.M804231200

Buscher, A. Z., Grass, S., Heuser, J., Roth, R., and St Geme, J. W. III. (2006). Surface anchoring of a bacterial adhesin secreted by the two-partner secretion pathway. *Mol. Microbiol.* 61, 470–483. doi: 10.1111/j.1365-2958.2006.05236.x

Charbonneau, M. E., Girard, V., Nikolakakis, A., Campos, M., Berthiaume, F., Dumas, F., et al. (2007). O-linked glycosylation ensures the normal conformation of the autotransporter adhesin involved in diffuse adherence. *J. Bacteriol.* 189, 8880–8889. doi: 10.1128/JB.00969-07

Charbonneau, M. E., and Mourez, M. (2008). The *Escherichia coli* AIDA-I autotransporter undergoes cytoplasmic glycosylation independently of export. *Res. Microbiol.* 159, 537–544. doi: 10.1016/j.resmic.2008.06.009

Chevalier, N., Moser, M., Koch, H. G., Schimz, K. L., Willery, E., Locht, C., et al. (2004). Membrane targeting of a bacterial virulence factor harbouring an extended signal peptide. *J. Mol. Microbiol. Biotechnol.* 8, 7–18. doi: 10.1159/000082076

Choi, P. S., and Bernstein, H. D. (2009). Sequential translocation of an *Escherichia coli* two-partner secretion pathway exoprotein across the inner and outer membranes. *Mol. Microbiol.* 75, 440–451. doi: 10.1111/j.1365-2958.2009.06993.x

Choi, P. S., Dawson, A. J., and Bernstein, H. D. (2007). Characterization of a novel two-partner secretion system in *Escherichia coli* O157:H7. *J. Bacteriol.* 189, 3452–3461. doi: 10.1128/JB.01751-06

Clantin, B., Delattre, A. S., Rucktooa, P., Saint, N., Meli, A. C., Locht, C., et al. (2007). Structure of the membrane protein FhaC: a member of the Omp85-TpsB transporter superfamily. *Science* 317, 957–961. doi: 10.1126/science.1143860

Clantin, B., Hodak, H., Willery, E., Locht, C., Jacob-Dubuisson, F., and Villeret, V. (2004). The crystal structure of filamentous hemagglutinin secretion domain and its implications for the two-partner secretion pathway. *Proc. Natl. Acad. Sci. U.S.A.* 101, 6194–6199. doi: 10.1073/pnas.0400291101

Cooley, R. B., Smith, T. J., Leung, W., Tierney, V., Borlee, B. R., O'Toole, G. A., et al. (2015). Cyclic Di-GMP-regulated periplasmic proteolysis of a *Pseudomonas aeruginosa* type Vb secretion system substrate. *J. Bacteriol.* 198, 66–76. doi: 10.1128/JB.00369-15

Cope, L. D., Thomas, S. E., Latimer, J. L., Slaughter, C. A., Müller-Eberhard, U., and Hansen, E. J. (1994). The 100-kDa haem:hemopexin-binding protein of *Haemophilus influenzae*: structure and localization. *Mol. Microbiol.* 13, 863–873.

Cope, L. D., Yogev, R., Muller-Eberhard, U., and Hansen, E. J. (1995). A gene cluster involved in the utilization of both free heme and heme:hemopexin by *Haemophilus influenzae* type b. *J. Bacteriol.* 177, 2644–2653.

Côté, J. P., Charbonneau, M. E., and Mourez, M. (2013). Glycosylation of the *Escherichia coli* TibA self-associating autotransporter influences the conformation and the functionality of the protein. *PLoS ONE* 8:e80739. doi: 10.1371/journal.pone.0080739

Cotter, S. E., Surana, N. K., and St Geme, J. W. III. (2005). Trimeric autotransporters: a distinct subfamily of autotransporter proteins. *Trends Microbiol.* 13, 199–205. doi: 10.1016/j.tim.2005.03.004

Coutte, L., Antoine, R., Drobecq, H., Locht, C., and Jacob-Dubuisson, F. (2001). Subtilisin-like autotransporter serves as maturation protease in a bacterial secretion pathway. *EMBO J.* 20, 5040–5048. doi: 10.1093/emboj/20.18.5040

Coutte, L., Willery, E., Antoine, R., Drobecq, H., Locht, C., and Jacob-Dubuisson, F. (2003). Surface anchoring of bacterial subtilisin important for maturation function. *Mol. Microbiol.* 49, 529–539.

da Mata Madeira, P. V., Zouhir, S., Basso, P., Neves, D., Laubier, A., Salacha, R., et al. (2016). Structural basis of lipid targeting and destruction by the type V secretion system of *Pseudomonas aeruginosa*. *J. Mol. Biol.* 428, 1790–1803. doi: 10.1016/j.jmb.2016.03.012

Darsonval, A., Darrasse, A., Durand, K., Bureau, C., Cesbron, S., and Jacques, M. A. (2009). Adhesion and fitness in the bean phyllosphere and transmission to seed of *Xanthomonas fuscans* subsp. *fuscans*. *Mol. Plant Microbe Interact.* 22, 747–757. doi: 10.1094/MPMI-22-6-0747

Delattre, A. S., Clantin, B., Saint, N., Locht, C., Villeret, V., and Jacob-Dubuisson, F. (2010). Functional importance of a conserved sequence motif in FhaC, a prototypic member of the TpsB/Omp85 superfamily. *FEBS J.* 277, 4755–4765. doi: 10.1111/j.1742-4658.2010.07881.x

Delattre, A. S., Saint, N., Clantin, B., Willery, E., Lippens, G., Locht, C., et al. (2011). Substrate recognition by the POTRA domains of TpsB transporter FhaC. *Mol. Microbiol.* 81, 99–112. doi: 10.1111/j.1365-2958.2011.07680.x

Depperschmidt, A., Ketterer, N., and Pfaffelhuber, P. (2013). A Brownian ratchet for protein translocation including dissociation of ratcheting sites. *J. Math. Biol.* 66, 505–534. doi: 10.1007/s00285-012-0519-8

Desvaux, M., Cooper, L. M., Filenko, N. A., Scott-Tucker, A., Turner, S. M., Cole, J. A., et al. (2006). The unusual extended signal peptide region of the type V secretion system is phylogenetically restricted. *FEMS Microbiol. Lett.* 264, 22–30. doi: 10.1111/j.1574-6968.2006.00425.x

Desvaux, M., Scott-Tucker, A., Turner, S. M., Cooper, L. M., Huber, D., Nataro, J. P., et al. (2007). A conserved extended signal peptide region directs posttranslational protein translocation via a novel mechanism. *Microbiology* 153, 59–70. doi: 10.1099/mic.0.29091-0

Di Venanzio, G., Stepanenko, T. M., and García Véscosi, E. (2014). *Serratia marcescens* ShlA pore-forming toxin is responsible for early induction of autophagy in host cells and is transcriptionally regulated by RcsB. *Infect. Immun.* 82, 3542–3554. doi: 10.1128/IAI.01682-14

Diner, E. J., Beck, C. M., Webb, J. S., Low, D. A., and Hayes, C. S. (2012). Identification of a target cell permissive factor required for contact-dependent growth inhibition (CDI). *Genes Dev.* 26, 515–525. doi: 10.1101/gad.1823 45.111

Dobrindt, U., Blum-Oehler, G., Nagy, G., Schneider, G., Johann, A., Gottschalk, G., et al. (2002). Genetic structure and distribution of four pathogenicity islands (PAI I(536) to PAI IV(536)) of uropathogenic *Escherichia coli* strain 536. *Infect. Immun.* 70, 6365–6372.

Dodd, D. A., Worth, R. G., Rosen, M. K., Grinstein, S., van Oers, N. S., and Hansen, E. J. (2014). The *Haemophilus ducreyi* LspA1 protein inhibits phagocytosis by using a new mechanism involving activation of C-terminal Src kinase. *MBio* 5, e01178–e01114. doi: 10.1128/mBio.01178-14

Domenighini, M., Relman, D., Capiau, C., Falkow, S., Prugnola, A., Scarlato, V., et al. (1990). Genetic characterization of *Bordetella pertussis* filamentous hemagglutinin: a protein processed from an unusually large precursor. *Mol. Microbiol.* 4, 787–800.

Drobnak, I., Braselmann, E., and Clark, P. L. (2015). Multiple driving forces required for efficient secretion of autotransporter virulence proteins. *J. Biol. Chem.* 290, 10104–10116. doi: 10.1074/jbc.M114.629170

Duret, G., Szymanski, M., Choi, K. J., Yeo, H. J., and Delcour, A. H. (2008). The TpsB translocator HMW1B of *Haemophilus influenzae* forms a large conductance channel. *J. Biol. Chem.* 283, 15771–15778. doi: 10.1074/jbc.M708970200

Dwyer, R. S., Ricci, D. P., Colwell, L. J., Silhavy, T. J., and Wingreen, N. S. (2013). Predicting functionally informative mutations in *Escherichia coli* BamA using evolutionary covariance analysis. *Genetics* 195, 443–455. doi: 10.1534/genetics.113.155861

Elsen, S., Huber, P., Bouillot, S., Coute, Y., Fournier, P., Dubois, Y., et al. (2014). A type III secretion negative clinical strain of *Pseudomonas aeruginosa* employs a two-partner secreted exolysin to induce hemorrhagic pneumonia. *Cell Host Microbe* 15, 164–176. doi: 10.1016/j.chom.2014.01.003

Emsley, P., Charles, I. G., Fairweather, N. F., and Isaacs, N. W. (1996). Structure of *Bordetella pertussis* virulence factor P.69 pertactin. *Nature* 381, 90–92.

Fairman, J. W., Dautin, N., Wojtowicz, D., Liu, W., Noinaj, N., Barnard, T. J., et al. (2012). Crystal structures of the outer membrane domain of intimin and invasin from enterohemorrhagic *E. coli* and enteropathogenic *Y. pseudotuberculosis*. *Structure* 20, 1233–1243. doi: 10.1016/j.str.2012.04.011

Fan, E., Chauhan, N., Udatha, D. B., Leo, J. C., and Linke, D. (2016). Type V secretion systems in bacteria. *Microbiol. Spectr.* 4:VMBF-0009-2015. doi: 10.1128/microbiolspec.VMBF-0009-2015

Fan, E., Fiedler, S., Jacob-Dubuisson, F., and Müller, M. (2012). Two-partner secretion of gram-negative bacteria: a single beta-barrel protein enables transport across the outer membrane. *J. Biol. Chem.* 287, 2591–2599. doi: 10.1074/jbc.M111.293068

Faure, L. M., Garvis, S., de Bentzmann, S., and Bigot, S. (2014). Characterization of a novel two-partner secretion system implicated in the virulence of *Pseudomonas aeruginosa*. *Microbiology* 160, 1940–1952. doi: 10.1099/mic.0.079616-0

Fleckenstein, J. M., Roy, K., Fischer, J. F., and Burkitt, M. (2006). Identification of a two-partner secretion locus of enterotoxigenic *Escherichia coli*. *Infect. Immun.* 74, 2245–2258. doi: 10.1128/IAI.74.4.2245-2258.2006

Fournier, C., Smith, A., and Delepelaire, P. (2011). Haem release from haemopexin by HxuA allows *Haemophilus influenzae* to escape host nutritional immunity. *Mol. Microbiol.* 80, 133–148. doi: 10.1111/j.1365-2958.2011.07562.x

Fuller, T. E., Kennedy, M. J., and Lowery, D. E. (2000). Identification of *Pasteurella multocida* virulence genes in a septicemic mouse model using signature-tagged mutagenesis. *Microb. Pathog.* 29, 25–38. doi: 10.1006/mpat.2000.0365

Gal-Mor, O., Gibson, D. L., Baluta, D., Vallance, B. A., and Finlay, B. B. (2008). A novel secretion pathway of *Salmonella enterica* acts as an antivirulence modulator during salmonellosis. *PLoS Pathog.* 4:e1000036. doi: 10.1371/journal.ppat.1000036

Garcia, E. C., Anderson, M. S., Hagar, J. A., and Cotter, P. A. (2013). *Burkholderia* BcpA mediates biofilm formation independently of interbacterial contact-dependent growth inhibition. *Mol. Microbiol.* 89, 1213–1225. doi: 10.1111/mmi.12339

Garcia, E. C., Perault, A. I., Marlatt, S. A., and Cotter, P. A. (2016). Interbacterial signaling via *Burkholderia* contact-dependent growth inhibition system proteins. *Proc. Natl. Acad. Sci. U.S.A.* 113, 8296–8301. doi: 10.1073/pnas.1606323113

Garnett, J. A., Muhl, D., Douse, C. H., Hui, K., Busch, A., Omisore, A., et al. (2015). Structure-function analysis reveals that the *Pseudomonas aeruginosa* Tps4 two-partner secretion system is involved in CupB5 translocation. *Protein Sci.* 24, 670–687. doi: 10.1002/pro.2640

Gatzeva-Topalova, P. Z., Warner, L. R., Pardi, A., and Sousa, M. C. (2010). Structure and flexibility of the complete periplasmic domain of BamA: the protein insertion machine of the outer membrane. *Structure* 18, 1492–1501. doi: 10.1016/j.str.2010.08.012

Gessmann, D., Chung, Y. H., Danoff, E. J., Plummer, A. M., Sandlin, C. W., Zaccai, N. R., et al. (2014). Outer membrane beta-barrel protein folding is physically controlled by periplasmic lipid head groups and BamA. *Proc. Natl. Acad. Sci. U.S.A.* 111, 5878–5883. doi: 10.1073/pnas.1322473111

Gottig, N., Garavaglia, B. S., Garofalo, C. G., Orellano, E. G., and Ottado, J. (2009). A filamentous hemagglutinin-like protein of *Xanthomonas axonopodis* pv. citri, the phytopathogen responsible for citrus canker, is involved in bacterial virulence. *PLoS ONE* 4:e4358. doi: 10.1371/journal.pone.0004358

Grass, S., and St Geme, J. W. III. (2000). Maturation and secretion of the non-typable *Haemophilus influenzae* HMW1 adhesin: roles of the N-terminal and C-terminal domains. *Mol. Microbiol.* 36, 55–67.

Grass, S., Buscher, A. Z., Swords, W. E., Apicella, M. A., Barenkamp, S. J., Ozchlewski, N., et al. (2003). The *Haemophilus influenzae* HMW1 adhesin is glycosylated in a process that requires HMW1C and phosphoglucomutase, an enzyme involved in lipooligosaccharide biosynthesis. *Mol. Microbiol.* 48, 737–751.

Grass, S., Lichti, C. F., Townsend, R. R., Gross, J., and St Geme, J. W. III. (2010). The *Haemophilus influenzae* HMW1C protein is a glycosyltransferase that transfers hexose residues to asparagine sites in the HMW1 adhesin. *PLoS Pathog.* 6:e1000919. doi: 10.1371/journal.ppat.1000919

Grass, S., Rempe, K. A., and St Geme, J. W. III. (2015). Structural determinants of the interaction between the TpsA and TpsB proteins in the *Haemophilus influenzae* HMW1 two-partner secretion system. *J. Bacteriol.* 197, 1769–1780. doi: 10.1128/JB.00039-15

Grijpstra, J., Arenas, J., Rutten, L., and Tommassen, J. (2013). Autotransporter secretion: varying on a theme. *Res. Microbiol.* 164, 562–582. doi: 10.1016/j.resmic.2013.03.010

Gross, J., Grass, S., Davis, A. E., Gilmore-Erdmann, P., Townsend, R. R., and St Geme, J. W. III. (2008). The *Haemophilus influenzae* HMW1 adhesin is a glycoprotein with an unusual N-linked carbohydrate modification. *J. Biol. Chem.* 283, 26010–26015. doi: 10.1074/jbc.M801819200

Grosskinsky, U., Schütz, M., Fritz, M., Schmid, Y., Lamparter, M. C., Szczesny, P., et al. (2007). A conserved glycine residue of trimeric autotransporter domains plays a key role in *Yersinia adhesin* a autotransport. *J. Bacteriol.* 189, 9011–9019. doi: 10.1128/JB.00985-07

Gruss, F., Zähringer, F., Jakob, R. P., Burmann, B. M., Hiller, S., and Maier, T. (2013). The structural basis of autotransporter translocation by TamA. *Nat. Struct. Mol. Biol.* 20, 1318–1320. doi: 10.1038/nsmb.2689

Gu, Y., Li, H., Dong, H., Zeng, Y., Zhang, Z., Paterson, N. G., et al. (2016). Structural basis of outer membrane protein insertion by the BAM complex. *Nature* 531, 64–69. doi: 10.1038/nature17199

Guédin, S., Willery, E., Locht, C., and Jacob-Dubuisson, F. (1998). Evidence that a globular conformation is not compatible with FhaC-mediated secretion of the *Bordetella pertussis* filamentous haemagglutinin. *Mol. Microbiol.* 29, 763–774.

Guédin, S., Willery, E., Tommassen, J., Fort, E., Drobecq, H., Locht, C., et al. (2000). Novel topological features of FhaC, the outer membrane transporter involved in the secretion of the *Bordetella pertussis* filamentous hemagglutinin. *J. Biol. Chem.* 275, 30202–30210. doi: 10.1074/jbc.M005515200

Guérin, J., Baud, C., Touati, N., Saint, N., Willery, E., Locht, C., et al. (2014). Conformational dynamics of protein transporter FhaC: large-scale motions of plug helix. *Mol. Microbiol.* 92, 1164–1176. doi: 10.1111/mmi.12585

Guerin, J., Saint, N., Baud, C., Meli, A. C., Etienne, E., Locht, C., et al. (2015). Dynamic interplay of membrane-proximal POTRA domain and conserved loop L6 in Omp85 transporter FhaC. *Mol. Microbiol.* 98, 490–501. doi: 10.1111/mmi.13137

Guilhabert, M. R., and Kirkpatrick, B. C. (2005). Identification of *Xylella fastidiosa* antivirulence genes: hemagglutinin adhesins contribute a biofilm maturation to *X. fastidios* and colonization and attenuate virulence. *Mol. Plant Microbe Interact.* 18, 856–868. doi: 10.1094/MPMI-18-0856

Hagan, C. L., Silhavy, T. J., and Kahne, D. (2011). beta-Barrel membrane protein assembly by the Bam complex. *Annu. Rev. Biochem.* 80, 189–210. doi: 10.1146/annurev-biochem-061408-144611

Haines, S., Arnaud-Barbe, N., Poncet, D., Reverchon, S., Wawrzyniak, J., Nasser, W., et al. (2015). IscR regulates synthesis of colonization factor antigen I fimbriae in response to iron starvation in enterotoxigenic *Escherichia coli*. *J. Bacteriol.* 197, 2896–2907. doi: 10.1128/JB.00214-15

Han, L., Zheng, J., Wang, Y., Yang, X., Liu, Y., Sun, C., et al. (2016). Structure of the BAM complex and its implications for biogenesis of outer-membrane proteins. *Nat. Struct. Mol. Biol.* 23, 192–196. doi: 10.1038/nsmb.3181

Hartmann, M. D., Ridderbusch, O., Zeth, K., Albrecht, R., Testa, O., Woolfson, D. N., et al. (2009). A coiled-coil motif that sequesters ions to the hydrophobic core. *Proc. Natl. Acad. Sci. U.S.A.* 106, 16950–16955. doi: 10.1073/pnas.0907256106

Heinz, E., and Lithgow, T. (2014). A comprehensive analysis of the Omp85/TpsB protein superfamily structural diversity, taxonomic occurrence, and evolution. *Front. Microbiol.* 5:370. doi: 10.3389/fmicb.2014.00370

Heinz, E., Stubenrauch, C. J., Grinter, R., Croft, N. P., Purcell, A. W., Strugnell, R. A., et al. (2016). Conserved features in the structure, mechanism, and biogenesis of the inverse autotransporter protein family. *Genome Biol. Evol.* 8, 1690–1705. doi: 10.1093/gbe/evw112

Hertle, R., Hilger, M., Weingardt-Kocher, S., and Walev, I. (1999). Cytotoxic action of *Serratia marcescens* hemolysin on human epithelial cells. *Infect. Immun.* 67, 817–825.

Hirono, I., Tange, N., and Aoki, T. (1997). Iron-regulated haemolysin from *Edwardsiella tarda*. *Mol. Microbiol.* 24, 851–856.

Hodak, H., and Jacob-Dubuisson, F. (2007). Current challenges in autotransport and two-partner protein secretion pathways. *Res. Microbiol.* 158, 631–637. doi: 10.1016/j.resmic.2007.08.001

Hodak, H., Clantin, B., Willery, E., Villeret, V., Locht, C., and Jacob-Dubuisson, F. (2006). Secretion signal of the filamentous haemagglutinin, a model two-partner secretion substrate. *Mol. Microbiol.* 61, 368–382. doi: 10.1111/j.1365-2958.2006.05242.x

Hoiczyk, E., Roggenkamp, A., Reichenbecher, M., Lupas, A., and Heesemann, J. (2000). Structure and sequence analysis of *Yersinia* YadA and *Moraxella* UspAs reveal a novel class of adhesins. *EMBO J.* 19, 5989–5999. doi: 10.1093/emboj/19.22.5989

Iadanza, M. G., Higgins, A. J., Schiffrin, B., Calabrese, A. N., Brockwell, D. J., Ashcroft, A. E., et al. (2016). Lateral opening in the intact beta-barrel assembly machinery captured by cryo-EM. *Nat. Commun.* 7:12865. doi: 10.1038/ncomms12865

Ieva, R., and Bernstein, H. D. (2009). Interaction of an autotransporter passenger domain with BamA during its translocation across the bacterial outer membrane. *Proc. Natl. Acad. Sci. U.S.A.* 106, 19120–19125. doi: 10.1073/pnas.0907912106

Ieva, R., Skillman, K. M., and Bernstein, H. D. (2008). Incorporation of a polypeptide segment into the beta-domain pore during the assembly of a bacterial autotransporter. *Mol. Microbiol.* 67, 188–201. doi: 10.1111/j.1365-2958.2007.06048.x

Ieva, R., Tian, P., Peterson, J. H., and Bernstein, H. D. (2011). Sequential and spatially restricted interactions of assembly factors with an autotransporter beta domain. *Proc. Natl. Acad. Sci. U.S.A.* 108, E383–E391. doi: 10.1073/pnas.1103827108

Jacob-Dubuisson, F., Buisine, C., Willery, E., Renauld-Mongenie, G., and Locht, C. (1997). Lack of functional complementation between *Bordetella pertussis* filamentous hemagglutinin and *Proteus mirabilis* HpmA hemolysin secretion machineries. *J. Bacteriol.* 179, 775–783.

Jacob-Dubuisson, F., Fernandez, R., and Coutte, L. (2004). Protein secretion through autotransporter and two-partner pathways. *Biochim. Biophys. Acta* 1694, 235–257. doi: 10.1016/j.bbamcr.2004.03.008

Jacob-Dubuisson, F., Guerin, J., Baelen, S., and Clantin, B. (2013). Two-partner secretion: as simple as it sounds? *Res. Microbiol.* 164, 583–595. doi: 10.1016/j.resmic.2013.03.009

Jacob-Dubuisson, F., Locht, C., and Antoine, R. (2001). Two-partner secretion in Gram-negative bacteria: a thrifty, specific pathway for large virulence proteins. *Mol. Microbiol.* 40, 306–313.

Jacob-Dubuisson, F., Villeret, V., Clantin, B., Delattre, A. S., and Saint, N. (2009). First structural insights into the TpsB/Omp85 superfamily. *Biol. Chem.* 390, 675–684. doi: 10.1515/BC.2009.099

Jain, S., and Goldberg, M. B. (2007). Requirement for YaeT in the outer membrane assembly of autotransporter proteins. *J. Bacteriol.* 189, 5393–5398. doi: 10.1128/JB.00228-07

Jones, A. M., Garza-Sanchez, F., So, J., Hayes, C. S., and Low, D. A. (2017). Activation of contact-dependent antibacterial tRNase toxins by translation elongation factors. *Proc. Natl. Acad. Sci. U.S.A.* 114, E1951–E1957. doi: 10.1073/pnas.1619273114

Julio, S. M., and Cotter, P. A. (2005). Characterization of the filamentous hemagglutinin-like protein FhaS in *Bordetella bronchiseptica*. *Infect. Immun.* 73, 4960–4971. doi: 10.1128/IAI.73.8.4960-4971.2005

Junker, M., and Clark, P. L. (2010). Slow formation of aggregation-resistant beta-sheet folding intermediates. *Proteins* 78, 812–824. doi: 10.1002/prot.22609

Junker, M., Besingi, R. N., and Clark, P. L. (2009). Vectorial transport and folding of an autotransporter virulence protein during outer membrane secretion. *Mol. Microbiol.* 71, 1323–1332. doi: 10.1111/j.1365-2958.2009.06607.x

Junker, M., Schuster, C. C., McDonnell, A. V., Sorg, K. A., Finn, M. C., Berger, B., et al. (2006). Pertactin beta-helix folding mechanism suggests common themes for the secretion and folding of autotransporter proteins. *Proc. Natl. Acad. Sci. U.S.A.* 103, 4918–4923. doi: 10.1073/pnas.0507923103

Kachalova, G. S., Rogulin, E. A., Yunusova, A. K., Artyukh, R. I., Perevyazova, T. A., Matvienko, N. I., et al. (2008). Structural analysis of the heterodimeric type IIS restriction endonuclease R.BspD6I acting as a complex between a monomeric site-specific nickase and a catalytic subunit. *J. Mol. Biol.* 384, 489–502. doi: 10.1016/j.jmb.2008.09.033

Kajava, A. V., and Steven, A. C. (2006a). The turn of the screw: variations of the abundant beta-solenoid motif in passenger domains of Type V secretory proteins. *J. Struct. Biol.* 155, 306–315. doi: 10.1016/j.jsb.2006.01.015

Kajava, A. V., and Steven, A. C. (2006b). Beta-rolls, beta-helices, and other beta-solenoid proteins. *Adv. Protein Chem.* 73, 55–96. doi: 10.1016/S0065-3233(06)73003-0

Kajava, A. V., Cheng, N., Cleaver, R., Kessel, M., Simon, M. N., Willery, E., et al. (2001). Beta-helix model for the filamentous haemagglutinin adhesin of *Bordetella pertussis* and related bacterial secretory proteins. *Mol. Microbiol.* 42, 279–292.

Kang'ethe, W., and Bernstein, H. D. (2013a). Stepwise folding of an autotransporter passenger domain is not essential for its secretion. *J. Biol. Chem.* 288, 35028–35038. doi: 10.1074/jbc.M113.515635

Kang'ethe, W., and Bernstein, H. D. (2013b). Charge-dependent secretion of an intrinsically disordered protein via the autotransporter pathway. *Proc. Natl. Acad. Sci. U.S.A.* 110, E4246–E4255. doi: 10.1073/pnas.1310345110

Kaundal, S., Uttam, M., and Thakur, K. G. (2016). Dual role of a biosynthetic enzyme, CysK, in contact dependent growth inhibition in bacteria. *PLoS ONE* 11:e0159844. doi: 10.1371/journal.pone.0159844

Kida, Y., Higashimoto, Y., Inoue, H., Shimizu, T., and Kuwano, K. (2008). A novel secreted protease from *Pseudomonas aeruginosa* activates NF-kappaB through protease-activated receptors. *Cell. Microbiol.* 10, 1491–1504. doi: 10.1111/j.1462-5822.2008.01142.x

Kida, Y., Shimizu, T., and Kuwano, K. (2011). Cooperation between LepA and PlcH contributes to the *in vivo* virulence and growth of *Pseudomonas aeruginosa* in mice. *Infect. Immun.* 79, 211–219. doi: 10.1128/IAI.01053-10

Kim, D. S., Chao, Y., and Saier, M. H. Jr. (2006). Protein-translocating trimeric autotransporters of gram-negative bacteria. *J. Bacteriol.* 188, 5655–5667. doi: 10.1128/JB.01596-05

Kim, S., Malinverni, J. C., Sliz, P., Silhavy, T. J., Harrison, S. C., and Kahne, D. (2007). Structure and function of an essential component of the outer membrane protein assembly machine. *Science* 317, 961–964. doi: 10.1126/science.1143993

Klee, S. R., Nassif, X., Kusecek, B., Merker, P., Beretti, J. L., Achtman, M., et al. (2000). Molecular and biological analysis of eight genetic islands that distinguish *Neisseria meningitidis* from the closely related pathogen *Neisseria gonorrhoeae*. *Infect. Immun.* 68, 2082–2095.

Knowles, T. J., Scott-Tucker, A., Overduin, M., and Henderson, I. R. (2009). Membrane protein architects: the role of the BAM complex in outer membrane protein assembly. *Nat. Rev. Microbiol.* 7, 206–214. doi: 10.1038/nrmicro2069

Konninger, U. W., Hobbie, S., Benz, R., and Braun, V. (1999). The haemolysin-secreting ShlB protein of the outer membrane of *Serratia marcescens*: determination of surface-exposed residues and formation of ion-permeable pores by ShlB mutants in artificial lipid bilayer membranes. *Mol. Microbiol.* 32, 1212–1225.

Labandeira-Rey, M., Dodd, D. A., Brautigam, C. A., Fortney, K. R., Spinola, S. M., and Hansen, E. J. (2013). The *Haemophilus ducreyi* Fis protein is involved in controlling expression of the lspB-lspA2 operon and other virulence factors. *Infect. Immun.* 81, 4160–4170. doi: 10.1128/IAI.00714-13

Labandeira-Rey, M., Mock, J. R., and Hansen, E. J. (2009). Regulation of expression of the *Haemophilus ducreyi* LspB and LspA2 proteins by CpxR. *Infect. Immun.* 77, 3402–3411. doi: 10.1128/IAI.00292-09

Lehr, U., Schutz, M., Oberhettinger, P., Ruiz-Perez, F., Donald, J. W., Palmer, T., et al. (2010). C-terminal amino acid residues of the trimeric autotransporter adhesin YadA of *Yersinia enterocolitica* are decisive for its recognition and assembly by BamA. *Mol. Microbiol.* 78, 932–946. doi: 10.1111/j.1365-2958.2010.07377.x

Leo, J. C., Grin, I., and Linke, D. (2012). Type V secretion: mechanism(s) of autotransport through the bacterial outer membrane. *Philos. Trans. R. Soc. Lond. B Biol. Sci.* 367, 1088–1101. doi: 10.1098/rstb.2011.0208

Leo, J. C., Oberhettinger, P., Chaubey, M., Schutz, M., Kuhner, D., Bertsche, U., et al. (2015a). The Intimin periplasmic domain mediates dimerisation and binding to peptidoglycan. *Mol. Microbiol.* 95, 80–100. doi: 10.1111/mmi.12840

Leo, J. C., Oberhettinger, P., Schutz, M., and Linke, D. (2015b). The inverse autotransporter family: intimin, invasin and related proteins. *Int. J. Med. Microbiol.* 305, 276–282. doi: 10.1016/j.ijmm.2014.12.011

Leonard-Rivera, M., and Misra, R. (2012). Conserved residues of the putative L6 Loop of *Escherichia coli* BamA play a critical role in the assembly of beta-barrel outer membrane proteins, including that of BamA itself. *J. Bacteriol.* 194, 4662–4668. doi: 10.1128/JB.00825-12

Leyton, D. L., Rossiter, A. E., and Henderson, I. R. (2012). From self sufficiency to dependence: mechanisms and factors important for autotransporter biogenesis. *Nat. Rev. Microbiol.* 10, 213–225. doi: 10.1038/nrmicro2733

Lin, C. S., Horng, J. T., Yang, C. H., Tsai, Y. H., Su, L. H., Wei, C. F., et al. (2010). RssAB-FlhDC-ShlBA as a major pathogenesis pathway in *Serratia marcescens*. *Infect. Immun.* 78, 4870–4881. doi: 10.1128/IAI.00661-10

Linke, D., Riess, T., Autenrieth, I. B., Lupas, A., and Kempf, V. A. (2006). Trimeric autotransporter adhesins: variable structure, common function. *Trends Microbiol.* 14, 264–270. doi: 10.1016/j.tim.2006.04.005

Llamas, M. A., van der Sar, A., Chu, B. C., Sparrius, M., Vogel, H. J., and Bitter, W. (2009). A novel extracytoplasmic function (ECF) sigma factor regulates virulence in *Pseudomonas aeruginosa*. *PLoS Pathog.* 5:e1000572. doi: 10.1371/journal.ppat.1000572

Locht, C., Bertin, P., Menozzi, F. D., and Renauld, G. (1993). The filamentous haemagglutinin, a multifaceted adhesin produced by virulent *Bordetella* spp. *Mol. Microbiol.* 9, 653–660.

Maier, T., Clantin, B., Gruss, F., Dewitte, F., Delattre, A. S., Jacob-Dubuisson, F., et al. (2015). Conserved Omp85 lid-lock structure and substrate recognition in FhaC. *Nat. Commun.* 6:7452. doi: 10.1038/ncomms8452

Makhov, A. M., Hannah, J. H., Brennan, M. J., Trus, B. L., Kocsis, E., Conway, J. F., et al. (1994). Filamentous hemagglutinin of *Bordetella pertussis*. A bacterial adhesin formed as a 50-nm monomeric rigid rod based on a 19-residue repeat motif rich in beta strands and turns. *J. Mol. Biol.* 241, 110–124.

Matlack, K. E., Misselwitz, B., Plath, K., and Rapoport, T. A. (1999). BiP acts as a molecular ratchet during posttranslational transport of prepro-alpha factor across the ER membrane. *Cell* 97, 553–564.

Mazar, J., and Cotter, P. A. (2006). Topology and maturation of filamentous haemagglutinin suggest a new model for two-partner secretion. *Mol. Microbiol.* 62, 641–654. doi: 10.1111/j.1365-2958.2006.05392.x

Melvin, J. A., Scheller, E. V., Noel, C. R., and Cotter, P. A. (2015). New insight into filamentous hemagglutinin secretion reveals a role for full-length FhaB in *Bordetella* virulence. *mBio* 6:e01189-15. doi: 10.1128/mBio.01189-15

Meng, G., Surana, N. K., St Geme, J. W. III, and Waksman, G. (2006). Structure of the outer membrane translocator domain of the *Haemophilus influenzae* Hia trimeric autotransporter. *EMBO J.* 25, 2297–2304. doi: 10.1038/sj.emboj.7601132

Menozzi, F. D., Boucher, P. E., Riveau, G., Gantiez, C., and Locht, C. (1994). Surface-associated filamentous hemagglutinin induces autoagglutination of *Bordetella pertussis*. *Infect. Immun.* 62, 4261–4269.

Mercy, C., Ize, B., Salcedo, S. P., de Bentzmann, S., and Bigot, S. (2016). Functional characterization of *Pseudomonas* contact dependent growth inhibition (CDI) systems. *PLoS ONE* 11:e0147435. doi: 10.1371/journal.pone.0147435

Mogensen, J. E., and Otzen, D. E. (2005). Interactions between folding factors and bacterial outer membrane proteins. *Mol. Microbiol.* 57, 326–346. doi: 10.1111/j.1365-2958.2005.04674.x

Molina, M. A., Ramos, J. L., and Espinosa-Urgel, M. (2006). A two-partner secretion system is involved in seed and root colonization and iron uptake by *Pseudomonas putida* KT2440. *Environ. Microbiol.* 8, 639–647. doi: 10.1111/j.1462-2920.2005.00940.x

Monteiro-Neto, V., Bando, S. Y., Moreira-Filho, C. A., and Giron, J. A. (2003). Characterization of an outer membrane protein associated with haemagglutination and adhesive properties of enteroaggregative *Escherichia coli* O111:H12. *Cell. Microbiol.* 5, 533–547.

Moon, C. P., Zaccai, N. R., Fleming, P. J., Gessmann, D., and Fleming, K. G. (2013). Membrane protein thermodynamic stability may serve as the energy sink for sorting in the periplasm. *Proc. Natl. Acad. Sci. U.S.A.* 110, 4285–4290. doi: 10.1073/pnas.1212527110

Moormann, C., Benz, I., and Schmidt, M. A. (2002). Functional substitution of the TibC protein of enterotoxigenic *Escherichia coli* strains for the autotransporter adhesin heptosyltransferase of the AIDA system. *Infect. Immun.* 70, 2264–2270.

Morse, R. P., Nikolakakis, K. C., Willett, J. L., Gerrick, E., Low, D. A., Hayes, C. S., et al. (2012). Structural basis of toxicity and immunity in contact-dependent growth inhibition (CDI) systems. *Proc. Natl. Acad. Sci. U.S.A.* 109, 21480–21485. doi: 10.1073/pnas.1216238110

Moslavac, S., Mirus, O., Bredemeier, R., Soll, J., von Haeseler, A., and Schleiff, E. (2005). Conserved pore-forming regions in polypeptide-transporting proteins. *FEBS J.* 272, 1367–1378. doi: 10.1111/j.1742-4658.2005.04569.x

Neil, R. B., and Apicella, M. A. (2009). Role of HrpA in biofilm formation of *Neisseria meningitidis* and regulation of the hrpBAS transcripts. *Infect. Immun.* 77, 2285–2293. doi: 10.1128/IAI.01502-08

Nelson, K. M., Young, G. M., and Miller, V. L. (2001). Identification of a locus involved in systemic dissemination of *Yersinia enterocolitica*. *Infect. Immun.* 69, 6201–6208. doi: 10.1128/IAI.69.10.6201-6208.2001

Ni, D., Wang, Y., Yang, X., Zhou, H., Hou, X., Cao, B., et al. (2014). Structural and functional analysis of the beta-barrel domain of BamA from *Escherichia coli*. *FASEB J.* 28, 2677–2685. doi: 10.1096/fj.13-248450

Noel, C. R., Mazar, J., Melvin, J. A., Sexton, J. A., and Cotter, P. A. (2012). The prodomain of the *Bordetella* two-partner secretion pathway protein FhaB remains intracellular yet affects the conformation of the mature C-terminal domain. *Mol. Microbiol.* 86, 988–1006. doi: 10.1111/mmi.12036

Noinaj, N., Kuszak, A. J., Balusek, C., Gumbart, J. C., and Buchanan, S. K. (2014). Lateral opening and exit pore formation are required for BamA function. *Structure* 22, 1055–1062. doi: 10.1016/j.str.2014.05.008

Noinaj, N., Kuszak, A. J., Gumbart, J. C., Lukacik, P., Chang, H., Easley, N. C., et al. (2013). Structural insight into the biogenesis of beta-barrel membrane proteins. *Nature* 501, 385–390. doi: 10.1038/nature12521

Noinaj, N., Rollauer, S. E., and Buchanan, S. K. (2015). The beta-barrel membrane protein insertase machinery from Gram-negative bacteria. *Curr. Opin. Struct. Biol.* 31, 35–42. doi: 10.1016/j.str.2014.05.008

Norell, D., Heuck, A., Tran-Thi, T. A., Gotzke, H., Jacob-Dubuisson, F., Clausen, T., et al. (2014). Versatile *in vitro* system to study translocation and functional integration of bacterial outer membrane proteins. *Nat. Commun.* 5:5396. doi: 10.1038/ncomms6396

Oberhettinger, P., Schutz, M., Leo, J. C., Heinz, N., Berger, J., Autenrieth, I. B., et al. (2012). Intimin and invasin export their C-terminus to the bacterial cell surface using an inverse mechanism compared to classical autotransport. *PLoS ONE* 7:e47069. doi: 10.1371/journal.pone.0047069

Ogier, J. C., Duvic, B., Lanois, A., Givaudan, A., and Gaudriault, S. (2016). A new member of the growing family of contact-dependent growth inhibition systems in *Xenorhabdus doucetiae*. *PLoS ONE* 11:e0167443. doi: 10.1371/journal.pone.0167443

Oliver, D. C., Huang, G., Nodel, E., Pleasance, S., and Fernandez, R. C. (2003). A conserved region within the *Bordetella pertussis* autotransporter BrkA is necessary for folding of its passenger domain. *Mol. Microbiol.* 47, 1367–1383.

Oomen, C. J., Van Ulsen, P., Van Gelder, P., Feijen, M., Tommassen, J., and Gros, P. (2004). Structure of the translocator domain of a bacterial autotransporter. *EMBO J.* 23, 1257–1266. doi: 10.1038/sj.emboj.7600148

Otto, B. R., Sijbrandi, R., Luirink, J., Oudega, B., Heddle, J. G., Mizutani, K., et al. (2005). Crystal structure of hemoglobin protease, a heme binding autotransporter protein from pathogenic *Escherichia coli*. *J. Biol. Chem.* 280, 17339–17345. doi: 10.1074/jbc.M412885200

Palmer, K. L., and Munson, R. S. J. (1995). Cloning and characterization of the genes encoding the haemolysin of *Haemophilus ducreyi*. *Mol. Microbiol.* 18, 821–830.

Pavlova, O., Peterson, J. H., Ieva, R., and Bernstein, H. D. (2013). Mechanistic link between beta barrel assembly and the initiation of autotransporter secretion. *Proc. Natl. Acad. Sci. U.S.A.* 110, E938–E947. doi: 10.1073/pnas.1219076110

Pei, J., Kim, B. H., and Grishin, N. V. (2008). PROMALS3D: a tool for multiple protein sequence and structure alignments. *Nucleic Acids Res.* 36, 2295–2300. doi: 10.1093/nar/gkn072

Perez, A., Merino, M., Rumbo-Feal, S., Alvarez-Fraga, L., Vallejo, J. A., Beceiro, A., et al. (2016). The FhaB/FhaC two-partner secretion system is involved in adhesion of *Acinetobacter baumannii* AbH12O-A2 strain. *Virulence* 18, 1–16. doi: 10.1080/21505594.2016.1262313

Peterson, J. H., Szabady, R. L., and Bernstein, H. D. (2006). An unusual signal peptide extension inhibits the binding of bacterial presecretory proteins to the signal recognition particle, trigger factor, and the SecYEG complex. *J. Biol. Chem.* 281, 9038–9048. doi: 10.1074/jbc.M508681200

Peterson, J. H., Tian, P., Ieva, R., Dautin, N., and Bernstein, H. D. (2010). Secretion of a bacterial virulence factor is driven by the folding of a C-terminal segment. *Proc. Natl. Acad. Sci. U.S.A.* 107, 17739–17744. doi: 10.1073/pnas.1009491107

Plamondon, P., Luke, N., and Campagnari, A. (2007). Identification of a novel two-partner secretion locus in *Moraxella catarrhalis*. *Infect. Immun.* 75, 2929–2936. doi: 10.1128/IAI.00396-07

Pohlner, J., Halter, R., Beyreuther, K., and Meyer, T. F. (1987). Gene structure and extracellular secretion of *Neisseria gonorrheae* IgA protease. *Nature* 325, 458–462.

Poole, K., and Braun, V. (1988). Iron regulation of *Serratia marcescens* hemolysin gene expression. *Infect. Immun.* 56, 2967–2971.

Poole, K., Schiebel, E., and Braun, V. (1988). Molecular characterization of the hemolysin determinant of *Serratia marcescens*. *J. Bacteriol.* 170, 3177–3188.

Renauld-Mongénie, G., Cornette, J., Mielcarek, N., Menozzi, F. D., and Locht, C. (1996). Distinct roles of the N-terminal and the C-terminal precursor domains in the biogenesis of the *Bordetella pertussis* filamentous hemagglutinin. *J. Bacteriol.* 178, 1053–1060.

Renn, J. P., and Clark, P. L. (2008). A conserved stable core in the passenger domain beta-helix of autotransporter virulence proteins. *Biopolymers* 89, 420–427. doi: 10.1002/bip.20924

Renn, J. P., Junker, M., Besingi, R. N., Braselmann, E., and Clark, P. L. (2012). ATP-independent control of autotransporter virulence protein transport via the folding properties of the secreted protein. *Chem. Biol.* 19, 287–296. doi: 10.1016/j.chembiol.2011.11.009

Ricci, D. P., and Silhavy, T. J. (2012). The Bam machine: a molecular cooper. *Biochim. Biophys. Acta* 1818, 1067–1084. doi: 10.1016/j.bbamem.2011.08.020

Rigel, N. W., Ricci, D. P., and Silhavy, T. J. (2013). Conformation-specific labeling of BamA and suppressor analysis suggest a cyclic mechanism for beta-barrel assembly in *Escherichia coli*. *Proc. Natl. Acad. Sci. U.S.A.* 110, 5151–5156. doi: 10.1073/pnas.1302662110

Rojas, C. M., Ham, J. H., Deng, W. L., Doyle, J. J., and Collmer, A. (2002). HecA, a member of a class of adhesins produced by diverse pathogenic bacteria, contributes to the attachment, aggregation, epidermal cell killing, and virulence phenotypes of *Erwinia chrysanthemi* EC16 on *Nicotiana clevelandii* seedlings. *Proc. Natl. Acad. Sci. U.S.A.* 99, 13142–13147. doi: 10.1073/pnas.2023 58699

Roy, K., Hilliard, G. M., Hamilton, D. J., Luo, J., Ostmann, M. M., and Fleckenstein, J. M. (2009). Enterotoxigenic *Escherichia coli* EtpA mediates adhesion between flagella and host cells. *Nature* 457, 594–598. doi: 10.1038/nature07568

Ruhe, Z. C., Low, D. A., and Hayes, C. S. (2013). Bacterial contact-dependent growth inhibition. *Trends Microbiol.* 21, 230–237. doi: 10.1016/j.tim.2013.02.003

Ruhe, Z. C., Nguyen, J. Y., Chen, A. J., Leung, N. Y., Hayes, C. S., and Low, D. A. (2016). CDI Systems are stably maintained by a cell-contact mediated surveillance mechanism. *PLoS Genet.* 12:e1006145. doi: 10.1371/journal.pgen.1006145

Ruhe, Z. C., Townsley, L., Wallace, A. B., King, A., Van der Woude, M. W., Low, D. A., et al. (2015). CdiA promotes receptor-independent intercellular adhesion. *Mol. Microbiol.* 98, 175–192. doi: 10.1111/mmi.13114

Rybtke, M., Berthelsen, J., Yang, L., Hoiby, N., Givskov, M., and Tolker-Nielsen, T. (2015). The LapG protein plays a role in *Pseudomonas aeruginosa* biofilm formation by controlling the presence of the CdrA adhesin on the cell surface. *Microbiologyopen* 4, 917–930. doi: 10.1002/mbo3.301

Salacha, R., Kovacic, F., Brochier-Armanet, C., Wilhelm, S., Tommassen, J., Filloux, A., et al. (2010). The *Pseudomonas aeruginosa* patatin-like protein PlpD is the archetype of a novel Type V secretion system. *Environ. Microbiol.* 12, 1498–1512. doi: 10.1111/j.1462-2920.2010.02174.x

Sauri, A., Soprova, Z., Wickstrom, D., de Gier, J. W., Van der Schors, R. C., Smit, A. B., et al. (2009). The Bam (Omp85) complex is involved in secretion of the autotransporter haemoglobin protease. *Microbiology* 155, 3982–3991. doi: 10.1099/mic.0.034991-0

Scarlato, V., Arico, B., Prugnola, A., and Rappuoli, R. (1991). Sequential activation and environmental regulation of virulence genes in *Bordetella pertussis*. *EMBO J.* 10, 3971–3975.

Schiebel, E., Schwarz, H., and Braun, V. (1989). Subcellular localization and unique secretion of the hemolysin of *Serratia marcescens*. *J. Biol. Chem.* 264, 16311–16320.

Schmitt, C., Turner, D., Boesl, M., Abele, M., Frosch, M., and Kurzai, O. (2007). A functional two-partner secretion system contributes to adhesion of *Neisseria meningitidis* to epithelial cells. *J. Bacteriol.* 189, 7968–7976. doi: 10.1128/JB.00851-07

Schönherr, R., Tsolis, R., Focareta, T., and Braun, V. (1993). Amino acid replacements in the *Serratia marcescens* haemolysin ShlA define sites involved in activation and secretion. *Mol. Microbiol.* 9, 1229–1237.

Sen, K., Hellman, J., and Nikaido, H. (1988). Porin channels in intact cells of *Escherichia coli* are not affected by Donnan potentials across the outer membrane. *J. Biol. Chem.* 263, 1182–1187.

Serra, D. O., Conover, M. S., Arnal, L., Sloan, G. P., Rodriguez, M. E., Yantorno, O. M., et al. (2012). FHA-mediated cell-substrate and cell-cell adhesions are critical for *Bordetella pertussis* biofilm formation on abiotic surfaces and in the mouse nose and the trachea. *PLoS ONE* 6:e28811. doi: 10.1371/journal.pone.0028811

Shahid, S. A., Bardiaux, B., Franks, W. T., Krabben, L., Habeck, M., van Rossum, B. J., et al. (2012). Membrane-protein structure determination by solid-state NMR spectroscopy of microcrystals. *Nat. Methods* 9, 1212–1217. doi: 10.1038/nmeth.2248

Siddaramappa, S., Challacombe, J. F., Duncan, A. J., Gillaspy, A. F., Carson, M., Gipson, J., et al. (2011). Horizontal gene transfer in *Histophilus somni* and its role in the evolution of pathogenic strain 2336, as determined by comparative genomic analyses. *BMC Genomics* 12:570. doi: 10.1186/1471-2164-12-570

Simon, S. M., Peskin, C. S., and Oster, G. F. (1992). What drives the translocation of proteins? *Proc. Natl. Acad. Sci. U.S.A.* 89, 3770–3774.

St Geme, J. W. III, and Grass, S. (1998). Secretion of the *Haemophilus influenzae* HMW1 and HMW2 adhesins involves a periplasmic intermediate and requires the HMWB and HMWC proteins. *Mol. Microbiol.* 27, 617–630.

St Geme, J. W. III, and Yeo, H. J. (2009). A prototype two-partner secretion pathway: the *Haemophilus influenzae* HMW1 and HMW2 adhesin systems. *Trends Microbiol.* 17, 355–360. doi: 10.1016/j.tim.2009.06.002

Strauss, E. J., Ghori, N., and Falkow, S. (1997). An *Edwardsiella tarda* strain containing a mutation in a gene with homology to *shlB* and *hpmB* is defective for entry into epithelial cells in culture. *Infect. Immun.* 65, 3924–3932.

Surana, N. K., Grass, S., Hardy, G. G., Li, H., Thanassi, D. G., and Geme, J. W. III. (2004). Evidence for conservation of architecture and physical properties of Omp85-like proteins throughout evolution. *Proc. Natl. Acad. Sci. U.S.A.* 101, 14497–14502. doi: 10.1073/pnas.0404679101

Szabady, R. L., Peterson, J. H., Skillman, K. M., and Bernstein, H. D. (2005). An unusual signal peptide facilitates late steps in the biogenesis of a bacterial autotransporter. *Proc. Natl. Acad. Sci. U.S.A.* 102, 221–226. doi: 10.1073/pnas.0406055102

Szczesny, P., and Lupas, A. (2008). Domain annotation of trimeric autotransporter adhesins–daTAA. *Bioinformatics* 24, 1251–1256. doi: 10.1093/bioinformatics/btn118

Tala, A., Progida, C., De Stefano, M., Cogli, L., Spinosa, M. R., Bucci, C., et al. (2008). The HrpB-HrpA two-partner secretion system is essential for intracellular survival of *Neisseria meningitidis*. *Cell. Microbiol.* 10, 2461–2482. doi: 10.1111/j.1462-5822.2008.01222.x

Tsai, J. C., Yen, M. R., Castillo, R., Leyton, D. L., Henderson, I. R., and Saier, M. H. Jr. (2010). The bacterial intimins and invasins: a large and novel family of secreted proteins. *PLoS ONE* 5:e14403. doi: 10.1371/journal.pone.0014403

Tuanyok, A., Leadem, B. R., Auerbach, R. K., Beckstrom-Sternberg, S. M., Beckstrom-Sternberg, J. S., Mayo, M., et al. (2008). Genomic islands from five strains of *Burkholderia pseudomallei*. *BMC Genomics* 9:566. doi: 10.1186/1471-2164-9-566

Tumapa, S., Holden, M. T., Vesaratchavest, M., Wuthiekanun, V., Limmathurotsakul, D., Chierakul, W., et al. (2008). *Burkholderia pseudomallei* genome plasticity associated with genomic island variation. *BMC Genomics* 9:190. doi: 10.1186/1471-2164-9-190

Uphoff, T. S., and Welch, R. A. (1990). Nucleotide sequencing of the *Proteus mirabilis* calcium-independent hemolysin genes (*hpmA* and *hpmB*) reveals sequence similarity with the *Serratia marcescens* hemolysin genes (*shlA* and *shlB*). *J. Bacteriol.* 172, 1206–1216.

Uphoff, T. S., and Welch, R. A. (1994). "Structural and functional analysis of HpmA hemolysin of *Proteus mirabilis*," in *Molecular Mechanisms of Bacterial Virulence*, eds C. I. Kado and J. H. Crosa (Kluwer Academics Publishers), 283–292.

ur Rahman, S., and van Ulsen, P. (2013). System specificity of the TpsB transporters of coexpressed two-partner secretion systems of *Neisseria meningitidis*. *J. Bacteriol.* 195, 788–797. doi: 10.1128/JB.01355-12

ur Rahman, S., Arenas, J., Ozturk, H., Dekker, N., and van Ulsen, P. (2014). The polypeptide transport-associated (POTRA) domains of TpsB transporters determine the system specificity of two-partner secretion systems. *J. Biol. Chem.* 289, 19799–19809. doi: 10.1074/jbc.M113.544627

Vakevainen, M., Greenberg, S., and Hansen, E. J. (2003). Inhibition of phagocytosis by *Haemophilus ducreyi* requires expression of the LspA1 and LspA2 proteins. *Infect. Immun.* 71, 5994–6003.

van den Berg, B. M. (2010). Crystal structure of a full-length autotransporter. *J. Mol. Biol.* 396, 627–633. doi: 10.1016/j.jmb.2009.12.061

van Ulsen, P., Rahman, S., Jong, W., Daleke-Schermerhorn, M., and Luirink, J. (2014). Type V secretion: from biogenesis to biotechnology. *Biochim. Biophys. Acta* 1843, 1592–1611. doi: 10.1016/j.bbamcr.2013.11.006

van Ulsen, P., Rutten, L., Feller, M., Tommassen, J., and van der Ende, A. (2008). Two-partner secretion systems of *Neisseria meningitidis* associated with invasive clonal complexes. *Infect. Immun.* 76, 4649–4658. doi: 10.1128/IAI.00393-08

Walker, G., Hertle, R., and Braun, V. (2004). Activation of *Serratia marcescens* hemolysin through a conformational change. *Infect. Immun.* 72, 611–614.

Wang, F., Zhang, M., Hu, Y., Zhang, W., and Sun, L. (2009). Regulation of the *Edwardsiella tarda* hemolysin gene and luxS by EthR. *J. Microbiol. Biotechnol.* 19, 765–773.

Wang, X., Wang, Q., Xiao, J., Liu, Q., Wu, H., and Zhang, Y. (2010). Hemolysin EthA in *Edwardsiella tarda* is essential for fish invasion *in vivo* and *in vitro* and regulated by two-component system EsrA-EsrB and nucleoid protein HhaEt. *Fish Shellfish Immunol.* 29, 1082–1091. doi: 10.1016/j.fsi.2010.08.025

Ward, C. K., Latimer, J. L., Nika, J., Vakevainen, M., Mock, J. R., Deng, K., et al. (2003). Mutations in the lspA1 and lspA2 genes of *Haemophilus ducreyi* affect the virulence of this pathogen in an animal model system. *Infect. Immun.* 71, 2478–2486.

Ward, C. K., Lumbley, S. R., Latimer, J. L., Cope, L. D., and Hansen, E. J. (1998). *Haemophilus ducreyi* secretes a filamentous hemagglutinin-like protein. *J. Bacteriol.* 180, 6013–6022.

Weaver, T. M., Hocking, J. M., Bailey, L. J., Wawrzyn, G. T., Howard, D. R., Sikkink, L. A., et al. (2009). Structural and functional studies of truncated hemolysin a from *Proteus mirabilis*. *J. Biol. Chem.* 284, 22297–22309. doi: 10.1074/jbc.M109.014431

Webb, C. T., Heinz, E., and Lithgow, T. (2012). Evolution of the beta-barrel assembly machinery. *Trends Microbiol.* 20, 612–620. doi: 10.1016/j.tim.2012.08.006

Webb, J. S., Nikolakakis, K. C., Willett, J. L., Aoki, S. K., Hayes, C. S., and Low, D. A. (2013). Delivery of CdiA nuclease toxins into target cells during contact-dependent growth inhibition. *PLoS ONE* 8:e57609. doi: 10.1371/journal.pone.0057609

Willems, R. J., Geuijen, C., van der Heide, H. G., Renauld, G., Bertin, P., van den Akker, W. M., et al. (1994). Mutational analysis of the *Bordetella pertussis fim/fha* gene cluster: identification of a gene with sequence similarities to haemolysin accessory genes involved in export of FHA. *Mol. Microbiol.* 11, 337–347.

Willett, J. L., Gucinski, G. C., Fatherree, J. P., Low, D. A., and Hayes, C. S. (2015a). Contact-dependent growth inhibition toxins exploit multiple independent cell-entry pathways. *Proc. Natl. Acad. Sci. U.S.A.* 112, 11341-11346. doi: 10.1073/pnas.1512124112

Willett, J. L., Ruhe, Z. C., Goulding, C. W., Low, D. A., and Hayes, C. S. (2015b). Contact-dependent growth inhibition (CDI) and CdiB/CdiA two-partner secretion proteins. *J. Mol. Biol.* 427, 3754–3765. doi: 10.1016/j.jmb.2015.09.010

Wimmer, M. R., Woods, C. N., Adamczak, K. J., Glasgow, E. M., Novak, W. R., Grilley, D. P., et al. (2015). Sequential unfolding of the hemolysin two-partner secretion domain from *Proteus mirabilis*. *Protein Sci.* 24, 1841–1855. doi: 10.1002/pro.2791

Wong, H. C., and Lee, Y. S. (1994). Regulation of iron on bacterial growth and production of thermostable direct hemolysin by *Vibrio parahaemolyticus* in intraperitoneal infected mice. *Microbiol. Immunol.* 38, 367–371.

Yeo, H. J., Yokoyama, T., Walkiewicz, K., Kim, Y., Grass, S., and St Geme, J. W. III. (2007). The structure of the *Haemophilus influenzae*

HMW1 pro-piece reveals a structural domain essential for bacterial two-partner secretion. *J. Biol. Chem.* 282, 31076–31084. doi: 10.1074/jbc.M705750200

Yoder, M. D., Keen, N. T., and Jurnak, F. (1993). New domain motif: the structure of pectate lyase C, a secreted plant virulence factor. *Science* 260, 1503–1507.

Zambolin, S., Clantin, B., Chami, M., Hoos, S., Haouz, A., Villeret, V., et al. (2016). Structural basis for haem piracy from host haemopexin by *Haemophilus influenzae*. *Nat. Commun.* 7:11590. doi: 10.1038/ncomms11590

Zhai, Y., Zhang, K., Huo, Y., Zhu, Y., Zhou, Q., Lu, J., et al. (2011). Autotransporter passenger domain secretion requires a hydrophobic cavity at the extracellular entrance of the beta-domain pore. *Biochem. J.* 435, 577–587. doi: 10.1042/BJ20101548

Zhang, D., Iyer, L. M., and Aravind, L. (2011). A novel immunity system for bacterial nucleic acid degrading toxins and its recruitment in various eukaryotic and DNA viral systems. *Nucleic Acids Res.* 39, 4532–4552. doi: 10.1093/nar/gkr036

Zwihart, K., and Welch, R. (1990). Cytotoxic activity of the *Proteus* hemolysin HpmA. *Infect. Immun.* 58, 1861–1869.

9

Identification of a Contact-Dependent Growth Inhibition (CDI) System that Reduces Biofilm Formation and Host Cell Adhesion of *Acinetobacter baumannii* DSM30011 Strain

Morgane Roussin[1], Sedera Rabarioelina[1], Laurence Cluzeau[1], Julien Cayron[2], Christian Lesterlin[2], Suzana P. Salcedo[1†] and Sarah Bigot[1,2*†]*

[1] Cell Biology of Bacterial Pathogenicity Team, Laboratory of Molecular Microbiology and Structural Biochemistry, CNRS UMR 5086, University of Lyon, Lyon, France, [2] Cell to Cell DNA Transfer Team, Laboratory of Molecular Microbiology and Structural Biochemistry, CNRS UMR 5086, University of Lyon, Lyon, France

***Correspondence:**
Suzana P. Salcedo
suzana.salcedo@ibcp.fr
Sarah Bigot
sarah.bigot@ibcp.fr

Acinetobacter baumannii is a multidrug-resistant nosocomial opportunistic pathogen that is becoming a major health threat worldwide. In this study, we have focused on the *A. baumannii* DSM30011 strain, an environmental isolate that retains many virulence-associated traits. We found that its genome contains two loci encoding for contact-dependent growth inhibition (CDI) systems. These systems serve to kill or inhibit the growth of non-sibling bacteria by delivering toxins into the cytoplasm of target cells, thereby conferring the host strain a significant competitive advantage. We show that one of the two toxins functions as a DNA-damaging enzyme, capable of inducing DNA double-stranded breaks to the chromosome of *Escherichia coli* strain. The second toxin has unknown catalytic activity but stops the growth of *E. coli* without bactericidal effect. In our conditions, only one of the CDI systems was highly expressed in the *A. baumannii* DSM30011 strain and was found to mediate interbacterial competition. Surprisingly, the absence of this CDI system promotes adhesion of *A. baumannii* DSM30011 to both abiotic and biotic surfaces, a phenotype that differs from previously described CDI systems. Our results suggest that a specific regulation mediated by this *A. baumannii* DSM30011 CDI system may result in changes in bacterial physiology that repress host cell adhesion and biofilm formation.

Keywords: type V secretion system, contact-dependent growth inhibition, *Acinectobacter baumannii*, biofilm, cell adhesion ability

INTRODUCTION

In Gram-negative bacteria, the two-partner secretion (TPS) pathway, also known as type Vb secretion system (T5bSS), mediates the translocation across the outer membrane of large, mostly virulence-related, TpsA proteins (Guérin et al., 2017). Functions of the TpsA secreted through the TPS pathway are diverse ranging from cytolysis, adhesion, and iron acquisition to contact-dependent growth inhibition (CDI) (van Ulsen et al., 2014). CDI system was the first secretion system identified to deliver toxin into neighboring cells, arming bacteria with a killing mechanism for outcompeting non-kin cells and establishment of self-communities (Aoki et al., 2005). Growth inhibition involves direct physical contact between bacteria and depends on the production of toxin–antitoxin pairs (Willett et al., 2015). This mechanism exploits the CdiA/CdiB subfamily of TPS systems to export CdiA to the surface through the cognate CdiB transporter and deliver into the cytosol of the target bacterium the last ~300 C-terminal toxic residues of the CdiA proteins, called CdiA-CT. The C-terminal domain is delimited by conserved motifs of unknown function such as (Q/E)LYN in *Burkholderia*, VENN in most bacteria, or yet other motifs in *Pseudomonas* (Aoki et al., 2005; Anderson et al., 2012; Mercy et al., 2016). The presence of the cytoplasmic immunity protein CdiI protects CDI^+ bacteria by interacting with the cognate CdiA-CT toxin and neutralizing its toxic activity. CdiA-CT is highly variable and shows various folds and activities (tRNase, DNase, and pore forming), allowing for a wide diversity of distinct toxins to be deployed to target bacteria (Zhang et al., 2011).

Contact-dependent growth inhibition systems are widespread among Gram-negative bacteria, as *cdi* gene clusters are found in several α-, β-, and γ-proteobacteria. They have been extensively studied in Enterobacteria and *Burkholderia* species, and recent work investigated their role in *Acinetobacter* species (Harding et al., 2017). *Acinetobacter baumannii* can be found associated with severe infections in humans, exhibiting multidrug resistance and causing fatal infections in susceptible hosts, such as patients in intensive care units. *A. baumannii* resists desiccation and forms biofilms that may contribute to its persistence in the clinical devices, causing acute infections. The molecular mechanisms implicated in infection by *A. baumannii* and the virulence factors associated with this process are still unclear. Recent studies investigated the potential implication of TPS systems in *A. baumannii* pathogenesis. The TpsA proteins characterized in strains *A. baumannii* ATCC 19606(T) and clinical AbH12O-A2 are both adhesins that mediate adherence to eukaryotic cells (Darvish Alipour Astaneh et al., 2014; Pérez et al., 2016), and TpsA of *A. baumannii* AbH12O-A2 was shown to contribute to virulence in models of mouse systemic infection and *Caenorhabditis elegans* (Pérez et al., 2016). Interestingly, our *in silico* analysis revealed that these two adhesins associated with their respective CdiB and CdiI partners constitute putative CDI systems, suggesting a potential involvement of these systems in the virulence of *A. baumannii*. This is in line with studies in other organisms suggesting a role for CDI systems beyond bacterial competition. Indeed, several CdiA promotes bacterial auto-aggregation and biofilm formation in *Escherichia coli*, *Pseudomonas aeruginosa*, and *Burkholderia thailandensis* (Garcia et al., 2013; Ruhe et al., 2015; Mercy et al., 2016), as well as intracellular escape and immune evasion of *Neisseria meningitidis* (Talà et al., 2008), functions that are required for the virulence of several pathogens (Gallagher and Manoil, 2001; Rojas et al., 2002; Guilhabert and Kirkpatrick, 2005; Gottig et al., 2009). Recently, *in silico* analysis revealed the identification of more than 40 different CDI systems in pathogenic *Acinetobacter* genomes that have been sorted into type I and II groups (De Gregorio et al., 2019). While sequencing the genome from *A. baumannii* DSM30011 strain (Repizo et al., 2017), we have also identified two *cdiBAI* loci potentially encoding type I and II CDI systems. *A. baumannii* DSM30011, an environmental strain isolated in 1944 from resin-producing guayule plants, has many of the characteristics of clinical strains and was shown to use a type 6 secretion system (T6SS) for bacterial competition and colonization in the model organism *Galleria mellonella* (Repizo et al., 2015). In this study, we used live-cell microscopy to characterize the function of CdiA-CT toxins when produced in *E. coli* cells. Using transcriptional fusions, we show that only one CDI system is expressed in *A. baumannii* DSM30011 and promotes interbacterial competition but is surprisingly a limiting factor for the adhesion process.

RESULTS

The *Acinetobacter baumannii* DSM30011 Genome Contains Two Predicted CDI Systems

In the course of this study, we performed a bioinformatic search to obtain the global repartition and representation of TPS systems among *A. baumannii* species. Each subset of TpsA was used to blast against the *A. baumannii* sequence database. Based on their sequence, TpsA proteins can be phylogenetically classified into at least five subfamilies with distinct functions: (i) the CDI CdiA proteins (Aoki et al., 2005), (ii) the hemolysins/cytolysins such as ShlA of *Serratia marcescens* (Braun et al., 1992), (iii) the adhesins such as filamentous hemagglutinin (FHA) of *Bordetella pertussis* (Relman et al., 1989), (iv) HxuA-type proteins involved in iron acquisition (Fournier et al., 2011), and (v) TpsA with unknown specific activities (Faure et al., 2014). The blast search revealed that the CDI system subfamily is predominantly represented within *A. baumannii* strains with the exception of some genomes comprising Hxu system homologues. We detected two loci in our *A. baumannii* DSM30011 laboratory model strain containing gene organization related to the "*Escherichia coli*"-type CDI systems (**Figure 1A**). We renamed them as $cdi_1^{Ab30011}$ (encoding proteins PNH15603.1, PNH15604.1, and PNH15605.1) and $cdi_2^{Ab30011}$ (encoding proteins PNH14818.1, PNH14817.1, and PNH14816.1). The CdiA proteins of these systems share only 9.6% identity overall, but both contain the highly conserved VENN motif (PF04829) that delimits the N- and C-terminal (CT) domains. The sequence analysis of $CdiA_1$ revealed that the N-terminal domain of this very large protein (532 kDa) harbors long stretches of imperfect repeats predicted to form β-helix folds, that is, β-strand structure organized in fibrous (Kajava et al., 2001), which classifies it as a type II CdiA protein (De Gregorio et al., 2019). $CdiA_1$-CT does not contain any conserved domain. The smaller $CdiA_2$ protein (204 kDa) belongs to the type I CdiA and its $CdiA_2$-CT preceded by the small-helical DUF637 domain found in many CdiA proteins (Iyer et al., 2011) contains a Tox-REase7 nuclease domain. Three potential orphan *cdiI* genes encoding the PNH15606.1,

PNH15607.1, and PNH15608.1 proteins are located downstream of the *cdi*$_1$ locus. Indeed, PNH15606.1 and PNH15607.1 proteins contain an Imm23 domain, and PNH15608.1 protein has a Smi1/Knr4 superfamily domain typically found in immunity proteins present in bacterial polymorphic toxin systems (Iyer et al., 2011; Zhang et al., 2011).

CdiA$_1$-CT/CdiI$_1$ and CdiA$_2$-CT/CdiI$_2$ Are Two Non-interchangeable Toxin–Antitoxin Pairs

To address the toxicity of CT domains, we generated pBAD33 plasmid derivatives producing each CdiA-CT (from the VENN motif to the stop codon) in the presence of arabinose. To assess the CdiI immunity property, nucleotide sequences encoding CdiI fused to 6xHis tag were introduced in pTrc99a plasmid and induced with isopropyl-β-D-1-thiogalactopyranoside (IPTG). The production of CdiA$_1$-CT alone stops the growth of the *E. coli* DH5α strain after 4 h of induction (**Figure 1B**). Unlike CdiA$_1$-CT, CdiA$_2$-CT is highly toxic in *E. coli* where its induction inhibits the growth (**Figure 1C**). Cells coproducing CdiI$_1$ and CdiA$_1$-CT or CdiI$_2$ and CdiA$_2$-CT are protected from the toxic effect of the toxins and exhibited growth equivalent to that of cells containing the empty vector (**Figures 1B,C**). In contrast, the production of CdiI$_1$ or CdiI$_2$ with CdiA$_2$-CT or CdiA$_1$-CT, respectively, does not suppress toxicity. Both CdiI-6xHis were detected in *E. coli* cells in the presence or absence of CdiA-CT using Western blot experiment (**Figure 1D**) showing that the inability to rescue the growth defect caused by a non-cognate CdiA-CT is not due to a lack of CdiI production. CdiA$_1$-CT/CdiI$_1$ and CdiA$_2$-CT/CdiI$_2$ therefore function as pairs of toxin–antitoxin, and these systems are not interchangeable.

CdiA$_2$-CT^{Ab30011} Toxin Induces DNA Damage in *E. coli*

CdiA$_2$-CT contains a restriction endonuclease-like domain belonging to the Tox-REase7 family (Pfam PF15649) mostly found in CdiA of *Pseudomonas* and *Acinetobacter* species (Zhang et al., 2012; Mercy et al., 2016). To determine whether CdiA$_2$-CT displays nuclease activity when expressed in *E. coli* cells, we performed real-time microscopy visualization of the nucleoid-associated HU protein after induction of the toxin. HU is a widely conserved histone-like protein very abundant in the bacterial cytoplasm that binds to DNA in a non-specific manner. Owing to its nucleoid association, HU localization reveals the global organization of the chromosome and potential alterations. We grew a CdiA$_2$-CT-producing *E. coli* MG1655 strain in which the *hupA* gene encoding the α-subunit of HU is fused to the *mcherry* gene at the endogenous locus. Twenty minutes after CdiA$_2$-CT induction, the majority of the cells contain organized and well-segregated nucleoids (**Figure 2** and **Supplementary Movie S1**). However, after 60 min, the nucleoids condense as a dense mass at midcell of the bacteria or show a diffused localization pattern. This global nucleoid disorganization is followed by cell filamentation indicative of cell division inhibition. These chromosome alterations are associated with cell death, as CdiA$_2$-CT-producing cells are not able to form viable colony units (**Supplementary Figure S1A**). No filamentation is observed after induction of the CdiA$_2$-CT in *recA*- cells showing that cell division arrest depends on the homologous recombination RecA protein (**Supplementary Figure S1B**). In contrast to bacteria producing only CdiA$_2$, cells coproducing the CdiI$_2$ immunity protein suffer no loss of viability and retain normal chromosome organization and cell division (**Figure 2**, **Supplementary Movie S2**, and **Supplementary Figure S1A**). The perturbation of DNA organization together with the RecA-dependent filamentation observed in the presence of CdiA$_2$-CT suggests that this toxin induces DNA damage to the chromosomal DNA. To test this hypothesis, we examined the localization pattern of the RecA protein, which has been reported to polymerize into large intracellular structures in response to DNA lesions (Lesterlin et al., 2014). To do so, we used an *E. coli* MG1655 strain expressing a carboxy-terminal fusion of RecA to green fluorescent protein (GFP) and wild-type (wt) RecA, both expressed from wt chromosome *recA* promoters. Before induction of CdiA$_2$-CT, RecA-GFP fluorescence appears uniformly distributed in most cells (**Figure 3**; $t = 0$ h and **Supplementary Movie S3**). From 20 min after production of CdiA$_2$-CT, fluorescent RecA-GFP structures form in the majority of cells, and we observed the formation of RecA bundles reported to promote homologous recombination repair between distant regions of homology (Lesterlin et al., 2014). As expected, RecA-GFP fluorescence is diffuse when CdiA$_2$-CT is co-expressed with CdiI$_2$, reflecting the absence of DNA damage (**Figure 3** and **Supplementary Movie S4**). Altogether, these results demonstrate that CdiA$_2$-CT creates multiple DNA breaks that cannot be repaired by the cells leading to growth inhibition, loss of chromosome organization, and eventual cell death.

CdiA$_1$-CT Toxin Inhibits the Growth of *E. coli*

In order to get insight into the mechanism of growth inhibition generated by the production of CdiA$_1$-CT in *E. coli* (**Figure 1B**), we analyzed in real-time microscopy the localization pattern of the recombinant HU-mCherry and RecA-GFP proteins after induction of CdiA$_1$-CT in the presence or absence of its cognate CdiI$_1$ immunity protein. Microscopy analysis showed no diffusion of the HU-mCherry in CdiA$_1$-CT-producing cells and RecA-GFP formed no spot or bundle, indicating that the toxin does not induce nucleoid disruption nor DNA damage (**Figure 4A** and **Supplementary Movies S5–S8**). However, we noticed CdiA$_1$-CT production led to increased cell size (**Figure 4B**) and division arrest in more than half of the cell population (**Figure 4C**). These results are consistent with the observed cell viability decrease 2 h post production of the CdiA$_1$-CT followed by a plateau of the number of colony-forming unit (CFU)/ml indicating a cell growth defect (**Supplementary Figure S2A**). To assess if these arrested cells are alive, we used the Live/Dead assay on the basis of the green fluorescent SYTO9 entering all cells to stain nucleic acid and the propidium iodide entering only dead cells with damaged cytoplasmic membranes. Our results showed the CdiA$_1$-CT-producing cells are not dying once they have stopped growing and that the percentage of cell

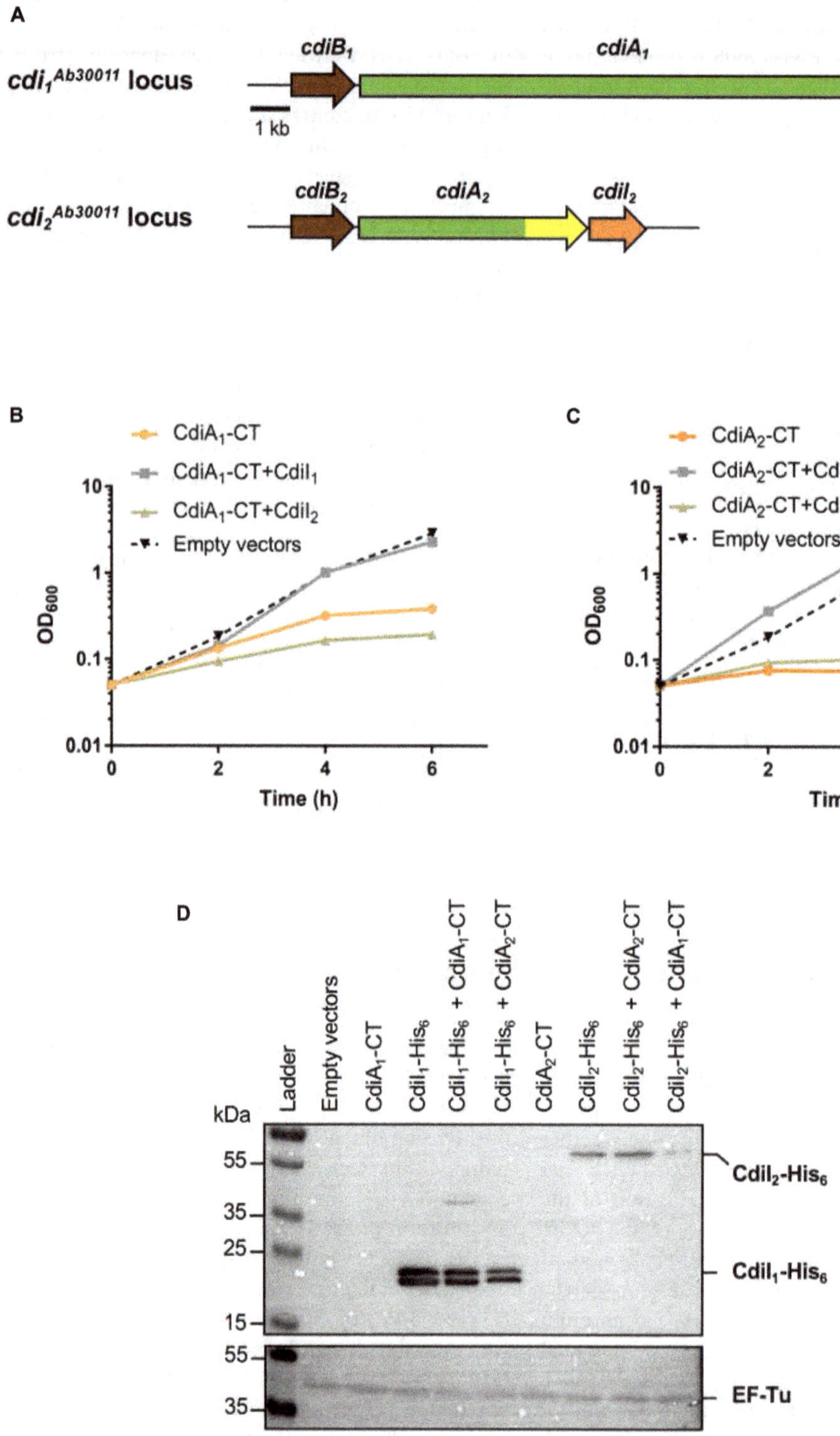

FIGURE 1 | The production of CT domains of $CdiA_1$ or $CdiA_2$ in *Escherichia coli* is toxic, and *cdiI* genes encode immunity proteins. **(A)** Schematic of the $cdi_1^{Ab30011}$ and $cdi_2^{Ab30011}$ loci. Genes encoding putative CdiB transporters, CdiA exoproteins, and CdiI immunity proteins are colored, respectively, in brown, green, and orange. Gray arrows represent putative orphan immunity genes. The highly variable nucleotide regions encoding CdiA-CT domains are highlighted in yellow. Black bar represents the 1-kb scale. Based on sequenced *Acinetobacter baumannii* DSM30011 genome (Repizo et al., 2017), $CdiB_1$, $CdiA_1$, and $CdiI_1$ correspond, respectively, to PNH15603.1, PNH15604.1, and PNH15605.1 proteins and $CdiB_2$, $CdiA_2$, and $CdiI_2$ to PNH14818.1, PNH14817.1, and PNH14816.1 proteins. **(B,C)** Effect of $CdiA_1$-CT **(B)** or $CdiA_2$-CT **(C)** production in *E. coli* DH5α strain. CdiA-CT production was induced at 0 min with or without CdiI, and growth was monitored by measuring the optical density at 600 nm (OD_{600}). **(D)** After 6 h of culture, *E. coli* cell extracts containing an indicated set of produced proteins were analyzed to probe the production of CdiI-His_6 and the cytoplasmic EF-Tu control using the anti-pentaHis (top panel) and anti-EF-Tu monoclonal antibodies (bottom panel). Molecular weight marker (kDa) is indicated on the left.

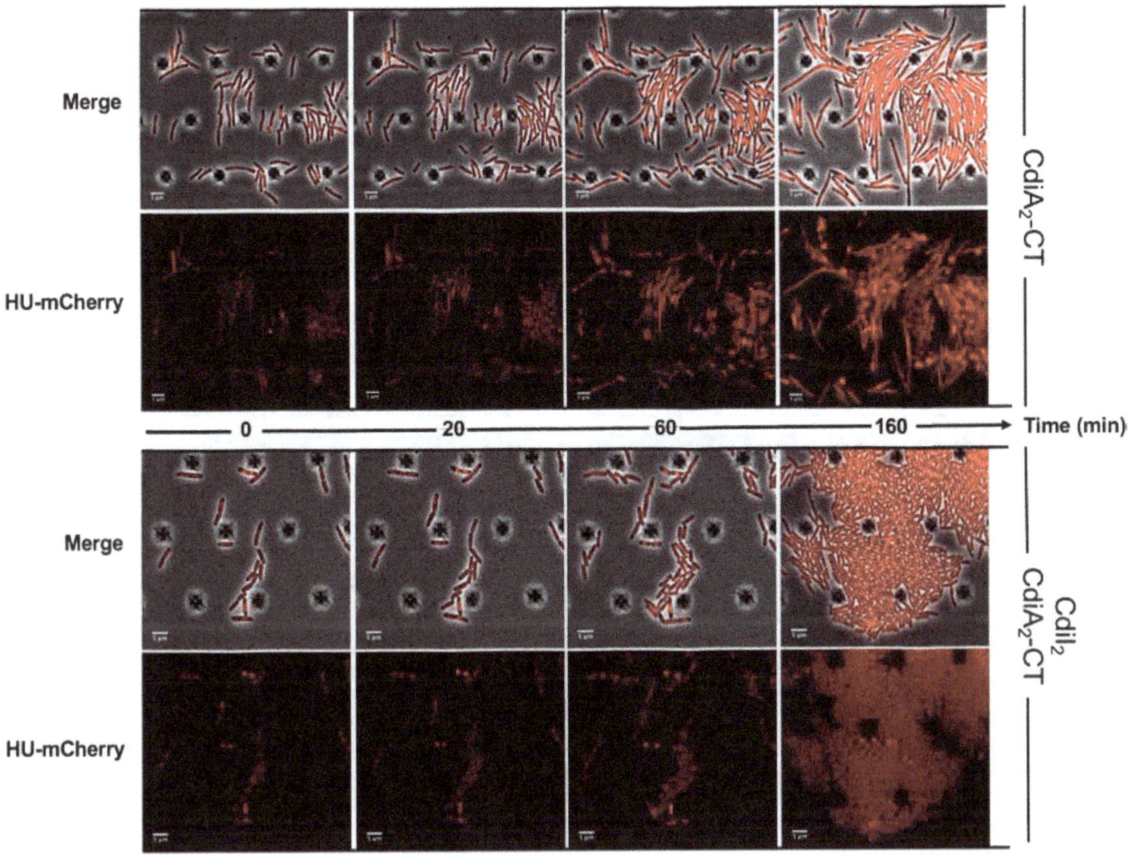

FIGURE 2 | The production of $CdiA_2$-CT in *Escherichia coli* disorganizes the nucleoid localization. Time-lapse fluorescence microscopy of the recombinant HU-mCherry protein produced by *E. coli* MG1655 strain after induction of the $CdiA_2$-CT in the absence or in presence of its cognate $CdiI_2$ immunity protein. The scale bar corresponds to 5 μm.

death was similar to that of cells producing $CdiA_1$-CT in the presence of $CdiI_1$ (**Supplementary Figure S2B**).

Unlike the *cdiBAI*$_2$ Locus, the *cdiBAI*$_1$ Genes Are Expressed in *A. baumannii* DSM30011

Most of the *cdi* genes are not expressed in laboratory growth conditions (Cope et al., 1994; Rojas et al., 2002; Mercy et al., 2016). In order to get insight into the expression profile of *cdi* genes present in *A. baumannii* DSM30011, we constructed plasmids containing transcriptional fusions between DNA region upstream of these genes and the *gfp* reporter. *A. baumannii* DSM30011 reporter strains were grown in liquid Luria–Bertani (LB)-rich medium at 37°C with agitation and static conditions, and the GFP fluorescence intensity was measured at 6 and 8 h, respectively. Equivalent results were obtained for each growth condition (**Figure 5A**). The level of GFP fluorescence of P*cdiB*$_2$, P*cdiA*$_2$, and P*cdiI*$_2$ fusions is identical to that of the promoterless fusion, indicating that DNA regions upstream of these genes do not have any promoter activity and that the *cdi*$_2$ locus might not be expressed under the growth conditions tested (**Figure 5A**). In contrast, the P*cdiB*$_1$ fusion produces a really high level of GFP compared to the regions upstream the *cdiA*$_1$ and *cdiI*$_1$ genes that do not exhibit any promoter activity (**Figure 5A**). In addition, the GFP fluorescence is quite homogeneous within the population, as all individual bacteria produce high levels of GFP fluorescence (**Figure 5B**). In order to determine whether $CdiA_1$ is produced in the tested conditions, we tried to detect this protein using sodium dodecyl sulfate polyacrylamide gel electrophoresis (SDS-PAGE). Overnight cultures were fractionated to analyze the protein profile of the whole cell lysate and secreted fraction. A band with a slower mobility than 250-kDa molecular weight marker was detected in the secreted fraction of the wt strain, which was identified as $CdiA_1$ protein by mass spectrometry (**Figure 5C**). For controls, we confirmed that this band disappeared in the Δ*cdiA*$_1$ mutant and that the $CdiA_1$ transport required $CdiB_1$ because no $CdiA_1$ is secreted in a Δ*cdiB*$_1$ mutant probably owing to the instability of the protein that is trapped in the periplasm, which is consistent with previous reports on FHA undergoing a rapid proteolytic degradation in the periplasm in the absence of its transporter FhaC (Jacob-Dubuisson et al., 1997; Guédin et al., 1998). Furthermore, the secretion of $CdiA_1$ is not due to cell lysis, as the cytoplasmic EF-Tu protein is only found in the whole cell fraction and Hcp, identified by mass spectrometry, the main component of the T6SS, is detected in the secreted fraction

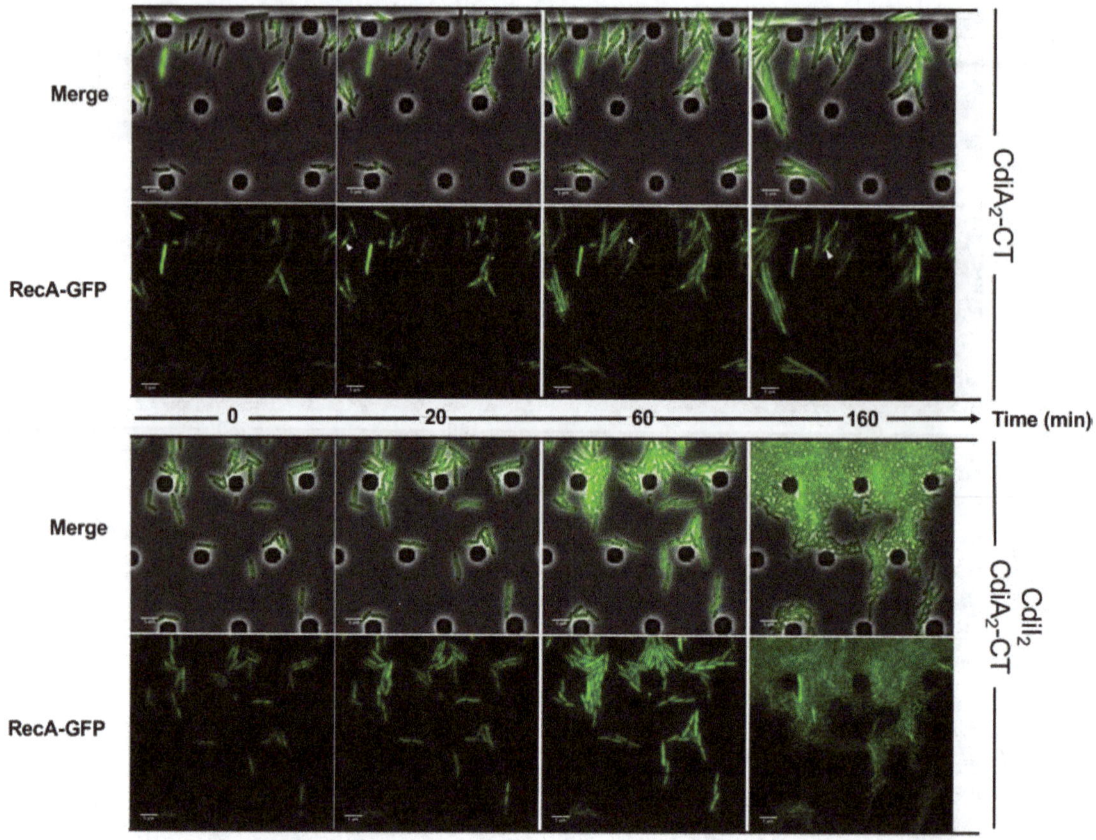

FIGURE 3 | The production of $CdiA_2$-CT in *Escherichia coli* induces DNA damages. Time-lapse fluorescence microscopy of the recombinant RecA-GFP protein produced by *E. coli* MG1655 strain after induction of the $CdiA_2$-CT in the absence or in the presence of its cognate $CdiI_2$ immunity protein. White arrows indicate examples of bundles of RecA-GFP. The scale bar corresponds to 5 μm. GFP, green fluorescent protein.

(**Figure 5C**). Knowing that $CdiA_1$ is highly produced and can be visualized by Coomassie blue staining, this suggests that the three *cdiBAI*$_1$ genes are transcribed as a polycistronic mRNA from the same promoter upstream *cdiB*$_1$.

The *cdiBAI*$_1$ Locus Mediates Bacterial Competition

As only the CDI_1 system is turned on under the tested conditions and we have not yet determined the regulatory pathway of the *cdi*$_2$ locus, we pursued in *A. baumannii* the characterization of the *cdiBAI*$_1$ system. To determine whether this system functions as a CDI system, the entire locus was replaced by a kanamycin cassette or deleted generating the Δ*cdiBAI*$_1$:*kn* and Δ*cdiBAI*$_1$ mutants. Next, we performed competition experiments by mixing the wt or Δ*cdiBAI*$_1$ attacker strains with the Δ*cdiBAI*$_1$:*kn* target strain and measure the CFU/ml of the target over time. As seen in **Figure 6**, wt strain inhibits the growth of the isogenic Δ*cdiBAI*$_1$:*kn* target strain by ~1 log after 6 h of growth competition, whereas no growth inhibition is observed with the Δ*cdiBAI*$_1$ attacker strain. No significant viability defect between the wt and mutant strains was observed, indicating that the ability of wt strain to outcompete the Δ*cdiBAI*$_1$ is not due to a growth rate difference (**Supplementary Figure S3**).

cdi$_1$ Locus Decreases *A. baumannii* DSM30011 Biofilm Formation and Adhesion to Epithelial Cells

CdiA proteins can promote biofilm formation and/or attachment to eukaryotic cells (Rojas et al., 2002; Plamondon et al., 2007; Schmitt et al., 2007; Gottig et al., 2009; Neil and Apicella, 2009; Garcia et al., 2013; Ruhe et al., 2015; Mercy et al., 2016). To investigate whether *cdi*$_1$ locus contributes to biofilm formation, we quantified in 96-well polystyrene plates over a 24-h time period the biofilm biomass formed by the wt and *cdiBAI*$_1$ mutant strains. After 3 h, the capacity to form biofilm of the mutant was lower than that of the wt (**Figure 7A**). Surprisingly, *cdiBAI*$_1$ mutant generated twice as much biofilm mass as the wt after 5 and 24 h (**Figure 7A**). Analysis of the depth bacterial growth on glass-bottom slides by confocal microscopy confirmed that the *cdiBAI*$_1$ mutant exhibited the highest ability to form a bacterial 3D structured layer especially after 5 h (**Figure 7B** and **Supplementary Figure S4**). To determine whether the *cdi*$_1$ locus is also implicated in the adhesion of *A. baumannii* DSM30011 to biotic surfaces, we compared the adhesiveness of wt and isogenic *cdiBAI*$_1$ mutant strains to A549 epithelial cells by CFU measurement and confocal microscopy analysis to directly visualize *A. baumannii* strains and confirm CFU

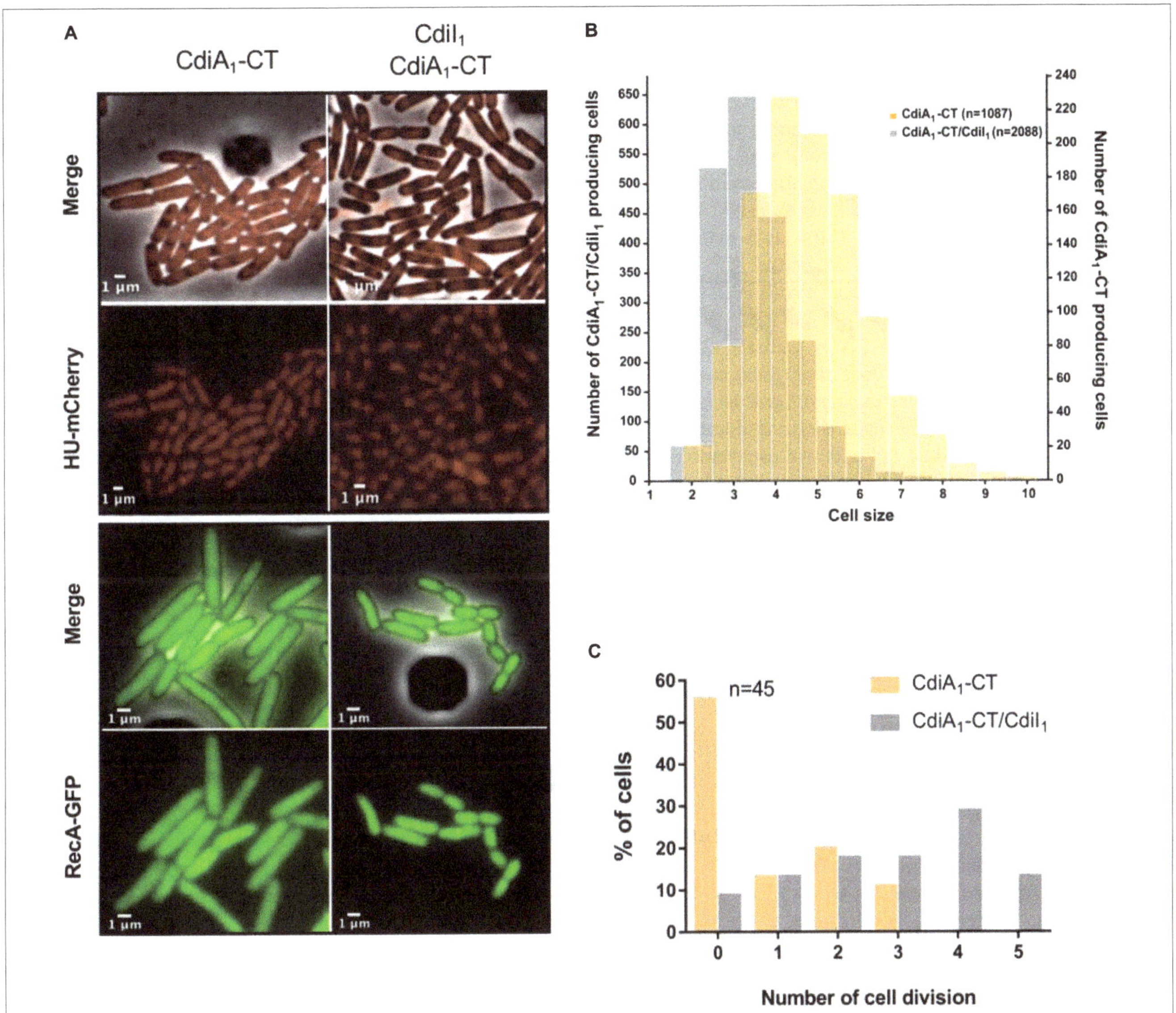

FIGURE 4 | The $CdiA_1$-CT toxin stops the growth of *Escherichia coli*. **(A)** Fluorescence microscopy of recombinant HU-mCherry or RecA-GFP produced by *E. coli* MG1655 strains 130 min after induction of $CdiA_1$-CT in the absence or in the presence of its cognate $CdiI_1$ immunity protein. The scale bar is indicated on the lower left. **(B)** Cell length analysis of RecA-GFP producing *E. coli* MG1655 strains 3 h after induction of $CdiA_1$-CT in the absence or in the presence of its cognate $CdiI_1$ immunity protein. *n* indicates the number of analyzed cells. **(C)** HU-mCherry producing *E. coli* MG1655 strains were grown in M9-casa after induction of $CdiA_1$-CT with or without $CdiI_1$, and real-time microscopy was performed in order to calculate the number of division over 45 single bacteria. GFP, green fluorescent protein.

counts. No difference between strains was observed after 2 h of infection with exponential cultures grown in LB liquid medium (**Figure 7C**; exponential). The biofilm increase is a late phenotype (**Figure 7A**), and we noticed that on agar plate the Δ*cdiBAI*$_1$ colonies were slightly smaller than those of the wt, reflecting a potential change in physiology depending on the growth condition. For these reasons, we directly analyzed the capacity of bacteria scratched from the agar plate to bind to host cells. As seen in **Figure 7C** (solid), the deletion of the *cdi*$_1$ locus led to a significant 2.5-fold increase in the proportion of cell-associated bacteria 2-h post infection. Furthermore, the number of cell-attached bacteria detected by immunofluorescence using an anti-*Acinetobacter* antibody was also higher for the *cdiBAI*$_1$ mutant (**Figure 7D**). Z-stack reconstruction confirmed that the bacteria are well attached to the cell surface and not endocyted by the host cells (**Supplementary Figure S5**).

DISCUSSION

The knowledge on virulence mechanisms and factors contributing to the pathogenic potential of *Acinetobacter baumannii* is limited, and a deeper understanding of its infection mechanisms may shed light on new strategies for drug development. On the basis of recent studies that characterized the potential implication of secretion systems including the TPS

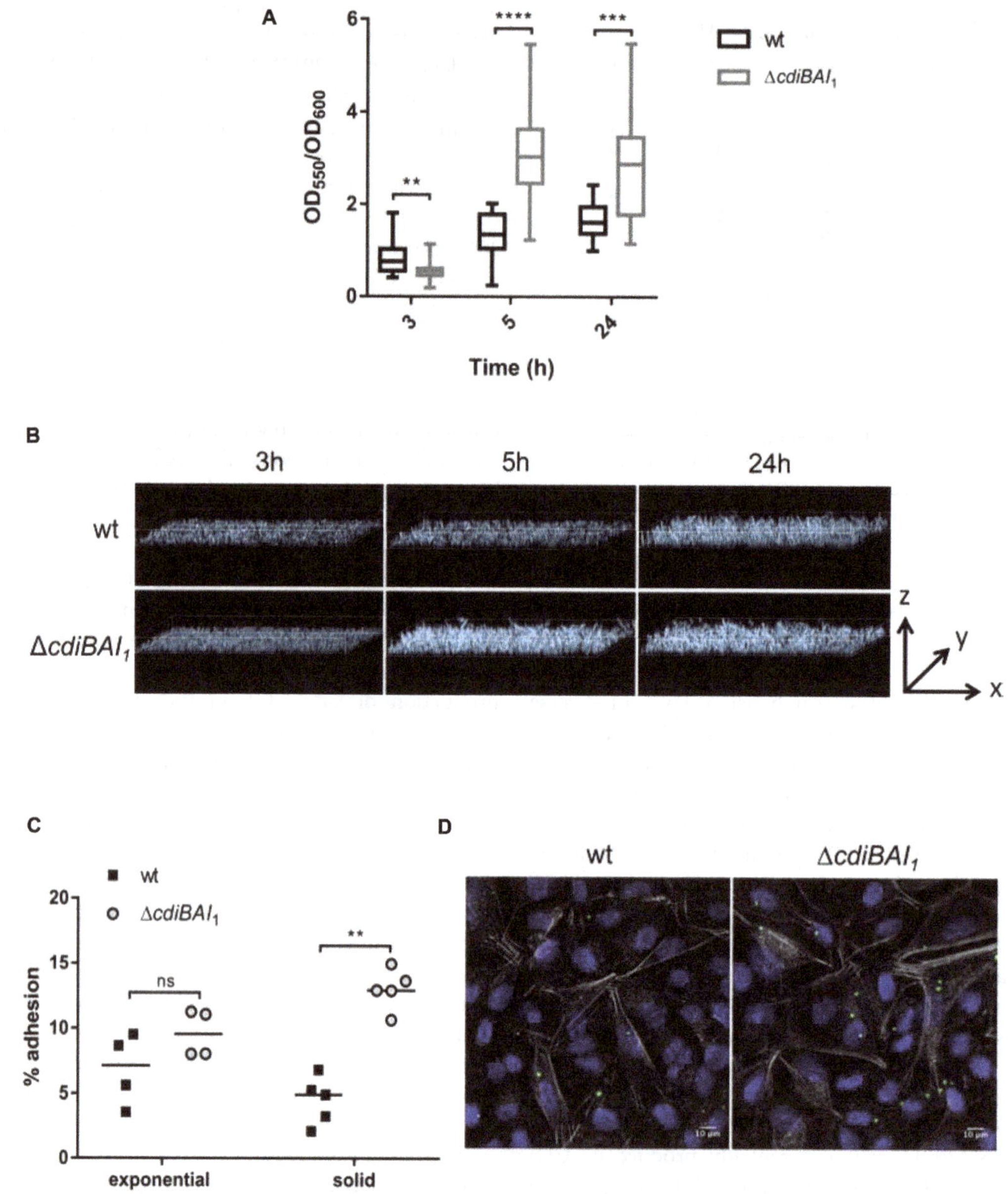

FIGURE 7 | The adhesive properties of *Acinetobacter baumannii* DSM30011 is enhanced in the absence of *cdiBAI*$_1$ locus. **(A)** Biofilm formation assayed by crystal violet staining. *A. baumannii* DSM30011 wild-type (wt) and Δ*cdiBAI*$_1$ strains were statically grown at 37°C for 3, 5, and 24 h. The biofilm biomass was estimated by calculating the OD_{550}/OD_{600} ratio from three independent experimental replicates. For statistical analyses, a non-parametric Mann–Whitney test was performed. $^{**}p = 0.0045$, $^{***}p = 0.0004$, $^{****}p < 0.0001$. **(B)** Confocal microscopy of biofilm formed by the wild-type and Δ*cdiBAI*$_1$ strains grown on glass-bottom slides in static conditions. Images correspond to the depth analysis of a 3D reconstruction of z-stacks obtained for the different strains at 3, 5, and 24 h. The height of the *z* axis is between 0 and 10 μm. Bacteria were labeled with DAPI. **(C)** Adhesion assay in which A549 cells were infected with *A. baumannii* DSM30011 wt or Δ*cdiBAI*$_1$ strains at a MOI of 100 for 2 h. Data are expressed as a percentage of *A. baumannii* adhesion obtained from the ratio between CFU/ml before and after infection. For statistical analyses, a non-parametric Mann–Whitney test was performed. $^{**}p = 0.0079$, ns: not significant. **(D)** Representative immunofluorescence images obtained by confocal microscopy and analyzed with ImageJ of A549 cells infected with bacteria grown in solid. Images correspond to Z-projections at average intensity. *A. baumannii* strains were detected with an anti-*A. baumannii* antibody (green). The actin cytoskeleton and nucleus were labeled with phalloidin (white) and DAPI (blue), respectively. MOI, multiplicity of infection.

behavior between sibling immune cells. In *P. aeruginosa*, the deletion of *cdi* locus increases the production of cyanide and swarming motility potentially via post-transcriptional regulation (Melvin et al., 2017). *Burkholderia* uses the contact-dependent signaling (CDS) mechanism to modulate gene expression in immune recipient bacteria that are dependent on the activity of the CdiA-CT toxin but independent of CDI growth inhibitory function (Garcia et al., 2016); and in *E. coli*, CDI modulates the cellular (p)ppGpp levels to increase the number of persister cells (Ghosh et al., 2018). It is therefore possible that the *A. baumannii*

CDI_1 system could also impact overall bacterial physiology by fine-tuning cellular responses.

EXPERIMENTAL PROCEDURES

Growth Conditions, Strains, Plasmids, and Primers

Strains/plasmids and primers used in this study are listed in **Supplementary Tables S1, S2**, respectively. *Acinetobacter baumannii* and *Escherichia coli* strains were grown in LB, EZ-Rich Defined Medium (RDM), or M9 medium containing 0.2% glucose and 0.4% casamino acid (M9-casa) supplemented with appropriate antibiotics: 30 μg/ml of chloramphenicol (Cm), 50 μg/ml of ampicillin (Amp), 50 μg/ml of kanamycin (Kn), 15 μg/ml of gentamycin (Gm), and 50 (liquid) or 200 μg/ml (solid) of carbenicillin (Cb).

Strain Construction

Gene insertion in the *E. coli* chromosome was performed by λRed recombination (Datsenko and Wanner, 2000; Yu et al., 2000). Mutant alleles were transferred by phage P1 transduction to generate the final strains. The *kan* and *cat* genes were removed using site-specific recombination induced by expression of the Flp recombinase from plasmid pCP20 (Datsenko and Wanner, 2000).

$cdiBAI_1$ mutants were constructed following the Tucker et al. (2014) protocol. Briefly, the FRT (Flippase Recognition Target) site-flanked kanamycin resistance cassette was amplified from the pKD4 plasmid with primers containing 100-nt extension with homology to the flanking regions of *cdiBAI* locus. After the PCR product was electroporated into *A. baumannii* competent cells carrying pAT02 plasmid, which produces the $RecA_b$ recombinase, mutants were selected on Kn 50 μg/ml, and the presence of integrated kanamycin cassette was verified by PCR. The *kan* gene was removed using site-specific recombination induced by expression of the Flp recombinase from plasmid pFLP2 (Hoang et al., 2000).

$cdiA_1$ and *$cdiB_1$* mutants were constructed by amplifying 2 kb with homology to the flanking regions of the genes. PCR products were combined by overlapping extension PCR and cloned into pUC18T-mini-Tn7-Ap *SacI*/*Bam*HI. The apramycin (Apr) resistance cassette was then amplified from pMHL2-2 and cloned between the 2-kb-flanking regions with *NcoI*/*SacI* restriction site. Then, the 2-kb-flanked apramycin cassette was amplified by PCR and electroporated into *A. baumannii* competent cells, and mutants were selected on Apr 50 μg/ml. The presence of integrated cassette was verified by PCR.

Toxicity Assays in *E. coli*

CdiA-CT domains were cloned with the artificial Shine-Dalgarno sequence into the pBAD33 plasmid using *SacI* and *SalI*. The *cdiI* genes were PCR amplified with a reverse primer encoding a 6xHis C-terminal tag and cloned into the pTrc99a plasmid using *NcoI* and *Bam*HI. Plasmid cloning was verified by Sanger sequencing (GATC Biotech). To perform toxicity assay, an overnight culture in LB with 0.5% glucose was washed in LB and diluted to an OD_{600} ~ 0.05 in LB with 100 μM of IPTG and 1% arabinose to produce the immunity protein and the CdiA-CT domain, respectively. At indicated time of culture at 37°C, cells were washed in LB, and CFU/ml was calculated by plating onto LB agar plates containing Cm, Amp, and glucose 0.5%. The production of immunity proteins was verified by Western blot analyses. Briefly, the cell extract was separated on 12% SDS-PAGE, transferred onto polyvinylidene difluoride (PVDF) membranes, and probed with primary mouse anti-pentaHis (Qiagen) or anti EF-Tu.

Live-Cell Microscopy Experiment

Live and Dead Assay

Overnight cultures in RDM supplemented with 0.5% glucose were washed and diluted to OD_{600} of 0.05 with 100 μM of IPTG and 1% arabinose and grown further at 37°C for 3 h 30 min before treatment with the LIVE/DEAD® BacLight™ Bacterial Viability Kit. To control the functionality of the Live/Dead assay, we treated the samples with ethanol to kill the bacteria, and as expected, the percentage of cell death reaches ~100% in this condition (**Supplementary Figure S2B**). Cells were stained for 20 min, washed, resuspended in RDM, and spread over a RDM or M9-casa 1% agarose pad.

Time-Lapse Experiments

Overnight cultures in RDM or M9-casa media supplemented with 0.5% glucose were diluted to OD_{600} of 0.05 with 0.5% glucose and grown further to OD_{600} = 0.1. Cultures were loaded to B04A microfluidic chamber (ONIX, CellASIC®) with 5 psi for 1 min. Medium supplemented with 1% arabinose was maintained at 1 psi with a constant temperature of 37°C. Cells were imaged every 10 min for 6 h.

Image Acquisition and Analysis

Conventional wide-field fluorescence microscopy imaging was carried out on an Eclipse Ti-E microscope (Nikon), equipped with ×100/1.45 oil Plan Apo Lambda phase objective, FLash4 V2 CMOS camera (Hamamatsu), and using NIS software for image acquisition. Acquisition setting was 10 ms for Syto9, 100 ms for GFP, 10 ms for propidium iodide, and 100 ms for mCherry, using 50% power of a fluo LED Spectra X light source at 488- and 560-nm excitation wavelengths, respectively. Cell counting and length analysis were performed using MicrobeJ (Ducret et al., 2016).

Quantification of Promoter Activities

The P_{empty} transcriptional fusion was constructed by cloning the *gfpmut2* gene from pUA66 plasmid as an *Eco*RI/*Bgl*II PCR fragment cloned into pWH1266. To construct transcriptional fusions, 500 bp corresponding to the putative promoter regions was amplified as a *Bam*HI/*SacI* PCR fragment and cloned into pWH1266-P_{empty}-*gfp*. To quantify promoter activities, overnight cultures in LB were diluted to an OD_{600} of 0.05 and grown at 37°C for 6 h. Two hundred microliters of cells was transferred into well of a black 96-well plate (Greiner), and the absorbance at 600 nm and fluorescence (excitation 485 nm, emission 530 nm) were measured using TECAN Spark multimode plate reader. The relative fluorescence was expressed as the intensity of fluorescence divided by the absorbance at 600 nm after subtracting the values of blank sample. Fluorescence repartition of the P*cdiB*$_1$-*gfp* was performed by diluting an overnight culture in RDM to an OD_{600} of 0.05 and grown further at 37°C to an $OD_{600} \sim 0.8$ before spreading the cells over a RDM 1% agarose pad. The analysis was performed using MicrobeJ (Ducret et al., 2016).

Detection of CdiA$_1$

Cell extract and secreted fractions were prepared as follows. Bacterial cells from overnight culture grown in LB were harvested by centrifugation at 4,000 × *g* for 20 min, and pellets (cell extracts) were resuspended in loading buffer. The supernatant fraction was centrifuged at 13,000 × *g* for 20 min at 4°C. Proteins from the supernatant (secreted fraction) were then precipitated with 12% (w/v) trichloroacetic acid (TCA), washed with acetone, air-dried, and resuspended in loading buffer. The protein samples were then heated to 95°C for 10 min, separated by SDS-PAGE, and revealed by Coomassie blue staining or immunoblotting.

Growth Competition Assays

The attackers and target strains were grown overnight separately in LB medium without antibiotic at 37°C. Overnight cultures were diluted to an OD_{600} of 0.05 in LB medium without antibiotic and grown at 37°C with shaking to an $OD_{600} \sim 0.35$. Strains were then mixed at an attacker to target cell ratio of 4:1, and the mixed bacteria were grown at 37°C with agitation at 160 rpm. At indicated times, the mix was serially diluted and plated onto kanamycin-containing LB agar plates to determine the CFU/ml of the target strain.

Biofilm Assays

Biofilm assays were performed following the O'Toole (2011) protocol. Briefly, overnight cultures were inoculated into LB at a final OD_{600} of 0.1. One hundred microliters of culture was added to 96-well polystyrene plates and incubated over a 5-h period without shaking. At the indicated times, cells in suspension were removed, and the wells washed twice with distilled water. One hundred twenty-five microliters of 0.1% crystal violet was then added to the wells, incubated for 10 min, and washed three times with 125 μl of distilled water. To solubilize the crystal violet, 125 μl of 30% acetic acid was added and the absorbance measured at 550 nm. The ratio OD_{550}/OD_{600} was calculated to normalize the biofilm formation due to variation in bacterial growth.

For biofilm imaging, bacteria were grown in BM2 minimal medium (Repizo et al., 2015) supplemented with 10 mM of potassium glutamate (BM2G) as carbon source in a glass-bottom 24-well μ-plate. Cultures were inoculated at an initial OD_{600} of 0.1 from an overnight culture grown in LB and then incubated at 37°C under static conditions. At indicated times, the biofilm was labeled with DAPI, and images were taken with a confocal Zeiss LSM800 Airyscan microscope and analyzed with ImageJ and Imaris software.

A. baumannii Infection of A549 Cells

A549 cells were grown in Dulbecco's modified Eagle medium (DMEM) supplemented with 10% of fetal calf serum and 1% L-glutamine at 37°C with 5% CO_2 atmosphere. For adhesion assays and microscopy analysis, A549 cells were first seeded into 24-well tissue culture plates at 5 × 10^5 cells/well to obtain a monolayer. *A. baumannii* strains were grown on LB agar plate for 24 h at 37°C to form a "lawn" covering. Bacteria were scraped from the agar surface and resuspended in 1 ml of LB to form a homogeneous suspension of $\sim 10^8$ CFU/ml. Cells were then infected at a multiplicity of infection (MOI) of 100 of *A. baumannii* in 500 μl of complete medium per well. Plates were centrifuged at 400 × *g* for 5 min and then incubated for 2 h at 37°C with 5% CO_2 atmosphere. Cells were then washed five times with phosphate-buffered saline (PBS) 1 × and either lysed with 0.1% sodium deoxycholate (5-min incubation) or fixed with 3% paraformaldehyde (15 min incubation). The number of CFU/ml before and after infection was determined to calculate the percentage of bacterial adhesion. The number of CFU/ml of the inocula was also used to verify the MOI and ensure equivalent numbers of bacteria were used for wt and mutant strains.

Immunofluorescence Labeling and A549 Cell Microscopy

After fixation, cells were incubated at room temperature for 1 h in a PBS 1 × 0.1% saponin and 10% horse serum solution for permeabilization and blocking. Cells were then labeled at room temperature with primary rabbit anti-*Acinetobacter* antibody mix diluted at 1/20,000 in the same solution for 1 h followed by two washes in PBS 1 × 0.1% saponin. Secondary antibodies (anti-rabbit Alexa-488 [1/1,000], phalloidin-568 [1/250], and DAPI nuclear dye [1/1,000] to label *A. baumannii*, actin cytoskeleton, and host cell nucleus, respectively) were then mixed and incubated for 45 min, followed by two washes in PBS 1 × 0.1% saponin, one wash in PBS 1×, and one wash in distilled water before mounting with ProLong Gold. Coverslips were examined on a Zeiss LSM800 laser scanning confocal microscopes and analyzed with ImageJ software (Schindelin et al., 2012). Z-stack tool and Z-projection for maximum intensity were used for image presentation.

AUTHOR CONTRIBUTIONS

MR performed the majority of the experiments. SR, LC, JC, and CL also conducted the experiments. MR, SS, and CL participated in the experimental design and data analysis. SB conceived the project, designed and undertook experiments, interpreted data, and wrote the manuscript. All authors read and approved the manuscript.

FUNDING

This work was funded by a FINOVI young principal investigator grant awarded to SS. MR has a Ph.D. fellowship from the French

Ministry of Research. JC was funded by the FINOVI Foundation in partnership to the ATIP-Avenir grant to CL. SS and CL was supported by an INSERM staff scientist contract. SB was supported by the CNRS staff scientist contract.

ACKNOWLEDGMENTS

We thank E. Gueguen at the MAP, University of Lyon, for helpful discussions and support and for providing pUA66 plasmid. We are grateful to B. Davies at the University of Texas at Austin for providing the pAT02 plasmid, to X. Charpentier at the CIRI (INSERM, University of Lyon, CNRS, ENS) for the pMHL2-2 plasmid, and to R. Voulhoux at the CNRS-Aix-Marseille University for the anti EF-Tu antibody. We thank the proteomic facility of the Protein Science Facility of the SFR Biosciences for the mass spectrometry.

REFERENCES

Allsopp, L. P., Wood, T. E., Howard, S. A., Maggiorelli, F., Nolan, L. M., Wettstadt, S., et al. (2017). RsmA and AmrZ orchestrate the assembly of all three type VI secretion systems in *Pseudomonas aeruginosa*. *Proc. Natl. Acad. Sci. U.S.A.* 114, 7707–7712. doi: 10.1073/pnas.1700286114

Anderson, M. S., Garcia, E. C., and Cotter, P. A. (2012). The burkholderia bcpAIOB genes define unique classes of two-partner secretion and contact dependent growth inhibition systems. *PLoS Genet.* 8:e1002877. doi: 10.1371/journal.pgen.1002877

Aoki, S. K., Diner, E. J., de Roodenbeke, C., Burgess, B. R., Poole, S. J., Braaten, B. A., et al. (2010). A widespread family of polymorphic contact-dependent toxin delivery systems in bacteria. *Nature* 468, 439–442. doi: 10.1038/nature09490

Aoki, S. K., Pamma, R., Hernday, A. D., Bickham, J. E., Braaten, B. A., and Low, D. A. (2005). Contact-dependent inhibition of growth in *Escherichia coli*. *Science* 309, 1245–1248. doi: 10.1126/science.1115109

Aoki, S. K., Webb, J. S., Braaten, B. A., and Low, D. A. (2009). Contact-dependent growth inhibition causes reversible metabolic downregulation in *Escherichia coli*. *J. Bacteriol.* 191, 1777–1786. doi: 10.1128/JB.01437-1438

Balder, R., Hassel, J., Lipski, S., and Lafontaine, E. R. (2007). *Moraxella* catarrhalis strain O35E expresses two filamentous hemagglutinin-like proteins that mediate adherence to human epithelial cells. *Infect. Immun.* 75, 2765–2775. doi: 10.1128/IAI.00079-77

Braun, V., Hobbie, S., and Ondraczek, R. (1992). *Serratia marcescens* forms a new type of cytolysin. *FEMS Microbiol. Lett.* 100, 299–305. doi: 10.1016/0378-1097(92)90225-d

Carruthers, M. D., Nicholson, P. A., Tracy, E. N., and Munson, R. S. (2013). *Acinetobacter baumannii* utilizes a type VI secretion system for bacterial competition. *PLoS One* 8:e59388. doi: 10.1371/journal.pone.0059388

Cope, L. D., Thomas, S. E., Hrkal, Z., and Hansen, E. J. (1998). Binding of heme-hemopexin complexes by soluble HxuA protein allows utilization of this complexed heme by *Haemophilus influenzae*. *Infect. Immun.* 66, 4511–4516.

Cope, L. D., Thomas, S. E., Latimer, J. L., Slaughter, C. A., Müller-Eberhard, U., and Hansen, E. J. (1994). The 100 kDa haem:haemopexin-binding protein of *Haemophilus influenzae*: structure and localization. *Mol. Microbiol.* 13, 863–873. doi: 10.1111/j.1365-2958.1994.tb00478.x

Cope, L. D., Yogev, R., Muller-Eberhard, U., and Hansen, E. J. (1995). A gene cluster involved in the utilization of both free heme and heme:hemopexin by *Haemophilus influenzae* type b. *J. Bacteriol.* 177, 2644–2653. doi: 10.1128/jb.177.10.2644-2653.1995

Darvish Alipour Astaneh, S., Rasooli, I., and Mousavi Gargari, S. L. (2014). The role of filamentous hemagglutinin adhesin in adherence and biofilm formation in *Acinetobacter baumannii* ATCC19606(T). *Microb. Pathog.* 74, 42–49. doi: 10.1016/j.micpath.2014.07.007

Datsenko, K., and Wanner, B. (2000). One-step inactivation of chromosomal genes in *Escherichia coli* K-12 using PCR products. *Proc. Natl. Acad. Sci. U.S.A.* 97, 6640–6645. doi: 10.1073/pnas.120163297

De Gregorio, E., Zarrilli, R., and Di Nocera, P. P. (2019). Contact-dependent growth inhibition systems in acinetobacter. *Sci. Rep.* 9:154. doi: 10.1038/s41598-018-36427-36428

Ducret, A., Quardokus, E. M., and Brun, Y. V. (2016). MicrobeJ, a tool for high throughput bacterial cell detection and quantitative analysis. *Nat. Microbiol.* 1:16077. doi: 10.1038/nmicrobiol.2016.77

Faure, L. M., Garvis, S., de Bentzmann, S., and Bigot, S. (2014). Characterization of a novel two-partner secretion system implicated in the virulence of *Pseudomonas aeruginosa*. *Microbiol. Read. Engl.* 160, 1940–1952. doi: 10.1099/mic.0.079616-79610

Faure, L. M., Llamas, M. A., Bastiaansen, K. C., de Bentzmann, S., and Bigot, S. (2013). Phosphate starvation relayed by PhoB activates the expression of the *Pseudomonas aeruginosa* σvreI ECF factor and its target genes. *Microbiol. Read. Engl.* 159, 1315–1327. doi: 10.1099/mic.0.067645-67640

Fournier, C., Smith, A., and Delepelaire, P. (2011). Haem release from haemopexin by HxuA allows *Haemophilus influenzae* to escape host nutritional immunity: HxuA releases haem from haemopexin. *Mol. Microbiol.* 80, 133–148. doi: 10.1111/j.1365-2958.2011.07562.x

Gallagher, L. A., and Manoil, C. (2001). *Pseudomonas aeruginosa* PAO1 kills *Caenorhabditis elegans* by cyanide poisoning. *J. Bacteriol.* 183, 6207–6214. doi: 10.1128/JB.183.21.6207-6214.2001

Garcia, E. C., Anderson, M. S., Hagar, J. A., and Cotter, P. A. (2013). BcpA mediates biofilm formation independently of interbacterial contact-dependent growth inhibition: CDI system protein-mediated biofilm. *Mol. Microbiol.* 89, 1213–1225. doi: 10.1111/mmi.12339

Garcia, E. C., Perault, A. I., Marlatt, S. A., and Cotter, P. A. (2016). Interbacterial signaling via burkholderia contact-dependent growth inhibition system proteins. *Proc. Natl. Acad. Sci. U.S.A.* 113, 8296–8301. doi: 10.1073/pnas.1606323113

Ghosh, A., Baltekin, Ö, Wäneskog, M., Elkhalifa, D., Hammarlöf, D. L., Elf, J., et al. (2018). Contact-dependent growth inhibition induces high levels of antibiotic-tolerant persister cells in clonal bacterial populations. *EMBO J.* 37:e98026. doi: 10.15252/embj.201798026

Gottig, N., Garavaglia, B. S., Garofalo, C. G., Orellano, E. G., and Ottado, J. (2009). A filamentous hemagglutinin-like protein of *Xanthomonas axonopodis* pv. citri, the phytopathogen responsible for citrus canker, is involved in bacterial virulence. *PloS One* 4:e4358. doi: 10.1371/journal.pone.0004358

Guédin, S., Willery, E., Locht, C., and Jacob-Dubuisson, F. (1998). Evidence that a globular conformation is not compatible with FhaC-mediated secretion of the *Bordetella pertussis* filamentous haemagglutinin. *Mol. Microbiol.* 29, 763–774. doi: 10.1046/j.1365-2958.1998.00970.x

Guérin, J., Bigot, S., Schneider, R., Buchanan, S. K., and Jacob-Dubuisson, F. (2017). Two-partner secretion: combining efficiency and simplicity in the secretion of large proteins for bacteria-host and bacteria-bacteria interactions. *Front. Cell. Infect. Microbiol.* 7:148. doi: 10.3389/fcimb.2017.00148

Guilhabert, M. R., and Kirkpatrick, B. C. (2005). Identification of Xylella fastidiosa antivirulence genes: hemagglutinin adhesins contribute a biofilm maturation to X. fastidios and colonization and attenuate virulence. *Mol. Plant Microb. Interact. MPMI* 18, 856–868. doi: 10.1094/MPMI-18-0856

Harding, C. M., Pulido, M. R., Di Venanzio, G., Kinsella, R. L., Webb, A. I., Scott, N. E., et al. (2017). Pathogenic acinetobacter species have a functional type i secretion system and contact-dependent inhibition systems. *J. Biol. Chem.* 292, 9075–9087. doi: 10.1074/jbc.M117.781575

Hoang, T. T., Kutchma, A. J., Becher, A., and Schweizer, H. P. (2000). Integration-proficient plasmids for *Pseudomonas aeruginosa*: site-specific integration and use for engineering of reporter and expression strains. *Plasmid* 43, 59–72. doi: 10.1006/plas.1999.1441

Iyer, L. M., Zhang, D., Rogozin, I. B., and Aravind, L. (2011). Evolution of the deaminase fold and multiple origins of eukaryotic editing and mutagenic nucleic acid deaminases from bacterial toxin systems. *Nucleic Acids Res.* 39, 9473–9497. doi: 10.1093/nar/gkr691

Jacob-Dubuisson, F., Buisine, C., Willery, E., Renauld-Mongénie, G., and Locht, C. (1997). Lack of functional complementation between Bordetella pertussis filamentous hemagglutinin and *Proteus mirabilis* HpmA hemolysin secretion machineries. *J. Bacteriol.* 179, 775–783. doi: 10.1128/jb.179.3.775-783.1997

Jacob-Dubuisson, F., Locht, C., and Antoine, R. (2001). Two-partner secretion in Gram-negative bacteria: a thrifty, specific pathway for large virulence proteins. *Mol. Microbiol.* 40, 306–313. doi: 10.1046/j.1365-2958.2001.02278.x

Kajava, A. V., Cheng, N., Cleaver, R., Kessel, M., Simon, M. N., Willery, E., et al. (2001). Beta-helix model for the filamentous haemagglutinin adhesin of Bordetella pertussis and related bacterial secretory proteins. *Mol. Microbiol.* 42, 279–292. doi: 10.1046/j.1365-2958.2001.02598.x

Lesterlin, C., Ball, G., Schermelleh, L., and Sherratt, D. J. (2014). RecA bundles mediate homology pairing between distant sisters during DNA break repair. *Nature* 506, 249–253. doi: 10.1038/nature12868

Melvin, J. A., Gaston, J. R., Phillips, S. N., Springer, M. J., Marshall, C. W., Shanks, R. M. Q., et al. (2017). *Pseudomonas aeruginosa* contact-dependent growth inhibition plays dual role in host-pathogen interactions. *mSphere* 2, e336–e317. doi: 10.1128/mSphere.00336-317

Mercy, C., Ize, B., Salcedo, S. P., de Bentzmann, S., and Bigot, S. (2016). Functional characterization of *Pseudomonas* contact dependent growth inhibition (CDI) systems. *PLoS One* 11:e0147435. doi: 10.1371/journal.pone.0147435

Neil, R. B., and Apicella, M. A. (2009). Role of HrpA in biofilm formation of *Neisseria meningitidis* and regulation of the hrpBAS transcripts. *Infect. Immun.* 77, 2285–2293. doi: 10.1128/IAI.01502-1508

O'Toole, G. A. (2011). Microtiter dish biofilm formation assay. *J. Vis. Exp.* 47, e2437. doi: 10.3791/2437

Pérez, A., Merino, M., Rumbo-Feal, S., Álvarez-Fraga, L., Vallejo, J. A., Beceiro, A., et al. (2016). The FhaB/FhaC two-partner secretion system is involved in adhesion of *Acinetobacter baumannii* AbH12O-A2 strain. *Virulence* 8, 959–974. doi: 10.1080/21505594.2016.1262313

Perez, F., Hujer, A. M., Hujer, K. M., Decker, B. K., Rather, P. N., and Bonomo, R. A. (2007). Global challenge of multidrug-resistant *Acinetobacter baumannii*. *Antimicrob. Agents Chemother.* 51, 3471–3484. doi: 10.1128/AAC.01464-1466

Plamondon, P., Luke, N. R., and Campagnari, A. A. (2007). Identification of a novel two-partner secretion locus in *Moraxella catarrhalis*. *Infect. Immun.* 75, 2929–2936. doi: 10.1128/IAI.00396-397

Relman, D. A., Domenighini, M., Tuomanen, E., Rappuoli, R., and Falkow, S. (1989). Filamentous hemagglutinin of Bordetella pertussis: nucleotide sequence and crucial role in adherence. *Proc. Natl. Acad. Sci. U.S.A.* 86, 2637–2641. doi: 10.1073/pnas.86.8.2637

Repizo, G. D., Gagné, S., Foucault-Grunenwald, M.-L., Borges, V., Charpentier, X., Limansky, A. S., et al. (2015). Differential Role of the T6SS in *Acinetobacter baumannii* virulence. *PLoS One* 10:e0138265. doi: 10.1371/journal.pone.0138265

Repizo, G. D., Viale, A. M., Borges, V., Cameranesi, M. M., Taib, N., Espariz, M., et al. (2017). The environmental *Acinetobacter baumannii* isolate DSM30011 reveals clues into the preantibiotic era genome diversity, virulence potential, and niche range of a predominant nosocomial pathogen. *Genome Biol. Evol.* 9, 2292–2307. doi: 10.1093/gbe/evx162

Rojas, C. M., Ham, J. H., Deng, W.-L., Doyle, J. J., and Collmer, A. (2002). HecA, a member of a class of adhesins produced by diverse pathogenic bacteria, contributes to the attachment, aggregation, epidermal cell killing, and virulence phenotypes of erwinia chrysanthemi EC16 on *Nicotiana clevelandii* seedlings. *Proc. Natl. Acad. Sci. U.S.A.* 99, 13142–13147. doi: 10.1073/pnas.202358699

Ruhe, Z. C., Townsley, L., Wallace, A. B., King, A., Van der Woude, M. W., Low, D. A., et al. (2015). CdiA promotes receptor-independent intercellular adhesion. *Mol. Microbiol.* 98, 175–192. doi: 10.1111/mmi.13114

Schindelin, J., Arganda-Carreras, I., Frise, E., Kaynig, V., Longair, M., Pietzsch, T., et al. (2012). Fiji: an open-source platform for biological-image analysis. *Nat. Methods* 9, 676–682. doi: 10.1038/nmeth.2019

Schmitt, C., Turner, D., Boesl, M., Abele, M., Frosch, M., and Kurzai, O. (2007). A functional two-partner secretion system contributes to adhesion of *Neisseria meningitidis* to epithelial cells. *J. Bacteriol.* 189, 7968–7976. doi: 10.1128/JB.00851-857

Talà, A., Progida, C., De Stefano, M., Cogli, L., Spinosa, M. R., Bucci, C., et al. (2008). The HrpB-HrpA two-partner secretion system is essential for intracellular survival of *Neisseria meningitidis*. *Cell. Microbiol.* 10, 2461–2482. doi: 10.1111/j.1462-5822.2008.01222.x

Tucker, A. T., Nowicki, E. M., Boll, J. M., Knauf, G. A., Burdis, N. C., Trent, M. S., et al. (2014). Defining gene-phenotype relationships in *Acinetobacter baumannii* through one-step chromosomal gene inactivation. *mBio* 5, e1313–e1314. doi: 10.1128/mBio.01313-1314

van Ulsen, P., Rahman, S. U., Jong, W. S. P., Daleke-Schermerhorn, M. H., and Luirink, J. (2014). Type V secretion: from biogenesis to biotechnology. *Biochim. Biophys. Acta* 1843, 1592–1611. doi: 10.1016/j.bbamcr.2013.11.006

Willett, J. L. E., Ruhe, Z. C., Goulding, C. W., Low, D. A., and Hayes, C. S. (2015). Contact-dependent growth inhibition (CDI) and CdiB/CdiA Two-Partner Secretion Proteins. *J. Mol. Biol.* 427, 3754–3765. doi: 10.1016/j.jmb.2015.09.010

Yu, D., Ellis, H. M., Lee, E. C., Jenkins, N. A., Copeland, N. G., and Court, D. L. (2000). An efficient recombination system for chromosome engineering in *Escherichia coli*. *Proc. Natl. Acad. Sci. U.S.A.* 97, 5978–5983. doi: 10.1073/pnas.100127597

Zhang, D., de Souza, R. F., Anantharaman, V., Iyer, L. M., and Aravind, L. (2012). Polymorphic toxin systems: comprehensive characterization of trafficking modes, processing, mechanisms of action, immunity and ecology using comparative genomics. *Biol. Direct.* 7:18. doi: 10.1186/1745-6150-7-18

Zhang, D., Iyer, L. M., and Aravind, L. (2011). A novel immunity system for bacterial nucleic acid degrading toxins and its recruitment in various eukaryotic and DNA viral systems. *Nucleic Acids Res.* 39, 4532–4552. doi: 10.1093/nar/gkr036

10

A New Strain Collection for Improved Expression of Outer Membrane Proteins

Ina Meuskens [1,2], Marcin Michalik [1], Nandini Chauhan [1], Dirk Linke [1] and Jack C. Leo [1*]*

[1] Section for Evolution and Genetics, Department of Biosciences, University of Oslo, Oslo, Norway, [2] Interfaculty Institute for Biochemistry, Eberhard Karls University, Tübingen, Germany

Almost all integral membrane proteins found in the outer membranes of Gram-negative bacteria belong to the transmembrane β-barrel family. These proteins are not only important for nutrient uptake and homeostasis, but are also involved in such processes as adhesion, protein secretion, biofilm formation, and virulence. As surface exposed molecules, outer membrane β-barrel proteins are also potential drug and vaccine targets. High production levels of heterologously expressed proteins are desirable for biochemical and especially structural studies, but over-expression and subsequent purification of membrane proteins, including outer membrane proteins, can be challenging. Here, we present a set of deletion mutants derived from *E. coli* BL21(DE3) designed for the over-expression of recombinant outer membrane proteins. These strains harbor deletions of four genes encoding abundant β-barrel proteins in the outer membrane (OmpA, OmpC, OmpF, and LamB), both single and in all combinations of double, triple, and quadruple knock-outs. The sequences encoding these outer membrane proteins were deleted completely, leaving only a minimal scar sequence, thus preventing the possibility of genetic reversion. Expression tests in the quadruple mutant strain with four test proteins, including a small outer membrane β-barrel protein and variants thereof as well as two virulence-related autotransporters, showed significantly improved expression and better quality of the produced proteins over the parent strain. Differences in growth behavior and aggregation in the presence of high salt were observed, but these phenomena did not negatively influence the expression in the quadruple mutant strain when handled as we recommend. The strains produced in this study can be used for outer membrane protein production and purification, but are also uniquely useful for labeling experiments for biophysical measurements in the native membrane environment.

***Correspondence:**
Dirk Linke
dirk.linke@ibv.uio.no
Jack C. Leo
j.c.leo@ibv.uio.no

Keywords: outer membrane, β-barrel protein, recombinant protein expression, P1 transduction, production strain

INTRODUCTION

The envelope of Gram-negative bacteria such as, *Escherichia coli* consists of two membranes, the inner and the outer membrane. This double membrane system protects the bacteria from environmental insult and makes them resistant to many antibiotics and host immune defenses, but allows the efficient uptake of nutrients. The outer membrane is permeable to small hydrophilic molecules due to the presence of porins. Porins, and almost all other transmembrane outer membrane proteins (OMPs), are composed of a transmembrane β-barrel domain (Fairman et al., 2011). β-barrels consist of an antiparallel β-sheet that closes in on itself; the proteins thus adopt a cylindrical shape, with hydrophobic residues facing the membrane environment and mostly hydrophilic residues lining the inside of the β-barrel, which in the case of porins acts as an aqueous channel permitting the diffusion of water and other nutrients through the outer membrane (Delcour, 2009). Other OMPs act as secretion pores, transporting a variety of macromolecules across the outer membrane, such as, lipopolysaccharide (Dong et al., 2014), biofilm matrix components (Hufnagel et al., 2015), other proteins (Chagnot et al., 2013), or, in the case of autotransporters, parts of the same polypeptide chain (Leo et al., 2012). OMPs are further involved in such functions as self-recognition (Aoki et al., 2005, 2008), protein hydrolysis (Haiko et al., 2009), and virulence (Monteiro et al., 2016).

All β-barrel OMPs in Gram-negative bacteria are homologous (Remmert et al., 2010), and follow a conserved route of membrane insertion. OMPs are transported across the inner membrane via the Sec machinery in an unfolded conformation (Walther et al., 2009b). In the periplasm, chaperones such as, SurA, Skp, and DegP help to keep the OMPs in an unfolded state (Goemans et al., 2014). Insertion of OMPs into the outer membrane is accomplished by the β-barrel assembly machinery or BAM complex (Bakelar et al., 2016; Gu et al., 2016; Han et al., 2016). A recent study has shown that OMPs are inserted into the outer membrane at discreet sites near the cell center and move laterally toward the cell poles (Rassam et al., 2015). As the periplasm is devoid of adenosine triphosphate and ionic gradients cannot be maintained across the outer membrane, the energy for insertion into the outer membrane must be provided by the folding of the β-barrel itself (Moon et al., 2013).

Insertion of OMPs is thus dependent on the two constitutive membrane insertase/translocase systems, the Sec, and the BAM. For efficient recombinant production of properly folded OMPs, sufficient capacity is required for both systems to process the additional burden of heterologously expressed protein. When the BAM copy number is reduced, OMPs are inefficiently integrated into the outer membrane, though cell viability is not significantly affected (Aoki et al., 2008). Thus, under OMP over-expression conditions, the BAM may become congested, resulting in a bottleneck for efficient OMP integration. In addition to misfolding, this may also lead to induction of the envelope stress response, and thus indirectly to induction of protease expression (Alba and Gross, 2004) including the periplasmic protease DegP (Grosskinsky et al., 2007).

The Sec system is also prone to saturation, based e.g., on observations that, in some over-expression conditions, cytosolic inclusion bodies are formed where the signal peptide was not properly processed, or periplasmic inclusion bodies are observed due to follow-up problems of improper processing (Georgiou and Segatori, 2005). Over-expression of inner membrane proteins leads to accumulation of cytoplasmic inclusion bodies and aggregates, but also reduces the amount of proteins secreted into the periplasm and outer membrane (Wagner et al., 2007). Congestion of the Sec machinery further affects cell viability and the maximum rate at which heterologous OMPs can be transported into the periplasm (Schlegel et al., 2013). The Sec machinery also transports soluble periplasmic proteins, lipoproteins, integral inner membrane proteins, and several types of secreted proteins in addition to OMPs (Kudva et al., 2013). Therefore, for over-expression of heterologous OMPs in *E. coli*, it would be advisable to knock out abundant but non-essential OMPs to relieve some of the burden on the BAM and Sec machineries. In addition, removing these abundant proteins from the membrane leaves more space for recombinant proteins, potentially influencing the maximum yield per cell; limited membrane area can be a bottleneck for the over-production of membrane proteins (Arechaga et al., 2000; Wagner et al., 2006).

Koebnik and coworkers have previously developed such a set of strains derived from the common expression strain BL21(DE3) (Prilipov et al., 1998b). These strains lack one or more of the most abundant OMPs: OmpA, OmpC, OmpF, or LamB (maltoporin). We have successfully used some of these strains for expression and purification of OMPs, especially BL21 Omp2 and BL21 Omp8 (Wollmann et al., 2006; Arnold et al., 2007; Leo et al., 2011; Mikula et al., 2012; Oberhettinger et al., 2012; Shahid et al., 2012), but also for NMR experiments using native membranes (Shahid et al., 2015). However, in our hands these strains have proven to be genetically unstable and prone to sudden lysis, possibly due to mobilization of the Tn*5* transposon under stress conditions, used in generating these knock-out strains (Prilipov et al., 1998b; Supplementary Figure 1).

In this work, we present a series of knock-out strains lacking one, two, three, or all four of the genes encoding the proteins OmpA, OmpC, OmpF, and LamB. These strains are designed for use in over-expression of recombinant OMPs, and are equivalent to some of the strains produced earlier (Prilipov et al., 1998b). However, our series is more complete than that produced by Prilipov et al. and we used a different strategy to produce our knock-outs resulting in genetically more stable strains. Particularly, we have not observed spontaneous lysis of our quadruple knock-out strain lacking all four abundant OMPs (similar to the Omp8 strain produced earlier) when handled as we recommend. We also demonstrate that the quadruple mutant strain shows improved levels of four test proteins in the outer membrane compared to the BL21(DE3) parent strain.

MATERIALS AND METHODS

Bacteria, Media, and Growth Conditions

The *E. coli* strains produced in this work are derivatives of the commonly used expression strain BL21(DE3) (Studier and Moffatt, 1986). In addition to being widely utilized for expression, this strain also lacks the outer membrane protease OmpT, which we reasoned would be beneficial for over-expression of OMPs in particular. For transductions, we used the generally transducing bacteriophage P1 *vir*. The donor strains harboring the kanamycin cassettes for gene deletion were from the Keio collection (Baba et al., 2006). The K-12 reference strain was BW25113 (Datsenko and Wanner, 2000).

Bacteria were grown in lysogeny broth (LB) unless stated otherwise. For most experiments, we used the "Lennox" formulation: 10 g tryptone, 5 g yeast extract, and 5 g NaCl per liter. In the text below, we mean this formulation when referring to LB. For growth curves, we also used the "Miller" formulation (10 g tryptone, 5 g yeast extract, and 10 g NaCl per liter)—we refer to this as LB-Miller. Where necessary, media were supplemented with kanamycin (kan) or ampicillin (amp) at 25 μg/ml and 100 μg/ml, respectively. SOC medium was used after transformations as described elsewhere (Hanahan, 1983). As a defined medium, we used the minimal medium M9 (Miller, 1972) supplemented with glucose 0.2% (w/v) and 18 amino acids (all except cysteine and tyrosine) at 0.1 mg/ml each. Bacteria were usually grown at 37°C, unless harboring the plasmid pCP20, in which case they were grown either at 30°C for plasmid maintenance or 42°C to cure the plasmid. Some of the *omp* deletion strains, such as, the quadruple mutant BL21ΔABCF, grew significantly better at 30°C than at 37°C, and these were thus propagated at 30°C.

Plasmids

Plasmid pCP20 encoding the FLP recombinase (Flippase) was used for excising the kanamycin cassette after transduction into the knock-out strains (Cherepanov and Wackernagel, 1995). For λ red recombination, we employed the plasmid pKD46 (Datsenko and Wanner, 2000). The expression constructs used for testing our strains have been described previously: pET3b containing the genes encoding *ompX* and variants thereof (Arnold et al., 2007), pASK-IBA2 with *Yersinia enterocolitica* YadA membrane anchor domain (YadAM) (Wollmann et al., 2006) or Intimin (Oberhettinger et al., 2012). pET3b-OmpX was also modified for the purpose of this study by inserting a double haemagglutinin (HA)-tag with GSG linkers (GSGYPYDVPDYAGSGYPYDVPDYAGSG) in the position between S53 and S54 of OmpX for easier detection (pET3b-OmpX-HA). The insertion was created by site-directed mutagenesis (Byrappa et al., 1995) using the primers given in **Table 1**.

P1 Phage Transduction

P1 phage transduction was performed essentially as described (Thomason et al., 2007). Briefly, the *E. coli* strains from the Keio collection were grown in LB medium to an optical density at 600 nm (OD_{600}) of 1.0 and infected with P1 *vir* phages at various dilutions (e.g., 10^{-5}, 10^{-6}, 10^{-7}), mixed with 3 ml liquid top agar and poured onto pre-warmed LB plates. The following day, a semi-confluent plate was chosen and the top agar scraped off. This was mixed with 2 ml LB medium supplemented with a drop of chloroform, vortexed for 2 min and centrifuged for 10 min at 5,000 × g. Another drop of chloroform added to the supernatant, which was then stored at 4°C. The parent strain *E. coli* BL21(DE3) was infected with dilution series of each P1 phage lysate and the titer of the lysates was calculated from the number of plaques formed on the plates.

For the transduction experiments, *E. coli* BL21(DE3) and derivatives were grown in LB medium overnight, diluted 1:100 in the morning and grown until an OD_{600} of ~1.0, and then supplemented with 10 mM $CaCl_2$ and mixed the P1 phage lysate harboring the kan cassette specific for the desired knock-out at a multiplicity of infection (MOI) of 0.5, assuming 10^9 bacteria/ml culture. After incubating for 20 min at 37°C, the infection was stopped by addition of 100 mM sodium citrate pH 5.5. The mix was centrifuged for 2 min at 5,000 × *g*. The pellet was washed in LB medium supplemented with 100 mM sodium citrate and centrifuged as before. This washing step was repeated twice and then the bacteria were incubated for ~1 h at 37°C in LB containing 100 mM sodium citrate. Finally, the bacteria were centrifuged for 2 min at 4,000 × *g* diluted in 100 μl LB medium and streaked out on LB agar plates supplemented with kanamycin and 10 mM sodium citrate.

Introduction of the Kan Cassette by λ Red Recombination

To delete the *ompF* locus, we amplified the FLP recognition target (FRT)-kanamycin cassette flanked by sequence directly outside the sequence coding for OmpF, using the Keio collection Δ*ompF* strain and the same primer sequences described in that study (Baba et al., 2006). Insertion of the kan cassette was achieved by λ red recombination, essentially as described (Datsenko and Wanner, 2000): the plasmid pKD46 was transformed into recipient strains by electroporation, and transformants were selected for by plating on ampicillin and growing at 30°C. To introduce the kan cassette into the *ompF* locus, the pKD46-containing bacteria were grown to mid-log phase at 30°C, at which time the λ red genes were induced by the addition of 1 mM L-arabinose. After 1 h of induction, the cells were harvested and made electrocompetent. One hundred nanograms of PCR product was transformed into the cells by electroporation, after which cells were allowed to recover for 1 h at 30°C in SOC medium supplemented with 1 mM L-arabinose. Transformants were then selected for by growing on LB with kanamycin at 30°C. To remove pKD46, bacteria were grown on LB + kan at 37°C, and then tested for ampicillin sensitivity. Insertion of the kan cassette into the *ompF* locus was verified by colony PCR.

Excision of the Kan Cassette

For excision of the kan cassette, kan-resistant transductants were transformed with the conditionally replicating plasmid pCP20 encoding the FLP recombinase by electroporation, following the procedure suggested by Baba et al. (2006). After electroporation the cells were quickly mixed with 1 ml SOC medium and incubated for 1 h at 30°C. The bacteria were then plated on LB agar plates with ampicillin and incubated overnight at 30°C. To cure pCP20, one amp-resistant colony was streaked out onto an LB agar plate and incubated at 42°C overnight. To screen for mutants strains, colonies were streaked out on LB plates containing kan, amp, and no antibiotic, respectively, using a grid, and then incubated at 37°C overnight. Clones sensitive to both kan and amp were chosen, and correct deletions were verified using colony PCR.

Colony PCR

For verification of the right gene deletions in our mutants PCR with primers specific for the upstream and downstream region of the gene to be deleted was used. The primers sequences are given in **Table 1**. Colony PCR was performed using Taq polymerase

TABLE 1 | Primers used in this study.

COLONY PCR		
Gene	**Direction**	**Sequence (5′ → 3′)**
ompA	Forward	ATTTTGGATGATAACGAGGCGCAAAAAATG
ompA	Reverse	GAACTTAAGCCTGCGGCTGAGTTAC
lamB	Forward	AAAAGAAAAGCAATGACTCAGGAGATAGAATG
lamB	Reverse	GGTTTTGCTATTACCACCAGATTTCCATCTG
ompF	Forward	AGGTGTCATAAAAAAAACCATGAGGGTAATAAATAAT
ompF	Reverse	GAGGTGTGCTATTAGAACTGGTAAACGATACC
ompC (common)	Forward	CAATCGGTGCAAATGCCAGATAAGACAC
ompC (*E. coli* K-12)	Forward	GCAAATAAAGGCATATAACAGAGGGTTAATAACATG
ompC	Reverse	ATATCAATCGAGATTAGAACTGGTAAACCAGACC
MUTAGENESIS		
Product	**Direction**	**Sequence (5′ → 3′)**
HA-OmpX	Forward	GTTATCCATACGACGTACCTGATTACGCAGGTTCTGGGTCTGGTGACTACAACAAAAACCAG
HA-OmpX	Reverse	CTGAGCCCGCATAATCCGGAACATCATACGGGTAACCAGAACCGCTTGCAGTACGGCTTTTCTC

(New England Biolabs) and 20 pmol of primer per reaction. A typical colony PCR program was as follows: initial denaturation for 3 min at 94°C, followed by 25 cycles of denaturation (30 s at 94°C), annealing (20 s 50°C), and extension [1.5 min (or 5 min with *ompC* common primers) at 70°C]. After a final extension of 5 min at 70°C, samples were mixed with loading buffer and applied to a 1% agarose gel (0.8% for *ompC* common primers). The primer pair used amplified the coding sequences of each locus are indicated in **Table 1**.

Outer Membrane Preparations

Outer membrane isolations were performed essentially as described in Leo et al. (2015). Briefly, 20 ml of an overnight culture at OD_{600} 1.0 were pelleted and washed with 10 mM HEPES buffer at pH 7.4. To promote lysis, 0.1 mg/ml lysozyme was added, along with $MgCl_2$ and $MnCl_2$ to 10 mM and a pinch of DNase I (Sigma). The cells were then disrupted using a bead beater (SpeedMill Plus from Analytik Jena, Germany). The lysates were centrifuged at 15,600 × *g* for 30 s in a tabletop centrifuge and the supernatant was then moved to a fresh 2 ml microcentrifuge tube and centrifuged at 15,600 × *g* for another 30 min. The supernatant was decanted and the brownish membrane pellet resuspended in 400 μl 10 mM HEPES pH 7.4 with 1% (w/v) *N*-lauroyl sarcosine. The inner membranes were solubilized at room temperature (RT) for 30 min. Following this, the tubes were centrifuged at 15,600 × *g* for 30 min to pellet the outer membrane. The pellet was washed with 10 mM HEPES pH 7.4 and then resuspended in 30 μl HEPES buffer. For SDS-PAGE, 10 μl of 4 × non-reducing SDS sample buffer was added. Fifteen percentage SDS-PAGE gels were used for experimental verification of the knockout mutants at the protein level. For Coomassie G-250 (colloidal) staining of polyacrylamide gels, 12 μl of the outer membrane samples were used. For silver staining (Nesterenko et al., 1994), 8 μl of the outer membrane prep samples were run in a polyacrylamide gel and for Western blots 6 μl of the outer membrane prep samples were used.

Growth Curves

To draw growth curves, starter cultures were grown in 5 ml LB or supplemented M9 medium and the OD_{600} values were measured. The bacteria were then diluted to an OD_{600} value of 0.01 and 5 μl of this suspension was added to 200 μl of medium (LB, LB-Miller, or supplemented M9) in a sterile microtiter plate. For blanks, no bacteria were added. The plates were sealed with a BreathEasy® membrane (from Sigma-Aldrich). The plates were incubated in a Biotek Synergy plate reader with controlled temperature and orbital rotation at the "slow" setting; absorbance at 600 nm was recorded at 20-min intervals. For plotting, values from four biological replicates were averaged.

Aggregation Assays

For sedimentation assays, an overnight culture was diluted 1:100 in fresh LB (total volume 10 ml). The cultures were grown with shaking at 30°C in a flask till late log phase (OD_{600} ~1.0), at which point $MgCl_2$ or $CaCl_2$ were added to 10 mM to some of the cultures. After a further hour of incubation at 30°C with shaking, the bacteria were transferred carefully to 18 mm tubes so as not to disrupt any floccules. The tubes were then incubated statically at RT. One hundred and fifty microliter samples were taken from the very top of the cultures at 5-min intervals for 20 min and the absorbance at 600 nm was measured using a microcuvette (light path 1 cm). To estimate autoaggregation, the absorbance at each time point was compared to the absorbance at time point zero and expressed as a percentage:

$$(A_t * 100)/A_0,$$

where A_t is the absorbance at the relevant time point and A_0 is the absorbance at time point zero. For plotting, three biological replicates were used.

For photography, 5 ml cultures were grown to late log phase ($OD_{600} \approx 0.8$) and $MgCl_2$ or $CaCl_2$ were added as above. After a further hour of shaking, the tubes were incubated statically at RT and photographed after 20 min and 2 h.

Recombinant Protein Expression and Detection

For inducing recombinant protein production, plasmids encoding the test proteins were transform into the quadruple mutant strain (BL21ΔABCF). For production, a 5 ml overnight culture of a transformed clone was diluted 1:100 in fresh LB and grown at 30°C till mid-log phase (OD_{600} ~0.5). The culture was then induced with either isopropyl thiogalactoside (at 1 mM) or anhydrotetracycline (at 50 ng/ml). The cultures were incubated at 30°C for a further 2 h, after which the cells were harvested and outer membranes were isolated. The OMPs were separated by SDS-PAGE. Over-expressed YadAM, OmpX, and its duplicated variant OmpX88 were detected by colloidal Coomassie G-250 staining. Overexpression of a HA-tagged variant of OmpX and Intimin was detected by immunoblotting. The proteins were transferred to a 0.45 μm polyvinylidine difluoride membrane (Thermo Scientific) using a semi-dry transfer unit (Hoefer TE70X). The membranes were blocked with 2% skimmed milk powder dissolved in phosphate-buffered saline (PBS; 20 mM sodium phosphate pH 7.4, 150 mMNaCl) for 1 h at RT or overnight at 4°C. This was followed by incubation for an hour with primary antibodies; 1:2,000 dilution of rabbit anti-HA tag antibody (for OmpX-HA) and 1:5000 dilution of rabbit anti-Intimin antibody (Oberhettinger et al., 2012). The membrane was washed three times with PBS+0.05% Tween20 followed by incubation with a 1:10,000 dilution of goat anti-rabbit IgG horseradish peroxidase-conjugate (Santa Cruz Biotech) in PBS+2% skimmed milk powder for an hour. The membrane was washed three times with PBS+0.05% Tween20. The bands were detected using enhanced chemiluminescence (Pierce ECL western blotting substrate) and a Kodak 4000R Image station.

Whole-Cell ELISAs

For quantitative examination of Intimin and OmpX-HA expression, we performed whole-cell enzyme-linked immunosorbent assays (ELISAs). Bacteria transformed with the corresponding plasmids were grown overnight at 30°C in 5 ml LB medium with ampicillin. The following day, the bacteria were diluted 1:10 in fresh medium (5 ml, with amp) and grown till mid-log (OD_{600} ~0.5; about 2 h), at which time they were induced with anhydrotetracycline or isopropyl thiogalactoside as in the section on Recombinant Protein Expression and Detection. The bacteria were grown at 30°C for another 2 h. The OD_{600} of the cultures was measured and the bacteria were diluted in PBS to an OD_{600} value of 0.2. One hundred microliters of this suspension were applied to the wells of a polystyrene microtiter plate and bacteria were allowed to adhere to the surface of the well for 1 h at RT. The wells were washed three times with 200 μl washing buffer [PBS + 0.1% bovine serum albumin (BSA, from VWR)] and then blocked for 1 h with PBS + 2% BSA. The wells were washed once with 200 μl washing buffer, and 100 μl of the primary antibody diluted into blocking buffer was applied. The antibodies were the same as in the section on Recombinant Protein Expression and Detection, anti-HA (1:2,000), and anti-Intimin (1:1,000). After an hour's incubation, the wells were washed three times as above, and the secondary antibody (anti-rabbit-HRP, from Agrisera) was added, diluted 1:2,000 in blocking buffer. The plate was incubated for 1 h at RT, after which the wells were washed three times as above. Detection was performed using the colorimetric HRP substrate ABTS (ThermoScientific) according to the manufacturer's instructions. After color development (40 min) the reactions were stopped with 1% SDS and absorbances were recorded at 405 nm.

RESULTS

Production of Knock-Out Strains

To avoid the problems we had encountered with the strains from Prilipov et al. we pursued a different strategy in making our knock-out strains. We decided to delete the entire coding sequences for the four genes encoding the OMPs lacking in the Omp8 strain of Prilipov et al. namely *ompA*, *ompC*, *ompF*, and *lamB* (Prilipov et al., 1998b). We reasoned that this strategy would prevent the possibility of a genetic reversion, thus improving the genetic stability of the newly generated knock-out strains. BL21 strains probably do not express *ompC* naturally, due to an insertion element-mediated deletion of the upstream region of the *ompC* locus, including the signal peptide of OmpC (Pugsley and Rosenbusch, 1983; Studier et al., 2009; Han et al., 2012). Nevertheless, we decided to delete the entire *ompC* coding sequence to fully prevent the possibility of reversion, e.g., by a recombination event restoring a functional signal peptide. To make the deletions, we employed the Keio collection, a set of 3,985 single-gene deletions in *E. coli*, where virtually the entire coding sequence of the deleted genes is replaced by a kanamycin resistance cassette (Baba et al., 2006). This cassette is flanked by sequences targeted by the FLP recombinase; thus, when FLP is supplied in trans, the kan cassette can be excised from the genome leaving only a ~100 bp-long scar sequence.

We produced the single knock-outs in *E. coli* BL21(DE3) by phage P1 transduction: a phage lysate was produced from the Keio strains harboring the desired OMP gene deletions. This lysate was used to infect the recipient strain, and kan-resistant transductants were then selected for by plating on kanamycin plates. To remove the kan cassette, we introduced the FLP-containing plasmid pCP20 into the kan-resistant bacteria and selected for amp-resistant colonies without the addition of kanamycin. To cure pCP20, clones were plated onto LB (no selection) and grown at 42°C. Clones that were sensitive to both amp and kan were chosen for PCR screening to verify the loss of the kan cassette and the loss of the wild-type allele. Using this strategy, we produced the four individual knock-outs, and then by re-iterating the process, we obtained five double knock-outs, three triple knock-outs, and the quadruple knock-out strain (**Table 2**).

We experienced particular problems producing the *ompA*-*ompF* double knock-out and the *ompA-ompF-ompC* triple knock-out. The *ompA* and *ompF* loci are situated relatively close to each other in the *E. coli* genome (distance ~32 kb; P1 can transduce fragments ~ three times this size); therefore, we often obtained revertants for one mutant while trying to produce the other. To circumvent this problem, we employed a different strategy: we amplified the FRT-kan cassette from the Keio Δ*ompF* strain by PCR, with 50 bp overhangs identical to

TABLE 2 | Knock-out strains produced in this study.

Knock-outs	Strain	Genes deleted	Addgene ID
SINGLE KNOCK-OUTS			
	BL21ΔA	*ompA*	102256
	BL21ΔB	*lamB*	102257
	BL21ΔC	*ompC*	102258
	BL21ΔF	*ompF*	102259
DOUBLE KNOCK-OUTS			
	BL21ΔAB	*ompA, lamB*	102260
	BL21ΔAC	*ompA, ompC*	102261
	BL21ΔAF	*ompA, ompF*	102262
	BL21ΔBC	*lamB, ompC*	102263
	BL21ΔBF	*lamB, ompF*	102264
	BL21ΔCF	*ompC, ompF*	102265
TRIPLE KNOCK-OUTS			
	BL21ΔABC	*ompA, lamB, ompC*	102266
	BL21ΔABF	*ompA, lamB,ompF*	102267
	BL21ΔACF	*ompA, ompC, ompF*	102268
	BL21ΔBCF	*lamB, ompC, ompF*	102269
QUADRUPLE KNOCK-OUT			
	BL21ΔABCF	*ompA, lamB, ompC, ompF*	102270

All strains are derived from BL21(DE3).

the sequence flanking the *ompF* coding region, as was used to make the *ompF* mutant in the original Keio collection (Baba et al., 2006). We then produced the BL21ΔAF and BL21ΔACF strains by λ red recombination in the BL21ΔA and BL21ΔAC strains (Datsenko and Wanner, 2000). We then selected for kan-resistant colonies and subsequently removed the kan cassette as described for the transduction experiments. Indeed, this strategy proved successful.

Verification of the Knock-Out Mutant Strains

To verify that the correct gene had been deleted, we amplified the target coding sequence by colony PCR. Using primers specific for each of the four loci, we could show that the mutant strains had lost the wild-type allele (**Figure 1A**). The sequences remaining in the deletion mutants correspond to ~150 bp, the size of the scar sequence and flanking regions, indicating that the gene was actually replaced by the kan cassette, which in turn was excised by FLP. The size of the wild-type coding sequence is 1041 bp for *ompA*, 1089 bp for *ompF*, 1104 bp for *ompC*, and 1341 bp for *lamB*. These sizes are consistent with the PCR products obtained from the parent strain BL21(DE3). For verification of the *ompC* deletion, another forward primer binding downstream the *rcsC* locus was used due to the fact that in *E. coli* BL21 the upstream region of *ompC* is deleted (Studier et al., 2009). Thus, the forward primer amplifying the *ompC* locus in *E. coli* K-12 strains does not produce a product in B strains. The common forward primer, which binds downstream of the *rscC* gene, produces a product in both strains when combined with the same reverse primer used for amplifying the K-12 locus (**Table 1**). In BL21(DE3), this results in a product of ~1.9 kb. In K-12, the product also contains the region deleted in BL21(DE3), so the total length of the product is ~5.3 kb. For the mutants, where the *ompC* coding sequence is deleted within the K-12 context, the product is ~4.2 kb (**Figure 1B**). These results confirm that the kan cassette had correctly replaced the *ompC* sequence of BL21(DE3).

In order to show that the PCR-positive knock-out strains lack the corresponding proteins, we prepared outer membrane samples from all the strains and analyzed these by SDS-PAGE and silver staining (**Figure 1C**). *E. coli* BL21(DE3) was included as a positive sample showing outer membrane protein bands of interest. Maltoporin (LamB) has a size of ~49 kDa. OmpC and OmpF are approximately the same size and run as a single band at ~39 kDa, and OmpA has the smallest size of ~35 kDa. All of these protein bands are visible in the parent strain. The single knock-out strain BL21ΔA shows all bands of interest except the 35 kDa OmpA band indicating that this protein is lacking in this strain. The ΔB strain shows the bands of interest at 35 kDa for OmpA and at 37 kDa for OmpC and OmpF but no band at 49 kDa. As a note, maltoporin is not well expressed in *E. coli* B strains, including BL21, which makes the confirmation of the *lamB* knock-out difficult on the protein level (Ronen and Raanan-Ashkenazi, 1971; Han et al., 2012); thus, the *lamB* knock-outs could only be fully confirmed by PCR. Single *ompC* and *ompF* knock-outs show a reduction in band intensity at 39 kDa, and only the double knock-outs lack the band at 39 kDa completely, suggesting that our strategy of knocking out *ompC* was a reasonable approach to make sure the gene is entirely inactivated. A possible explanation for a residual band at 39 kDa (e.g. for BL21ΔF) is expression of the cryptic porin OmpN (Prilipov et al., 1998a). Taken together, the PCR results and OMP profiles of the strains show that we have successfully deleted the genes encoding the major OMPs, either singly or in all combinations.

Growth Properties of the Quadruple Knock-Out Strain BL21ΔABCF

While working with the new strains, it became obvious that by altering the outer membrane protein composition the growth behavior changed. BL21ΔABCF grew significantly more slowly than the parent strain BL21(DE3). The strain grew initially faster at 37°C than at 30°C, but the culture at 37°C saturated at a lower OD_{600} (**Figure 2A**). However, even at 30°C, BL21ΔABCF did not reach the same OD_{600} value as BL21(DE3).

We also observed that when using the Miller formulation of LB (with 10 g sodium chloride per liter), BL21ΔABCF grew significantly slower than in our standard LB (5 g NaCl/l), also at 30°C, whereas BL21(DE3) showed no significant differences in growth in the two media (**Figure 2B**). We do not currently have an explanation for this phenomenon; perhaps BL21ΔABCF is unable to compensate efficiently for the increased osmolarity of LB-Miller.

We also tested the growth of BL21ΔABCF in defined medium (**Figure 2C**). For this, we used minimal medium M9 supplemented with 18 amino acids. Though growth was slower than in LB, BL21ΔABCF reached higher optical densities than in the rich, undefined medium. It apparently also reached a higher density than BL21(DE3); however, part of the higher

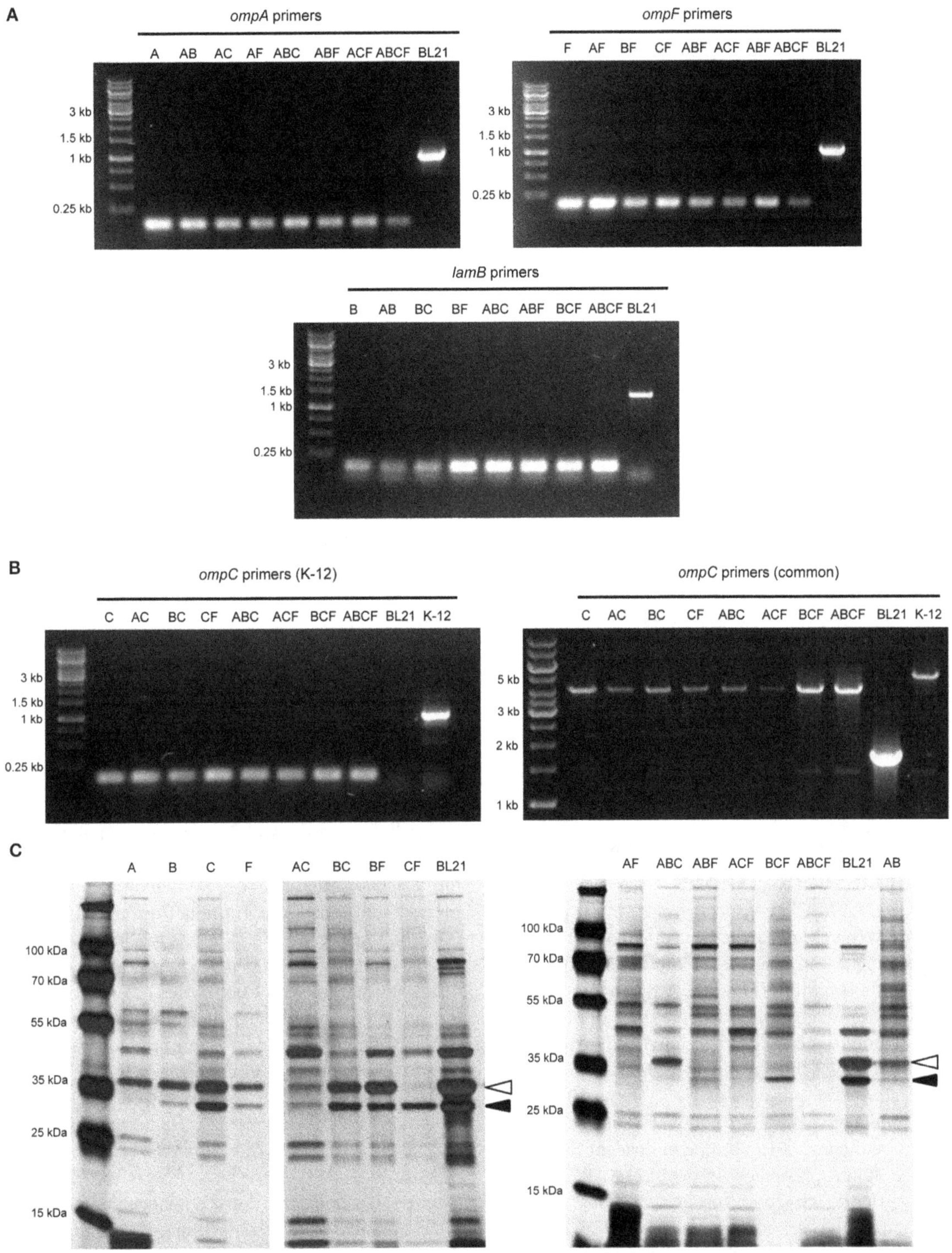

FIGURE 1 | Verification of the BL21 OMP knock-out strains. **(A)** Colony PCR results with primers for *ompA*, *ompF*, and *lamB* showing that in the mutant strains only a scar sequence (130–150 bp) remains at the locus. BL21 = parent strain BL21(DE3) control (expected sizes: *ompA* 1072, *ompF* 1135, *lamB* 1380 bp). **(B)** Colony PCR results of *ompC*. On the left, results using primers specific for the K-12 *ompC* locus are shown, where BL21(DE3) does not give a product and the deletion strains show just a short scar sequence (~150 bp). The expected size for K-12 *ompC is* 1101 bp. On the right, results using common primers amplifying a larger region around the *ompC* locus in both BL21 and K-12. Here, the expected product for BL21(DE3) is 1.9 kb, the size expected for *E. coli* K-12 product is 5.3 kb and for the deletion strains 4.2 kb. **(C)** Silver-stained 15% polyacrylamide gel of BL21 OMP knock-out strains. The positions of OmpA (black arrowhead) and OmpC/F (open arrowhead) bands are indicated for the parent strain control (BL21). LamB is poorly expressed in *E. coli* B strains when grown at temperatures above 30°C and in the presence of other carbon sources (Ronen and Raanan-Ashkenazi, 1971), so this protein is not evident in most of the samples. Note that the Δ symbol has been omitted in the figure texts due to space constraints.

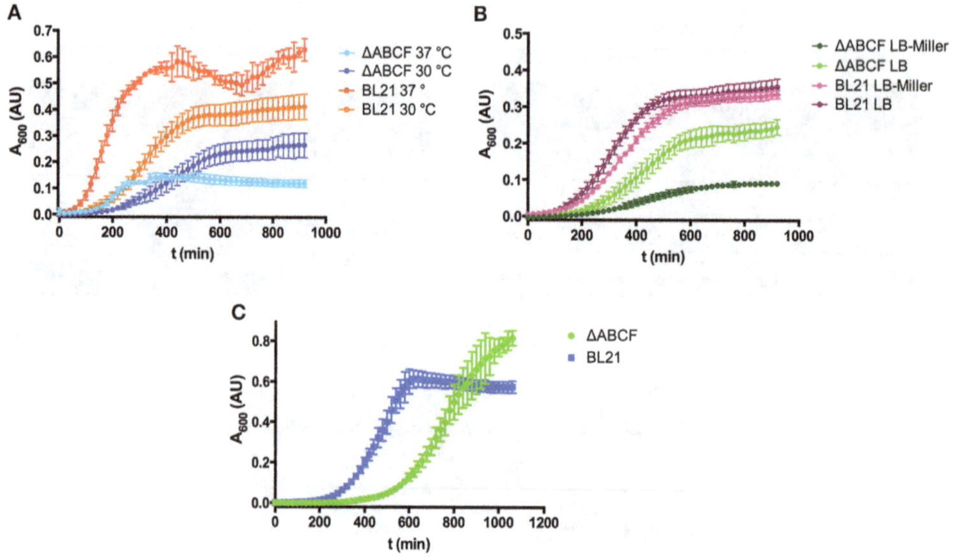

FIGURE 2 | Growth properties of the quadruple mutant BL21ΔABCF. **(A)** Growth of BL21ΔABCF in LB medium at 30 and 37°C. The parent strain BL21(DE3) is shown for comparison. Data points are the mean of four biological replicates; error bars denote the standard deviation. **(B)** Growth of BL21ΔABCF in LB (0.5% NaCl) and LB-Miller (1% NaCl) medium at 30°C. The parent strain BL21(DE3) is shown for comparison. Data points are the mean of four biological replicates; error bars denote the standard deviation. **(C)** Growth of BL21ΔABCF in supplemented M9 medium at 30°C. The parent strain BL21(DE3) is shown for comparison. Data points are the mean of four biological replicates; error bars denote the standard deviation. Note that the absorbance values shown here are not directly comparable to those measured with a 1 cm cuvette, due to the difference in light path length.

absorbance readings of the quadruple mutant cultures could be attributed to the tendency of BL21ΔABCF to clump in the defined medium, presumably due to the relatively high concentration of magnesium (2 mM; see section Aggregation of BL21ΔABCF in the Presence of Divalent Cations).

Aggregation of BL21ΔABCF in the Presence of Divalent Cations

As noted above, BL21ΔABCF tends to aggregate in the presence of divalent cations. When Mg^{2+} or Ca^{2+} is added to the medium, BL21ΔABCF flocculates and settles rapidly at the bottom of the tube under static condition (**Figures 3A,B**). In contrast, the parent strain does not aggregate in the presence of either ion during the short time frame of the experiment (**Figures 3A,C**). However, upon prolonged incubation (>1 h), also BL21(DE3) began to flocculate in the presence of Ca^{2+} (**Figure 3D**). The reason for the rapid aggregation of BL21ΔABCF is not clear. A possibility might be the increased binding of divalent cations by the more exposed lipid A phosphates in the BL21ΔABCF strain, leading to electrostatic attraction through bridging divalent cations. In principle, the aggregation caused by $CaCl_2$ might cause problems when preparing chemically competent cells; however, in our hands BL21ΔABCF can be made competent and transformed efficiently using the standard $CaCl_2$ protocol (data not shown).

BL21ΔABCF Is Superior in Producing Recombinant OMPs

To qualitatively test the performance of our new quadruple mutant strain, we over-expressed four test proteins from our laboratory. For comparison, we used the parent strain *E. coli* BL21 (DE3). The test proteins were OmpX, a native OMP of *E. coli*, a duplicated variant of this protein with 16 β-strands rather than the usual eight (Arnold et al., 2007), and another OmpX variant containing a HA tag in one of the extracellular loops. Additionally, we tested the expression of two autotransporter proteins: the membrane anchor domain of the *Yersinia* adhesin YadA (Wollmann et al., 2006) and the inverse autotransporter Intimin from enteropathogenic *E. coli* (Oberhettinger et al., 2012).

The expression of wild-type OmpX can be seen as a band at 15 kDa when stained with Coomassie G-250 (**Figure 4A**). The band is more intense for BL21ΔABCF than for the parent strain. Other bands of native proteins, for example the band at 18 kDa that presumably represents OmpW, show that the same amount of sample was loaded. Note that there is no clear difference between the strains for the duplicated variant OmpX88 (~37 kDa). The OmpX-HA construct was also expressed in BL21(DE3) and BL21ΔABCF. A Western blot of outer membrane preparations (**Figure 4B**) shows that for the quadruple knock-out strain, the total amount of expressed OmpX-HA is higher compared to the parent strain BL21(DE3). An additional band was detected at an increased molecular weight (~25 kDa) that we originally attributed to non-denatured OmpX-HA (**Figure 4B**, right panel), similar to previous findings on OmpX gel shifts (Arnold et al., 2007), Based on the OMP gel shift phenomenon (Rosenbusch, 1974; Schweizer et al., 1978), we know that native and denatured forms of OMPs can migrate differently in SDS-PAGE. However, when comparing heated and unheated samples, the band did not change, suggesting that it is an artifact yet to be explained (data

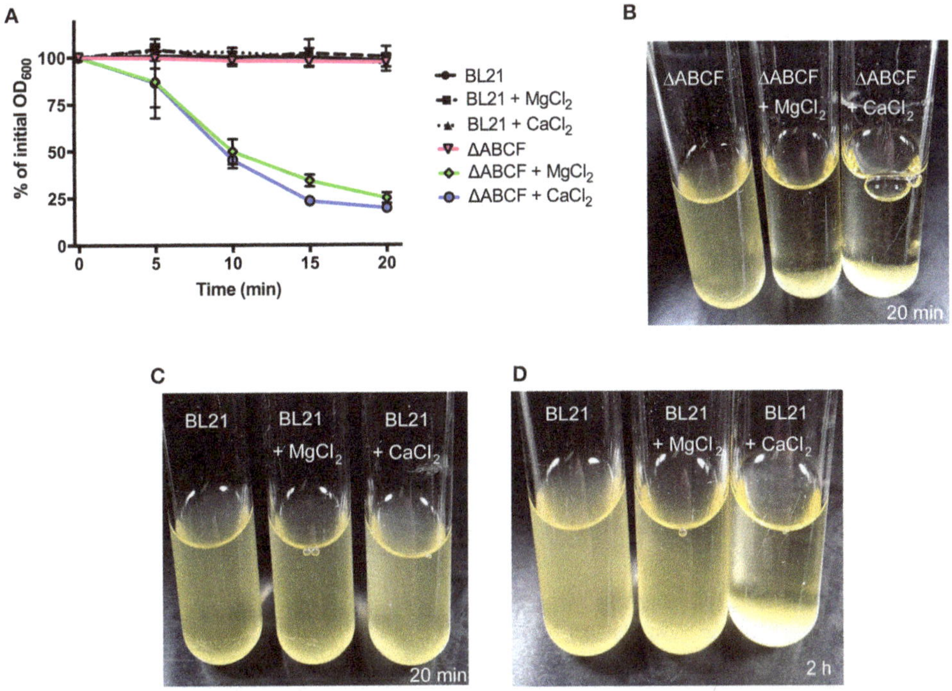

FIGURE 3 | Divalent cation-mediated aggregation of BL21ΔABCF. **(A)** Quantitative sedimentation assay. Cultures of BL21ΔABCF or the parent strain were cultured in LB medium (with or without the addition of $MgCl_2$ or $CaCl_2$ at 10 mM) at 30°C with shaking (200 rpm). For the sedimentation assay, the cultures were incubated statically and the OD_{600} value was measured from the very top of the culture at 5-min intervals. The data points represent the percentage of the initial OD_{600} value as the mean of three biological replicates; error bars denote standard deviations. **(B)** Photograph of BL21ΔABCF cultures after 20 min of static incubation. In the presence of 10 mM $MgCl_2$ or $CaCl_2$, BL21ΔABCF flocculates and rapidly settles at the bottom of the tube, leaving the medium clear. **(C)** Photograph of BL21(DE3) cultures after 20 min of static incubation. Turbidity is not reduced by the addition of 10 mM $MgCl_2$ or $CaCl_2$ to cultures of BL21(DE3). **(D)** Photograph of BL21(DE3) cultures after 2 h of static incubation. In the presence of $CaCl_2$, also BL21(DE3) flocculates.

not shown). The third specific band at ~50 kDa is presumably a folded dimer of OmpX at very low concentration (Chaturvedi and Mahalakshmi, 2013).

YadA is an obligate homotrimer and an adhesin of enteropathogenic *Yersiniae* (Mühlenkamp et al., 2015). It is an extremely stable protein which remains trimeric in the presence of denaturants such as, SDS and urea (Wollmann et al., 2006). In SDS-PAGE, YadAM (membrane anchor domain of YadA) migrates at an apparent molecular weight of 45 kDa (Wollmann et al., 2006). The expression of YadAM in BL21(DE3) and BL21ΔABCF is shown in **Figure 4C**. The colloidal Coomassie G250-stained gel shows better expression of YadAM in BL21ΔABCF than BL21(DE3). As mentioned above, many native outer membrane protein bands (e.g., ~30 kDa and ~60 kDa) are absent in the ΔABCF strain.

The expression of Intimin is shown in **Figure 4D**. Here, a construct including a StrepII tag was used and its expression visualized specifically in a Western blot using an anti-Intimin antibody (Oberhettinger et al., 2012). The blot shows two bands for the parent strain: one at ~95 kDa corresponding to the molecular weight of Intimin and a second band at ~120 kDa. This latter band is sometimes observed in Intimin blots, though its provenance is not clear (Heinz et al., 2016; Leo et al., 2016). For the ΔABCF strain, the 95 kDa band is more intense, and the ~120 kDa band fainter, suggesting better membrane insertion. In addition, some apparent degradation product can be seen for the quadruple mutant (band at ~70 kDa). The superiority of the BL21ΔABCF strain is demonstrated by a higher yield of the "correct" Intimin band and less of the (presumably mis-incorporated) 120 kDa band.

To gain a more quantitative view of OMP production in BL21ΔABCF and to assess reproducibility between culture batches, we performed whole-cell ELISA on bacteria expressing OmpX-HA and Intimin. We compared expression of these two proteins in BL21(DE3), BL21ΔABCF, and the Prilipov strain BL21 Omp8. We also tested the expression of YadAM in these strains, but due to technical problems with detecting the StrepII tag on the bacterial surface combined with the tendency of YadAM-expressing cells to clump, we did not obtain reliable results (data not shown). In this construct, only a short stretch of YadAM is exposed to the surface, so the StrepII tag is presumably not fully accessible to antibodies (Shahid et al., 2012).

BL21ΔABCF produced both Intimin and OmpX-HA at higher amounts than the parent strain BL21(DE3) (**Figure 5**). Somewhat unexpectedly, BL21ΔABCF also outperformed the Omp8 strain, though the difference is not large. The ELISA also demonstrate that the variability between biological replicates is low, though for Intimin there is more variability between replicates. Incidentally, in the whole-cell assays the detected proteins must be surface-exposed, showing that the detected species must be correctly processed and inserted into the membrane.

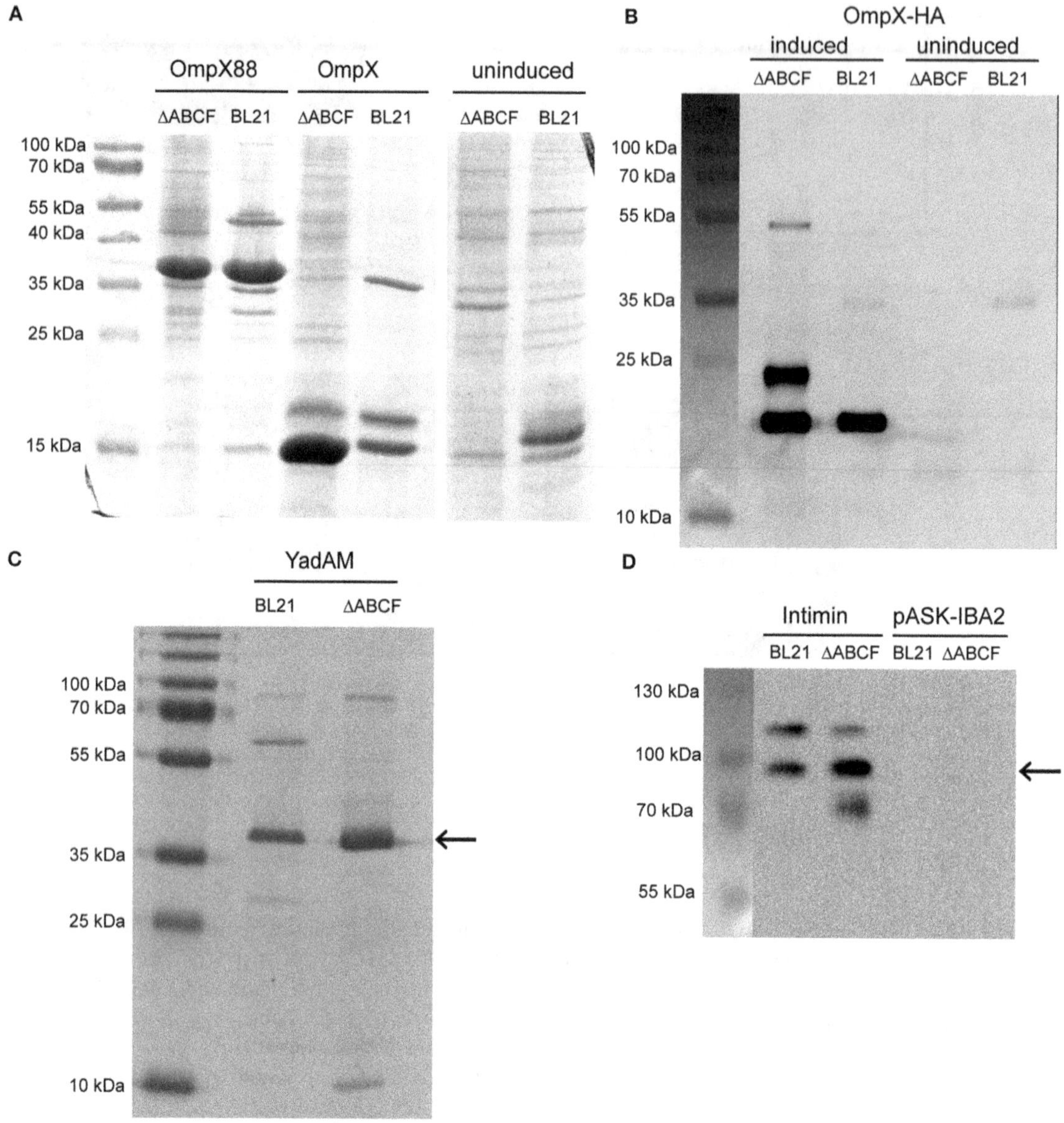

FIGURE 4 | Improved over-production of recombinant OMPs in BL21ΔABCF. **(A)** Coomassie-stained 15% polyacrylamide gel showing production levels of recombinant OmpX and duplicated OmpX (OmpX88) in BL21(DE3) and BL21ΔABCF. Uninduced cultures of the OmpX construct are shown as a control. Note that the artificial construct OmpX88 does not show significantly improved expression, while the expression of OmpX is massively improved in the BL21ΔABCF strain. **(B)** Western blot of OmpX-HA produced in both BL21(DE3) and BL21ΔABCF probed with an anti-HA antibody. An equal amount of cells (based on OD_{600} measurement) was lysed by heating in sample buffer and loaded onto the gel. Uninduced samples are shown as controls. A picture showing the positions of the pre-stained molecular weight marker bands on the blotting membrane is shown on the left. **(C)** Colloidal Coomassie G250-stained 15% polyacrylamide gel showing production levels of the YadA membrane anchor (YadAM; position denoted by the arrow) produced in both BL21 and BL21ΔABCF. **(D)** Western blot of Intimin produced in both BL21 and BL21ΔABCF probed with an anti-Intimin antibody. An equal amount of cells (based on OD600 measurement) was lysed by heating in sample buffer and loaded onto the gel. Strains with the empty vector (pASK-IBA2) serve as controls. The arrow shows the position of the main Intimin band (~95 kDa). A picture showing the positions of the pre-stained molecular weight marker bands on the blotting membrane is shown on the left.

DISCUSSION

We have produced a series of *E. coli* knock-out strains for use in over-expressing OMPs with deletions of at least one of four abundant OMP protein genes. Our series contains the four single deletions, all combinations of double and triple deletions, and the quadruple deletion strain BL21ΔABCF. The strains all contain the DE3 lysogen and can therefore be used with vectors requiring the T7 polymerase for expression.

We noted some unusual properties when culturing the quadruple mutant strain BL21ΔABCF: the strain grows poorly at 37°C and does not tolerate high salt concentrations. In addition, BL21ΔABCF aggregates in the presence of divalent cations. We therefore recommend that BL21ΔABCF be grown at 30°C in

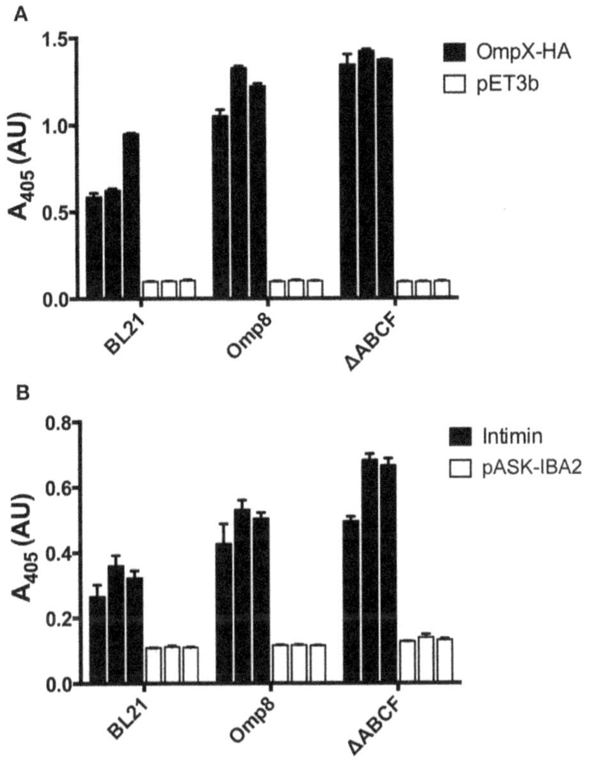

FIGURE 5 | Quantitative assessment of recombinant OMP production by BL21 ΔABCF **(A)** Whole-cell ELISA of bacteria producing OmpX-HA. Bacteria were coated onto wells of a microtiter plate and probed with an anti-HA tag antibody. The primary antibody was detected with a HRP-conjugated secondary antibody and colorimetric staining using the substrate ABTS. Black bars denote the biological replicates (three for each strain) expressing OmpX-HA; white bars show values for empty vector controls. Each bar represent the mean of three technical replicates; error bars denote the standard deviation of three technical replicates. **(B)** Whole-cell ELISA of bacteria producing Intimin. The experimental set up was similar to **(A)**; the primary antibody was an anti-Intimin antibody. Black bars denote biological replicates expressing Intimin, white bars represent vector controls. Each bar represent the mean of three technical replicates; error bars denote the standard deviation of three technical replicates.

medium with low sodium chloride ($\leq$5 g/l) and without excess divalent cations.

We demonstrated the superiority of the quadruple mutant strain in producing four different test proteins (OmpX, artificial OmpX variants, YadA, and Intimin) compared with BL21(DE3). This strain has mutations in the same genes as the Omp8 strain previously produced (Prilipov et al., 1998b), and we assumed that there would be no major differences between these two strains regarding OMP production capability. However, our whole-cell ELISAs showed that BL21ΔABCF is slightly better at over-expressing OMPs than Omp8, and significantly better than the parent strain BL21(DE3). In addition, as our strain lacks the transposon found in Omp8, and the full deletion of the OMP coding sequences prevents any reversion to wild-type, it is more stable than the Omp8 strain has proven to be, at least in our hands. A second advantage of the ΔABCF strain is the lack of any intrinsic antibiotic resistance markers, allowing it to host a broader choice of vector plasmids.

An additional advantage of these OMP deletion strains, similarly to the strains of Prilipov et al., is the low level of endogenous OMPs. Especially the ΔABCF strain can be used for *in situ* studies of OMP functions, without interference from endogenous proteins, where efficient labeling of the protein of interest against a low background is required. The power of such approaches can be seen in work where YadA was expressed in the original Omp8 strain in isotope-labeled medium for nuclear magnetic resonance (NMR) studies, where it was then possible to directly measure NMR spectra of the protein in native membranes (Shahid et al., 2015). This would not have been possible using wild-type *E. coli* due to the high background from other abundant OMPs.

Furthermore, the lack of all major naturally occurring OMPs in this strain may aid in purifying heterologous OMPs for functional or structural studies. As the amount of competing OMPs is low, heterologous OMPs can be purified efficiently and simply with e.g., ion exchange chromatography, without the need to introduce affinity tags, which might compromise protein function. This applies even to transmembrane β-barrel proteins of eukaryotic origin, some of which have been produced in bacteria (Walther et al., 2009a).

AUTHOR CONTRIBUTIONS

DL conceived the project; JL and DL designed the project; IM and JL performed the recombinant DNA work; IM, JL, MM, and NC performed the strain characterization; and all authors were involved in analyzing the data and writing the manuscript.

FUNDING

This work was funded by an Erasmus student exchange fellowship (to IM), FriMedBio funding by the Research Council of Norway (to DL), and a grant from VISTA, a basic research program funded by Statoil in collaboration with the NorwegianAcademy of Science and Letters (to JL).

ACKNOWLEDGMENTS

We thank Sophie Krauss, Pao Jané, and Hawzeen Salah Khalil for technical assistance. The strains from the Keio collection were obtained from the National BioResource Project (NIG, Japan): *E. coli*.

REFERENCES

Alba, B. M., and Gross, C. A. (2004). Regulation of the *Escherichia coli* sigma(E)-dependent envelope stress response. *Mol. Microbiol.* 52, 613–619. doi: 10.1111/j.1365-2958.2003.03982.x

Aoki, S. K., Malinverni, J. C., Jacoby, K., Thomas, B., Pamma, R., Trinh, B. N., et al. (2008). Contact-dependent growth inhibition requires the essential outer membrane protein BamA (YaeT) as the receptor and the inner membrane transport protein AcrB. *Mol. Microbiol.* 70, 323–340. doi: 10.1111/j.1365-2958.2008.06404.x

Aoki, S. K., Pamma, R., Hernday, A. D., Bickham, J. E., Braaten, B. A., and Low, D. A. (2005). Contact-dependent inhibition of growth in *Escherichia coli*. *Science* 309, 1245–1248. doi: 10.1126/science.1115109

Arechaga, I., Miroux, B., Karrasch, S., Huijbregts, R., de Kruijff, B., Runswick, M. J., et al. (2000). Characterisation of new intracellular membranes in *Escherichia coli* accompanying large scale over-production of the b subunit of F(1)F(o) ATP synthase. *FEBS Lett.* 482, 215–219. doi: 10.1016/S0014-5793(00)02054-8

Arnold, T., Poynor, M., Nussberger, S., Lupas, A. N., and Linke, D. (2007). Gene duplication of the eight-stranded beta-barrel OmpX produces a functional pore: a scenario for the evolution of transmembrane β-barrels. *J. Mol. Biol.* 366, 1174–1184. doi: 10.1016/j.jmb.2006.12.029

Baba, T., Ara, T., Hasegawa, M., Takai, Y., Okumura, Y., Baba, M., et al. (2006). Construction of *Escherichia coli* K-12 in-frame, single-gene knockout mutants: the Keio collection. *Mol. Syst. Biol.* 2:2006.0008. doi: 10.1038/msb4100050

Bakelar, J., Buchanan, S. K., and Noinaj, N. (2016). The structure of the β-barrel assembly machinery complex. *Science* 351, 180–186. doi: 10.1126/science.aad3460

Byrappa, S., Gavin, D. K., and Gupta, K. C. (1995). A highly efficient procedure for site-specific mutagenesis of full-length plasmids using Vent DNA polymerase. *Genome Res.* 5, 1–5. doi: 10.1101/gr.5.4.404

Chagnot, C., Zorgani, M. A., Astruc, T., and Desvaux, M. (2013). Proteinaceous determinants of surface colonization in bacteria: bacterial adhesion and biofilm formation from a protein secretion perspective. *Front. Microbiol.* 4:303. doi: 10.3389/fmicb.2013.00303

Chaturvedi, D., and Mahalakshmi, R. (2013). Methionine mutations of outer membrane protein X influence structural stability and beta-barrel unfolding. *PLoS ONE* 8:e79351. doi: 10.1371/journal.pone.0079351

Cherepanov, P. P., and Wackernagel, W. (1995). Gene disruption in *Escherichia coli*: TcR and KmR cassettes with the option of Flp-catalyzed excision of the antibiotic-resistance determinant. *Gene* 158, 9–14. doi: 10.1016/0378-1119(95)00193-A

Datsenko, K. A., and Wanner, B. L. (2000). One-step inactivation of chromosomal genes in *Escherichia coli* K-12 using PCR products. *Proc. Natl. Acad. Sci. U.S.A.* 97, 6640–6645. doi: 10.1073/pnas.120163297

Delcour, A. H. (2009). Outer membrane permeability and antibiotic resistance. *Biochim. Biophys. Acta.* 1794, 808–816. doi: 10.1016/j.bbapap.2008.11.005

Dong, H., Xiang, Q., Gu, Y., Wang, Z., Paterson, N. G., Stansfeld, P. J., et al. (2014). Structural basis for outer membrane lipopolysaccharide insertion. *Nature* 511, 52–56. doi: 10.1038/nature13464

Fairman, J. W., Noinaj, N., and Buchanan, S. K. (2011). The structural biology of β-barrel membrane proteins: a summary of recent reports. *Curr. Opin. Struct. Biol.* 21, 523–531. doi: 10.1016/j.sbi.2011.05.005

Georgiou, G., and Segatori, L. (2005). Preparative expression of secreted proteins in bacteria: status report and future prospects. *Curr. Opin. Biotechnol.* 16, 538–545. doi: 10.1016/j.copbio.2005.07.008

Goemans, C., Denoncin, K., and Collet, J. F. (2014). Folding mechanisms of periplasmic proteins. *Biochim. Biophys. Acta* 1843, 1517–1528. doi: 10.1016/j.bbamcr.2013.10.014

Grosskinsky, U., Schütz, M., Fritz, M., Schmid, Y., Lamparter, M. C., Szczesny, P., et al. (2007). A conserved glycine residue of trimeric autotransporter domains plays a key role in *Yersinia* adhesin A autotransport. *J. Bacteriol.* 189, 9011–9019. doi: 10.1128/JB.00985-07

Gu, Y., Li, H., Dong, H., Zeng, Y., Zhang, Z., Paterson, N. G., et al. (2016). Structural basis of outer membrane protein insertion by the BAM complex. *Nature* 531, 64–69. doi: 10.1038/nature17199

Haiko, J., Suomalainen, M., Ojala, T., Lähteenmäki, K., and Korhonen, T. K. (2009). Breaking barriers–attack on innate immune defences by omptin surface proteases of enterobacterial pathogens. *Innate Immun.* 15, 67–80. doi: 10.1177/1753425909102559

Han, L., Zheng, J., Wang, Y., Yang, X., Liu, Y., Sun, C., et al. (2016). Structure of the BAM complex and its implications for biogenesis of outer-membrane proteins. *Nat. Struct. Mol. Biol.* 23, 192–196. doi: 10.1038/nsmb.3181

Han, M. J., Lee, S. Y., and Hong, S. H. (2012). Comparative analysis of envelope proteomes in *Escherichia coli* B and K-12 strains. *J. Microbiol. Biotechnol.* 22, 470–478. doi: 10.4014/jmb.1110.10080

Hanahan, D. (1983). Studies on transformation of *Escherichia coli* with plasmids. *J. Mol. Biol.* 166, 557–580. doi: 10.1016/S0022-2836(83)80284-8

Heinz, E., Stubenrauch, C. J., Grinter, R., Croft, N. P., Purcell, A. W., Strugnell, R. A., et al. (2016). Conserved features in the structure, mechanism, and biogenesis of the inverse autotransporter protein family. *Genome Biol. Evol.* 8, 1690–1705. doi: 10.1093/gbe/evw112

Hufnagel, D. A., Depas, W. H., and Chapman, M. R. (2015). The biology of the *Escherichia coli* extracellular matrix. *Microbiol. Spectr.* 3:249. doi: 10.1128/microbiolspec.MB-0014-2014

Kudva, R., Denks, K., Kuhn, P., Vogt, A., Müller, M., and Koch, H. G. (2013). Protein translocation across the inner membrane of gram-negative bacteria: the Sec and Tat dependent protein transport pathways. *Res. Microbiol.* 164, 505–534. doi: 10.1016/j.resmic.2013.03.016

Leo, J. C., Grin, I., and Linke, D. (2012). Type V secretion: mechanism(s) of autotransport through the bacterial outer membrane. *Philos. Trans. R. Soc. Lond. B Biol. Sci.* 367, 1088–1101. doi: 10.1098/rstb.2011.0208

Leo, J. C., Lyskowski, A., Hattula, K., Hartmann, M. D., Schwarz, H., Butcher, S. J., et al. (2011). The structure of *E. coli* IgG-binding protein D suggests a general model for bending and binding in trimeric autotransporter adhesins. *Structure* 19, 1021–1030. doi: 10.1016/j.str.2011.03.021

Leo, J. C., Oberhettinger, P., and Linke, D. (2015). Assessing the outer membrane insertion and folding of multimeric transmembrane β-barrel proteins. *Methods Mol. Biol.* 1329, 157–167. doi: 10.1007/978-1-4939-2871-2_12

Leo, J. C., Oberhettinger, P., Yoshimoto, S., Udatha, D. B., Morth, P. J., Schütz, M., et al. (2016). Secretion of the intimin passenger domain is driven by protein folding. *J. Biol. Chem.* 291, 20096–20112. doi: 10.1074/jbc.M116.731497

Mikula, K. M., Leo, J. C., Łyskowski, A., Kedracka-Krok, S., Pirog, A., and Goldman, A. (2012). The translocation domain in trimeric autotransporter adhesins is necessary and sufficient for trimerization and autotransportation. *J. Bacteriol.* 194, 827–838. doi: 10.1128/JB.05322-11

Miller, J. H. (1972). *Experiments in Bacterial Genetics*. Cold Spring Harbor, NY: Cold Spring Harbor Laboratory.

Monteiro, R., Ageorges, V., Rojas-Lopez, M., Schmidt, H., Weiss, A., Bertin, Y., et al. (2016). A secretome view of colonisation factors in Shiga toxin-encoding *Escherichia coli* (STEC): from enterohaemorrhagic *E. coli* (EHEC) to related enteropathotypes. *FEMS Microbiol. Lett.* 363:fnw179. doi: 10.1093/femsle/fnw179

Moon, C. P., Zaccai, N. R., Fleming, P. J., Gessmann, D., and Fleming, K. G. (2013). Membrane protein thermodynamic stability may serve as the energy sink for sorting in the periplasm. *Proc. Natl. Acad. Sci. U.S.A.* 110, 4285–4290. doi: 10.1073/pnas.1212527110

Mühlenkamp, M., Oberhettinger, P., Leo, J. C., and Linke, D. (2015). Yersinia adhesin A (YadA)-beauty & beast. *Int. J. Med. Microbiol.* 305, 252–258. doi: 10.1016/j.ijmm.2014.12.008

Nesterenko, M. V., Tilley, M., and Upton, S. J. (1994). A simple modification of Blum's silver stain method allows for 30 minute detection of proteins in polyacrylamide gels. *J. Biochem. Biophys. Methods* 28, 239–242. doi: 10.1016/0165-022X(94)90020-5

Oberhettinger, P., Schütz, M., Leo, J. C., Heinz, N., Berger, J., Autenrieth, I. B., et al. (2012). Intimin and invasin export their C-terminus to the bacterial cell surface using an inverse mechanism compared to classical autotransport. *PLoS ONE* 7:e47069. doi: 10.1371/annotation/cb7e47be-dd4b-46cd-b4e5-18b7077f64df

Prilipov, A., Phale, P. S., Koebnik, R., Widmer, C., and Rosenbusch, J. P. (1998a). Identification and characterization of two quiescent porin genes, *nmpC* and *ompN*, in *Escherichia coli* BE. *J Bacteriol* 180, 3388–3392.

Prilipov, A., Phale, P. S., Van Gelder, P., Rosenbusch, J. P., and Koebnik, R. (1998b). Coupling site-directed mutagenesis with high-level expression: large scale production of mutant porins from *E. coli*. *FEMS Microbiol. Lett.* 163, 65–72. doi: 10.1111/j.1574-6968.1998.tb13027.x

Pugsley, A. P., and Rosenbusch, J. P. (1983). OmpF porin synthesis in *Escherichia coli* strains B and K-12 carrying heterologous ompB and/or ompF loci. *FEMS Microbiol. Lett.* 16, 143–148. doi: 10.1111/j.1574-6968.1983.tb00275.x

Rassam, P., Copeland, N. A., Birkholz, O., Tóth, C., Chavent, M., Duncan, A. L., et al. (2015). Supramolecular assemblies underpin turnover of outer membrane proteins in bacteria. *Nature* 523, 333–336. doi: 10.1038/nature14461

Remmert, M., Biegert, A., Linke, D., Lupas, A. N., and Söding, J. (2010). Evolution of outer membrane β-barrels from an ancestral ββ hairpin. *Mol. Biol. Evol.* 27, 1348–1358. doi: 10.1093/molbev/msq017

Ronen, A., and Raanan-Ashkenazi, O. (1971). Temperature sensitivity of maltose utilization and lambda resistance in *Escherichia coli* B. *J. Bacteriol.* 106, 791–796.

Rosenbusch, J. P. (1974). Characterization of the major envelope protein from *Escherichia coli*. regular arrangement on the peptidoglycan and unusual dodecyl sulfate binding. *J. Biol. Chem.* 249, 8019–8029.

Schlegel, S., Rujas, E., Ytterberg, A. J., Zubarev, R. A., Luirink, J., and de Gier, J. W. (2013). Optimizing heterologous protein production in the periplasm of *E. coli* by regulating gene expression levels. *Microb. Cell Fact.* 12:24. doi: 10.1186/1475-2859-12-24

Schweizer, M., Hindennach, I., Garten, W., and Henning, U. (1978). Major proteins of the *Escherichia coli* outer cell envelope membrane. Interaction of protein ii with lipopolysaccharide. *Eur. J. Biochem.* 82, 211–217. doi: 10.1111/j.1432-1033.1978.tb12013.x

Shahid, S. A., Bardiaux, B., Franks, W. T., Krabben, L., Habeck, M., van Rossum, B.-J., et al. (2012). Membrane-protein structure determination by solid-state NMR spectroscopy of microcrystals. *Nat. Methods* 9, 1212–1217. doi: 10.1038/nmeth.2248

Shahid, S. A., Nagaraj, M., Chauhan, N., Franks, T. W., Bardiaux, B., Habeck, M., et al. (2015). Solid-state NMR study of the YadA membrane-anchor domain in the bacterial outer membrane. *Angew. Chem. Int. Ed. Engl.* 54, 12602–12606. doi: 10.1002/anie.201505506

Studier, F. W., and Moffatt, B. A. (1986). Use of bacteriophage T7 RNA polymerase to direct selective high-level expression of cloned genes. *J. Mol. Biol.* 189, 113–130. doi: 10.1016/0022-2836(86)90385-2

Studier, F. W., Daegelen, P., Lenski, R. E., Maslov, S., and Kim, J. F. (2009). Understanding the differences between genome sequences of *Escherichia coli* B strains REL606 and BL21(DE3) and comparison of the *E. coli* B and K-12 genomes. *J. Mol. Biol.* 394, 653–680. doi: 10.1016/j.jmb.2009.09.021

Thomason, L. C., Costantino, N., and Court, D. L. (2007). *E. coli* genome manipulation by P1 transduction. *Curr. Protoc. Mol. Biol.* 79, 1.17.1–1.17.8. doi: 10.1002/0471142727.mb0117s79

Wagner, S., Baars, L., Ytterberg, A. J., Klussmeier, A., Wagner, C. S., Nord, O., et al. (2007). Consequences of membrane protein overexpression in *Escherichia coli*. *Mol. Cell. Proteomics* 6, 1527–1550. doi: 10.1074/mcp.M600431-MCP200

Wagner, S., Bader, M. L., Drew, D., and de Gier, J. W. (2006). Rationalizing membrane protein overexpression. *Trends Biotechnol.* 24, 364–371. doi: 10.1016/j.tibtech.2006.06.008

Walther, D. M., Bos, M. P., Rapaport, D., and Tommassen, J. (2009a). The mitochondrial porin, VDAC, has retained the ability to be assembled in the bacterial outer membrane. *Mol. Biol. Evol.* 27, 887–895. doi: 10.1093/molbev/msp294

Walther, D. M., Rapaport, D., and Tommassen, J. (2009b). Biogenesis of β-barrel membrane proteins in bacteria and eukaryotes: evolutionary conservation and divergence. *Cell. Mol. Life Sci.* 66, 2789–2804. doi: 10.1007/s00018-009-0029-z

Wollmann, P., Zeth, K., Lupas, A. N., and Linke, D. (2006). Purification of the YadA membrane anchor for secondary structure analysis and crystallization. *Int. J. Biol. Macromol.* 39, 3–9. doi: 10.1016/j.ijbiomac.2005.11.009

11

Redundancy and Specificity of Type VI Secretion *vgrG* Loci in Antibacterial Activity of *Agrobacterium tumefaciens* 1D1609 Strain

Mary Nia M. Santos[1,2,3], *Shu-Ting Cho*[1], *Chih-Feng Wu*[1†], *Chun-Ju Chang*[1], *Chih-Horng Kuo*[1,2,4] *and Erh-Min Lai*[1,2,4*]

[1] *Institute of Plant and Microbial Biology, Academia Sinica, Taipei, Taiwan,* [2] *Molecular and Biological Agricultural Sciences Program, Taiwan International Graduate Program, National Chung Hsing University and Academia Sinica, Taipei, Taiwan,* [3] *Graduate Institute of Biotechnology, National Chung Hsing University, Taichung, Taiwan,* [4] *Biotechnology Center, National Chung Hsing University, Taichung, Taiwan*

Correspondence:
Erh-Min Lai
emlai@gate.sinica.edu.tw

Type VI secretion system (T6SS) is a contractile nanoweapon employed by many Proteobacteria to deliver effectors to kill or inhibit their competitors. One T6SS gene, *vgrG,* encodes a spike protein for effector translocation and is often present as multiple copies in bacterial genomes. Our phylogenomic analyses sampled 48 genomes across diverse Proteobacteria lineages and found ~70% of them encode multiple VgrGs, yet only four genomes have nearly identical paralogs. Among these four, *Agrobacterium tumefaciens* 1D1609 has the highest *vgrG* redundancy. Compared to *A. tumefaciens* model strain C58 which harbors two *vgrG* genes, 1D1609 encodes four *vgrG* genes (i.e., *vgrGa-d*) with each adjacent to different putative effector genes. Thus, 1D1609 was selected to investigate the functional redundancy and specificity of multiple *vgrG* genes and their associated effectors. Secretion assay of single and multiple *vgrG* deletion mutants demonstrated that these four *vgrG*s are functionally redundant in mediating T6SS secretion. By analyzing various *vgrG* mutants, we found that all except for the divergent *vgrGb* could contribute to 1D1609's antibacterial activity. Further characterizations of putative effector-immunity gene pairs revealed that *vgrGa*-associated gene 2 (*v2a*) encodes an AHH family nuclease and serves as the major antibacterial toxin. Interestingly, C58's VgrG2 shares 99% amino acid sequence identity with 1D1609's VgrGa, VgrGc and VgrGd. This high sequence similarity allows 1D1609 to use an exogenous VgrG delivered from C58 to kill another competing bacterium. Taken together, *Agrobacterium* can use highly similar VgrGs, either produced endogenously or injected from its close relatives, for T6SS-mediated interbacterial competition.

Keywords: type VI secretion system, VgrG, effector, antibacterial, functional redundancy, *Agrobacterium tumefaciens*

INTRODUCTION

Bacteria have evolved many survival strategies, including pathogenesis, competition, and cooperation, to thrive in diverse and changing environments. One of the weapons that they use is type VI secretion system (T6SS), a machinery that delivers effectors to both eukaryotic and prokaryotic target cells. Its coding genes are present in approximately 25% of the Gram-negative bacterial genomes sequenced (Bingle et al., 2008).

T6SS has an important role in interbacterial competition and provides T6SS-possessing bacteria with competitive advantage in microbial community. It can deliver a variety of effectors such as nuclease, amidase, phospholipase, peptidoglycan hydrolase, muramidase, glycosidase, NADase, and ADP-ribosyltransferase into the target bacterial cell by a contractile machinery (Russell et al., 2014; Tang et al., 2018; Ting et al., 2018). Contraction of the sheath-like structure drives the inner tube composed of Hcp tipped by VgrG-PAAR and the associated effectors across bacterial membranes to extracellular milieu or into the target cell. After firing, the structure is immediately disassembled into its individual components, which can be recycled to assemble new machinery for continuous firing (Zoued et al., 2014).

The spike component VgrG is homologous to the gp27/gp5 complex or the tail spike of bacteriophage T4 and assembles into a trimeric complex (Leiman et al., 2009). Current knowledge based on studies from several bacterial systems suggests that VgrG is specifically required for delivery of cognate effector(s) encoded in the same *vgrG* genetic module (Hachani et al., 2014; Whitney et al., 2014). Furthermore, the C-terminal variable region of VgrG is the molecular determinant conferring specificity of effector delivery by binding to its cognate effector directly or via adaptor/chaperone that interacts with a specific effector (Bondage et al., 2016; Flaugnatti et al., 2016). T6SS adaptors/chaperones including DUF4123-, DUF1795-, and DUF2169-containing proteins are required for loading a specific effector onto the cognate VgrG for delivery (Lien and Lai, 2017).

Agrobacterium tumefaciens is a soil Alphaproteobacterium that infects a broad range of dicotyledonous plants and transfers T-DNA, an oncogenic DNA fragment, to plant's nuclear chromosomes (Gelvin, 2000; Hwang et al., 2017). *A. tumefaciens* strain C58 encodes a single T6SS gene cluster and is equipped with three toxins namely type VI amidase effector (Tae), type VI DNase effector 1 and 2 (Tde1 and Tde2), in which its toxin activity can be neutralized by its cognate immunity. Tde is a major antibacterial weapon during *in planta* interbacterial competition and its associated VgrG is specifically required for Tde1/2-dependent bacterial killing (Ma et al., 2014; Bondage et al., 2016). A gene which encodes DUF2169 is always found between *vgrG2* and *tde2* orthologs across many Proteobacterial classes (Bondage et al., 2016). In *A. tumefaciens* strain C58, a DUF2169-containing protein encoded upstream of *tde2* is required to stabilize Tde2 and for Tde2-mediated antibacterial activity. For *vgrG1*-associated Tde1, Tap1 (encoded upstream of *tde1*) is the specific chaperone/adaptor interacting with Tde1 prior to loading to VgrG1 for formation of Tde1-Tap1-VgrG-PAAR secretion complex (Bondage et al., 2016).

Aside from the representative *A. tumefaciens* model strain C58, there is little knowledge of T6SS available for other *A. tumefaciens* strains. Our recent comparative analysis of T6SS gene clusters from 11 *A. tumefaciens* strains with complete genome sequences revealed that T6SS is present in all sequenced strains belonging to different genomospecies (Wu et al., 2019b). The *imp* operon (*impA-N*) encoding core structural or regulatory components and the first five genes (*clpV, tai, tae, hcp, vgrG*) encoded in the *hcp* operon are highly conserved but the *vgrG*-associated downstream genes are variable. While all strains only harbor one *vgrG* gene encoded in the main T6SS gene cluster, additional orphan *vgrG* genes not genetically linked to the main T6SS gene cluster were often identified in some strains.

A T6SS-harboring bacterium can encode one to multiple VgrG proteins, in which several of them were demonstrated to be specifically required for delivery of cognate effector(s) encoded in the same *vgrG* genetic module (Hachani et al., 2014; Whitney et al., 2014). However, the prevalence and biological significance of *vgrG* redundancy has not been tackled. In this study, *A. tumefaciens* 1D1609 which has the highest number of nearly identical *vgrG* genes among all sampled Proteobacteria lineages was chosen to address this question. We investigated the functional redundancy and specificity of multiple VgrG in the effector delivery strategies of T6SS in the context of interbacterial competition. We generated single to multiple in-frame deletion of *vgrG* mutants to characterize the role of paralogous VgrG proteins and its associated effectors in 1D1609. We found that the four *vgrGs* are functionally redundant in mediating Hcp secretion but also exert both redundancy and specificity in mediating effector delivery for interbacterial competition. We also demonstrated that 1D1609 employs a nuclease effector as the major antibacterial toxin. Importantly, we provided experimental evidence that *A. tumefaciens* can use T6SS in the context of interbacterial competition to exchange VgrG as an effector carrier between its close siblings.

RESULTS

Majority of T6SS-Possessing Proteobacterial Genomes Harbor Multiple *vgrG* Genes

To survey the number of *vgrG* genes in T6SS-encoding bacterial genomes, 48 representative Proteobacteria harboring T6SS gene cluster(s) were selected for phylogenetic analysis. The result revealed that 33 of these genomes (~70%) encode multiple *vgrG* genes. The *vgrG* copy numbers have no strong tie to the phylogenetic placement of individual genomes (**Figure 1**), suggesting that the copy number evolution is highly dynamic, even at the intra-genus level (e.g., *Agrobacterium* in Alphaproteobacteria or *Pseudomonas* in Gammaproteobacteria). The *vgrG* gene tree (**Supplementary Figure S1**) is not congruent with the species tree (**Figure 1**) and the patterns suggest that horizontal gene transfers across different classes are not rare events. Nonetheless, the species with multiple VgrG homologs mostly (~64%) form a monophyletic clade at family levels.

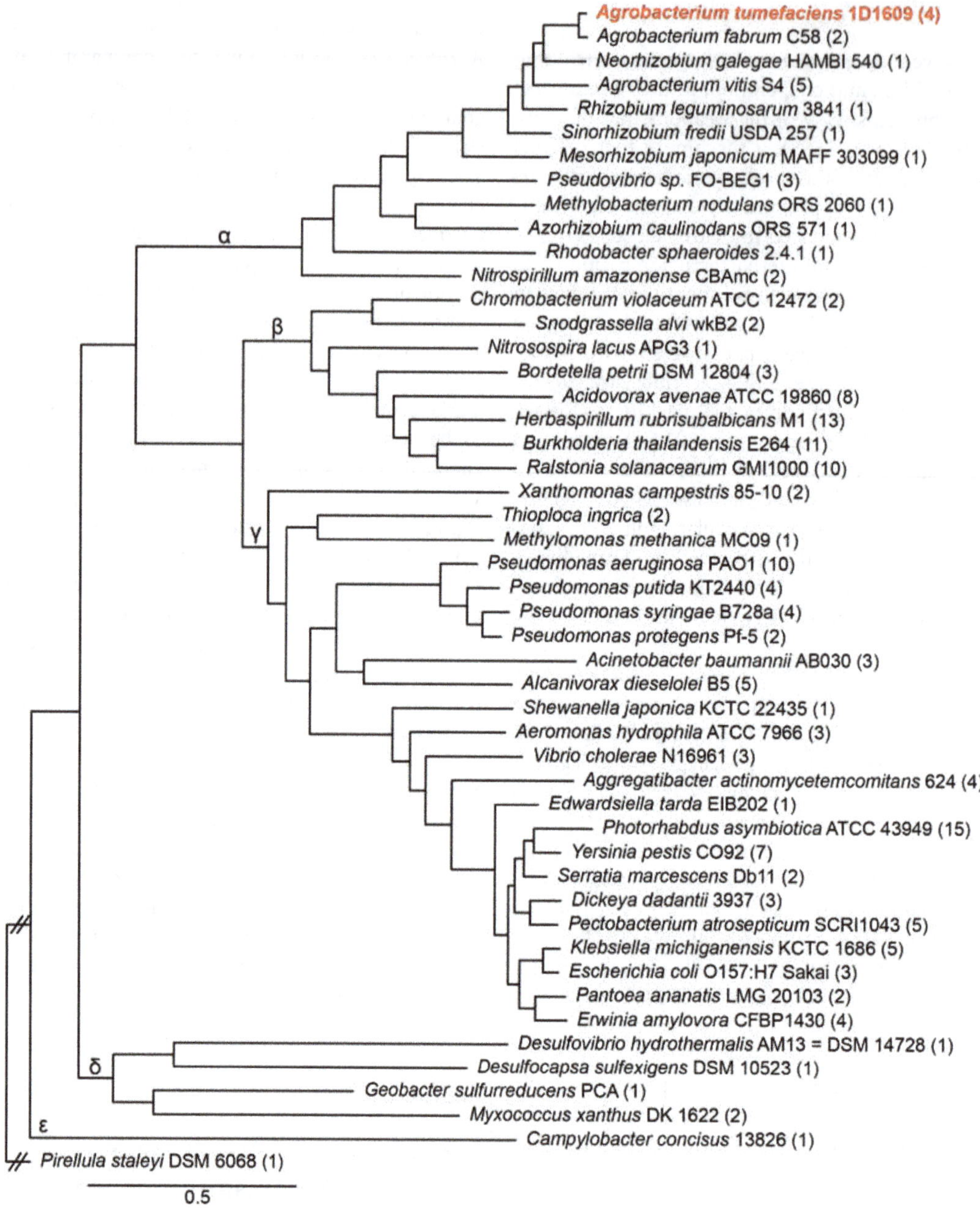

FIGURE 1 | Bayesian phylogeny of representative Proteobacteria based on 120 shared single-copy genes. The labels on the branches indicate the five classes within this phylum: Alphaproteobacteria (α), Betaproteobacteria (β), Deltaproteobacteria (δ), Epsilonproteobacteria (ε) and Gammaproteobacteria (γ). The numbers in parentheses after strain names indicate the *vgrG* copy numbers.

The genome of all the sampled Rhizobiaceae lineages harbors only one main T6SS gene cluster and forms a monophyletic clade except for *Sinorhizobium fredii* (**Supplementary Figure S1**) (Bladergroen et al., 2003; Wu et al., 2019b). This pattern suggests that gene duplication could be the major driving force for copy number increase within families.

We further asked, when there are multiple *vgrG* homologs in a genome, how often can we find highly similar genes that are likely to be functionally redundant. Using protein sequence identity ≥ 95% as the cut-off, only four genomes met the criteria (**Supplementary Table S1**). These include Alphaproteobacterium *A. tumefaciens* strain 1D1609 (three out of four with 99% identity, the remaining one is 93–94% identical), Betaproteobacterium *Acidovorax avenae subsp. avenae* ATCC 19860 (two out of eight with 99% identity), Gammaproteobacterium *Aggregatibacter actinomycetemcomitans* strain 624 (four copies belonging to two types: within-type = 99–100% identity, between-type = 90% identity), and Gammaproteobacterium *Dickeya dadantii* strain

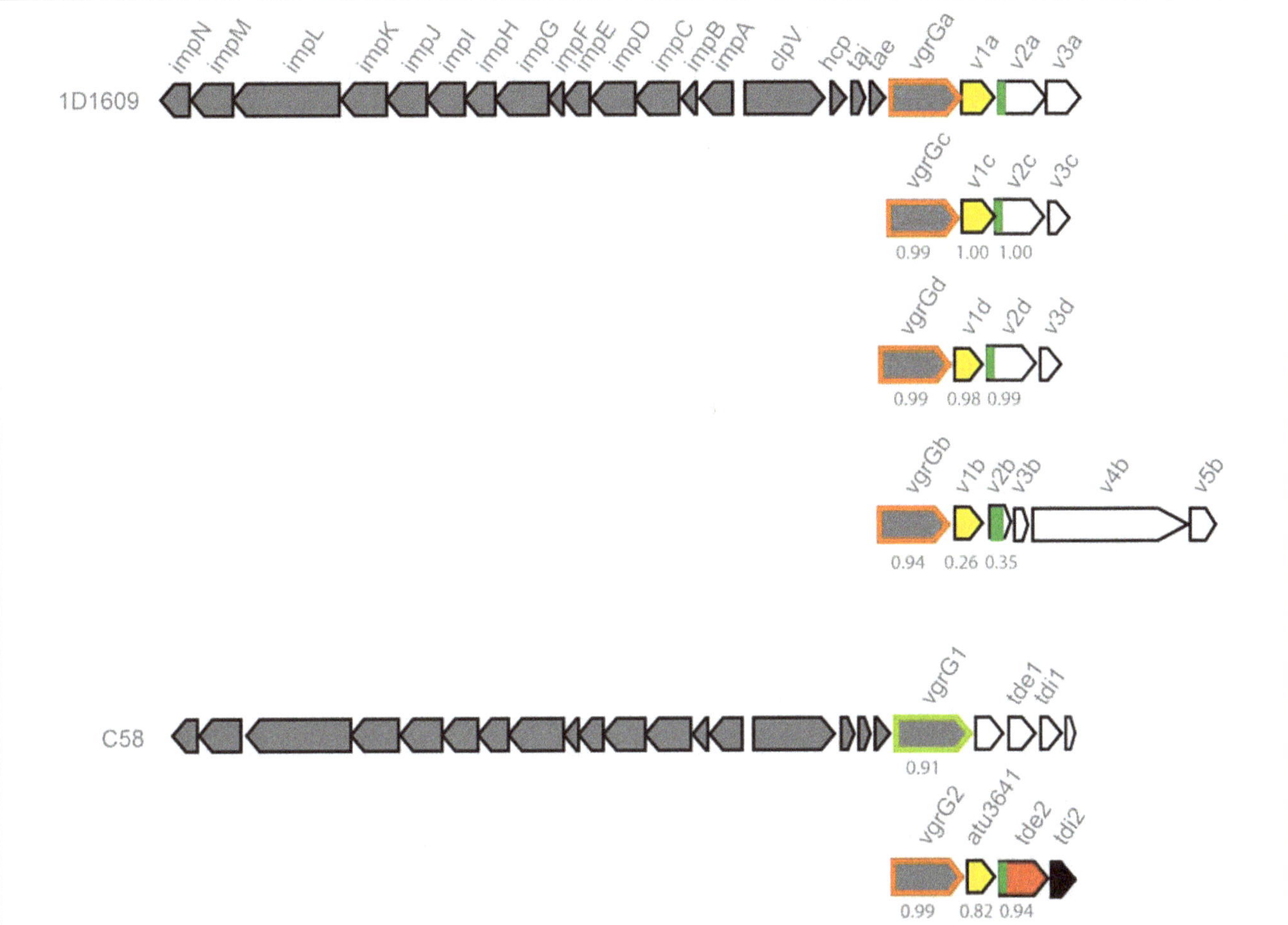

FIGURE 2 | 1D1609 encodes four *vgrG* genes, each is genetically linked with different potential effector gene(s). Genetic organization of *A. tumefaciens* 1D1609 and C58 T6SS gene cluster and *vgrG* genetic modules. C58 *vgrG1* is outlined with green and C58 *vgrG2* and 1D1609's four *vgrG* genes are outlined in orange. The gene encoding DUF2169 domain is highlighted in yellow and DUF4150 (PAAR-like) domain is shown in dark green. The *vgrG-associated genes* (*v*) are numbered according to their position from *vgrG*. The percentage identity, which corresponds to **Supplementary Table S3** is indicated below the gene cluster.

3937 (two out of three with 97% identity, the remaining one is 78% identical). Among them 1D1609 has the highest redundancy.

1D1609 Has Four *vgrG* Genes With Each Genetically Linked to Specific Putative Effector Gene(s)

1D1609 genome encodes one main T6SS gene cluster including *vgrGa* (At1D1609_RS23245) that is encoded in *hcp* operon within the T6SS main gene cluster. The other three *vgrGs* – *vgrGb* (At1D1609_RS26290), *vgrGc* (At1D1609_RS22460) and *vgrGd* (At1D1609_RS18895) are encoded in different loci elsewhere (**Figure 2**). All four *vgrG* genes are genetically linked with distinct potential effector gene(s) and associated genes predicted to function as adaptor/chaperone or immunity (Wu et al., 2019b). The four *vgrG* genetic modules consist of the first three genes with conserved domain and same gene order encoding VgrG-DUF2169-DUF4150. The *vgrGa-*, *vgrGc-*, and *vgrGd-*associated genes (*v2a, v2c, v2d*) encode N-terminal PAAR-like DUF4150 domain followed by C-terminal putative effector domain. The *vgrGb*-linked *v2b* does not encode obvious effector domain and instead followed by downstream genes encoding putative effector domain, as predicted by Phyre or NCBI CDD search and BLASTP (Boratyn et al., 2013; Kelley et al., 2015; Marchler-Bauer et al., 2017) (**Supplementary Table S2**). The *vgrGc*-associated putative effector gene *v2c* does not encode any conserved domain, while the one (*v2d)* associated with *vgrGd* encodes a putative GH25 muramidase domain. Genes encoding DUF2169 domain are commonly found downstream of *vgrG* and upstream of DUF4150-containing effector genes. This gene order in *vgrG* genetic module is highly conserved in the *vgrG2* locus of C58, in which DUF2169-containing protein (Atu3641) may function as adaptor/chaperone of Tde2 due to its requirement for Tde2 stability and Tde2-dependent bacterial killing (Bondage et al., 2016). Thus, DUF2169-containing V1 protein is likely to function as a chaperone/adaptor required for delivery of cognate effectors in conjunction with the associated VgrG.

Unlike VgrG1 and VgrG2 which share 92% identity and are highly divergent at their C-terminus (Bondage et al., 2016), we found that the three VgrG proteins - VgrGa, VgrGc and VgrGd in 1D1609 share 99% overall amino acid sequence identity (and 100% identity in the C-terminal region). These are also highly similar with VgrG2 of C58 (**Figure 2** and **Supplementary Table S3**). VgrGb shares 93–94% overall identity to the other three VgrGs and has a highly divergent C-terminal region (**Supplementary Figure S2** and **Supplementary Table S3**). Consistent with the VgrG comparisons, the DUF2169 and DUF4150 proteins with *vgrGa/c/d* also share 98–100% and 99–100% amino acid sequence identity, respectively (**Supplementary Table S3**). In contrast, VgrGb-associated DUF2169 and DUF4150 share only 26 and 35% sequence identities to those encoded in the other three *vgrG* loci respectively. The four predicted effector domains fused to DUF4150 or Rhs do not share high sequence similarity to each other or to known effectors, which could equip 1D1609 with diverse effector activities to fight with a wide range of competing bacteria. Homologs of *vgrGa-*, *vgrGb-*, *vgrGc-*, and *vgrGd*-associated effector genes are widely found in species belonging to Rhizobiales, suggesting that these are common effectors in this group.

Four VgrG Proteins Are Functionally Redundant in Mediating Hcp Secretion

In C58, VgrG1 and VgrG2 are functionally redundant in mediating Hcp secretion but specifically required for delivery of the cognate effectors Tde1 and Tde2, respectively (Lin et al., 2013; Bondage et al., 2016). Each of in-frame deletion mutants of *vgrGa*, *vgrGb*, *vgrGc* and *vgrGd* were generated to determine their functions in mediating Hcp secretion, a hallmark of a functional T6SS assembly. The Δ*tssL* mutant, with deletion of gene encoding the essential T6SS membrane component TssL, is used as a negative control. The secretion assay showed that all single *vgrG* deletion mutants remain active in Hcp secretion, suggesting that they are functionally redundant for assembly of a functional T6SS (**Figure 3A**). We are able to detect secretion of VgrG proteins from 1D1609 using polyclonal antibody against VgrG1 protein of C58, which can recognize all four VgrG proteins produced in 1D1609 and VgrG2 of C58. The Hcp and VgrG proteins are secreted in a T6SS-dependent manner because no Hcp and VgrG signals are detected in the secretion fraction of Δ*tssL* and RpoA (RNA polymerase α-subunit), a non-secreted protein, is not detectable in any secretion fraction. Hcp secretion remains active in double and triple *vgrG* deletion mutants but is only completely abolished when all four *vgrG* genes was deleted (**Figure 3B**). The overexpression of each of all four *vgrG* on a plasmid in the quadruple *vgrG* mutant restores Hcp secretion (**Figure 3C**). Furthermore, trans complementation of each 1D1609 *vgrG* constitutively expressed on a plasmid can also restore Hcp secretion in C58 double *vgrG* deletion mutant (Δ*vgrG*1,2) (**Figure 3D**). This is consistent with a previous study that either VgrG1 or VgrG2 is sufficient in mediating the secretion of Hcp in C58 (Lin et al., 2013). Indeed, all triple *vgrG* mutants wherein only one VgrG is present remains capable of mediating Hcp and VgrG secretion (**Figure 3E**). In Δ*vgrGabd* mutant, wherein only VgrGc is produced, Hcp secretion level is at lesser amount as compared to WT. The transcript expression level of *vgrGc* is also low compared to the other *vgrG*s (Haryono et al., 2019). Altogether, our comprehensive secretion assays demonstrated that the four VgrGs are functionally redundant in mediating Hcp secretion. Single *vgrG* is sufficient for assembly of a functional T6SS although the degree of assembly efficiency may not be the same due to expression level or sequence divergence.

T6SS-Dependent Antibacterial Activity Against *Escherichia coli* Is Mainly Contributed by *vgrGa* and *vgrGd*

We previously showed that all tested *A. tumefaciens* strains including 1D1609 exhibit T6SS-mediated antibacterial activity against T6SS-negative *E. coli* (Wu et al., 2019b). Here, we further investigated the role of the four *vgrG* genes in interbacterial competition against *E. coli*. As a positive control, ~10x reduction of surviving *E. coli* target cells was observed when co-cultured with 1D1609 WT as compared to that of Δ*tssL*. However, each of single *vgrG* deletion mutants remains to have similar antibacterial activity to WT (**Figure 4A**). Further antibacterial activity assay of double, triple and quadruple *vgrG* mutants showed that the antibacterial activity of 1D1609 is completely lost in Δ*Gacd*, Δ*Gabd*, or Δ*Gabcd*, while Δ*Gbcd* and Δ*Gabc* triple *vgrG* mutants remain similar antibacterial activity to that of WT 1D1609 (**Figures 4B,C**). These results suggest that *vgrGa* and *vgrGd* alone is sufficient to contribute to the antibacterial activity of 1D1609. In contrast, *vgrGb* or *vgrGc* alone cannot exert any detectable antibacterial activity even though either *vgrG* alone (Δ*Gacd*, Δ*Gabd*) is sufficient in mediating Hcp and VgrG secretion (**Figure 3E**). However, when each single *vgrG* is constitutively overexpressed on a plasmid in quadruple *vgrG* mutant, *vgrGa*, *vgrGc*, and *vgrGd* but not *vgrGb* is able to partially restore antibacterial activity (**Figure 4D**). These results strongly suggest that endogenous *vgrGa* and *vgrGd* indeed play important roles for antibacterial activity while *vgrGb* plays no role in antibacterial activity to *E. coli*. The data that endogenous *vgrGc* plays no role but can exert its function in antibacterial activity when overexpressed are consistent with its low endogenous expression and high amino acid sequence identity to VgrGa and VgrGd.

The *vgrGa-* and *vgrGd*-Associated EI Pairs Are Responsible for Antibacterial Activity of 1D1609 and V2a Is a Nuclease of HNH/ENDO VII Superfamily

We also generated deletion mutants of each putative effector-immunity (EI) gene pairs individually and mutants with deletions in multiple putative EI pairs. Due to failure in generating the *vgrGc*-associated *v2c-v3c* EI pair deletion mutant after several attempts, we instead generated the deletion of the whole *vgrGc* cluster to assay the antibacterial effect of *vgrGc*-associated effector. Deletion of *vgrGa-* and *vgrGd*-associated EI pair partially compromised antibacterial activity against *E. coli* while deletion of *vgrGb*-associated EI pair or *vgrGc* cluster/associated toxin has no effect in compromising 1D1609's killing activity to *E. coli*, as compared to WT (**Figure 5A**). Importantly, any mutant minimally deleting both *vgrGa-* and *vgrGd*-associated EI pairs (Δ*2EIad*, Δ*3EIabd*, or Δ*4EIabcd*) completely abolished the

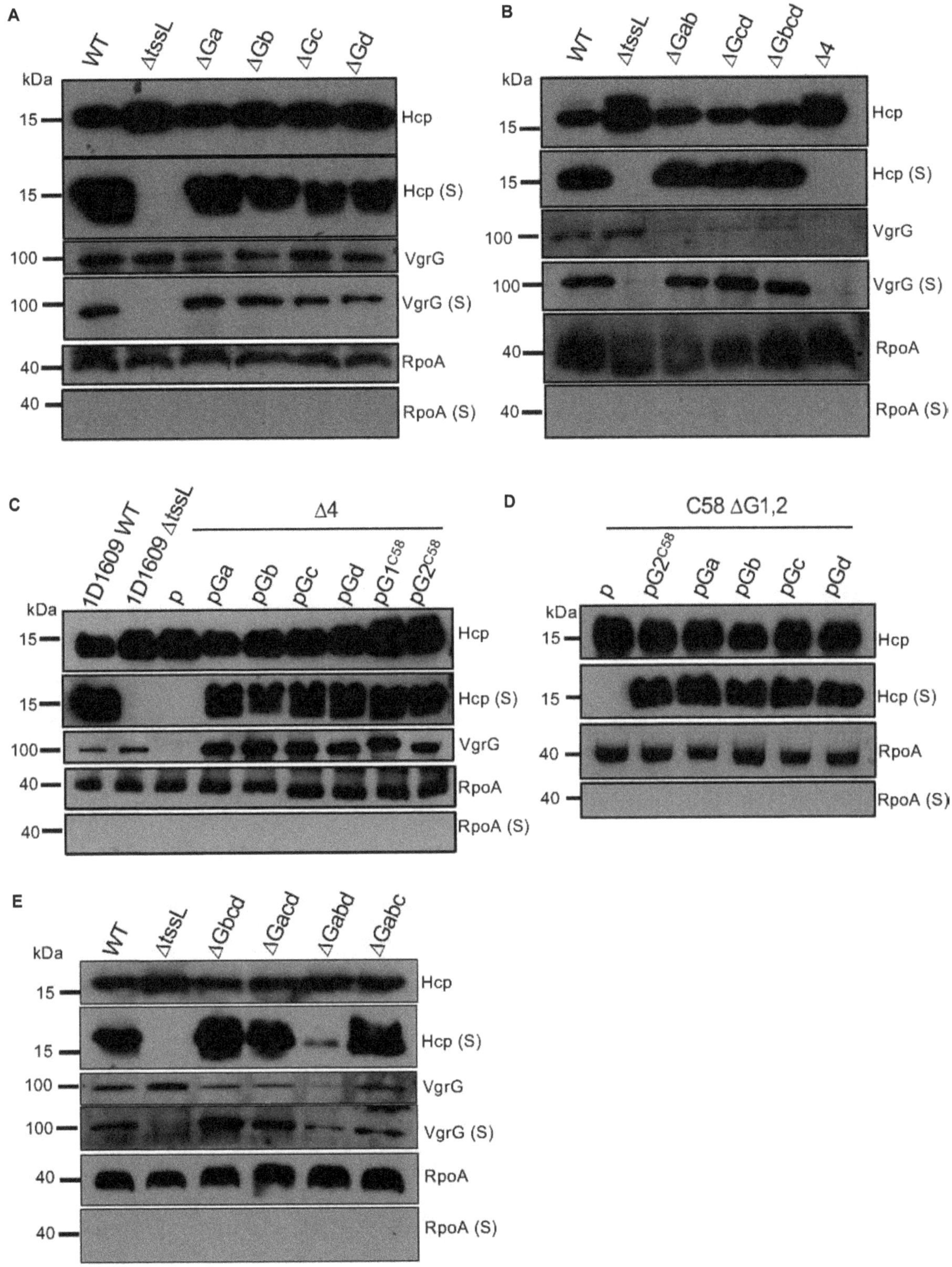

FIGURE 3 | The four VgrG proteins of 1D1609 are functionally redundant for Hcp secretion. Western blot analysis of cellular and secreted (S) proteins from single *vgrG* deletion mutants **(A)**, multiple *vgrG* deletion mutants **(B)**, overexpression of VgrG in 1D1609 quadruple *vgrG* mutant (Δ4) **(C),** and in C58 double *vgrG* deletion mutant (ΔG1,2) **(D),** and triple *vgrG* deletion mutants **(E)**. Various *A. tumefaciens* strains were cultured in LB **(A,B,E)** or AK **(C,E)** broth at 25°C and cellular and secreted (S) fractions were subjected to western blotting using anti-Hcp, anti-VgrG, and RpoA as indicated. The T6SS inactive mutant Δ*tssL* is a negative control and RpoA serves as a non-secreted protein control. Protein markers (in kDa) are indicated on the left. Similar results were obtained from 2–4 independent experiments.

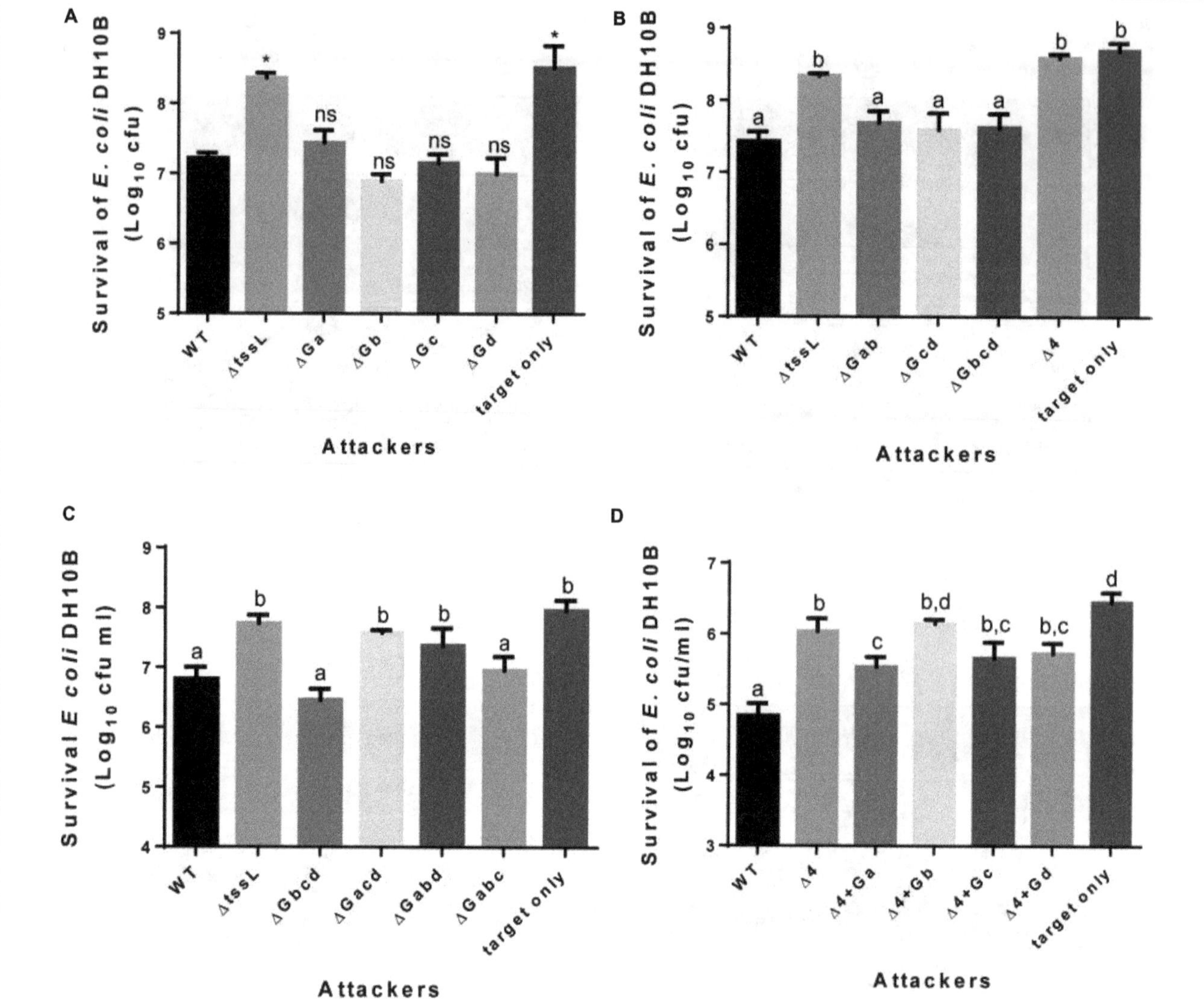

FIGURE 4 | *vgrGa* and *vgrGd* contributes to antibacterial activity of 1D1609. Each of various *A. tumefaciens* 1D1609 strains (indicated in the *x* axis) was mixed with *E. coli* DH10B cells expressing pRL662 to confer gentamicin resistance at 30:1 ratio in LB **(A,B)** or AK **(C,D)** media for 18 h. The survival of *E. coli* cells was quantified as cfu as shown on the *y* axis. **(A)** Antibacterial activity of single *vgrG* deletion mutants. Data are mean ± SEM of three biological replicates, similar results were obtained from three independent experiments. Two-tailed Student's *t*-test was used for statistical analyses. $^*p < 0.01$. **(B)** Antibacterial activity in multiple *vgrG* deletion mutants. **(C)** Antibacterial activity using triple *vgrG* mutants. **(D)** Single *vgrG* expressed *in trans* using pRLBla in quadruple *vgrG* mutant (Δ4). Data are mean ± SEM of three biological replicates **(B)** or four biological replicates from two independent experiments **(C,D)**. Different letters above the bar indicate statistically different groups of strains ($P < 0.05$) determined by Tukey's HSD test, based on cfu of surviving *E. coli* cells.

antibacterial activity against *E. coli* (**Figure 5B**). These results suggest that *vgrGa*- and *vgrGd*-associated EI pairs contribute to antibacterial activity to *E. coli*.

Since single deletion of *vgrGa*-associated EI pair (Δ*EIa*) or in combination with additional EI-pair/s showed reduced or abolished antibacterial activity (**Figures 5A,B**), we considered *vgrGa*-associated effector V2a as the primary toxin and characterized its function. The putative effector gene *v2a* was expressed by an arabinose inducible promoter on plasmid pJN105 and its putative cognate immunity gene *v3a* was expressed constitutively on plasmid pTrc200 in *E. coli*. The results showed that the bacterial growth is inhibited when *v2a* is induced as compared to the vector control whereas co-expression with *v3a* restores the growth (**Figure 5C**), indicating their toxin-immunity relationship.

V2a is 522-aa in length and contains a N-terminal PAAR-like DUF4150 domain and a C-terminal nuclease domain belonging to HNH/ENDOVII superfamily (pfam14412) of the treble cleft fold (Marchler-Bauer et al., 2017) (**Figure 5D**). This nuclease family has a conserved motif AHH, which is a predicted toxin module found in bacterial polymorphic toxin systems. In the AHH motif, the first His forms one of the catalytic metal-chelating ligands and the second His contributes to the active site that directs the water for phosphoester hydrolysis (Zhang et al., 2011). Partial sequence alignment of representative nuclease family of HNH/ENDO

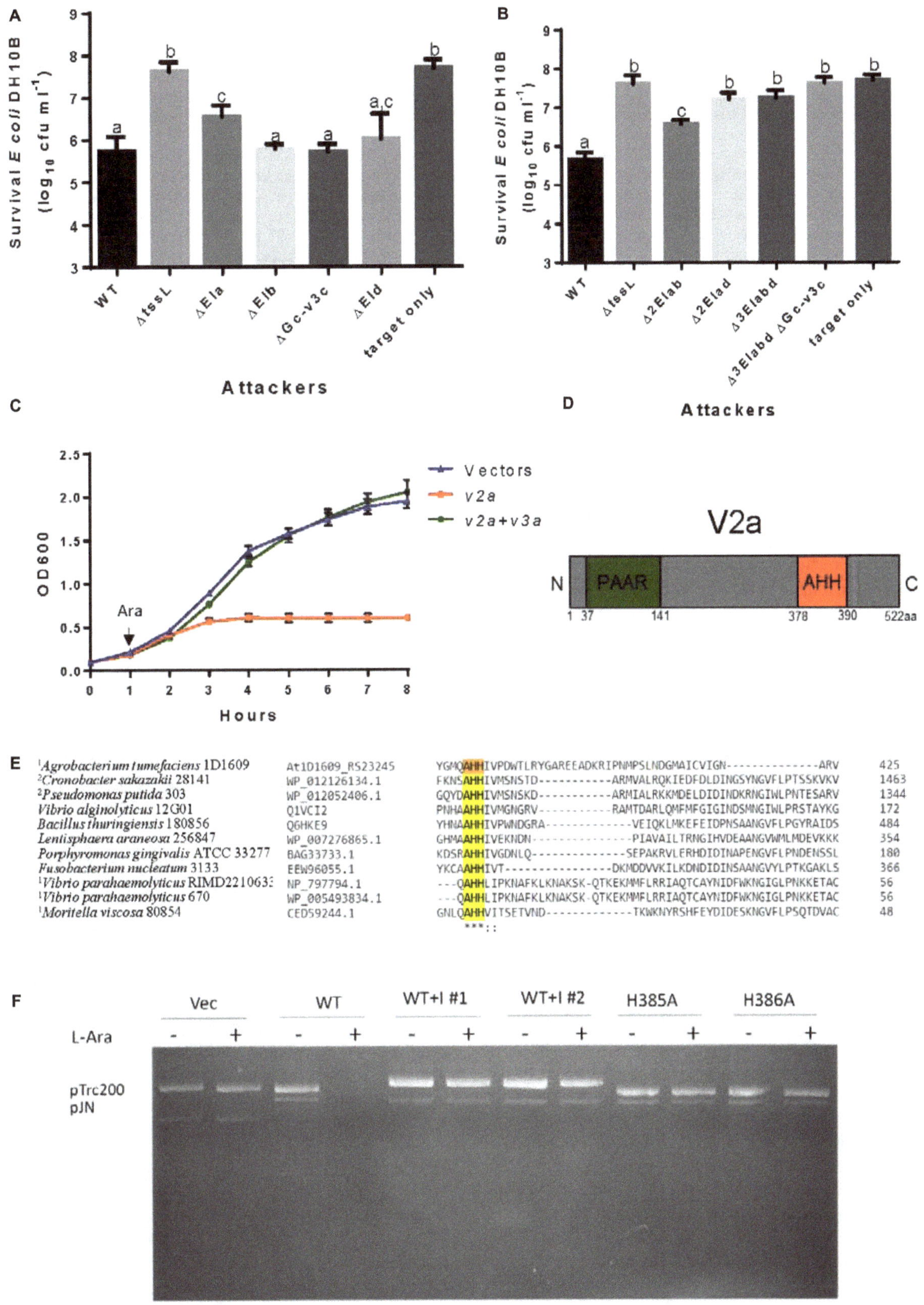

FIGURE 5 | Continued

FIGURE 5 | *vgrGa*- and *vgrGd*-associated EI pairs are responsible for antibacterial activity and V2a is a nuclease. *A. tumefaciens* 1D1609 strains (indicated in the *x* axis) was mixed with *E. coli* DH10B cells expressing pRL662 to confer Gentamicin resistance at 30:1 ratio in LB. The survival of *E. coli* cells was quantified as cfu as shown on the y axis when co-cultured with single **(A)** and multiple **(B)** EI pair deletion mutant. Data are mean ± SEM of four biological repeats from two independent experiments. Different letters above the bar indicate statistically different groups of strains ($P < 0.05$) determined by Tukey's HSD test, based on cfu of surviving *E. coli* cells. **(C)** *E. coli* growth inhibition analysis in *vgrGa*-associated EI pair. *E. coli* cultures were induced with 1 mM IPTG at 0 h for the expression of putative immunity protein expressed on pTrc200 plasmid followed by L-arabinose (Ara) induction at 1 hr to induce putative toxin gene from pJN105 plasmid. Cell growth was recorded every hour at OD_{600}. Empty vectors were used as controls. Data are mean ± SEM of three independent experiments. **(D)** Schematic diagram showing N-terminal PAAR region and C-terminal AHH nuclease domain of *vgrGa*-associated effector V2a. **(E)** Partial sequence alignment of representative nuclease family of HNH/ENDO VII superfamily with conserved AHH motif, modified from NCBI CDD sequence alignment of nuclease family of the HNH/ENDO VII superfamily with conserved AHH (pfam14412). The strain name and locus tag/accession number are on the left, and the conserved amino acid residues are indicated as * (identical) and: (similar) respectively. AHH motif is highlighted in yellow with the two His targeted for mutagenesis. AHH domain linked to DUF4150 domain[1] or Rhs[2] is indicted. **(F)** Nuclease activity assay. *E. coli* cells with pTrc200 and pJN105 plasmid (Vec) or derivatives expressing *v2a* (WT), WT with immunity protein (WT + I; #1 and #2 are two independent constructs) and catalytic site mutants (H385A, H386A) were induced with (+) or without (–) L-arabinose (L-Ara) for 2 h. Plasmid DNA was extracted and the degradation pattern was observed in agarose gel.

VII superfamily with conserved AHH motif is shown in **Figure 5E**.

To determine its nuclease activity, we examined the degradation of the plasmid DNA extracted from *E. coli* cells after *v2a* is induced by arabinose for 2 h. We showed that both pTrc200 and pJN-derived plasmids were not detectable from *v2a*-containing cells induced by arabinose, in contrast to the presence of both plasmids in vector control or *v2a*-containing cells not treated with arabinose (**Figure 5F**). The plasmid degradation is indeed caused by nuclease activity of V2a because the plasmid degradation is no longer detectable when the cells expressing the catalytic site (H385A and H386A) mutant or co-expression of *v3a* (**Figure 5F**). Taken together, we demonstrated that V2a is a T6SS effector that requires its AHH motif for nuclease activity. Moreover, this toxicity can be specifically neutralized by its cognate immunity protein. While this study was under way, a type VI nuclease effector Tse7 with GHH catalytic site (Tox-GHH2, pfam14412) from the same HNH/ENDO VII superfamily was reported in *P. aeruginosa* (Pissaridou et al., 2018). In conclusion, HNH nuclease superfamily appeared to be a widespread T6SS nuclease toxin family for antibacterial activity. These results strongly suggested the *v2a-v3a* toxin-immunity relationship, which supported their contribution to 1D1609's antibacterial activity to *E. coli.*

VgrG Can Be Exchanged Between C58 and 1D1609

Considering that VgrGa, VgrGc and VgrGd of 1D1609 and VgrG2 of C58 are highly similar with identical C-terminal region and their DUF2169 and DUF4150 share high sequence similarity (**Supplementary Table S3**), it is plausible that these VgrG proteins can substitute each other's role in effector delivery. Previous work showed that Hcp and VgrG can be exchanged between *Vibrio cholerae* cells in a T6SS-dependent manner and can be reused to assemble a new T6SS (Vettiger and Basler, 2016). Thus, we hypothesized that *Agrobacterium* may take advantage of having multiple, highly similar VgrG to receive or donate this effector carrier from/to its siblings and the donated VgrG can be used by the recipient cell to kill another competing bacterial cell. To test this hypothesis, we designed a tripartite interbacterial transfer system that will allow us to see the killing of the target *E. coli* cell only when there is a functionally exchangeable VgrG protein translocated from C58 to 1D1609. The nearly identical VgrGs ($G2^{C58}$ and Ga^{1D1609}) expressed on a non-transferable pRL662 plasmid in C58 $\Delta tdei1\Delta G1\Delta G2op$, a mutant deleting *vgrG1, tde1-tdi1, vgrG2* operon, serves as a donor cell. 1D1609 $\Delta 4$ with deletion of all four *vgrG* genes but is still armed with effectors is designated as a recipient cell as well as an attacker to kill *E. coli* (**Figure 6A**). Since no antibacterial activity can be detected in C58 $\Delta tdei1\Delta G1\Delta G2op$ (Ma et al., 2014) and 1D1609 $\Delta 4$ (**Figure 4B**), 1D1609 $\Delta 4$ can only exhibit antibacterial activity by obtaining VgrG proteins from C58 donor and using it for effector delivery to kill *E. coli.*

During this course of study, our group also discovered that Tde effector loading onto VgrG is critical for T6SS assembly and Hcp secretion (Wu et al., 2019a). Thus, aside from expressing $G2^{C58}$ or Ga^{1D1609} in C58 $\Delta tdei\Delta G1\Delta G2op$ donor strain, a plasmid expressing Tde2 with catalytic site mutation and its cognate DUF2169 chaperone/adaptor ($pTde2^M$) was also included to ensure effective T6SS assembly and firing. Hcp secretion and antibacterial activity assays confirmed that the $G2^{C58}$ or Ga^{1D1609} in C58 $\Delta tdei\Delta G1\Delta G2op$ donor strain remained active in Hcp secretion as WT level but completely lost the antibacterial activity against *E. coli* (**Figures 6B,C**). However, the donor-recipient-prey tripartite co-incubation showed that only the experimental set with C58 $\Delta tdei\Delta G1\Delta G2op$ donor strain harboring $G2^{C58}$ or Ga^{1D1609} in the presence of $pTde2^M$ can allow 1D1609 $\Delta 4$ to exhibit antibacterial activity to *E. coli* (**Figure 6D**). 1D1609 $\Delta 4$ co-cultured with donor strains C58 $\Delta tssL$, $\Delta tdei\Delta G1\Delta G2op$ harboring vector only, $G2^{C58}$ or Ga^{1D1609} alone do not exhibit detectable killing activity to *E. coli*. These results suggest that 1D1609 can use the $VgrG2^{C58}$ and $VgrGa^{1D1609}$ delivered from C58 to kill *E. coli* and $VgrG2^{C58}$ can function as an effector carrier in 1D1609.

DISCUSSION

Functional redundancy is a useful strategy for the pathogen to build a robust system (Galán, 2009). In this study, our phylogenomic analyses revealed that the majority of T6SS-harboring Proteobacteria encode multiple *vgrG* genes. Among them, *A. tumefaciens* strain 1D1609 is unique for having multiple VgrG paralogs (VgrGa, VgrGc, and VgrGd) with high sequence identity (99%). The three *vgrG* genetic modules have the

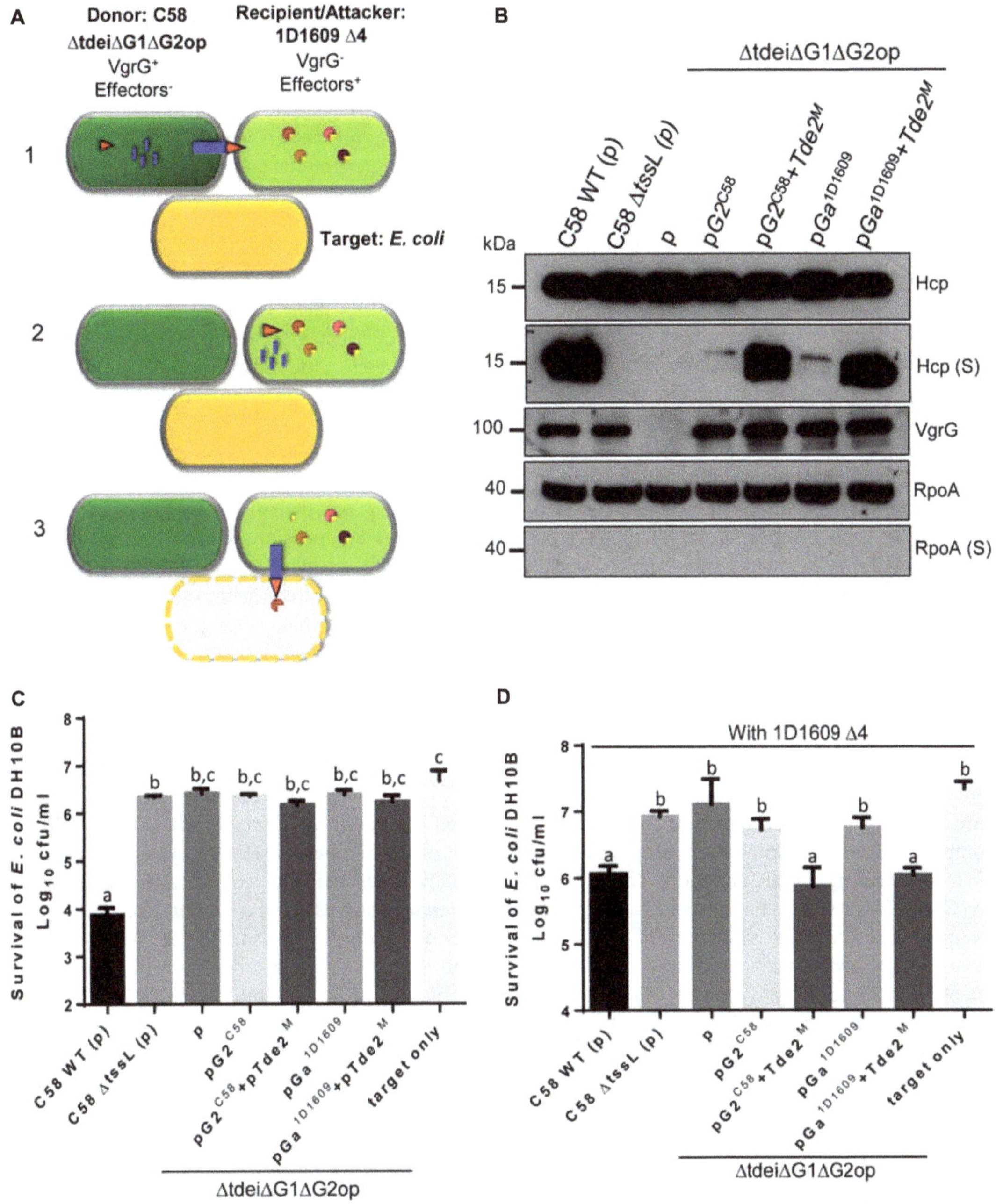

FIGURE 6 | VgrG can be exchanged between C58 and 1D1609 for executing antibacterial activity. **(A)** Schematic diagram for tripartite interaction assay to determine the VgrG exchange/killing of *E. coli* by the recipient *Agrobacterium*. The donor C58 *ΔtdeiΔG1ΔG2op* was co-cultured with recipient 1D1609 Δ4 and *E. coli* target. The "exchangeable" VgrGs ($G2^{C58}$ or Ga^{1D1609}) was expressed alone or co-expressed with Atu3641 and Tde2 with catalytic site mutation (named as $Tde2^{M}$) in donor C58 cells. The exchange/killing is divided in three steps: (1) Donor C58 expresses T6SS components without active toxin effectors and recipient 1D1609 expresses effectors complexed with cognate immunity proteins (EI pairs shown in circle with triangle) without T6SS assembly. T6SS is assembled in donor C58 for injecting Hcp (blue blocks) and VgrG (red triangle) into recipient 1D1609. (2) Recipient 1D1609 uses the translocated VgrG to assemble a new T6SS machine carrying 1D1609 effector. (3) Recipient 1D1609 injects the toxin effector and kills the target *E. coli.* **(B)** Hcp secretion in the donor C58. *A. tumefaciens* strain C58 or derivatives containing the plasmid only (p) or expressing the indicated genes were cultured in ABMES (pH 5.5) broth at 25°C and cellular and secreted (S) fractions were subjected to immunoblotting using anti-Hcp, anti-VgrG, and RpoA. The T6SS inactive mutant *ΔtssL* is a negative control and RpoA serves as a non-secreted protein control. **(C,D)** *A. tumefaciens* 1D1609 strains (indicated in the *x* axis) was mixed with *E. coli* DH10B cells expressing pRLBla to confer ampicillin resistance at 30:1 ratio in AK medium. The survival of *E. coli* cells was quantified as cfu as shown on the y axis when co-cultured with donor cells only **(C)** or with donor and recipient 1D1609 cells, at 1:10 ratio **(D)**. Data are mean ± SEM of four biological repeats from three independent experiments. Different letters above the bar indicate statistically different groups of strains ($P < 0.05$) determined by Tukey's HSD test, based on cfu of surviving *E. coli* cells.

same gene orders encoding highly conserved VgrG-DUF2169-DUF4150. However the DUF4150-linked effectors do not share significant sequence similarities suggesting that these effectors may have distinct functions. This study provided genetic evidence that these nearly identical VgrG paralogs can carry not only their genetically linked cognate effector but also non-genetically linked effectors sharing the highly similar DUF4150. The functional replacement or exchange can occur for these proteins produced in the same bacterial cells or those taking from its isogenic sibling or close relatives during T6SS attacks. Thus, such functional redundancy may be a beneficial strategy for agrobacteria to compete in their ecological niche.

While several studies clearly demonstrated that VgrG is specifically required for delivery of cognate effector(s) encoded in the same *vgrG* genetic module (Hachani et al., 2014; Whitney et al., 2014) and C-terminal variable region of VgrG is the molecular determinant (Bondage et al., 2016; Flaugnatti et al., 2016), only few studies reveal the roles of highly homologous VgrG proteins in effector delivery. *D. dadantii* 3937 also encodes two highly similar VgrG homologs ($VgrG_A$ and $VgrG_B$, **Supplementary Table S1**) which are both genetically linked to genes encoding homologous DUF1795-containing EagR chaperone and Rhs-linked effectors RhsA and RhsB (Koskiniemi et al., 2013). The homologous DUF1795 shares 97% amino acid sequence identity and RhsA and RhsB share 86% amino acid sequence identity with conserved N-terminal PAAR domain (99% identity). By sharing the highly similar chaperone and PAAR-Rhs regions, RhsA and RhsB effectors each harboring distinct C-terminal nuclease toxin domains could be delivered by not only its cognate but also non-cognate VgrG. Indeed, the competition assay revealed that either $vgrG_A$ or $vgrG_B$ is required for RhsB-mediated inhibition. The inhibitor cells without $vgrG_B$ in $\Delta rhsA/rhsB^+$ background can still have competitive advantage. The advantage is lost when both *vgrG*s are deleted and restored when $vgrG_B$ was expressed in double *vgrG* deletion mutant. Sharing the same VgrG carrier was also found in *Serratia marcescens* Db10, in which two different PAAR-domain containing Rhs effectors (RhS1 and RhS2) can functionally pair with the same VgrG protein (VgrG2) for delivery to target cells (Cianfanelli et al., 2016). The *rhs2* effector gene is not genetically linked to *vgrG2*, but both Rhs1 and Rhs2 have the same DUF1795 (EagR)-PAAR-Rhs gene organization. The EagR1 shares only 26% amino acid sequence identity with EagR2 and each specifically interacts with its cognate Rhs and is required for delivery (Alcoforado Diniz and Coulthurst, 2015; Cianfanelli et al., 2016). VgrG2 can form VgrG2-Rhs1-EagR1 or VgrG2-Rhs2-EagR2 complexes even though the N-terminal PAAR and full-length amino acid sequence of Rhs1 and Rhs2 share only 34 and 30% identity, respectively. In this case, high amino acid sequence identity in chaperone and PAAR is not required for functional exchange. However, they may share structural similarity that is sufficient for interacting with the same VgrG.

A recent study demonstrated that T6SS components, Hcp and VgrG, can be transferred and reused by *V. cholera* cells (Vettiger and Basler, 2016). An isogenic $LacZ^+$ reporter strain was used to measure the level of LacZ released for detection of cell lysis when the isogenic donor cells translocate Hcp and VgrG2 to isogenic recipient cells for T6SS assembly and firing. In our system, a tripartite interbacterial exchange/competition assay was designed to show evidence that highly similar VgrG proteins can be exchanged between two different *A. tumefaciens* genomospecies to kill the co-existing *E. coli*. Different *A. tumefaciens* genomospecies are known to co-exist in the same geographic area (Vogel et al., 2003). Several studies revealed that more than two genomospecies of *A. tumefaciens* can be found in the same crown gall or soil samples (Costechareyre et al., 2010; Bouri et al., 2016). Using tomato and maize seedlings, Gharsa et al. (2018) evaluated the competition of different *A. tumefaciens* genomospecies in soil and rhizosphere and concluded that related ecotypes can coexist. The initial competition alters the relative abundance, but does not eliminate the weaker strain. VgrG exchange may bring the advantages of sympatry and possessing different sets of T6SS gene clusters can maintain balance in sympatry. In *V. cholerae*, the bacterial strains that are incompatible (i.e., with different effector module sets), actively use their T6SS to kill susceptible strain during intra-species competition (Unterweger et al., 2014). However, in *A. tumefaciens* species, compatibility of T6SS EI pairs is not always predictive of competition outcomes (Wu et al., 2019b). C58 and 1D1609, which belongs to different genomospecies, can exhibit antibacterial activity against each other when the attacker is initiated with a higher relative abundance during an *in planta* interbacterial competition assay. However, C58 and 1D1609 can coexist with similar competitiveness when co-cultured at equal ratio despite their distinct EI pairs (**Supplementary Figure S4**). No significant difference of competitiveness (competitive index ~1) could be observed when C58 WT is co-inoculated with equal number of 1D1609 WT or $\Delta tssL$, or vice versa. This indicates that the two strains are proliferating equally *in planta* regardless of the presence or absence of a functional T6SS of *Agrobacterium* in different host plants. Interestingly, highly similar VgrGs are common in different *A. tumefaciens* genomospecies. In genomospecies 1 (G1), all (except 1D1108) share 100% identity while G8 (represented by C58 VgrG1 and two VgrGs in 1D132) share 95.7–99.8%. G7 (three VgrGs in 1D1609) and G8 (C58 VgrG2, 1D132 VgrG and three VgrGs in 1D1609) share 96.9–99.9% identity (**Supplementary Figure S3**). Thus, VgrG exchange might be common between different genomospecies, which may allow them to coexist and could in turn benefit *A. tumefaciens* sympatry in its ecological niche.

While not always evident by statistical analysis, deletion of single *vgrGa* ($\Delta vgrGa$) or its associated effector-immunity (ΔEIa), but not other single *vgrG* or *EI* pair mutants, showed reduction of antibacterial activity (**Figures 4A, 5A,B**). The data suggest that *vgrGa* genetic module play the primary role in antibacterial activity of 1D1609. The *vgrGa*-associated effector V2a belongs to different type of nuclease toxin distinct from the Tde1 and Tde2 nuclease toxins (toxin_43 domain with HxxD catalytic motif) identified in C58 (Ma et al., 2014). The use of enzymatic toxins such as nuclease is the most prominent theme in bacterial warfare (Galán, 2009). Using bioinformatics analysis, Ma et al. (2017) found that among more than 2,500 T6SS-dependent Rhs-CTs with N-terminal PAAR in 143 bacterial species, nuclease represents the major group. Among these, the Rhs-AHH is the most dominant nuclease found in 66 bacterial species. Effectors with predicted AHH nuclease has been reported with antibacterial activity in *V. parahaemolyticus* VP1415 (Salomon et al., 2014) and *Pectobacterium carotovorum subsp. brasiliense* strain PBR 1692 (Bellieny-Rabelo et al., 2019) but no nuclease activity has been tested. In *Acinetobacter baylyi*, it was shown that the genomic DNA was completely degraded when Rhs2 with C-terminal AHH motif is expressed in *E. coli* (Fitzsimons et al., 2018). In this study, we characterize further to show that the AHH motif is indeed responsible for the DNase activity (**Figure 5**). The other conserved motif of HNH/ENDO VII superfamily nuclease has been reported in *P. putida* KT2440 Tke2 (Rhs-Tox-HNH) and Tke4 (Rhs-Tox-SHH) (Bernal et al., 2017) and functional characterization was done only in Tox-GHH2 in Tse7 in *P. aeruginosa* (Pissaridou et al., 2018). Among the 100 Soft-rot Enterobacteriaceae (SRE) genomes surveyed by Bellieny-Rabelo et al. (2019), about a quarter encodes AHH, suggesting that this nuclease is a common weapon deployed by both plant and animal pathogenic bacteria in interbacterial competition.

Among the four *vgrG* clusters encoded in 1D1609, *vgrGb* is distinct from the other three. Our data suggest that *vgrGb* and *v4b* encoding a putative toxin does not seem to play a role in antibacterial activity (**Figures 4, 5A,B**). This may be due to low expression level of this gene. Alternatively, V4b may target eukaryotic cells because it contains a nuclear localization signal and has an extensive structural similarity to the insecticidal TcdB2-TccC3 toxin of *Photorhabdus luminescens* and YenC2 toxin of *Yersinia entomophaga* (**Supplementary Table S2**). The activity of the remaining effectors remains unknown and is currently under investigation.

In conclusion, *Agrobacterium* has developed a flexible mode of T6SS effector delivery, by using highly similar VgrGs, either produced endogenously or injected from its close relatives, for T6SS assembly and firing. VgrG and PAAR are among the least abundant T6SS components (Lin et al., 2019) and limiting VgrG can result in reduced number of T6SS assemblies (Vettiger and Basler, 2016). Therefore, it is plausible that having multiple highly similar VgrGs may enhance robustness and abundance of T6SS assemblies. This flexibility could allow them to be an ally to its sister cells and an effective weapon against distantly related bacterial competitors. The knowledge gained in this study can help advance the understanding of mechanisms and physiological roles of multiple VgrG proteins and associated effectors and may provide new insights for sympatric speciation.

MATERIALS AND METHODS

Bacterial Strains, Plasmids, and Growth Conditions

The bacterial strains, plasmids and primers used in this study are listed in **Supplementary Tables S4, S5**. *A. tumefaciens* strains were grown in 523 medium at 25°C while *E. coli* strains were grown in LB medium at 37°C. In-frame deletion mutants in *Agrobacterium* were generated using a suicide plasmid via double crossing over by electroporation or by conjugation (Ma et al., 2009). The mutants were confirmed by colony PCR and/or Southern blot analysis (**Supplementary Figure S5**). Site directed mutagenesis was done using overlapping PCR (Ho et al., 1989).

Phylogenetic and Sequence Analysis

All bioinformatics tools were used with the default parameters unless stated otherwise. The function of putative effectors were inferred from NCBI's Conserved Domain Database (CDD) based on BLASTP searches (Boratyn et al., 2013; Marchler-Bauer et al., 2017) and Protein Homology/analogy Recognition Engine (Phyre2) (Kelley et al., 2015). SignalP was used to predict signal peptides (Petersen et al., 2011). PSORTb version 3.0.2 was used to predict sub-cellular localization of proteins (Yu et al., 2010).

For the phylogenomic analysis to investigate the VgrG diversity among Proteobacteria, the VgrG homologs from five representatives (i.e., *A. tumefaciens* 1D1609, *Burkholderia thailandensis* E264, *Geobacter sulfurreducens* PCA, *Helicobacter cinaedi* CCUG 18818, and *P. aeruginosa* PAO1) were used as queries to run BLASTP searches against the NCBI non-redundant protein database (*e*-value cutoff = 1e-15, max target sequences = 100,000). Spurious hits, defined as hits with the high scoring pairs (HSP) accounting for <74% of the query sequence or sequence similarity <48% within the HSP, were removed. The resulting lists from different query species were combined to remove redundant hits. The combined list was further manually curated to keep only the targets with complete genome sequences available in GenBank. Based on the taxonomy information of the targets, the list was iteratively trimmed to achieve a balance taxon sampling with ~50 genomes to represent all major lineages within Proteobacteria. One Planctomycetes, *Pirellula staleyi* DSM 6068, was included as the outgroup to root the species phylogeny (**Figure 1**). In addition to the aforementioned data set for phylum-level (i.e., Proteobacteria) diversity, a second data set containing 11 *Agrobacterium* genomes (Wu et al., 2019b) was compiled to examine the genus-level VgrG diversity; *Neorhizobium galegae* HAMBI 540 was included as the outgroup for this second data set (**Supplementary Figure S3**).

After genome selection, the procedures for homologous gene identification and molecular phylogenetic analysis were based on those described in our previous studies (Lo et al., 2013; Lo and Kuo, 2017). Briefly, the homologous genes among all genomes were identified by using OrthoMCL (Li et al., 2003). The single-copy genes shared by all genomes were used for inferring the species phylogeny. Additionally, all *vgrG* homologs in these genomes, defined as the genes containing at least 80% of the VgrG domain (TIGR03361), were extracted for inferring the gene tree. The protein sequences were aligned using MUSCLE (Edgar, 2004) and the molecular phylogenies were inferred using MrBayes (Ronquist and Huelsenbeck, 2003). The amino acid substitution model was set to mix with gamma-distributed rate variation across sites and a proportion of invariable sites. The number of rate categories for the gamma distribution was set to four. The Markov chain Monte Carlo analysis was set to run for 1,000,000 generations and sampled every 100 generations. The first 25% of the samples were discarded as the burn-in. Furthermore, the protein sequence identity among all VgrG homologs were calculated using PROTDIST (Felsenstein, 1989). The amino acid sequence identity and similarity percentage of VgrG and VgrG-associated proteins were determined using Vector NTI Advance 11.5.4.

Secretion Assay

Secretion assay from liquid culture of *A. tumefaciens* grown in either LB rich medium or AB-MES minimal medium was done as previously described (Ma et al., 2009). Proteins from cellular and secreted fractions were resolved by SDS-PAGE and transferred onto a PVDF membrane by using a transfer apparatus (Bio-Rad). The membrane was probed with primary antibody against C58 VgrG1 (1:1,000), which recognizes the C58 VgrG2 and all four VgrGs of 1D1609, Hcp (1:2,500), and RpoA (1:7,500) (Lin et al., 2013), followed by incubation with horseradish peroxidase-conjugated anti-rabbit secondary antibody (1:30,000) and visualized with the ECL system (PerkinElmer).

Interbacterial Competition Assay

Escherichia coli killing assay was performed as described previously (Bondage et al., 2016). In brief, overnight culture of *A. tumefaciens* and *E. coli* strain were adjusted to OD_{600} 0.1 and incubated at 25°C for 4 h. *A. tumefaciens* and *E. coli* cells were mixed at a 30:1 ratio (OD 0.3:0.01) and spotted on LB agar (1.5%) plates. After 18 hr incubation at 25°C, the co-cultured cells were collected, serially diluted and plated on LB agar containing appropriate antibiotics to quantify surviving *E. coli* by counting colony forming unit (cfu). When enhanced killing activity is desired, an optimized growth medium, named as *Agrobacterium* Kill-triggering, AK medium (3 g K_2HPO_4, 1 g NaH_2PO_4, 1 g NH_4Cl, 0.15 g KCl, 9.76 g MES in 900 mL ddH20, pH5.5) modified from AB-MES medium and solidified by 2% (w/v) agar, was used instead. Data are expressed as mean ± SEM (standard error of the mean) from three independent experiments. Statistics was done using one-way ANOVA and Tukey's honestly significance difference (HSD) test[1].

In planta bacterial competition assay was performed as described previously (Ma et al., 2014). *A. tumefaciens* strain C58 transformed with gentamicin resistance-conferring pRL662 plasmid and strain 1D1609 conferring spectinomycin resistance were mixed at 1:1 (OD 1) ratio and infiltrated into 6- to 7-week-old *Nicotiana benthamiana* and *Medicago truncatula* leaves. The competition outcome was quantified at 0 h and 24 h by counting cfu on LB plates with appropriate antibiotics. 1D1609/C58 ratio at t = 24 h was divided by 1D1609/C58 ratio at t = 0h to calculate the competitive index.

Growth Inhibition Assay

Growth inhibition assay was performed as described previously (Ma et al., 2014). In brief, overnight cultures of *E. coli* DH10B strain with vectors or their derivatives were adjusted to OD_{600} 0.1. The expression of the tested immunity protein was induced by 1 mM IPTG for 1 h before L-arabinose (0.2% final concentration) was added to induce expression of the toxin.

Plasmid DNA Degradation Analysis in *E. coli* Cells

In vivo plasmid DNA degradation analysis was performed as described previously (Ma et al., 2014). In brief, overnight cultures of *E. coli* DH10B strain with empty vectors or derivatives expressing *v2a* and catalytic site mutant were harvested and adjusted to OD_{600} 0.3. L-arabinose (0.2%, final concentration) was added to induce the expression and cultured for 2 h. Equal amounts of cells were used for plasmid DNA extraction and equal volume of extracted DNA was resolved in agarose gel followed by ethidium bromide staining.

Southern Blot Hybridization

Southern blot hybridization was performed as described (Sambrook, 2001). In brief, genomic DNA (gDNA) was extracted from overnight cultures of selected strains using Genomic DNA purification Kit (Promega) as per manufacturer's instructions. About 35 μg of gDNA was digested using NEB restriction enzymes (NsiI and *Pvu*II) and resolved in 0.8% agarose gel, 50 V, 3 h. The DNA fragments were transferred to a positively charged nylon membrane (Roche Diagnostics). Nylon membranes were cross-linked and used for hybridization with DIG-labeled probe (Roche). Hybridization was done overnight at 65°C using hybridization solution (FastHyb-Hybridization solution, BioChain). The washing, blocking and detection were done using Roche Wash and Block Buffer Set and DIG DNA Labeling and Detection Kit, according to manufacturer's instructions (Roche). The membrane was exposed to X-ray for detection. The probe for the four *vgrGs* (*vgrGa*, *vgrGb*, *vgrGc*, and *vgrGd*) and putative toxin genes (*v2a*, *v2c*, *v2d*, and *v4b*) was prepared using the plasmid DNA *vgrGa*-pJN105, *v2d*-pJN105, and *v4b*-pJN105, respectively. The primer sets used are listed in **Supplementary Table S5**.

AUTHOR CONTRIBUTIONS

E-ML and MS conceptualized the study. MS, S-TC, and C-JC worked on the data curation. E-ML, C-HK, C-FW, and MS worked on the methodology. C-HK, S-TC, MS, and C-JC carried out the investigation. E-ML was responsible for project administration and resources. E-ML and C-HK supervised the study. MS, C-HK, and E-ML wrote the manuscript. All authors reviewed and approved the manuscript.

FUNDING

Funding for this project was provided by the Ministry of Science and Technology of Taiwan (MOST) Grant Nos. 104-2311-B-001-025-MY3 and 107-2311-B-001-019-MY3 to E-ML. The funders had no role in study design, data collection and analysis, decision to publish, or preparation of the manuscript. Open access publication fees will be paid by the Institute of Plant and Microbial Biology, Academia Sinica, Taiwan.

[1] http://astatsa.com/OneWay_Anova_with_TukeyHSD/

ACKNOWLEDGMENTS

We thank Manda Yu for sharing the recipes of AK medium for enhanced T6SS killing assay and members of Lai lab for their help, encouragement, and stimulating discussion. We are grateful for Genomic Technology Core of Institute of Plant and Microbial Biology for DNA sequencing. This manuscript has been released as a Pre-Print at bioRxiv 740209; doi: 10.1101/740209.

SUPPLEMENTARY MATERIAL

FIGURE S1 | Bayesian phylogeny of the VgrG homologs identified in the representative Proteobacteria genomes presented in **Figure 1**. The color coding is based on the class: Alphaproteobacteria (black), Betaproteobacteria (blue), Deltaproteobacteria (cyan), Epsilonproteobacteria (purple) and Gammaproteobacteria (green). Numbers on the branches indicate the support levels based on posterior probabilities, only values > 60% were shown.

FIGURE S2 | Multiple sequence alignment of VgrG amino acid sequences of 1D1609 and C58. All VgrG homologs were aligned and conserved amino acid residues are shaded in yellow and variable residues are in blue or green, while the C-terminal extension of C58 VgrG1 not homologous to the other VgrGs is unshaded. The red and blue lines indicate the predicted gp27 and gp5 domains, respectively. The amino acid residue number is indicated.

FIGURE S3 | VgrG tree of the 11 *A. tumefaciens* strains. All VgrG homologs in these 11 genomes were extracted for inferring the gene tree. The VgrG orthologs share ≥ 95% identity in amino acid sequence were highlighted. The genomospecies and strain name for each VgrG indicated by a locus tag are shown.

FIGURE S4 | *In planta* competition experiments between C58 and 1D1609 at 1:1 ratio. *A. tumefaciens* strain C58 harboring gentamicin resistance-conferring pRL662 and strain 1D1609 which was selected in spectinomycin plate were mixed at 1:1 ratio and infiltrated into leaves of 6- to 7-week-old *Nicotiana benthamiana* **(A)** and *Medicago truncatula* **(B)**. The competition outcome was quantified at 0 and 24 h post-infection by counting cfu on LB plates with appropriate antibiotics. Data are mean ± SEM, with each data point indicating the competitive index of 4–6 biological replicates from a total of 2–3 independent experiments. No statistical difference ($P > 0.05$) could be detected among different samples as determined by Tukey's HSD test.

FIGURE S5 | Southern blot analysis of mutants generated in this study. Schematic diagram showing probes used for Southern blotting, restriction enzyme cleavage sites and expected sizes. The genomic DNA is hybridized with **(A)** 821-bp *vgrG* probe with homology to all four *vgrG* genes (*vgrGabcd*) was used to confirm *vgrG* mutants; **(B)** 478-bp *v2* probe with homology to *v2acd* was used to confirm *v2a*, *v2c*, and *v2d* mutant and **(C)** 778-bp *v4b* probe was used to confirm *v4b* mutant. Each lane contains 30 μg of genomic DNA digested with *Nsi*I only or combined with *Pvu*II. The expected size (in bp) is indicated on the side of the blot.

TABLE S1 | Percentage identity of VgrG within genomes with highly identical multiple VgrGs. The locus tag of each homolog is shown in rows and column and highlight shows ≥ 95% identity.

TABLE S2 | Predicted functions/domains of toxin/s associated with each *vgrG* based on Phyre or NCBI CDD search and BLASTP.

TABLE S3 | Amino acid sequence similarity/identity among the protein homologs encoded in the *vgrG* genetic modules in *A. tumefaciens* strains C58 and 1D1609.

TABLE S4 | Bacterial strains and plasmids.

TABLE S5 | Primers used in this study.

REFERENCES

Alcoforado Diniz, J., and Coulthurst, S. J. (2015). Intraspecies competition in *Serratia marcescens* is mediated by type VI-secreted Rhs effectors and a conserved effector-associated accessory protein. *J. Bacteriol.* 197, 2350–2360. doi: 10.1128/JB.00199-15

Bellieny-Rabelo, D., Tanui, C. K., Miguel, N., Kwenda, S., Shyntum, D. Y., and Moleleki, L. N. (2019). Transcriptome and comparative genomics analyses reveal new functional insights on key determinants of pathogenesis and interbacterial competition in pectobacterium and *Dickeya* spp. *Appl. Environ. Microbiol.* 85: e02050-018. doi: 10.1128/AEM.02050-18

Bernal, P., Allsopp, L. P., Filloux, A., and Llamas, M. A. (2017). The *Pseudomonas* putida T6SS is a plant warden against phytopathogens. *ISME J.* 11, 972–987. doi: 10.1038/ismej.2016.169

Bingle, L. E., Bailey, C. M., and Pallen, M. J. (2008). Type VI secretion: a beginner's guide. *Curr. Opin. Microbiol.* 11, 3–8. doi: 10.1016/j.mib.2008.01.006

Bladergroen, M. R., Badelt, K., and Spaink, H. P. (2003). Infection-blocking genes of a symbiotic *Rhizobium leguminosarum* strain that are involved in temperature-dependent protein secretion. *Mol. Plant Microbe Interact.* 16, 53–64. doi: 10.1094/mpmi.2003.16.1.53

Bondage, D. D., Lin, J.-S., Ma, L.-S., Kuo, C.-H., and Lai, E.-M. (2016). VgrG C terminus confers the type VI effector transport specificity and is required for binding with PAAR and adaptor–effector complex. *Proc. Natl. Acad. Sci. U.S.A.* 113, E3931–E3940. doi: 10.1073/pnas.1600428113

Boratyn, G. M., Camacho, C., Cooper, P. S., Coulouris, G., Fong, A., Ma, N., et al. (2013). BLAST: a more efficient report with usability improvements. *Nucleic Acids Res.* 41, W29–W33. doi: 10.1093/nar/gkt282

Bouri, M., Chattaoui, M., Gharsa, H. B., McClean, A., Kluepfel, D., Nesme, X., et al. (2016). Analysis of Agrobacterium populations isolated from tunisian soils: genetic structure, avirulent-virulent ratios and characterization of tumorigenic strains. *J. Plant Pathol.* 98, 265–274.

Cianfanelli, F. R., Alcoforado Diniz, J., Guo, M., De Cesare, V., Trost, M., and Coulthurst, S. J. (2016). VgrG and PAAR proteins define distinct versions of a functional type VI secretion system. *PLoS Pathog.* 12:e1005735. doi: 10.1371/journal.ppat.1005735

Costechareyre, D., Rhouma, A., Lavire, C., Portier, P., Chapulliot, D., Bertolla, F., et al. (2010). Rapid and efficient identification of agrobacterium species by recA Allele analysis. *Microb. Ecol.* 60, 862–872. doi: 10.1007/s00248-010-9685-7

Edgar, R. C. (2004). MUSCLE: multiple sequence alignment with high accuracy and high throughput. *Nucleic Acids Res.* 32, 1792–1797. doi: 10.1093/nar/gkh340

Felsenstein, J. (1989). PHYLIP - phylogeny inference package (Version 3.2). *Cladistics* 5, 164–166.

Fitzsimons, T. C., Lewis, J. M., Wright, A., Kleifeld, O., Schittenhelm, R. B., Powell, D., et al. (2018). Identification of novel *Acinetobacter baumannii* Type VI secretion system antibacterial effector and immunity pairs. *Infect. Immun.* 86:e00297-18. doi: 10.1128/IAI.00297-18

Flaugnatti, N., Le, T. T., Canaan, S., Aschtgen, M. S., Nguyen, V. S., Blangy, S., et al. (2016). A phospholipase A1 antibacterial Type VI secretion effector interacts directly with the C-terminal domain of the VgrG spike protein for delivery. *Mol. Microbiol.* 99, 1099–1118. doi: 10.1111/mmi.13292

Galán, J. E. (2009). Common themes in the design and function of bacterial effectors. *Cell Host Microbe* 5, 571–579. doi: 10.1016/j.chom.2009.04.008

Gelvin, S. B. (2000). Agrobacterium and plant genes involved in t-dna transfer and integration. *Annu. Rev. Plant Physiol. Plant Mol. Biol.* 51, 223–256.

Gharsa, H. B., Bouri, M., Glick, B., Gannar, A., Mougou Hamdane, A., and Rhouma, A. (2018). Evaluation of the interspecific competition within *Agrobacterium* spp. in the soil and rhizosphere of tomato (Solanum lycopersicum) and maize (Zea mays). *J. Plant Pathol.* 100, 505–511. doi: 10.1007/s42161-018-0114-y

Hachani, A., Allsopp, L. P., Oduko, Y., and Filloux, A. (2014). The VgrG proteins are "à la Carte" delivery systems for bacterial type VI effectors. *J. Biol. Chem.* 289, 17872–17884. doi: 10.1074/jbc.M114.563429

Haryono, M., Cho, S.-T., Fang, M.-J., Chen, A.-P., Chou, S.-J., Lai, E.-M., et al. (2019). Differentiations in gene content and expression response to virulence induction between two *Agrobacterium* strains. *Front. Microbiol.* 10:1554. doi: 10.3389/fmicb.2019.01554

Ho, S. N., Hunt, H. D., Horton, R. M., Pullen, J. K., and Pease, L. R. (1989). Site-directed mutagenesis by overlap extension using the polymerase chain reaction. *Gene* 77, 51–59. doi: 10.1016/0378-1119(89)90358-2

Hwang, H.-H., Yu, M., and Lai, E.-M. (2017). Agrobacterium-mediated plant transformation: biology and applications. *Arabidop. Book* 15:e0186. doi: 10.1199/tab.0186

Kelley, L. A., Mezulis, S., Yates, C. M., Wass, M. N., and Sternberg, M. J. (2015). The Phyre2 web portal for protein modeling, prediction and analysis. *Nat. Protoc.* 10, 845–858. doi: 10.1038/nprot.2015.053

Koskiniemi, S., Lamoureux, J. G., Nikolakakis, K. C., t'Kint de Roodenbeke, C., Kaplan, M. D., Low, D. A., et al. (2013). Rhs proteins from diverse bacteria mediate intercellular competition. *Proc. Natl. Acad. Sci. U.S.A.* 110, 7032–7037. doi: 10.1073/pnas.1300627110

Leiman, P. G., Basler, M., Ramagopal, U. A., Bonanno, J. B., Sauder, J. M., Pukatzki, S., et al. (2009). Type VI secretion apparatus and phage tail-associated protein complexes share a common evolutionary origin. *Proc. Natl. Acad. Sci. U.S.A.* 106, 4154–4159. doi: 10.1073/pnas.0813360106

Li, L., Stoeckert, C. J., and Roos, D. S. (2003). OrthoMCL: identification of ortholog groups for eukaryotic genomes. *Genome Res.* 13, 2178–2189. doi: 10.1101/gr.1224503

Lien, Y. W., and Lai, E. M. (2017). Type VI secretion effectors: methodologies and biology. *Front. Cell. Infect. Microbiol.* 7:254. doi: 10.3389/fcimb.2017.00254

Lin, J.-S., Ma, L.-S., and Lai, E.-M. (2013). Systematic dissection of the agrobacterium type VI secretion system reveals machinery and secreted components for subcomplex formation. *PLoS One* 8:e67647. doi: 10.1371/journal.pone.0067647

Lin, L., Lezan, E., Schmidt, A., and Basler, M. (2019). Abundance of bacterial Type VI secretion system components measured by targeted proteomics. *Nat. Commun.* 10:2584. doi: 10.1038/s41467-019-10466-9

Lo, W.-S., Chen, L.-L., Chung, W.-C., Gasparich, G. E., and Kuo, C.-H. (2013). Comparative genome analysis of Spiroplasma melliferum IPMB4A, a honeybee-associated bacterium. *BMC Genomics* 14:22. doi: 10.1186/1471-2164-14-22

Lo, W.-S., and Kuo, C.-H. (2017). Horizontal acquisition and transcriptional integration of novel genes in mosquito-associated spiroplasma. *Genome Biol. Evol.* 9, 3246–3259. doi: 10.1093/gbe/evx244

Ma, J., Sun, M., Dong, W., Pan, Z., Lu, C., and Yao, H. (2017). PAAR-Rhs proteins harbor various C-terminal toxins to diversify the antibacterial pathways of type VI secretion systems. *Environ. Microbiol.* 19, 345–360. doi: 10.1111/1462-2920.13621

Ma, L.-S., Hachani, A., Lin, J.-S., Filloux, A., and Lai, E.-M. (2014). *Agrobacterium tumefaciens* deploys a superfamily of Type VI secretion DNase effectors as weapons for interbacterial competition in planta. *Cell Host Microbe* 16, 94–104. doi: 10.1016/j.chom.2014.06.002

Ma, L. S., Lin, J. S., and Lai, E. M. (2009). An IcmF family protein, ImpLM, is an integral inner membrane protein interacting with ImpKL, and its walker a motif is required for type VI secretion system-mediated Hcp secretion in *Agrobacterium tumefaciens*. *J. Bacteriol.* 191, 4316–4329. doi: 10.1128/JB.00029-09

Marchler-Bauer, A., Bo, Y., Han, L., He, J., Lanczycki, C. J., Lu, S., et al. (2017). CDD/SPARCLE: functional classification of proteins via subfamily domain architectures. *Nucleic Acids Res.* 45, D200–D203. doi: 10.1093/nar/gkw1129

Petersen, T. N., Brunak, S., von Heijne, G., and Nielsen, H. (2011). SignalP 4.0: discriminating signal peptides from transmembrane regions. *Nat. Methods* 8, 785–786. doi: 10.1038/nmeth.1701

Pissaridou, P., Allsopp, L. P., Wettstadt, S., Howard, S. A., Mavridou, D. A. I., and Filloux, A. (2018). The *Pseudomonas* aeruginosaT6SS-VgrG1b spike is topped by a PAAR protein eliciting DNA damage to bacterial competitors. *Proc. Natl. Acad. Sci. U.S.A.* 115, 12519–15524. doi: 10.1073/pnas.1814181115

Ronquist, F., and Huelsenbeck, J. P. (2003). MrBayes 3: Bayesian phylogenetic inference under mixed models. *Bioinformatics* 19, 1572–1574. doi: 10.1093/bioinformatics/btg180

Russell, A. B., Peterson, S. B., and Mougous, J. D. (2014). Type VI secretion system effectors: poisons with a purpose. *Nat. Rev. Micro.* 12, 137–148. doi: 10.1038/nrmicro3185

Salomon, D., Kinch, L. N., Trudgian, D. C., Guo, X., Klimko, J. A., Grishin, N. V., et al. (2014). Marker for type VI secretion system effectors. *Proc. Natl. Acad. Sci. U.S.A.* 111, 9271–9276. doi: 10.1073/pnas.1406110111

Sambrook, J. (2001). *Molecular Cloning: A Laboratory Manual*, 3rd Edn. Cold Spring Harbor, NY: Cold Spring Harbor Laboratory Press.

Tang, J. Y., Bullen, N. P., Ahmad, S., and Whitney, J. C. (2018). Diverse NADase effector families mediate interbacterial antagonism via the type VI secretion system. *J. Biol. Chem.* 293, 1504–1514. doi: 10.1074/jbc.RA117.000178

Ting, S.-Y., Bosch, D. E., Mangiameli, S. M., Radey, M. C., Huang, S., Park, Y.-J., et al. (2018). Bifunctional immunity proteins protect bacteria against FtsZ-Targeting ADP-Ribosylating Toxins. *Cell* 175, 1380.e–1392.e. doi: 10.1016/j.cell.2018.09.037

Unterweger, D., Miyata, S. T., Bachmann, V., Brooks, T. M., Mullins, T., Kostiuk, B., et al. (2014). The *Vibrio cholerae* type VI secretion system employs diverse effector modules for intraspecific competition. *Nat. Commun.* 5:3549. doi: 10.1038/ncomms4549

Vettiger, A., and Basler, M. (2016). Type VI secretion system substrates are transferred and reused among sister cells. *Cell* 167, 99.e12–110.e12. doi: 10.1016/j.cell.2016.08.023

Vogel, J., Normand, P., Thioulouse, J., Nesme, X., and Grundmann, G. L. (2003). Relationship between spatial and genetic distance in *Agrobacterium* spp. in 1 cubic centimeter of soil. *Appl. Environ. Microbiol.* 69, 1482–1487. doi: 10.1128/aem.69.3.1482-1487.2003

Whitney, J. C., Beck, C. M., Goo, Y. A., Russell, A. B., Harding, B. N., De Leon, J. A., et al. (2014). Genetically distinct pathways guide effector export through the type VI secretion system. *Mol. Microbiol.* 92, 529–542. doi: 10.1111/mmi.12571

Wu, C.-F., Lien, Y.-W., Bondage, D., Lin, J.-S., Pilhofer, M., Shih, Y.-L., et al. (2019a). Effector loading onto the VgrG carrier activates type VI secretion system assembly. *EMBO Rep.* e47961. doi: 10.15252/embr.201947961

Wu, C.-F., Santos, M. N. M., Cho, S.-T., Chang, H.-H., Tsai, Y.-M., Smith, D. A., et al. (2019b). Plant-pathogenic *Agrobacterium tumefaciens* strains have diverse type VI effector-immunity pairs and vary in in planta competitiveness. *Mol. Plant Microbe Interact.* 32, 961–971. doi: 10.1094/MPMI-01-19-0021-R

Yu, N. Y., Wagner, J. R., Laird, M. R., Melli, G., Rey, S., Lo, R., et al. (2010). PSORTb 3.0: improved protein subcellular localization prediction with refined localization subcategories and predictive capabilities for all prokaryotes. *Bioinformatics* 26, 1608–1615. doi: 10.1093/bioinformatics/btq249

Zhang, D., Iyer, L. M., and Aravind, L. (2011). A novel immunity system for bacterial nucleic acid degrading toxins and its recruitment in various eukaryotic and DNA viral systems. *Nucleic Acids Res.* 39, 4532–4552. doi: 10.1093/nar/gkr036

Zoued, A., Brunet, Y. R., Durand, E., Aschtgen, M.-S., Logger, L., Douzi, B., et al. (2014). Architecture and assembly of the Type VI secretion system. *Biochim. Biophys. Acta Mol. Cell Res.* 1843, 1664–1673. doi: 10.1016/j.bbamcr.2014.03.018

12

The Type IX Secretion System (T9SS): Highlights and Recent Insights into its Structure and Function

Anna M. Lasica [1,2], Miroslaw Ksiazek [1,3], Mariusz Madej [3] and Jan Potempa [1,3]**

[1] Department of Oral Immunology and Infectious Diseases, University of Louisville School of Dentistry, Louisville, KY, United States, [2] Department of Bacterial Genetics, Faculty of Biology, Institute of Microbiology, University of Warsaw, Warsaw, Poland, [3] Department of Microbiology, Faculty of Biochemistry, Biophysics, and Biotechnology, Jagiellonian University, Krakow, Poland

***Correspondence:**
Anna M. Lasica
alasica@biol.uw.edu.pl
Jan Potempa
jan.potempa@louisville.edu

Protein secretion systems are vital for prokaryotic life, as they enable bacteria to acquire nutrients, communicate with other species, defend against biological and chemical agents, and facilitate disease through the delivery of virulence factors. In this review, we will focus on the recently discovered type IX secretion system (T9SS), a complex translocon found only in some species of the *Bacteroidetes* phylum. T9SS plays two roles, depending on the lifestyle of the bacteria. It provides either a means of movement (called gliding motility) for peace-loving environmental bacteria or a weapon for pathogens. The best-studied members of these two groups are *Flavobacterium johnsoniae*, a commensal microorganism often found in water and soil, and *Porphyromonas gingivalis*, a human oral pathogen that is a major causative agent of periodontitis. In *P. gingivalis* and some other periodontopathogens, T9SS translocates proteins, especially virulence factors, across the outer membrane (OM). Proteins destined for secretion bear a conserved C-terminal domain (CTD) that directs the cargo to the OM translocon. At least 18 proteins are involved in this still enigmatic process, with some engaged in the post-translational modification of T9SS cargo proteins. Upon translocation across the OM, the CTD is removed by a protease with sortase-like activity and an anionic LPS is attached to the newly formed C-terminus. As a result, a cargo protein could be secreted into the extracellular milieu or covalently attached to the bacterial surface. T9SS is regulated by a two-component system; however, the precise environmental signal that triggers it has not been identified. Exploring unknown systems contributing to bacterial virulence is exciting, as it may eventually lead to new therapeutic strategies. During the past decade, the major components of T9SS were identified, as well as hints suggesting the possible mechanism of action. In addition, the list of characterized cargo proteins is constantly growing. The actual structure of the translocon, situated in the OM of bacteria, remains the least explored area; however, new technical approaches and increasing scientific attention have resulted in a growing body of data. Therefore, we present a compact up-to-date review of this topic.

Keywords: secretion, T9SS, *Porphyromonas gingivalis*, pathogenesis, gliding motility, proteins, virulence

INTRODUCTION

Secretion of hemolysin A by *E. coli*, described four decades ago, was the first protein secretion system discovered in Gram-negative bacteria (diderm bacteria; Goebel and Hedgpeth, 1982). Since then, eight other protein secretion pathways have been characterized in these prokaryotes, which have a cell envelope consisting of the inner membrane (IM) and the outer membrane (OM) separated by the periplasm. They are now referred to as type *x* secretion systems (T1SS–T9SS; reviewed in Abdallah et al., 2007; Gerlach and Hensel, 2007; Remaut et al., 2008; Desvaux et al., 2009; Goyal et al., 2014; Costa et al., 2015; Abby et al., 2016). Secretion systems in diderm bacteria are considered gateways through the OM that transport cargo with the help of either dedicated IM and periplasmic proteins or the Sec, Tat, and holins systems that first transport cargo to the periplasm. In fact, the Sec, Tat, and holins pathways, which transport proteins across the cytoplasmic membrane, are universal among bacteria, eukaryotes, and even archaea (Hutcheon and Bolhuis, 2003; Denks et al., 2014; Berks, 2015; Saier and Reddy, 2015). Therefore, secretion may be either a single-step process in which substrates (proteins or DNA) are translocated through a designated cell envelope-spanning structure (T1SS, T3SS, T4SS, and T6SS) or a two-step process in which the substrates first cross the IM into the periplasm using the Sec/Tat/holins systems, then are directed to the OM translocon. The final destinations of secreted cargos are diverse: they may stay attached to the surface of the OM, be released into the extracellular milieu, or be injected into the cytoplasm of a target cell (Costa et al., 2015; Abby et al., 2016).

Secretion systems perform numerous physiological functions essential for cell propagation and fitness within a specific ecological niche. They facilitate nutrient acquisition, communication with the environment, attachment to various surfaces, defense against host antimicrobial systems, and delivery of virulence factors at a precise location such as a eukaryotic cell (Letoffe et al., 1994; Henke and Bassler, 2004; Gerlach and Hensel, 2007; Rondelet and Condemine, 2013; Gaytan et al., 2016; Hachani et al., 2016; Majerczyk et al., 2016). However, none of the above adaptations can be assigned solely to one type of secretion.

The presence of protein secretion systems varies among phylogenetic lineages of diderm bacteria. *Proteobacteria* encode the broadest range of described secretion types, whereas other clades have a strong preference for only one or two types (e.g., *Fusobacteria* possess only T5SS; *Chlamydiae*, T3SS and T5SS). The most widespread systems are T1SS and T5SS; conversely, T2SS is rarely detected outside *Proteobacteria* (Abby et al., 2016).

In this review, we will cover the current knowledge regarding the recently discovered type IX secretion system (T9SS), also known as the Por secretion system (PorSS) or PerioGate. T9SS is exclusively present in the *Bacteroidetes* phylum, in a majority of its species (62% out of 97 genomes available; Sato et al., 2010; McBride and Zhu, 2013; Abby et al., 2016).

DISCOVERY OF T9SS

Uncovering and characterizing this unique secretion system was a gradual process over the last two decades and originated from studies of the Gram-negative, non-motile, anaerobic bacterium *Porphyromonas gingivalis. P. gingivalis* is a human oral pathogen that is a major causative agent of periodontitis, and, along with two other bacteria, *Tannerella forsythia* and *Treponema denticola*, forms the so-called red complex (Hajishengallis, 2015). Besides being a key pathogen in periodontitis, *P. gingivalis* is implicated in many systemic illnesses such as atherosclerosis (Kebschull et al., 2010), aspiration pneumonia (Benedyk et al., 2016), rheumatoid arthritis (RA; Laugisch et al., 2016), and even cancer (Whitmore and Lamont, 2014; Gao et al., 2016).

An important initial finding was that *P. gingivalis* produces potent proteolytic enzymes called gingipains (Kgp, RgpA, and RgpB; discussed in more detail later in this review; Pike et al., 1994; Pavloff et al., 1995; Curtis et al., 1999). Gingipains are essential virulence factors responsible for corrupting host innate defense mechanisms (Potempa et al., 2003; Hajishengallis, 2015). They are secreted in large amounts and are mainly attached to the surface of the OM, but are also partially released in a soluble form into the extracellular milieu (Pike et al., 1994; Rangarajan et al., 1997). Because none of the genes associated with known protein secretion systems could be found in the *P. gingivalis* genome, it was suspected that this bacterium had developed a unique OM translocon.

The search for this novel secretion system was greatly facilitated by the observation that colonies of *P. gingivalis* deficient in gingipain activity lack black pigmentation while growing on blood agar plates (**Figure 1**; Okamoto et al., 1998; Shi et al., 1999). Colony pigmentation results from the accumulation of heme on the surface of *P. gingivalis* cells, a process dependent on the proteolytic activity and hemagglutinin- and heme/hemoglobin-binding activity of gingipains (Smalley et al., 1998; Sroka et al., 2001). Spontaneous white/beige mutants were occasionally observed, and this phenotype was associated with, among other things, decreased cell surface-associated proteolytic activity (McKee et al., 1988; Shah et al., 1989). The discovery of the essential role of secreted, cell-bound gingipains in heme acquisition meant that pigmentation could be used as an easy screening tool for mutations blocking gingipain secretion. Of note, as potent virulence factors, gingipains were of particular interest for elucidating the role of *P. gingivalis* in the development of periodontitis.

Several high-throughput transposon mutagenesis studies were performed, resulting in the characterization of various pigment-less clones. Early studies associated this phenotype with the impaired activity of trypsin-like proteases and diminished hemagglutination and heme acquisition by mutants (Hoover and Yoshimura, 1994; Genco et al., 1995). Later investigations found aberrations in polysaccharide synthesis and disruption of *kgp* (one of the gingipains; Simpson et al., 1999; Chen et al., 2000; Abaibou et al., 2001; Shoji et al., 2002). Finally, Sato et al. (2005) identified in their transposon study *porT* (PG0751/PGN_0778), the first gene encoding a protein involved in the secretion of

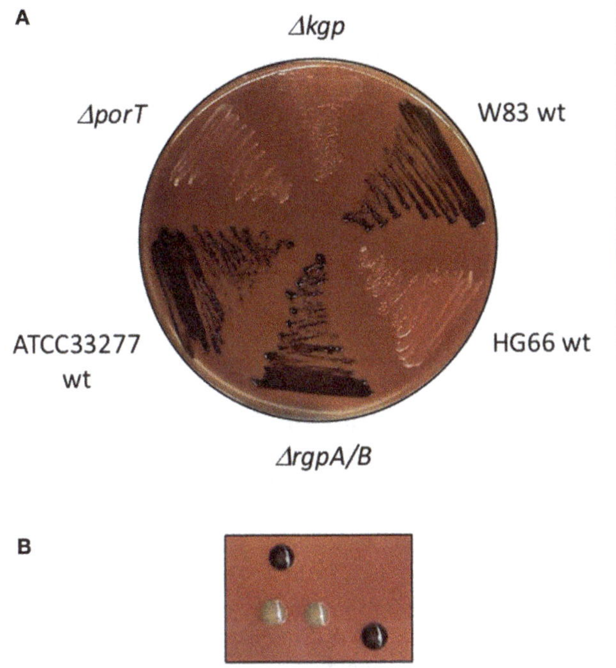

FIGURE 1 | Pigmentation of various *P. gingivalis* W83 strains. (A) The wild-type *P. gingivalis* W83 and ATCC33277 strains grown anaerobically on blood agar plates present brown/black pigmentation due to heme accumulation. This phenotype is in a great part dependent on Kgp gingipain activity on the cell surface. *P. gingivalis* strains deficient in Kgp activity yield beige colonies which darken over the time. Arginine gingipains (RgpA/B) are not involved in this process and their deletion does not influence pigmentation. Strains impaired in T9SS e.g., Δ*porT* lack pigmentation which is never restored. Due to the absence of A-LPS in the *P. gingivalis* HG66 strain all gingipains and other T9SS cargo proteins are not associated with the cell membrane, but secreted into extracellular milieu resulting in white phenotype. **(B)** Single colonies of *P. gingivalis* strains grown for 7 days showing black or white pigmentation.

gingipains. Their mutated, non-pigmented strain had impaired gingipain activity. Moreover, gingipains accumulated in the periplasm as enzymatically inactive proenzymes instead of being exported outside the cell. A database search (BLASTP) found that PorT is present only in some species of the *Bacteroidetes* phylum, such as *Porphyromonas gingivalis*, *Cytophaga hutchinsonii*, and *Prevotella intermedia*, and absent from many other phylum proteomes like *Bacteroides thetaiotaomicron* and *Bacteroides fragilis* (Sato et al., 2005). Two years later, another gene, *sov* (PG0809/PGN_0832), was implicated in the secretion of gingipains, showing a mutation phenotype identical to the one observed for the *porT* mutation (Saiki and Konishi, 2007).

Finally, the 2010 comparison of the *porT*-positive proteomes/genomes of *C. hutchinsonii* and *P. gingivalis* with the *porT*-negative species *B. thetaiotaomicron* resulted in a list of 55 genes (in addition to *porT*) potentially involved in the secretion mechanism. Subsequent isogenic mutagenesis of all selected genes resulted in the identification of 11 genes (including *porT* and *sov*) associated with gingipain transport across the OM and gingipain activation. Because these proteins do not have sequence similarity to components of any other known secretion system, it was assumed to be a novel secretion system and was originally called the Por secretion system (PorSS; Sato et al., 2010; Nakayama, 2015). To be consistent with the existing nomenclature of secretion systems in diderm bacteria, the system was later designated the type IX secretion system or T9SS.

NEW SECRETION SYSTEM: A DEADLY WEAPON OR A PEACEFUL TOOL?

The comparative analysis of genomes carried out in a search for *porT* homologs revealed that T9SS is exclusively present in the *Bacteroidetes* phylum (Sato et al., 2005). Numerous studies on *P. gingivalis* show that T9SS is involved in virulence factor secretion, which damages human tissues and dysregulates immune responses (Potempa et al., 2003; Yoshimura et al., 2008; Sato et al., 2013; Bielecka et al., 2014; Taguchi et al., 2015). In addition, *T. forsythia* and *Prevotella intermedia* (another oral pathogenic bacteria) use this secretion pathway to disseminate their effector proteins (Nguyen et al., 2007; Veith et al., 2013; Narita et al., 2014; Tomek et al., 2014; Ksiazek et al., 2015b). Consequently, it is plausible that more pathogens from the *Bacteroidetes* phylum carrying *porT* homologs are utilizing this mechanism for virulence factor secretion. Although no experimental data are available to support this, it is likely that T9SS is a molecular weapon aimed at various host cells, similar to many other secretion systems (especially T3SS and T6SS).

Among *Bacteroidetes*' *porT*-positive species, there are many non-pathogenic environmental microorganisms such as *C. hutchinsonii* and *F. johnsoniae*. Both bacteria are aerobes ubiquitously distributed in soil and are capable of digesting macromolecules such as cellulose and chitin, respectively (Stanier, 1942, 1947). They are motile microorganisms that use a movement mechanism called gliding motility (Jarrell and McBride, 2008; Nakane et al., 2013). Surprisingly, the core T9SS genes are a subset of those necessary for gliding (*gldK: ortholog of P. gingivalis porK*, *gldL/porL*, *gldM/porM*, *gldN/porN*, *sprA/sov*, *sprE/porW*, and *sprT/porT*; Sato et al., 2010; McBride and Zhu, 2013; Shrivastava et al., 2013; McBride and Nakane, 2015). Moreover, secretion of chitinase and cellulase requires T9SS, meaning the system functions as a non-invasive tool used for movement and food acquisition in these bacteria (Kharade and McBride, 2014; Zhu and McBride, 2014; Yang et al., 2016).

The detailed mechanisms and regulation of T9SS in gliding motility and food scavenging are still under investigation and may reveal additional functions (even in non-gliding species).

STRUCTURAL AND FUNCTIONAL COMPONENTS OF *P. gingivalis* T9SS

Presently, 18 genes from a total of 29 candidates have been proven essential for proper T9SS function in *P. gingivalis* by deletion mutagenesis studies (Heath et al., 2016). Deletion of any of these genes results in the white pigmentation phenotype and accumulation of cargos (e.g., gingipains) in the periplasm. Some of these proteins build the core structures in the IM and OM, some play regulatory or accessory roles, and others are involved in post-translationally modifying cargo proteins (**Table 1**). Many aspects of their functions have yet to be discovered.

Genes encoding T9SS components are scattered around the *P. gingivalis* genome. The exception is a group of five genes, *porP-porK-porL-porM-porN*, that are co-transcribed (Vincent et al., 2016). In many other *Bacteroidetes* species, the operon structure of these genes is conserved [databases: STRING (Snel et al., 2000), DOOR (Dam et al., 2007; Mao et al., 2009), ProOpDB (Taboada et al., 2012), OperonDB (Pertea et al., 2009)]. Orthologs of the *porP* gene (*sprP* in some gliding motility bacteria) show the most variation, as the gene can be located in different genomic loci (e.g., *F. johnsoniae Fjoh_3477* vs. *gldK/Fjoh_1853*), and, even if they precede *porK*, they remain as separate transcriptional units (e.g., *C. hutchinsonii sprP/CHU_0170* and *gldK/CHU_0171*; Zhu and McBride, 2014). The rest of the *P. gingivalis* T9SS genes are either single units or predicted to be in 2–5 gene operons (**Figure 2**) with genes unrelated to T9SS structure and function. In addition, none of the adjacent genes encode T9SS cargo proteins.

Cytoplasmic and IM Components

Presently, there is only one known T9SS-related protein residing entirely in the cytoplasm: PorX (PG0928/PGN_1019). It is a response regulator (RR) of a two-component system (TCS) involved in regulating the expression of several T9SS genes. Its sensor kinase partner, PorY (PG0052/PGN_2001), is an IM-anchored protein containing two transmembrane (TM) helices and a large cytoplasmic domain (~222 aa; Sato et al., 2010; Vincent et al., 2016). Both proteins will be discussed in more detail in the Regulation Section.

Two other essential components of T9SS, PorL (*PG0289 /PGN_1675*) and PorM (*PG0290/PGN_1674*), are also anchored in the IM. PorL possesses two TM helices located between residues 17–48 and 48–74, with both N- and C-termini in the cytoplasm. The precise locations of the helices (the exact amino acids) have not been determined (Vincent et al., 2017). The large cytoplasmic C-terminal domain (~236 residues) interacts *in vitro* with PorX (Vincent et al., 2016); thus it may be involved in regulating T9SS function. Moreover, PorL cytoplasmic domain forms a homotrimer in *E. coli* cells and the full-length protein was found in a complex with PorM both *in vitro* (Gorasia et al., 2016; Vincent et al., 2017) and *in vivo* (Sato et al., 2010). PorM is anchored in the IM by a single TM helix at its N-terminus (between residues 9 and 41), with the remaining residues (475) forming a domain facing the periplasm. In *E. coli* cells, the periplasmic part of PorM dimerizes and interacts with two other core T9SS proteins: PorK and PorN (Vincent et al., 2017). The recombinant periplasmic domain (amino acid residues 36–516) was crystallized, presenting with tetragonal crystals, but automatic model building failed to provide a realistic structure, thus leaving the nature of interactions unknown (Stathopulos et al., 2015). Nevertheless, a possible function for PorL/PorM, apart from the regulatory implications for PorL, has been suggested.

It was proposed that the two proteins form an energy transducer complex to provide energy for T9SS assembly and substrate translocation. The idea came from *F. johnsoniae*, which utilizes a proton-motive force for gliding motility (Nakane et al., 2013; Gorasia et al., 2016). It was further noted that the hydrophobic TM helixes of GldL (PorL ortholog), PorL, and PorM possess conserved glutamate residues characteristic of known energy transducers (Shrivastava et al., 2013; Vincent et al., 2017). These assumptions need experimental verification; nevertheless, they are compatible with mechanisms used by other secretion systems to provide the energy needed to drive substrate transport such as hydrolysis of ATP, proton-motive force, low-energy assembly, and entropy gradient (Costa et al., 2015).

Periplasmic Components

Four T9SS proteins are located in the periplasm: PorN (PG0291/PGN_1673), PorK (PG0288/PGN_1676), PorW (PG1947/PGN_1877), and PG1058/PGN_1296. All but one (PorN) are predicted or proven to be lipoproteins associated with membranes (Sato et al., 2010). PorW is the least investigated protein among the periplasmic elements of *P. gingivalis* secretion. Experimental work on PorW has only been performed on the *F. johnsoniae* PorW ortholog, SprE (Fjoh_1051), which is a predicted lipoprotein that localizes to a membrane fraction (most likely the OM). A mutant with a deleted *sprE* gene exhibits phenotypes in gliding bacteria typical of other T9SS function-deficient mutants, such as non-spreading colonies, defective gliding, and blocked secretion of chitinase (Rhodes et al., 2011; Kharade and McBride, 2015). Its subcellular localization and the effects of its mutation on the secretory/gliding phenotype suggest that SprE/PorW is yet another structural component of T9SS.

PG1058 is a multidomain protein necessary for T9SS function. The phenotype of *P. gingivalis* with an inactivated *PG1058* gene is typical of other T9SS mutants: colonies on blood agar lack pigmentation and inactive, unprocessed gingipains accumulate in the periplasm. The PG1058 protein is anchored by its lipid modification to the periplasmic surface of the OM. The predicted structure suggests the presence of four structural domains: a tetratricopeptide repeat (TPR) domain, a β-propeller domain, a carboxypeptidase regulatory domain-like fold (CRD), and an OmpA_C-like putative peptidoglycan-binding domain. TPR and β-propeller domains are involved in protein-protein interactions; hence, together with the *PG1058* mutant phenotype, it is plausible that PG1058 supports the T9SS translocon structure (Heath et al., 2016). Further, experiments are needed to verify this hypothesis.

PorN is a periplasmic protein that forms dimers *in vitro* and has the propensity to interact both *in vitro* and *in vivo* with IM protein PorM and periplasmic lipoprotein PorK (Gorasia et al., 2016; Vincent et al., 2017). The nature of the interaction with PorK is interesting, as both proteins form a ring-shaped structure with an external and internal diameter of 50 and 35 nm, respectively. It was proposed that they form a large complex in which PorN interacts in an almost 1:1 fashion (32–36 total subunits) with the PorK lipoprotein. The ring structure is anchored into the OM through the fatty acids of PorK. Consistent with detected interactions, PorN has a crucial role in stabilizing both PorL–PorM and PorN–PorK complexes, as deletion of the

TABLE 1 | T9SS components.

Locus Tag			*Porphyromonas gingivalis* W83					
W83 NC_002950.2		**ATCC33277 NC_010729.1**	**Protein accession number**	**Protein description**	**Mol weight (kDa)[a]**	**Interactions [b]*in vitro* [c]*in vivo***	**Homologs *T. forsythia* ATCC 43037–Tanf *F. johnsoniae* UW101-Fjoh**	**References[d]**
CYTOPLASMIC AND INNER MEMBRANE COMPONENTS								
PG_RS04080	PG0928	PGN_1019	WP_005875211.1	PorX; chemotaxis protein CheY, cytoplasmic protein	60.6	PorY[b], SigP[b], PorL[b]	Tanf_12330 Fjoh_2906	Sato et al., 2010; Kadowaki et al., 2016; Vincent et al., 2016
PG_RS00240	PG0052	PGN_2001	WP_005873974.1	PorY; sensor histidine kinase, inner membrane protein	44.6	PorX[b]	Tanf_13050 Fjoh_1592	
PG_RS01295	PG0289	PGN_1675	WP_012458450.1	PorL, inner membrane protein	34.8	PorM[b,c]	Tanf_02365 Fjoh_1854 (GldL)	Sato et al., 2010; Gorasia et al., 2016; Kadowaki et al., 2016; Vincent et al., 2016, 2017
PG_RS01300	PG0290	PGN_1674	WP_005874203.1	PorM, inner membrane protein	56.4	PorL/K/N[c]	Tanf_02370 Fjoh_1855 (GldM)	Sato et al., 2010; Gorasia et al., 2016; Kadowaki et al., 2016; Vincent et al., 2017
PERIPLASMIC COMPONENTS								
PG_RS01305	PG0291	PGN_1673	WP_005874243.1	PorN	41.3	PorP[b], PorK/L/M[c] PG0189[c]	Tanf_02375 Fjoh_1856 (GldN)	Sato et al., 2010; Gorasia et al., 2016; Kadowaki et al., 2016; Vincent et al., 2017
PG_RS01290	PG0288	PGN_1676	WP_043876477.1	PorK; lipoprotein	54.1	PorN[c], PorM/P[b]PG0189[c]	Tanf_02360 Fjoh_1853 (GldK)	Sato et al., 2010; Gorasia et al., 2016; Kadowaki et al., 2016; Vincent et al., 2017
PG_RS08590	PG1947	PGN_1877	WP_005873869.1	PorW; lipoprotein	132.1	n.d.[e]	Tanf_00060 Fjoh_1051 (SprE)	Sato et al., 2010
PG_RS04660	PG1058	PGN_1296	WP_005873448.1	Lipoprotein; TPRd, WD40d, CRDd, OmpA Family domain	74.9	n.d.	Tanf_02260 Fjoh_1647[f]	Heath et al., 2016
OUTER MEMBRANE AND SURFACE COMPONENTS								
PG_RS03550	PG0809	PGN_0832	WP_012457811.1[g]	Sov; β-barrel protein	281.1	n.d.	Tanf_04410 Fjoh_1653 (SprA)	Saiki and Konishi, 2007, 2010b; Sato et al., 2010; Kadowaki et al., 2016
PG_RS02670	PG0602	PGN_0645	WP_010956079.1	PorQ; β-barrel protein	37.9	n.d.	Tanf_12465 Fjoh_2755	Sato et al., 2010
PG_RS01285	PG0287	PGN_1677	WP_005874180.1	PorP; β-barrel protein	35.0	PorN/K[b]	Tanf_02355 Fjoh_3477[h]	Sato et al., 2010; Kadowaki et al., 2016; Vincent et al., 2017
PG_RS03295	PG0751	PGN_0778	WP_039417575.1	PorT; β-barrel protein	26.7	n.d.	Tanf_10520 Fjoh_1466 (SprT)	Sato et al., 2005, 2010; Nguyen et al., 2007; Kadowaki et al., 2016
PG_RS00125	PG0027	PGN_0023	WP_004583425.1	PorV (LptO); β-barrel protein	43.1	PorU[c]	Tanf_04220 Fjoh_1555	Ishiguro et al., 2009; Sato et al., 2010; Chen et al., 2011; Glew et al., 2012; Saiki and Konishi, 2014
PG_RS00870	PG0189	PGN_0297	WP_005874727.1	β-barrel protein	25.6	PorK/N[c]	Tanf_09815 Fjoh_1692	Gorasia et al., 2016
PG_RS02385	PG0534	PGN_1437	WP_005875072.1	TonB-dependent receptor; β-barrel protein	92.3	n.d.	Tanf_07980 Fjoh_0118	Saiki and Konishi, 2010a
PG_RS00885	PG0192	PGN_300	WP_043876475.1	Omp17; OmpH-like	19.6	n.d.	Tanf_09800 Fjoh_1689[i]	Taguchi et al., 2015

(Continued)

TABLE 1 | Continued

Locus Tag		*Porphyromonas gingivalis* W83					
W83 NC_002950.2	**ATCC33277 NC_010729.1**	**Protein accession number**	**Protein description**	**Mol weight (kDa)[a]**	**Interactions [b]*in vitro* [c]*in vivo***	**Homologs *T. forsythia* ATCC 43037-Tanf *F. johnsoniae* UW101-Fjoh**	**References[d]**
PG_RS00120 PG0026	PGN_0022	WP_005874469.1	PorU; surface C-terminal signal peptidase	128.2	PorV (LptO)[c]	Tanf_02580 Fjoh_1556	Sato et al., 2010; Glew et al., 2012; Saiki and Konishi, 2014; Gorasia et al., 2015
PG_RS07070 PG1604	PGN_0509	WP_010956350.1	PorZ; surface B-propeller protein	83.6	n.d.	Tanf_12435 Fjoh_0707	Glew et al., 2014; Lasica et al., 2016

[a]Calculated from amino acid sequence including a signal peptide.
[b]In vitro experiments.
[c]In vivo experiments.
[d]References to original papers pertinent only to P. gingivalis T9SS. Proteomic papers are not cited in the table but they are referred in the text.
[e]Not determined.
[f]F. johnsoniae possesses 5 proteins homologous to PG1058, the one with the highest score is given in the table. All 5 F. johnsoniae proteins (Fjoh_1647, Fjoh_4540, Fjoh_3950, Fjoh_3973, Fjoh_3476) range between 26–29% identities with 90–98% coverage comparing to PG1058 (assessed by NCBI BLAST).
[g]Accession number given in the table is for the Sov protein from P. gingivalis ATCC33277 due to miss-annotation in W83 genome as two separate ORFs (PG0809/PG0810; Saiki and Konishi, 2007).
[h]F. johnsoniae possesses numerous homologous proteins to PG0287 (PorP), the one with the highest score is given in the table. Five proteins with the highest overall score (Fjoh_3477, Fjoh_3951, Fjoh_1646, Fjoh_4539, Fjoh_2274) range between 25–29% identities with 86–93% coverage and gaps 3–9% comparing to PG0287 (PorP). The most explored PorP-like protein of F. johnsoniae is Fjoh_0978 (SprF; Rhodes et al., 2011) however, it has lower scores comparing to the proteins mentioned above (22% identities, 83% coverage, 18% gaps) as assessed by NCBI BLAST.
[i]The closest homolog in F. johnsoniae proteome is Fjoh_1689 is much larger protein than its equivalent in P. gingivalis (341 residues vs. 174; 32% identities, 95% PG0192 coverage assessed by NCBI BLAST).

porN gene resulted in the degradation of PorL, PorM, and PorK in *P. gingivalis* cells. By contrast, deletion of either *porL* or *porM* does not interfere with the stability of the PorN/K complex (Gorasia et al., 2016).

Further, studies on PorK,L,M,N interactions suggest the existence of a $PorK_2L_3M_2N_2$ complex that likely oligomerizes to form a superstructure with a final molecular mass of over 1.2 MDa (Gorasia et al., 2016; Vincent et al., 2017). Such a large complex was originally reported by Sato and colleagues, who identified all four proteins in a single spot on a blue-native electrophoresis gel (Sato et al., 2010). However, additional elements of the complex were recently identified: PG0189 and PorP (PG0287/PGN_1677). Because they are predicted to be integral OM β-barrel proteins, they are discussed in more detail in the following section.

OM and Surface Components

The vast majority of T9SS components are confined to the OM. In addition to the peripheral OM-associated and periplasmic proteins delineated above, seven others (Sov, PorQ, PorP, PorT, PorV, PG0189, and PG0534) are predicted to be integral OM β-barrel proteins. Furthermore, two proteins, PorU and PorZ, are associated with the bacterial surface. In addition, PG0192 was found in a membrane fraction, but its association with the OM needs further verification.

PorT and Sov were the first proteins found to be essential for *P. gingivalis* protein secretion, and the discovery led to intense research on T9SS (see Discovery Section; Sato et al., 2005, 2010; Saiki and Konishi, 2007). Despite this, we still know very little about the structure and function of these proteins a decade later. PorT is predicted to have eight anti-parallel, membrane-traversing β-strands, with four large loops facing the environment, and this topology has been experimentally confirmed (Nguyen et al., 2009). Sov was also described as an integral OM protein with its C-terminal region likely exposed to the extracellular milieu (Saiki and Konishi, 2007, 2010b). However, the precise roles of both proteins in T9SS structure and function remain unknown. Even less information is available concerning PorQ (PG0602/PGN_0645) as a T9SS component (Sato et al., 2010). In the genome annotation, it is described as a hypothetical protein with a β-barrel structure belonging to the porin superfamily (Nelson et al., 2003); thus it is assumed to localize to the OM.

Similarly, little is known about PG0534/PGN_1437 as a protein essential for T9SS function (Saiki and Konishi, 2010a). Interestingly, *PG0534* is upregulated in human gingival epithelial cells, suggesting its contribution to *P. gingivalis* eukaryotic cell invasion and/or intracellular survival (Park et al., 2004). *In silico* predictions run on the RaptorX server (Kallberg et al., 2012) modeled PG0534 as a β-barrel OM protein, with the pyochelin OM receptor FptA from *Pseudomonas aeruginosa* (Cobessi et al., 2005) as the best template (PDB: 1xkwA; *p*-value: 1.82e-23).

The next T9SS OM component, PG0192/PGN_300 (annotated as an OmpH-like protein), was found in the total membrane fraction. Due to its 17 kDa molecular mass, the protein is referred to as Omp17 (Taguchi et al., 2015). The best template prediction by the RaptorX server is a putative

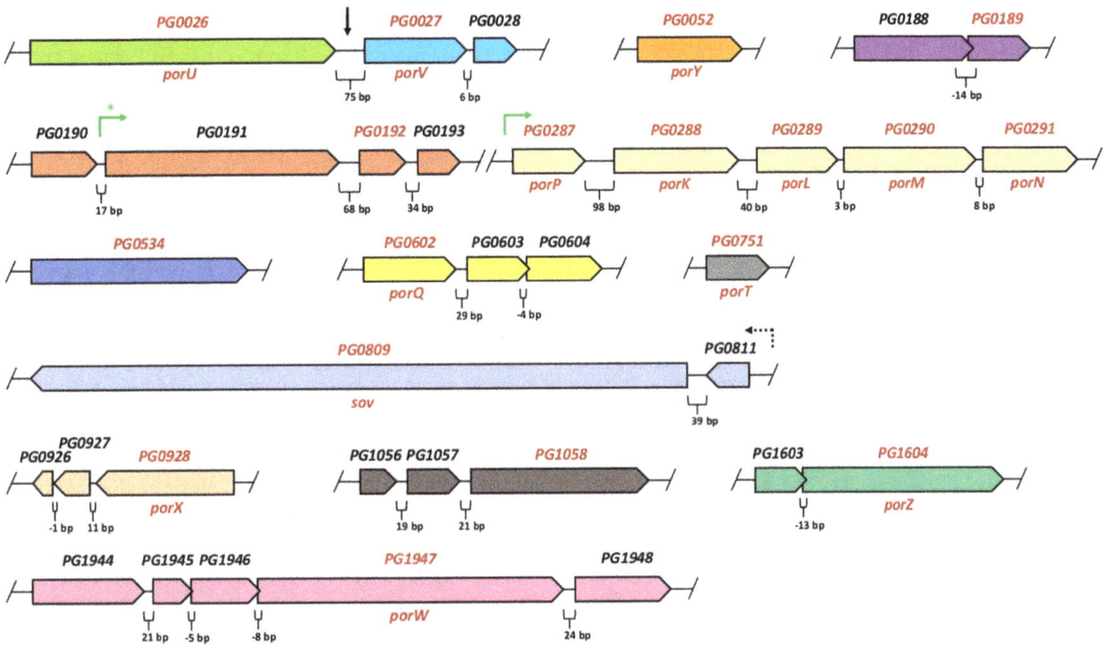

FIGURE 2 | Arrangement of *P. gingivalis* W83 genes encoding T9SS components. Genes are grouped according to *in silico* operon predictions, reflecting direction of transcripts (Dam et al., 2007; Mao et al., 2009; Pertea et al., 2009; Taboada et al., 2012). Gaps in the genome are indicated by the slashes. Intervals between adjacent genes or overlapping regions (in base pairs-bp) are marked below each section. Each transcription unit is shown in different color. Genes encoding T9SS components are depicted in red font. Black vertical arrow shows continuous region (75 bp) between *PG0026* (*porU*) and *PG0027* (*porV*) but the two genes were predicted to transcribe independently. Green arrows indicate operons that were confirmed experimentally (Taguchi et al., 2015; Vincent et al., 2017). Green asterisk denotes proved single transcription unit for the *PG0191-PG0192-PG0193* genes (in *P. gingivalis* ATCC33277 strain), however co-transcription of preceding the *PG0190* gene (17 bp interval) was not investigated (Taguchi et al., 2015). The *PG0809* (*Sov*) gene was re-sequenced and confirmed to consist of the two combined genes *PG0809* and *PG0810*, mis-annotated in W83 genome as separate ORFs (Saiki and Konishi, 2007). A dashed arrow denotes indirect evidence that *PG0809* (*Sov*) and *PG0811* may be co-transcribed. It was shown that sigma factor SigP (regulator of other *por* genes) binds to the region preceding *PG0811* but not the one before *PG0809* (Kadowaki et al., 2016).

OM chaperone (OmpH-like) from *Caulobacter crescentus* (PDB: 4kqtA; *p*-value: 6.78e-04). The phenotypic effects of *omp17* mutation are typical of other T9SS-defective mutants but with an interesting exception. The mutant is still able to secrete unprocessed T9SS cargo proteins, including pro-gingipains and CPG70, which accumulate in the periplasm in other secretion mutants (Taguchi et al., 2015). Of note, in the wild-type *P. gingivalis*, T9SS cargos remain attached to the bacterial surface through anionic lipopolysaccharide (A-LPS) anchoring (Shoji et al., 2002; Shoji and Nakayama, 2016). This modification is added by the surface-located PorU protein (Gorasia et al., 2015; for more details see the Mechanism Section). Taguchi and colleagues showed that A-LPS synthesis in the *omp17* mutant was not affected, suggesting the impairment of PorU function. Consistent with that, PorU was not detected in the *omp17*$^{-}$ cell envelope fraction, but was found in the cytoplasm/periplasm fraction. Moreover, the *omp17* mutant was less virulent than the wild type in the mouse subcutaneous model, which is consistent with the lack of gingipain activity (Taguchi et al., 2015).

As previously mentioned, PG0189 and PorP (a part of the *porPKLMN* operon) were detected in association with the PorKLMN complex. Specifically, a periplasmic loop of PG0189 interacts with both PorK and PorN, as shown by cross-linking experiments. Due to its low abundance, PG0189 is proposed to play an accessory role in secretion (Gorasia et al., 2016). The nature of the interaction of PorP with PorK and PorM is still enigmatic. The proteins co-precipitate *in vitro*; however, all tested proteins were produced in *E. coli* cells, and, so far, have not been detected in the native complex (Vincent et al., 2017).

Currently, the only OM β-barrel protein with an assigned function is PorV (PG0027/PGN_0023/LptO). The PorV-mutated strain retains inactive, unprocessed gingipains in the periplasm (Ishiguro et al., 2009) and fails to O-deacylate LPS, which might be a necessary step in post-translational processing during the secretion of cargo proteins (Chen et al., 2011; Glew et al., 2012). Yet another study indicated that PorV interacts *in vivo* with PorU (PG0026/PGN_0022), and it was proposed that PorV serves as an OM anchor for PorU (Saiki and Konishi, 2014). Indeed, PorU localizes to the surface of *P. gingivalis* cells and is involved in T9SS cargo processing (see the next section; Glew et al., 2012; Gorasia et al., 2015). Despite this relative abundance of knowledge on PorV, it remains unknown whether PorV is directly involved in LPS processing or if it is only an accessory protein for an unknown LPS O-deacylase. The secretion-deficient phenotype of the PorV mutant might be related to the lack of PorU immobilization on its surface.

The last known component of T9SS is a surface-located PorZ protein (PG1604/PGN_0509) recently characterized by our group (Lasica et al., 2016). The non-pigmented phenotype of the PorZ-mutant strain and its accumulation of unprocessed, inactive gingipains confirmed that PorZ is essential for the system. Interestingly, it was shown (through proteomics and mutagenesis studies) that PorZ is itself a cargo of T9SS and has the conserved C-terminal domain (CTD) (Glew et al., 2014; Lasica et al., 2016). The CTD works as a signal, directing T9SS cargo proteins to the OM translocon (see the next section; Shoji et al., 2011). However, unlike other cargos, the CTD of PorZ is not cleaved off upon secretion and the protein is not anchored in the OM in the same manner as other secreted proteins (Lasica et al., 2016). This phenomenon was observed for only one other protein, PorU, which is also both a functionally essential element and a cargo of T9SS (Glew et al., 2012). PorZ is currently the sole Por protein with a solved atomic structure. It is composed of two large β-propeller domains and a CTD, conforming to canonical β-sandwich architecture (de Diego et al., 2016; Lasica et al., 2016). Although the precise role of PorZ remains to be revealed, β-propeller domains are a good platform for protein-protein interactions and provide binding areas for small molecules (e.g., saccharides; Hunt et al., 1987; Zhang et al., 2014). Considering the structure and processing, we hypothesize that, like PorU, PorZ may be involved in post-translational maturation of T9SS cargo proteins during their translocation across the OM.

MECHANISM OF SECRETION

Protein secretion using T9SS is a two-step process. First, the cargo proteins are guided by a classical signal peptide to the Sec machinery in the IM. During translocation, the signal peptide is cleaved off by type I signal peptidase, and the cargo is released into the periplasm. Although, the Sec pathway has not been experimentally analyzed in *P. gingivalis*, the screening of *Bacteroidetes* genomes confirmed that the system is mostly conserved (McBride and Zhu, 2013). In the periplasm, transported proteins fold into a stable conformation, as indicated from the accumulation of their soluble forms in the periplasm of T9SS secretory mutants. Whether the cargo proteins require a chaperone(s) to assist in folding and/or guiding them to the OM translocon is still unknown.

A common feature of all T9SS cargo proteins is the conserved CTD that targets T9SS cargo proteins to the OM translocon. The function of the CTD was first recognized while studying the secretion and processing of the RgpB (PG0506/PGN_1466) gingipain. The protein without the C-terminal Ig-like domain of 72 amino acid residues was not secreted, but accumulated in the periplasm of the mutated *P. gingivalis* strain in its truncated form (Seers et al., 2006). A parallel study confirmed this observation, showing that the integrity of the CTD is essential for RgpB secretion, as even truncating the C-terminal by two residues hinders transport across the OM. The same effect is caused by mutating the highly conserved residues at the C-terminus of the CTD (Nguyen et al., 2007). The elegant follow-up investigations with CTDs from different *P. gingivalis* T9SS cargo proteins (HBP35/PG0616/PGN_0659, CPG70/PG0232/PGN_0335, P27/PG1795/no PGN, and RgpB) genetically fused to GFP found that GFP was secreted and post-translationally modified by *P. gingivalis* in the same way as the native T9SS cargos. The secretion/modification signal was narrowed down to the last 22 residues of the CTD domain (Shoji et al., 2011), and proteomic analysis revealed cleaved CTDs in the culture medium (Veith et al., 2013).

Taken together, these findings suggested the existence of a C-terminal-sorting peptidase responsible for the proteolytic removal of the CTD during the cargos' translocation across the OM. The postulated sortase was identified in *P. gingivalis* as PorU, a surface-located cysteine peptidase that shares significant sequence similarity with gingipains (see previous section; Glew et al., 2012). Analysis of the cleavage sites of T9SS cargos in *P. gingivalis* revealed a PorU preference toward polar or acidic amino acid residues (Ser, Thr, Asn, Asp) at the carbonyl site (P1′ position) and small amino acid residues (such as Gly, Ser, Ala) at the amide site (P1 position; Glew et al., 2012; Veith et al., 2013). This low specificity of PorU was confirmed when the amino acids surrounding the cleavage site (P1–P1′) in RgpB were mutated. Of note, this did not affect the secretion of the gingipain (Zhou et al., 2013).

Secretion Signal for T9SS Substrates Is Embedded in the Secondary Structure

Bioinformatic analysis of 21 fully sequenced genomes from the *Bacteroidetes* phylum revealed the presence of 663 predicted CTD-containing proteins (Veith et al., 2013). Alignment of the amino acid sequence of identified CTDs revealed up to five conserved sequential motifs (A–E) in different T9SS cargo proteins (Seers et al., 2006; Nguyen et al., 2007; Slakeski et al., 2011). Out of these, two sequential motifs, PxGxYVV and KxxxK, that reside in the last 22 amino acids of CTDs are the most conserved. This conservation is consistent with this fragment being sufficient for secretion in *P. gingivalis* (Shoji et al., 2011; Veith et al., 2013). Cumulatively, however, the limited sequence identity of CTDs suggests that the signal recognized by the T9SS machinery is not imprinted in the amino acid sequence but is formed by a specific fold of the CTD. This contention was confirmed by the atomic structure of the CTD from two *P. gingivalis* T9SS cargo proteins: RgpB and PorZ (de Diego et al., 2016; Lasica et al., 2016). Their CTDs consist of seven β-strands of similar length, generating a compact, sandwich-like fold typical of an immunoglobulin-superfamily (IgSF) domain. Analysis of the CTD of RgpB revealed a propensity of the protein to dimerize by swapping the last β-strand (de Diego et al., 2016). Of note, the last two β-strands overlap perfectly with the 22 amino acid residues essential for secretion of CTD proteins (Shoji et al., 2011). Despite the differences within the loops and the low amino acid sequence similarity, the PorZ-derived CTD structure is topologically equivalent to that of RgpB. This conclusion likely extends to the majority of identified CTDs, which share the fold of the IgSF domain. Therefore, the tertiary structure of the CTD, especially its two terminal β-strands, likely contains the signal recognized by the T9SS translocon (Lasica et al., 2016).

Secretion-Associated Modifications of T9SS Cargo Proteins

The characteristic feature of T9SS function is the retention of cargo proteins on the bacterial surface. SDS-PAGE analysis of OM-associated proteins produced diffuse bands about 20 kDa larger than that predicted from the primary structure of T9SS-secreted proteins (Veith et al., 2002). The difference is due to the presence of an A-LPS (Paramonov et al., 2005; Rangarajan et al., 2008) covalently attached to the cargo proteins imbedded into the OM, as indicated by western blot using specific antibodies (Abs). By contrast, the molecular mass of proteins accumulating in the periplasm of secretion mutants correlates well with the predicted molecular mass, and the proteins have no reactivity with anti-A-LPS Abs (Shoji et al., 2014). In addition, electron microscopy revealed that CTD-containing proteins (especially gingipains) form the electron-dense surface layer (EDSL) encapsulating *P. gingivalis* cells (Chen et al., 2011). Gorasia et al. (2015) found that the *wbaP* (PG1964/PGN_1896) mutant of *P. gingivalis*, which is defective in A-LPS synthesis, completely lacks the EDSL and releases T9SS cargos in soluble form into culture fluid. The proteins lack CTDs, suggesting normal PorU sortase activity, but are not A-LPS modified and therefore cannot be incorporated into the OM (Gorasia et al., 2015).

The mechanism of A-LPS attachment to CTD-containing proteins during secretion by T9SS is still unknown. The analysis of CTD proteins isolated from the growth media of the *wbaP* mutant revealed that peptides/amino acids derived from growth medium or glycine (if added in excess to the broth) were added to the proteins' C-termini via peptide bond. On the other hand, a 648 Da linker attached to C-termini by an isopeptide bond was identified in CTDs derived from the wild-type *P. gingivalis* strain (Gorasia et al., 2015). Such modification is reminiscent of a sortase-like mechanism of protein binding to peptidoglycan in Gram-positive bacteria. Sortases are cysteine proteases (C60 family) that have a catalytic Cys/His dyad, characteristic for many cysteine proteases, and possess a conserved Arg residue essential for sorting activity (Marraffini et al., 2004). This Arg is absent in gingipains, but is found in PorU sortase (Gorasia et al., 2015). All these findings suggest that PorU is a sortase, the first identified among Gram-negative bacteria. It cleaves the CTD and simultaneously attaches the A-LPS moiety to the newly generated C-terminus of a cargo protein via a linker of unknown structure. In this context, the T9SS mechanism resembles the covalent attachment of proteins to the cell wall in Gram-positive bacteria such as *S. aureus* (Schneewind and Missiakas, 2012).

REGULATION

Essential T9SS genes, including *porT*, *porV*, *sov*, *porP*, *porK*, *porL*, *porM*, and *porN*, are regulated at the transcriptional level by a signaling pathway composed of the PorXY two-component system (TCS) and an extracytoplasmic function (ECF) sigma factor (SigP/PG0162/PGN_0274; Kadowaki et al., 2016). In contrast to the majority of TCSs, in which the components are encoded within the same operon, the *porX* and *porY* genes occur at separate loci within the *P. gingivalis* chromosome. Despite this unusual genomic organization, the activation of the PorXY TCS is canonical. PorY has a modular architecture typical for a histidine kinase (HK) and undergoes autophosphorylation at His193, as shown by radiolabeled [^{32}P-γ]ATP. The phosphate group is then transferred to the conserved Asp58 residue in the receiver domain of PorX, which functions as the response regulator (RR). To compensate for the lack of a DNA-binding domain in the RR, PorX interacts with SigP, which directly binds the promotor regions of T9SS genes. The SigP protein level is very low in the *porX*-deletion mutant, suggesting a stabilizing function for PorX on SigP (Kadowaki et al., 2016). Disruption of the PorXY TCS results in the dysfunction of T9SS, which manifests as the decrease of Rgp and Kgp activity, as well as the impaired processing of gingipains (Sato et al., 2010).

PorX can also modulate the T9SS architecture directly by interacting with the cytoplasmic domain of PorL (Vincent et al., 2016). The N-terminal domain of PorX is similar to RRs belonging to the CheY family, which are involved in chemotaxis. After phosphorylation, the CheY protein binds to the C-ring of flagella, which changes the direction of flagellar movement (Roman et al., 1992; Sagi et al., 2003). Due to the fact that T9SS was proposed to be a rotary apparatus enabling the rotary movement of SprB adhesin in gliding bacteria (Shrivastava et al., 2015), it has been speculated that the PorX mechanism might be similar to that of CheY (Vincent et al., 2016). However, its role in *P. gingivalis* cells will likely be different as this bacterium is non-motile.

There are other studies reporting the changes in a T9SS protein's expression profile under specific circumstances. In a PorZ-deletion strain, some of the T9SS genes (including *porT*, *porV*, and *porN*), together with genes encoding CTD-cargo peptidases (RgpB, Kgp, and CPG70), are upregulated, whereas the expression of other T9SS genes (such as *porQ*, *porW*, *sov*, and *porU*) is not changed (Lasica et al., 2016). Additionally, the gliding motility protein GldN (orthologous of *P. gingivalis* PorN) of *Flavobacterium psychrophilum* is significantly upregulated under iron-limited growth conditions and *in vivo* (LaFrentz et al., 2009). The expression of T9SS proteins must be strictly regulated to fine-tune the energy-absorbing secretion of proteins into the environment. However, a precise environmental signal has not been identified and our knowledge about T9SS regulation is still limited.

PROTEIN EFFECTORS IN *P. gingivalis*

Only a few secretion systems are dedicated to carrying a single cargo protein; examples are HlyA in *E. coli* and HasA in *S. marcescens* for T1SS (Kanonenberg et al., 2013), and PulA in *K. oxytoca* and LT toxin in *E. coli* for T2SS (Rondelet and Condemine, 2013). The majority of secretion systems translocate many proteins of similar or diverse functions [e.g., T3SS; Gaytan et al., 2016]. In many respects, T9SS is one of the most robust secretion systems, which, in *P. gingivalis* alone, facilitates secretion of up to 35 cargos bearing the CTD (see **Table 2**), many of which are implicated in bacterial pathogenicity. In fact, experiments conducted to characterize the important virulence factors (the gingipains RgpA, RgpB, and Kgp) contributed to

TABLE 2 | T9SS cargo proteins.

Porphyromonas gingivalis[a]					
Locus Tag					
W83 NC_002950.2		**ATCC33277 NC_010729.1**	**Protein accession number**	**Protein description**	**References**
PG_RS00120	PG0026	PGN_0022	WP_005874469.1	PorU; surface C-terminal sortase	Glew et al., 2012; Veith et al., 2013; Gorasia et al., 2015
PG_RS00835	PG0182	PGN_0291	WP_010955943.1	Mfa5; VWA domain-containing protein [von Willebrand factor (vWF) type A domain]	Hasegawa et al., 2016
PG_RS00840	PG0183	no PGN	WP_043876389.1	Hypothetical protein containing VWA domain identical to that in PG0182 (circa 430 residues); lipoprotein	Found only by proteomic analysis[a]
PG_RS01060	PG0232	PGN_0335	WP_005873522.1	CPG70; zinc carboxypeptidase	Veith et al., 2004; Shoji et al., 2011; Zhou et al., 2013
PG_RS01560	PG0350	PGN_1611	WP_005873799.1	Internalin; hypothetical protein; leucine-rich repeats (x8)	Found only by proteomic analysis[a]
PG_RS01820	PG0410	no PGN	WP_005873803.1	Hypothetical gingipain-like peptidase C25	
PG_RS01825	PG0411	PGN_1556	WP_010956006.1	T9SS C-terminal target domain-containing protein	Found only by proteomic analysis[a]
PG_RS02195	PG0495	PGN_1476	WP_010956042.1	T9SS C-terminal target domain-containing protein	Found only by proteomic analysis[a]
PG_RS02240	PG0506	PGN_1466	WP_010956050.1	RgpB; arginine specific gingipain B, cysteine protease	Pike et al., 1994; Seers et al., 2006; Guo et al., 2010; de Diego et al., 2016
PG_RS02455	PG0553	PGN_1416	WP_010956068.1	PepK; lysine specific serine endopeptidase	Sato et al., 2013; Nonaka et al., 2014; Veith et al., 2014
PG_RS02700	PG0611	PGN_0654	WP_043876409.1	Hypothetical protein	Found only by proteomic analysis[a]
PG_RS02710	PG0614	PGN_0657	WP_005874506.1	Hypothetical protein	Found only by proteomic analysis[a]
PG_RS02720	PG0616	PGN_0659	WP_005874521.1	HBP35 (hemin binding protein 35)	Shoji et al., 2010, 2011
PG_RS02765	PG0626	no PGN	WP_005874512.1	T9SS C-terminal target domain-containing protein	Found only by proteomic analysis[a]
PG_RS02890	PG0654	PGN_0693	WP_005873571.1	T9SS C-terminal target domain-containing protein	Found only by proteomic analysis[a]; Glew et al., 2012
PG_RS03370	PG0769	PGN_0795	WP_010956121.1	Fibronectin; hypothetical protein[b]	Found only by proteomic analysis[a]; Sato et al., 2013
PG_RS03450	PG0787	PGN_0810	WP_005873930.1	T9SS C-terminal target domain-containing protein[c]	Found only by proteomic analysis[a]
PG_RS04535	PG1030	PGN_1321	WP_005874101.1	T9SS C-terminal target domain-containing protein	Found only by proteomic analysis[a]
PG_RS05835	PG1326	PGN_1115	WP_005875446.1	Hemagglutinin	Found only by proteomic analysis[a]
PG_RS06055	PG1374	PGN_0852	WP_005874331.1	T9SS C-terminal target domain-containing protein, leucine-rich repeats (x7)	Found only by proteomic analysis[a]; Glew et al., 2012
PG_RS06255	PG1424	PGN_0898	WP_005873463.1	PPAD; peptidylarginine deiminase	Sato et al., 2013; Koziel et al., 2014; Goulas et al., 2015
PG_RS06260	PG1427	PGN_0900	WP_005873781.1	Periodontain; peptidase C10; PrtT-related	Nelson et al., 1999
PG_RS06835	PG1548	PGN_0561	WP_043876505.1	PrtT; cystein protease (domain peptidase C10)	Madden et al., 1995; Gorasia et al., 2015
PG_RS07070	PG1604	PGN_0509	WP_010956350.1	PorZ; surface B-propeller protein	Lasica et al., 2016
PG_RS07920	PG1795	PGN_1770	WP_005874140.1	Hypothetical protein	Found only by proteomic analysis[a]
PG_RS07930	PG1798	PGN_1767	WP_005874135.1	T9SS C-terminal target domain-containing protein	Found only by proteomic analysis[a]
PG_RS08090	PG1837	PGN_1733	WP_043876452.1	HagA (hemagglutinin A, 8 HA domains)	Shi et al., 1999; Glew et al., 2012; Saiki and Konishi, 2014
PG_RS08105	PG1844	PGN_1728	WP_043876454.1	Kgp; lysine specific gingipain, cysteine protease	Pike et al., 1994; Veith et al., 2002
PG_RS08700	PG1969[d]	no PGN	WP_010956456.1	T9SS C-terminal target domain-containing protein	Found only by proteomic analysis[a]
PG_RS08940	PG2024	PGN_1970	WP_010956476.1	RgpA; arginine specific gingipain A; cysteine protease	Pike et al., 1994; Veith et al., 2002; Glew et al., 2012
PG_RS09310	PG2100	no PGN	WP_005873768.1	T9SS C-terminal target domain-containing protein; TapC	Kondo et al., 2010; Sato et al., 2013
PG_RS09320	PG2102	PGN_0152	WP_005873754.1	T9SS C-terminal target domain-containing protein; TapA	Kondo et al., 2010; Glew et al., 2012; Sato et al., 2013
PG_RS09640	PG2172	PGN_0123	WP_005874973.1	Hypothetical protein	Found only by proteomic analysis[a]; Glew et al., 2012
PG_RS09755	PG2198	PGN_2065	WP_005874281.1	Hypothetical protein; peptidase	Found only by proteomic analysis[a]

(Continued)

TABLE 2 | Continued

Porphyromonas gingivalis[a]				
Locus Tag				
W83 NC_002950.2	**ATCC33277 NC_010729.1**	**Protein accession number**	**Protein description**	**References**
PG_RS09850 PG2216	PGN_2080	WP_010956525.1	Hypothetical protein	Found only by proteomic analysis[a]; Glew et al., 2012
***Tannerella forsythia* ATCC43037**				
Tanf_03370		WP_046824918.1	TfsA (surface layer protein A), classical CTD	Tomek et al., 2014
Tanf_03375		WP_046824919.1	TfsB (surface layer protein B), classical CTD	Tomek et al., 2014
Tanf_04820		WP_046825062.1	BspA, cell surface antigen, leucine rich protein, classical CTD	Veith et al., 2009; Friedrich et al., 2015
Tanf_06225		WP_046825275.1	Forsilysin, metalloprotease, KLIKK-type CTD	Narita et al., 2014
Tanf_00450		WP_070098098.1	Mirolysin, metalloprotease, KLIKK-type CTD	Karim et al., 2010; Ksiazek et al., 2015a,b; Koneru et al., 2017
Tanf_06550		D0EM77.2	Karilysin, metalloprotease, KLIKK-type CTD	Karim et al., 2010; Narita et al., 2014; Ksiazek et al., 2015a; Koneru et al., 2017
Tanf_00440		AIZ49398.1	Mirolase, serine protease, KLIKK-type CTD	Karim et al., 2010; Ksiazek et al., 2015a,b; Koneru et al., 2017
Tanf_09450, Tanf_06530 (not merged in one contig)		AKG97061.1	Miropsin-1, serine protease, KLIKK-type CTD	Ksiazek et al., 2015b
Tanf_06530		WP_046825306.1	Miropsin-2, serine protease KLIKK-type CTD	Narita et al., 2014
***F. johnsoniae* UW101**[e]				
Fjoh_4555		WP_012026520.1	ChiA, chitinase	Rhodes et al., 2010; Kharade and McBride, 2014
Fjoh_0979		WP_012023065.1	SprB, surface adhesin, necessary for gliding motility	Rhodes et al., 2010; Shrivastava et al., 2013
Fjoh_0808		WP_052295174.1	RemA, mobile surface adhesin, necessary for gliding motility	Shrivastava et al., 2012, 2013

[a] *All P. gingivalis cargo proteins excluding PG0410 (no PGN) and PG1548 (PGN_0561) were originally found by Veith et al. (2013).*

[b] *PG0769 (PGN_0795) processing is unclear. Protein is devoid of N-terminal cleavage signal for periplasm transport (searched with SignalP and LipoP servers) as well as T9SS CTD domain.*

[c] *PG0787 (PGN_0810) is a very small peptide (80 aa) devoid of N-terminal cleavage signal for periplasm transport (searched in SignalP and LipoP servers), however its last 66 aa constitute a classical T9SS CTD domain.*

[d] *PG1969 processing is unclear. Protein is devoid of N-terminal cleavage signal for periplasm transport (searched with SignalP and LipoP servers) but contains T9SS CTD domain.*

[e] *Proteins listed are the best studied among other identified T9SS cargos of F. johnsoniae. For more information please see Kharade and McBride (2015).*

the discovery of T9SS. Below, we briefly describe only the most important cargos from the point of view of *P. gingivalis* virulence. References to other cargo proteins can be found in **Table 2**.

Gingipains and CPG70

There are three enzymes collectively termed gingipains: RgpA (PG2024/PGN_1970), RgpB (PG0506/PGN_1466), and Kgp (PG1844/PGN_1728). They are cysteine proteases that hydrolyze peptide bonds at the carboxyl group of arginine (RgpA/B: Arg–Xaa) or lysine residues (Kgp: Lys–Xaa; Pike et al., 1994). They are exported into the periplasm as inactive zymogens, with the N-terminal prodomain (NTP) functioning as a chaperone and maintaining the latency of the proteases (Mikolajczyk et al., 2003; Pomowski et al., 2017). After folding in the periplasm, they are transported to the bacterial surface, where they are subjected to extensive post-translational processing. The CTD is cleaved by PorU sortase during translocation, with the concomitant covalent attachment of A-LPS via an isopeptide bond to the newly formed carbonyl group (Glew et al., 2012; Gorasia et al., 2015). Then, the OM-anchored gingipains activate themselves by cleaving off the NTP. For RgpB, this is the end of processing, but the polypeptide chains of RgpA and Kgp are further fragmented to form a large, non-covalent complex of catalytic and hemagglutinin domains on the bacterial surface (Bhogal et al., 1997; Veith et al., 2002; Sztukowska et al., 2012). The activation and further processing are still not well-understood, and, in addition to trans- and cis-autoproteolysis, they also involve the removal of the C-terminal Arg and Lys residues by the Arg/Lys-specific carboxypeptidase CPG70 (PG0232/PGN_0335; Chen et al., 2002). Interestingly, CPG70 is a T9SS substrate itself (Veith et al., 2004; Zhou et al., 2013). Of note, the retention of gingipains, CPG70, and other T9SS cargos on the bacterial surface depends on the synthesis of A-LPS. The *P. gingivalis* strain HG66, which lacks the activity of an enzyme in the A-LPS synthesis pathway, secretes soluble gingipains into the media (Pike et al., 1994; Shoji et al., 2014; Siddiqui et al., 2014).

Gingipains are the most powerful weapon within the *P. gingivalis* arsenal of virulence factors, as they are responsible for nearly 85% of the total proteolytic activity (Potempa et al.,

1997). They are responsible for a variety of pathogenic functions such as colonization, nutrition, neutralization of host defenses, and alteration of the inflammatory response, which all lead to massive oral tissue destruction called periodontitis during prolonged infection (reviewed in Guo et al., 2010; Bostanci and Belibasakis, 2012; Hajishengallis, 2015). However, gingipains are not only directed against host proteins, but are also involved in processing other *P. gingivalis* proteins [e.g., long fimbriae (FimA)] (Nakayama et al., 1996; Xu et al., 2016). Interestingly, gingipains' activities rely on their local concentration, resulting in either activation of some pathways at low concentrations (specifically human complement) or destroying them upon accumulation (Krauss et al., 2010). Moreover, despite the cleavage specificity to a single C-terminal Arg or Lys residue, they can act in a precise and fastidious manner or as unlimited shredders (Potempa et al., 2000; Sroka et al., 2001; Goulet et al., 2004).

Considering the broad range of activities combined with cell surface localization, it is not surprising that gingipains are a tempting target for designing periodontitis treatments as well as preventive strategies (inhibitors and vaccines; Olsen and Potempa, 2014; Inaba et al., 2016; Wilensky et al., 2016).

Porphyromonas Peptidylarginine Deiminase (PPAD)

Porphyromonas peptidylarginine deiminase (PPAD), encoded by PG1424/PGN_0898, is a unique enzyme among prokaryotes. It is the first and only bacterial peptidylarginine deiminase (PAD) identified, and, moreover, its presence is limited to a single species: *P. gingivalis* (McGraw et al., 1999; Gabarrini et al., 2015).

PADs are well-described eukaryotic enzymes functioning in vertebrates as post-translational modifiers of proteins. Specifically, they citrullinate internal arginine residues, which changes the fold, function, and half-life of proteins and peptides (Vossenaar et al., 2003; Gyorgy et al., 2006). Dysregulation of this process, particularly the accumulation of citrullinated proteins, leads to inflammatory disorders and has been associated with numerous diseases such as Alzheimer's disease, multiple sclerosis, psoriasis, fibrosis, cancer, and rheumatoid arthritis (RA) (Vossenaar et al., 2003; Chang and Han, 2006; Baka et al., 2012; Gudmann et al., 2015). The latter develops through an autoimmune response against citrullinated proteins and is enhanced by a combination of environmental and genetic factors (MacGregor et al., 2000; McInnes and Schett, 2011). Currently, periodontal disease is an acknowledged RA risk factor, and the discovery of PPAD uncovered a missing mechanistic link between the two illnesses (Wegner et al., 2010; Koziel et al., 2014; Quirke et al., 2015; Laugisch et al., 2016).

PPAD was identified as a T9SS substrate through proteomics studies of a *porT* mutant (Sato et al., 2013); however, the enzyme was characterized mostly in relation to its function rather than secretion. It citrullinates C-terminal arginine residues in a calcium-independent manner, whereas eukaryotic PADs are Ca^{2+}-dependent (Takahara et al., 1986; McGraw et al., 1999; Abdallah et al., 2007; Wegner et al., 2010; Bielecka et al., 2014). Moreover, the C-terminal specificity of PPAD plays into the cleavage activities of RgpA/B (after Arg), which greatly enlarge the pool of citrullinated substrates from both bacterial and host origins as gingipains cleave numerous human proteins (Guo et al., 2010). Gingipain-null mutants (RgpA/B) are almost devoid of endogenous citrullination (Wegner et al., 2010). Furthermore, even the presence of PPAD (not only its activity) may elevate anti-citrullination immune responses, as it undergoes autocitrullination. Only this form triggers specific Abs in mice and was recognized by RA patients' sera (reviewed in Koziel et al., 2014).

Analysis of PPAD structure revealed that the enzyme is composed of four elements: a profragment, a catalytic domain (CD), an IgSF domain, and a CTD, resembling domains observed in gingipains. The CD has a flat 5-fold α/β-propeller architecture and includes a catalytic triad (C^{351}-H^{236}-N^{297}) also conserved in human PADs (Goulas et al., 2015; Montgomery et al., 2016). The crystal structure of substrate-free and substrate-bound forms confirmed that PPAD is efficient in accommodating and processing C-terminally situated Arg residues regardless of total chain length (peptide or protein; Goulas et al., 2015).

The surface location of PPAD and the availability of its detailed structure, combined with its important role in two prevalent human diseases (periodontitis and RA), should make PPAD a good target for therapeutic strategies; however, no such experiments have been reported.

T9SS IN *T. forsythia*

The mechanism of protein secretion by T9SS was mostly studied in *P. gingivalis* and gliding bacteria. Apart from a different subset of secreted proteins reflecting bacterial habitats, the mechanism of action is the same. Briefly, T9SS cargo proteins are directed to the T9SS machinery by the CTD, which is removed during secretion. Then, secreted proteins may be modified and attached to the surface by A-LPS (*P. gingivalis*), stay associated with the cell through polysaccharides, or be released (gliding bacteria; McBride and Nakane, 2015; Nakayama, 2015). However, analysis of T9SS in another member of the red complex, *T. forsythia*, revealed some interesting differences.

T. forsythia is covered with a two-dimensional crystalline surface (S-) layer that is thought to function as a protective coat, working as an external sieve and ion trap (Sleytr and Beveridge, 1999; Messner et al., 2010). It also mediates adhesion and subsequent invasion into human gingival epithelial cells (Sakakibara et al., 2007) and delays recognition of the bacterium by the host innate immune system (Sekot et al., 2012). The S-layer is composed of the glycosylated proteins TfsA (Tanf_03370) and TfsB (Tanf_03375). Deleting *porU* (Tanf_02580), *porT* (Tanf_10520), *sov* (Tanf_04410), or *porK* (Tanf_02360) results in the lack of an S-layer, which can be observed by transmission electron microscope (Narita et al., 2014; Tomek et al., 2014). In those mutants, both components of the S-layer are trapped within the periplasm, but, unlike in *P. gingivalis*, they are modified by O-glycosylation through the addition of multiple copies of a complex oligosaccharide using a general glycosylation pathway operating in *Bacteroidetes* (Coyne et al., 2013; Posch et al., 2013;

Tomek et al., 2014). Nevertheless, TfsA and TfsB trapped in the periplasm are much smaller than both proteins in the wild-type cells, indicating that, upon secretion, both proteins are modified by a second glycan attachment in a manner different than O-glycosylation. It is speculated that, as in *P. gingivalis*, it could be a variant of LPS (Tomek et al., 2014).

T9SS cargo proteins in *T. forsythia* have two different types of CTD. The "classical" CTD associated with proteins from other *Bacteroidetes* species is found in TfsA, TfsB, and leucine rich protein BspA (Veith et al., 2009; Tomek et al., 2014). By contrast, a family of six proteases, three metalloproteases (karilysin, mirolysin, and forsilysin) and three serine proteases (mirolase, miropsin-1, and miropsin-2), bear a nearly identical CTD that shares very limited sequence similarity with the classical CTD. Because these six CTDs end with a KLIKK sequential motif, the enzymes are referred to as KLIKK proteases (Ksiazek et al., 2015b). The KLIKK proteases possess a unique structure and undergo extensive autoproteolytic processing (Cerda-Costa et al., 2011; Lopez-Pelegrin et al., 2015). Their activities, such as degrading complement proteins and LL-37 (the crucial antimicrobial peptide in the human oral cavity), may contribute to *T. forsythia* virulence through evading innate immunity (Jusko et al., 2015; Koneru et al., 2017).

In stark contrast to the other CTD proteins of *T. forsythia*, KLIKK proteases seem to be secreted directly into the extracellular medium, as shown for miropsin-2 (Tanf_06530), karilysin (Tanf_06550), and forsilysin (Tanf_06225) (Narita et al., 2014). Supporting this, proteomic analysis of the *T. forsythia* OM identified 13 of 26 proteins bearing the classical CTD, including TfsA, TfsB, and BspA (Tanf_04820), but none of the KLIKK proteases (Veith et al., 2009). Conversely, four KLIKK proteases, forsilysin, miropsin-2 (Friedrich et al., 2015), mirolase (Tanf_00440), and karilysin (Veith et al., 2015), were found in outer membrane vesicles (OMVs), although with a low Mascot score. This discrepancy could be explained by the transient presence of these proteases in the periplasm before they enter the OM translocon of T9SS. Interestingly, all three of the KLIKK proteases characterized thus far (karilysin, mirolase, and mirolysin) can remove the CTD during autoprocessing (Karim et al., 2010; Ksiazek et al., 2015a; Koneru et al., 2017). Collectively, the available data suggest that the KLIKK proteases are secreted into the extracellular milieu without removal of the CTD. This finding is similar to the secretion of PorU and PorZ from *P. gingivalis*, where the CTD is also not removed during secretion, although proteins stay associated with the cell surface (Lasica et al., 2016).

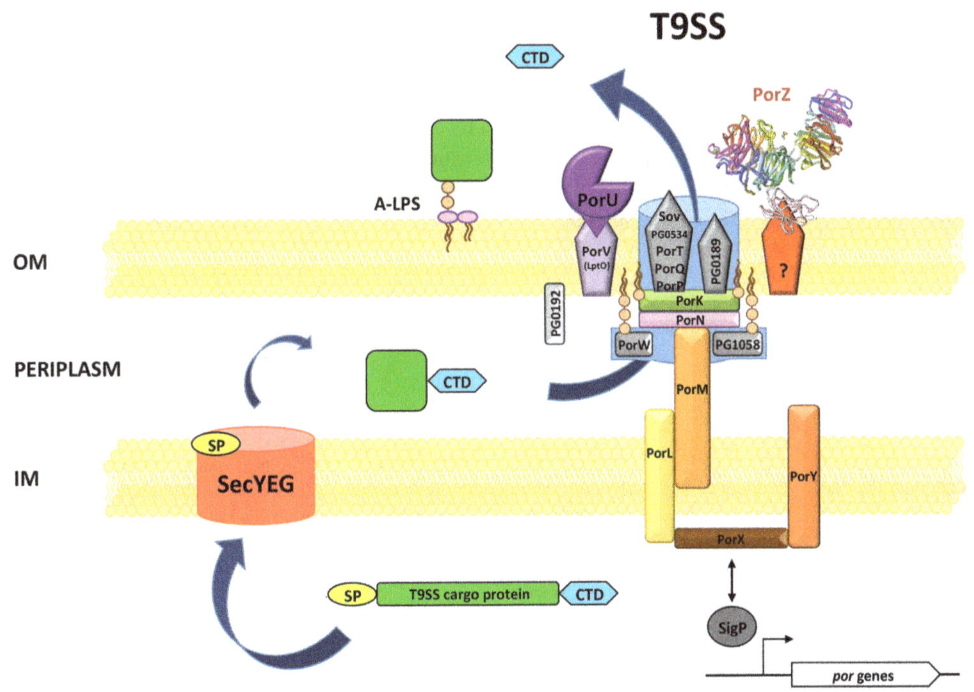

FIGURE 3 | Hypothetical model of the structure and function of *P. gingivalis* T9SS. The overall translocon structure and the protein(s) forming a pore in the OM (outer membrane) have not yet been characterized. Therefore, it is shown as a background blue shape accommodating known components. Interacting proteins are situated in close proximity. OM β-barrel proteins are depicted as pentagons. PorZ is presently the only T9SS protein with the known atomic structure. The mode of its association with the translocon is not yet defined. PorK, PorW, and PG1058 are lipoproteins anchored into the inner surface of the OM. PG0192 protein precise localization and possible interactions are not known. A T9SS cargo protein is equipped with two sorting signals: N-terminal signal peptide (SP) directing the protein to the general secretion system SecYEG and conserved C-terminal domain (CTD) recognized by T9SS. After translocation through the IM (inner membrane) most proteins acquire their proper fold in the periplasm. Next, CTD directs the protein for further translocation across the OM through T9SS. Finally, CTD is cleaved off by PorU sortase and a secreted protein is modified by attachment of A-LPS resulting in the anchorage of cargo protein to the cell surface. Two component system PorX/PorY and sigma factor SigP have regulatory effect on *por* genes. Although, they are not physical elements of T9SS, PorX was shown *in vitro* to interact with PorL.

CONCLUDING REMARKS

In this review, we summarized the biochemical and structural data concerning the recently discovered T9SS identified in a majority of the bacterial species belonging to the *Bacteroidetes* phylum (Sato et al., 2010; McBride and Zhu, 2013). The system has been investigated predominantly in human oral pathogens, such as *P. gingivalis* and *T. forsythia*, and environmental saprophytes, such as *F. johnsoniae* and *C. hutchinsonii*. It seems to be a major mechanism of protein secretion in these bacteria however, some families from *Bacteroidetes* were reported to possess other secretion systems e.g., T1SS or T6SS (Russell et al., 2014; Wilson et al., 2015; Abby et al., 2016; Chatzidaki-Livanis et al., 2016; Wexler et al., 2016; Ibrahim et al., 2017). Notably, both systems allow for direct substrate translocation from bacterial cytoplasm to the cell exterior, while T9SS cargos do not omit the periplasmic space during their secretion.

The role of T9SS is to ensure cell survival and fitness in response to the microorganisms' habitat by providing transportation of proteins necessary for, among other things, virulence, nutrition, and movement (gliding motility). Hence, the variety of secreted proteins even within a single species is large and comprises numerous adhesins and hydrolytic enzymes used for attachment and degradation of large organic compounds such as proteins, cellulose, and chitin (Guo et al., 2010; McBride and Nakane, 2015).

The cargo proteins of this system (**Table 2**) are equipped with the classical signal peptide for Sec-dependent translocation to the IM and the conserved CTD that directs them further to the secretion machinery in the OM. The recognition signal is mostly embedded within the IgSF-like tertiary structure of the CTD (de Diego et al., 2016; Lasica et al., 2016) and likely located within the 22 amino acid residues composing the sequential motifs of PxGxYVV and KxxxK in the two most C-terminal β-strands (Shoji et al., 2011; Veith et al., 2013).

Currently, for *P. gingivalis* cells, there are 16 proteins recognized as the structural and/or functional components of the translocon and two additional elements involved in T9SS regulation (**Table 1**). None of these proteins are fully characterized, so their structure, mode of reciprocal interactions, and precise roles in secretion are still obscure. Nevertheless, a contemporary general concept of T9SS structure and function based on available data is presented in **Figure 3**. Verification of this model requires extensive structural and functional investigations to elucidate the mechanism of CTD recognition and cleavage, passage of cargos though the OM translocon, attachment of a glucan moiety, and anchoring of cargos onto the cell surface, their release into the environment, or their assembly into gliding motility machinery.

AUTHOR CONTRIBUTIONS

AL analyzed literature, wrote the paper (excluding MK and MM sections), prepared the figures and tables. MK wrote the Mechanism of secretion and T9SS *T. forsythia* sections. MM wrote the Regulation section. JP edited the manuscript. All authors read and approved the full manuscript.

FUNDING

This work was supported by National Science Centre (NCN)—2012/04/A/NZ1/00051 to JP and UMO-2015/19/N/NZ1/00322 to MM; Polish Ministry of Science and Higher Education—1306/MOB/IV/2015/0 (Mobilnosc Plus) to MK and K/DSC/003690 to MM and National Institutes of Health (NIH)—DE 022597 to AL and JP.

REFERENCES

Abaibou, H., Chen, Z., Olango, G. J., Liu, Y., Edwards, J., and Fletcher, H. M. (2001). vimA gene downstream of recA is involved in virulence modulation in *Porphyromonas gingivalis* W83. *Infect. Immun.* 69, 325–335. doi: 10.1128/IAI.69.1.325-335.2001

Abby, S. S., Cury, J., Guglielmini, J., Neron, B., Touchon, M., and Rocha, E. P. (2016). Identification of protein secretion systems in bacterial genomes. *Sci. Rep.* 6:23080. doi: 10.1038/srep23080

Abdallah, A. M., Gey van Pittius, N. C., Champion, P. A., Cox, J., Luirink, J., Vandenbroucke-Grauls, C. M., et al. (2007). Type VII secretion–mycobacteria show the way. *Nat. Rev. Microbiol.* 5, 883–891. doi: 10.1038/nrmicro1773

Baka, Z., Gyorgy, B., Geher, P., Buzas, E. I., Falus, A., and Nagy, G. (2012). Citrullination under physiological and pathological conditions. *Joint Bone Spine* 79, 431–436. doi: 10.1016/j.jbspin.2012.01.008

Benedyk, M., Mydel, P. M., Delaleu, N., Plaza, K., Gawron, K., Milewska, A., et al. (2016). Gingipains: critical factors in the development of aspiration pneumonia caused by *Porphyromonas gingivalis*. *J. Innate Immun.* 8, 185–198. doi: 10.1159/000441724

Berks, B. C. (2015). The twin-arginine protein translocation pathway. *Annu. Rev. Biochem.* 84, 843–864. doi: 10.1146/annurev-biochem-060614-034251

Bhogal, P. S., Slakeski, N., and Reynolds, E. C. (1997). A cell-associated protein complex of *Porphyromonas gingivalis* W50 composed of Arg- and Lys-specific cysteine proteinases and adhesins. *Microbiology* 143(Pt 7), 2485–2495. doi: 10.1099/00221287-143-7-2485

Bielecka, E., Scavenius, C., Kantyka, T., Jusko, M., Mizgalska, D., Szmigielski, B., et al. (2014). Peptidyl arginine deiminase from *Porphyromonas gingivalis* abolishes anaphylatoxin C5a activity. *J. Biol. Chem.* 289, 32481–32487. doi: 10.1074/jbc.C114.617142

Bostanci, N., and Belibasakis, G. N. (2012). *Porphyromonas gingivalis*: an invasive and evasive opportunistic oral pathogen. *FEMS Microbiol. Lett.* 333, 1–9. doi: 10.1111/j.1574-6968.2012.02579.x

Cerda-Costa, N., Guevara, T., Karim, A. Y., Ksiazek, M., Nguyen, K. A., Arolas, J. L., et al. (2011). The structure of the catalytic domain of *Tannerella forsythia* karilysin reveals it is a bacterial xenologue of animal matrix metalloproteinases. *Mol. Microbiol.* 79, 119–132. doi: 10.1111/j.1365-2958.2010.07434.x

Chang, X., and Han, J. (2006). Expression of peptidylarginine deiminase type 4 (PAD4) in various tumors. *Mol. Carcinog.* 45, 183–196. doi: 10.1002/mc.20169

Chatzidaki-Livanis, M., Geva-Zatorsky, N., and Comstock, L. E. (2016). Bacteroides fragilis type VI secretion systems use novel effector and immunity proteins to antagonize human gut Bacteroidales species. *Proc. Natl. Acad. Sci. U.S.A.* 113, 3627–3632. doi: 10.1073/pnas.1522510113

Chen, T., Dong, H., Yong, R., and Duncan, M. J. (2000). Pleiotropic pigmentation mutants of *Porphyromonas gingivalis*. *Microb. Pathog.* 28, 235–247. doi: 10.1006/mpat.1999.0338

Chen, Y. Y., Cross, K. J., Paolini, R. A., Fielding, J. E., Slakeski, N., and Reynolds, E. C. (2002). CPG70 is a novel basic metallocarboxypeptidase with C-terminal polycystic kidney disease domains from *Porphyromonas gingivalis*. *J. Biol. Chem.* 277, 23433–23440. doi: 10.1074/jbc.M200811200

Chen, Y. Y., Peng, B., Yang, Q., Glew, M. D., Veith, P. D., Cross, K. J., et al. (2011). The outer membrane protein LptO is essential for the O-deacylation of LPS and the co-ordinated secretion and attachment of A-LPS and CTD proteins in *Porphyromonas gingivalis*. *Mol. Microbiol.* 79, 1380–1401. doi: 10.1111/j.1365-2958.2010.07530.x

Cobessi, D., Celia, H., and Pattus, F. (2005). Crystal structure at high resolution of ferric-pyochelin and its membrane receptor FptA from *Pseudomonas aeruginosa*. *J. Mol. Biol.* 352, 893–904. doi: 10.1016/j.jmb.2005.08.004

Costa, T. R., Felisberto-Rodrigues, C., Meir, A., Prevost, M. S., Redzej, A., Trokter, M., et al. (2015). Secretion systems in Gram-negative bacteria: structural and mechanistic insights. *Nat. Rev. Microbiol.* 13, 343–359. doi: 10.1038/nrmicro3456

Coyne, M. J., Fletcher, C. M., Chatzidaki-Livanis, M., Posch, G., Schaffer, C., and Comstock, L. E. (2013). Phylum-wide general protein O-glycosylation system of the Bacteroidetes. *Mol. Microbiol.* 88, 772–783. doi: 10.1111/mmi.12220

Curtis, M. A., Kuramitsu, H. K., Lantz, M., Macrina, F. L., Nakayama, K., Potempa, J., et al. (1999). Molecular genetics and nomenclature of proteases of *Porphyromonas gingivalis*. *J. Periodont. Res.* 34, 464–472. doi: 10.1111/j.1600-0765.1999.tb02282.x

Dam, P., Olman, V., Harris, K., Su, Z., and Xu, Y. (2007). Operon prediction using both genome-specific and general genomic information. *Nucleic Acids Res.* 35, 288–298. doi: 10.1093/nar/gkl1018

de Diego, I., Ksiazek, M., Mizgalska, D., Koneru, L., Golik, P., Szmigielski, B., et al. (2016). The outer-membrane export signal of *Porphyromonas gingivalis* type IX secretion system (T9SS) is a conserved C-terminal β-sandwich domain. *Sci. Rep.* 6:23123. doi: 10.1038/srep23123

Denks, K., Vogt, A., Sachelaru, I., Petriman, N. A., Kudva, R., and Koch, H. G. (2014). The Sec translocon mediated protein transport in prokaryotes and eukaryotes. *Mol. Membr. Biol.* 31, 58–84. doi: 10.3109/09687688.2014.907455

Desvaux, M., Hebraud, M., Talon, R., and Henderson, I. R. (2009). Secretion and subcellular localizations of bacterial proteins: a semantic awareness issue. *Trends Microbiol.* 17, 139–145. doi: 10.1016/j.tim.2009.01.004

Friedrich, V., Gruber, C., Nimeth, I., Pabinger, S., Sekot, G., Posch, G., et al. (2015). Outer membrane vesicles of *Tannerella forsythia*: biogenesis, composition, and virulence. *Mol. Oral Microbiol.* 30, 451–473. doi: 10.1111/omi.12104

Gabarrini, G., de Smit, M., Westra, J., Brouwer, E., Vissink, A., Zhou, K., et al. (2015). The peptidylarginine deiminase gene is a conserved feature of *Porphyromonas gingivalis*. *Sci. Rep.* 5:13936. doi: 10.1038/srep13936

Gao, S., Li, S., Ma, Z., Liang, S., Shan, T., Zhang, M., et al. (2016). Presence of *Porphyromonas gingivalis* in esophagus and its association with the clinicopathological characteristics and survival in patients with esophageal cancer. *Infect. Agents Cancer* 11, 3. doi: 10.1186/s13027-016-0049-x

Gaytan, M. O., Martinez-Santos, V. I., Soto, E., and Gonzalez-Pedrajo, B. (2016). Type three secretion system in attaching and effacing pathogens. *Front. Cell. Infect. Microbiol.* 6:129. doi: 10.3389/fcimb.2016.00129

Genco, C. A., Simpson, W., Forng, R. Y., Egal, M., and Odusanya, B. M. (1995). Characterization of a Tn4351-generated hemin uptake mutant of *Porphyromonas gingivalis*: evidence for the coordinate regulation of virulence factors by hemin. *Infect. Immun.* 63, 2459–2466.

Gerlach, R. G., and Hensel, M. (2007). Protein secretion systems and adhesins: the molecular armory of Gram-negative pathogens. *Int. J. Med. Microbiol.* 297, 401–415. doi: 10.1016/j.ijmm.2007.03.017

Glew, M. D., Veith, P. D., Chen, D., Seers, C. A., Chen, Y. Y., and Reynolds, E. C. (2014). Blue native-PAGE analysis of membrane protein complexes in *Porphyromonas gingivalis*. *J. Proteomics* 110, 72–92. doi: 10.1016/j.jprot.2014.07.033

Glew, M. D., Veith, P. D., Peng, B., Chen, Y. Y., Gorasia, D. G., Yang, Q., et al. (2012). PG0026 is the C-terminal signal peptidase of a novel secretion system of *Porphyromonas gingivalis*. *J. Biol. Chem.* 287, 24605–24617. doi: 10.1074/jbc.M112.369223

Goebel, W., and Hedgpeth, J. (1982). Cloning and functional characterization of the plasmid-encoded hemolysin determinant of *Escherichia coli*. *J. Bacteriol.* 151, 1290–1298.

Gorasia, D. G., Veith, P. D., Chen, D., Seers, C. A., Mitchell, H. A., Chen, Y. Y., et al. (2015). *Porphyromonas gingivalis* Type IX Secretion substrates are cleaved and modified by a sortase-like mechanism. *PLoS Pathog.* 11:e1005152. doi: 10.1371/journal.ppat.1005152

Gorasia, D. G., Veith, P. D., Hanssen, E. G., Glew, M. D., Sato, K., Yukitake, H., et al. (2016). Structural insights into the PorK and PorN components of the *Porphyromonas gingivalis* Type IX secretion system. *PLoS Pathog.* 12:e1005820. doi: 10.1371/journal.ppat.1005820

Goulas, T., Mizgalska, D., Garcia-Ferrer, I., Kantyka, T., Guevara, T., Szmigielski, B., et al. (2015). Structure and mechanism of a bacterial host-protein citrullinating virulence factor, *Porphyromonas gingivalis* peptidylarginine deiminase. *Sci. Rep.* 5:11969. doi: 10.1038/srep11969

Goulet, V., Britigan, B., Nakayama, K., and Grenier, D. (2004). Cleavage of human transferrin by *Porphyromonas gingivalis* gingipains promotes growth and formation of hydroxyl radicals. *Infect. Immun.* 72, 4351–4356. doi: 10.1128/IAI.72.8.4351-4356.2004

Goyal, P., Krasteva, P. V., Van Gerven, N., Gubellini, F., Van den Broeck, I., Troupiotis-Tsailaki, A., et al. (2014). Structural and mechanistic insights into the bacterial amyloid secretion channel CsgG. *Nature* 516, 250–253. doi: 10.1038/nature13768

Gudmann, N. S., Hansen, N. U., Jensen, A. C., Karsdal, M. A., and Siebuhr, A. S. (2015). Biological relevance of citrullinations: diagnostic, prognostic and therapeutic options. *Autoimmunity* 48, 73–79. doi: 10.3109/08916934.2014.962024

Guo, Y., Nguyen, K. A., and Potempa, J. (2010). Dichotomy of gingipains action as virulence factors: from cleaving substrates with the precision of a surgeon's knife to a meat chopper-like brutal degradation of proteins. *Periodontol. 2000* 54, 15–44. doi: 10.1111/j.1600-0757.2010.00377.x

Gyorgy, B., Toth, E., Tarcsa, E., Falus, A., and Buzas, E. I. (2006). Citrullination: a posttranslational modification in health and disease. *Int. J. Biochem. Cell Biol.* 38, 1662–1677. doi: 10.1016/j.biocel.2006.03.008

Hachani, A., Wood, T. E., and Filloux, A. (2016). Type VI secretion and anti-host effectors. *Curr. Opin. Microbiol.* 29, 81–93. doi: 10.1016/j.mib.2015.11.006

Hajishengallis, G. (2015). Periodontitis: from microbial immune subversion to systemic inflammation. *Nat. Rev. Immunol.* 15, 30–44. doi: 10.1038/nri3785

Hasegawa, Y., Iijima, Y., Persson, K., Nagano, K., Yoshida, Y., Lamont, R. J., et al. (2016). Role of Mfa5 in expression of Mfa1 fimbriae in *Porphyromonas gingivalis*. *J. Dent. Res.* 95, 1291–1297. doi: 10.1177/0022034516655083

Heath, J. E., Seers, C. A., Veith, P. D., Butler, C. A., Nor Muhammad, N. A., Chen, Y. Y., et al. (2016). PG1058 is a novel multidomain protein component of the bacterial Type IX secretion system. *PLoS ONE* 11:e0164313. doi: 10.1371/journal.pone.0164313

Henke, J. M., and Bassler, B. L. (2004). Quorum sensing regulates type III secretion in *Vibrio harveyi* and *Vibrio parahaemolyticus*. *J. Bacteriol.* 186, 3794–3805. doi: 10.1128/JB.186.12.3794-3805.2004

Hoover, C. I., and Yoshimura, F. (1994). Transposon-induced pigment-deficient mutants of *Porphyromonas gingivalis*. *FEMS Microbiol. Lett.* 124, 43–48. doi: 10.1111/j.1574-6968.1994.tb07259.x

Hunt, L. T., Barker, W. C., and Chen, H. R. (1987). A domain structure common to hemopexin, vitronectin, interstitial collagenase, and a collagenase homolog. *Protein Seq. Data Anal.* 1, 21–26.

Hutcheon, G. W., and Bolhuis, A. (2003). The archaeal twin-arginine translocation pathway. *Biochem. Soc. Trans.* 31(Pt 3), 686–689. doi: 10.1042/bst0310686

Ibrahim, M., Subramanian, A., and Anishetty, S. (2017). Comparative pan genome analysis of oral *Prevotella* species implicated in periodontitis. *Funct. Integr. Genomics.* doi: 10.1007/s10142-017-0550-3. [Epub ahead of print]. Available online at: http://link.springer.com/journal/10142/onlineFirst/page/1

Inaba, H., Tagashira, M., Kanda, T., Murakami, Y., Amano, A., and Matsumoto-Nakano, M. (2016). Apple- and Hop-polyphenols inhibit *Porphyromonas gingivalis*-mediated precursor of matrix metalloproteinase-9 activation and invasion of oral squamous cell carcinoma cells. *J. Periodontol.* 87, 1103–1111. doi: 10.1902/jop.2016.160047

Ishiguro, I., Saiki, K., and Konishi, K. (2009). PG27 is a novel membrane protein essential for a *Porphyromonas gingivalis* protease secretion system. *FEMS Microbiol. Lett.* 292, 261–267. doi: 10.1111/j.1574-6968.2009.01489.x

Jarrell, K. F., and McBride, M. J. (2008). The surprisingly diverse ways that prokaryotes move. *Nat. Rev. Microbiol.* 6, 466–476. doi: 10.1038/nrmicro1900

Jusko, M., Potempa, J., Mizgalska, D., Bielecka, E., Ksiazek, M., Riesbeck, K., et al. (2015). A metalloproteinase mirolysin of tannerella forsythia inhibits all pathways of the complement system. *J. Immunol.* 195, 2231–2240. doi: 10.4049/jimmunol.1402892

Kadowaki, T., Yukitake, H., Naito, M., Sato, K., Kikuchi, Y., Kondo, Y., et al. (2016). A two-component system regulates gene expression of the type IX secretion component proteins via an ECF sigma factor. *Sci. Rep.* 6:23288. doi: 10.1038/srep23288

Kallberg, M., Wang, H., Wang, S., Peng, J., Wang, Z., Lu, H., et al. (2012). Template-based protein structure modeling using the RaptorX web server. *Nat. Protoc.* 7, 1511–1522. doi: 10.1038/nprot.2012.085

Kanonenberg, K., Schwarz, C. K., and Schmitt, L. (2013). Type I secretion systems - a story of appendices. *Res. Microbiol.* 164, 596–604. doi: 10.1016/j.resmic.2013.03.011

Karim, A. Y., Kulczycka, M., Kantyka, T., Dubin, G., Jabaiah, A., Daugherty, P. S., et al. (2010). A novel matrix metalloprotease-like enzyme (karilysin) of the periodontal pathogen *Tannerella forsythia* ATCC 43037. *Biol. Chem.* 391, 105–117. doi: 10.1515/bc.2010.009

Kebschull, M., Demmer, R. T., and Papapanou, P. N. (2010). "Gum bug, leave my heart alone!"–epidemiologic and mechanistic evidence linking periodontal infections and atherosclerosis. *J. Dent. Res.* 89, 879–902. doi: 10.1177/0022034510375281

Kharade, S. S., and McBride, M. J. (2014). *Flavobacterium johnsoniae* chitinase ChiA is required for chitin utilization and is secreted by the type IX secretion system. *J. Bacteriol.* 196, 961–970. doi: 10.1128/JB.01170-13

Kharade, S. S., and McBride, M. J. (2015). *Flavobacterium johnsoniae* PorV is required for secretion of a subset of proteins targeted to the type IX secretion system. *J. Bacteriol.* 197, 147–158. doi: 10.1128/JB.02085-14

Kondo, Y., Ohara, N., Sato, K., Yoshimura, M., Yukitake, H., Naito, M., et al. (2010). Tetratricopeptide repeat protein-associated proteins contribute to the virulence of *Porphyromonas gingivalis*. *Infect. Immun.* 78, 2846–2856. doi: 10.1128/IAI.01448-09

Koneru, L., Ksiazek, M., Waligorska, I., Straczek, A., Lukasik, M., Madej, M., et al. (2017). Mirolysin, a LysargiNase from *Tannerella forsythia*, proteolytically inactivates the human cathelicidin, LL-37. *Biol Chem.* 398, 395–409. doi: 10.1515/hsz-2016-0267

Koziel, J., Mydel, P., and Potempa, J. (2014). The link between periodontal disease and rheumatoid arthritis: an updated review. *Curr. Rheumatol. Rep.* 16, 408. doi: 10.1007/s11926-014-0408-9

Krauss, J. L., Potempa, J., Lambris, J. D., and Hajishengallis, G. (2010). Complementary Tolls in the periodontium: how periodontal bacteria modify complement and Toll-like receptor responses to prevail in the host. *Periodontol. 2000* 52, 141–162. doi: 10.1111/j.1600-0757.2009.00324.x

Ksiazek, M., Karim, A. Y., Bryzek, D., Enghild, J. J., Thogersen, I. B., Koziel, J., et al. (2015a). Mirolase, a novel subtilisin-like serine protease from the periodontopathogen *Tannerella forsythia*. *Biol. Chem.* 396, 261–275. doi: 10.1515/hsz-2014-0256

Ksiazek, M., Mizgalska, D., Eick, S., Thogersen, I. B., Enghild, J. J., and Potempa, J. (2015b). KLIKK proteases of *Tannerella forsythia*: putative virulence factors with a unique domain structure. *Front. Microbiol.* 6:312. doi: 10.3389/fmicb.2015.00312

LaFrentz, B. R., LaPatra, S. E., Call, D. R., Wiens, G. D., and Cain, K. D. (2009). Proteomic analysis of *Flavobacterium psychrophilum* cultured *in vivo* and in iron-limited media. *Dis. Aquat. Org.* 87, 171–182. doi: 10.3354/dao02122

Lasica, A. M., Goulas, T., Mizgalska, D., Zhou, X., de Diego, I., Ksiazek, M., et al. (2016). Structural and functional probing of PorZ, an essential bacterial surface component of the type-IX secretion system of human oral-microbiomic *Porphyromonas gingivalis*. *Sci. Rep.* 6:37708. doi: 10.1038/srep37708

Laugisch, O., Wong, A., Sroka, A., Kantyka, T., Koziel, J., Neuhaus, K., et al. (2016). Citrullination in the periodontium–a possible link between periodontitis and rheumatoid arthritis. *Clin. Oral Investig.* 20, 675–683. doi: 10.1007/s00784-015-1556-7

Letoffe, S., Ghigo, J. M., and Wandersman, C. (1994). Secretion of the *Serratia marcescens* HasA protein by an ABC transporter. *J. Bacteriol.* 176, 5372–5377. doi: 10.1128/jb.176.17.5372-5377.1994

Lopez-Pelegrin, M., Ksiazek, M., Karim, A. Y., Guevara, T., Arolas, J. L., Potempa, J., et al. (2015). A novel mechanism of latency in matrix metalloproteinases. *J. Biol. Chem.* 290, 4728–4740. doi: 10.1074/jbc.M114.605956

MacGregor, A. J., Snieder, H., Rigby, A. S., Koskenvuo, M., Kaprio, J., Aho, K., et al. (2000). Characterizing the quantitative genetic contribution to rheumatoid arthritis using data from twins. *Arthritis Rheum* 43, 30–37. doi: 10.1002/1529-0131(200001)43:1<30::AID-ANR5>3.0.CO;2-B

Madden, T. E., Clark, V. L., and Kuramitsu, H. K. (1995). Revised sequence of the *Porphyromonas gingivalis* prtT cysteine protease/hemagglutinin gene: homology with streptococcal pyrogenic exotoxin B/streptococcal proteinase. *Infect. Immun.* 63, 238–247.

Majerczyk, C., Schneider, E., and Greenberg, E. P. (2016). Quorum sensing control of Type VI secretion factors restricts the proliferation of quorum-sensing mutants. *Elife* 5:e14712. doi: 10.7554/eLife.14712

Mao, F., Dam, P., Chou, J., Olman, V., and Xu, Y. (2009). DOOR: a database for prokaryotic operons. *Nucleic Acids Res.* 37, D459–D463. doi: 10.1093/nar/gkn757

Marraffini, L. A., Ton-That, H., Zong, Y., Narayana, S. V., and Schneewind, O. (2004). Anchoring of surface proteins to the cell wall of *Staphylococcus aureus*. A conserved arginine residue is required for efficient catalysis of sortase A. *J. Biol. Chem.* 279, 37763–37770. doi: 10.1074/jbc.M405282200

McBride, M. J., and Nakane, D. (2015). Flavobacterium gliding motility and the type IX secretion system. *Curr. Opin. Microbiol.* 28, 72–77. doi: 10.1016/j.mib.2015.07.016

McBride, M. J., and Zhu, Y. (2013). Gliding motility and Por secretion system genes are widespread among members of the phylum bacteroidetes. *J. Bacteriol.* 195, 270–278. doi: 10.1128/JB.01962-12

McGraw, W. T., Potempa, J., Farley, D., and Travis, J. (1999). Purification, characterization, and sequence analysis of a potential virulence factor from *Porphyromonas gingivalis*, peptidylarginine deiminase. *Infect. Immun.* 67, 3248–3256.

McInnes, I. B., and Schett, G. (2011). The pathogenesis of rheumatoid arthritis. *N. Engl. J. Med.* 365, 2205–2219. doi: 10.1056/NEJMra1004965

McKee, A. S., McDermid, A. S., Wait, R., Baskerville, A., and Marsh, P. D. (1988). Isolation of colonial variants of Bacteroides gingivalis W50 with a reduced virulence. *J. Med. Microbiol.* 27, 59–64. doi: 10.1099/00222615-27-1-59

Messner, P., Schaffer, C., Egelseer, E. M., and Sleytr, U. B. (2010). "Occurrence, structure, chemistry, genetics, morphogenesis, and functions of s-layers," in *Prokaryotic Cell Wall Compounds, Structure and Biochemistry*, eds H. König, H. Claus, and A. Varma (Berlin: Springer-Verlag), 53–109.

Mikolajczyk, J., Boatright, K. M., Stennicke, H. R., Nazif, T., Potempa, J., Bogyo, M., et al. (2003). Sequential autolytic processing activates the zymogen of Arg-gingipain. *J. Biol. Chem.* 278, 10458–10464. doi: 10.1074/jbc.M210564200

Montgomery, A. B., Kopec, J., Shrestha, L., Thezenas, M. L., Burgess-Brown, N. A., Fischer, R., et al. (2016). Crystal structure of *Porphyromonas gingivalis* peptidylarginine deiminase: implications for autoimmunity in rheumatoid arthritis. *Ann. Rheum. Dis.* 75, 1255–1261. doi: 10.1136/annrheumdis-2015-207656

Nakane, D., Sato, K., Wada, H., McBride, M. J., and Nakayama, K. (2013). Helical flow of surface protein required for bacterial gliding motility. *Proc. Natl. Acad. Sci. U.S.A.* 110, 11145–11150. doi: 10.1073/pnas.1219753110

Nakayama, K. (2015). *Porphyromonas gingivalis* and related bacteria: from colonial pigmentation to the type IX secretion system and gliding motility. *J. Periodont. Res.* 50, 1–8. doi: 10.1111/jre.12255

Nakayama, K., Yoshimura, F., Kadowaki, T., and Yamamoto, K. (1996). Involvement of arginine-specific cysteine proteinase (Arg-gingipain) in fimbriation of *Porphyromonas gingivalis*. *J. Bacteriol.* 178, 2818–2824. doi: 10.1128/jb.178.10.2818-2824.1996

Narita, Y., Sato, K., Yukitake, H., Shoji, M., Nakane, D., Nagano, K., et al. (2014). Lack of a surface layer in *Tannerella forsythia* mutants deficient in the type IX secretion system. *Microbiology* 160(Pt 10), 2295–2303. doi: 10.1099/mic.0.080192-0

Nelson, D., Potempa, J., Kordula, T., and Travis, J. (1999). Purification and characterization of a novel cysteine proteinase (periodontain) from Porphyromonas gingivalis. Evidence for a role in the inactivation of human alpha1-proteinase inhibitor. *J. Biol. Chem.* 274, 12245–12251. doi: 10.1074/jbc.274.18.12245

Nelson, K. E., Fleischmann, R. D., DeBoy, R. T., Paulsen, I. T., Fouts, D. E., Eisen, J. A., et al. (2003). Complete genome sequence of the oral pathogenic Bacterium *porphyromonas gingivalis* strain W83. *J. Bacteriol.* 185, 5591–5601. doi: 10.1128/JB.185.18.5591-5601.2003

Nguyen, K. A., Travis, J., and Potempa, J. (2007). Does the importance of the C-terminal residues in the maturation of RgpB from *Porphyromonas gingivalis* reveal a novel mechanism for protein export in a subgroup of Gram-Negative bacteria? *J. Bacteriol.* 189, 833–843. doi: 10.1128/JB.01530-06

Nguyen, K. A., Zylicz, J., Szczesny, P., Sroka, A., Hunter, N., and Potempa, J. (2009). Verification of a topology model of PorT as an integral outer-membrane protein in *Porphyromonas gingivalis*. *Microbiology* 155(Pt 2), 328–337. doi: 10.1099/mic.0.024323-0

Nonaka, M., Shoji, M., Kadowaki, T., Sato, K., Yukitake, H., Naito, M., et al. (2014). Analysis of a Lys-specific serine endopeptidase secreted via the type IX secretion system in *Porphyromonas gingivalis*. *FEMS Microbiol. Lett.* 354, 60–68. doi: 10.1111/1574-6968.12426

Okamoto, K., Nakayama, K., Kadowaki, T., Abe, N., Ratnayake, D. B., and Yamamoto, K. (1998). Involvement of a lysine-specific cysteine proteinase in hemoglobin adsorption and heme accumulation by *Porphyromonas gingivalis*. *J. Biol. Chem.* 273, 21225–21231. doi: 10.1074/jbc.273.33.21225

Olsen, I., and Potempa, J. (2014). Strategies for the inhibition of gingipains for the potential treatment of periodontitis and associated systemic diseases. *J. Oral Microbiol.* 6:24800. doi: 10.3402/jom.v6.24800

Paramonov, N., Rangarajan, M., Hashim, A., Gallagher, A., Aduse-Opoku, J., Slaney, J. M., et al. (2005). Structural analysis of a novel anionic polysaccharide from *Porphyromonas gingivalis* strain W50 related to Arg-gingipain glycans. *Mol. Microbiol.* 58, 847–863. doi: 10.1111/j.1365-2958.2005.04871.x

Park, Y., Yilmaz, O., Jung, I. Y., and Lamont, R. J. (2004). Identification of *Porphyromonas gingivalis* genes specifically expressed in human gingival epithelial cells by using differential display reverse transcription-PCR. *Infect. Immun.* 72, 3752–3758. doi: 10.1128/IAI.72.7.3752-3758.2004

Pavloff, N., Potempa, J., Pike, R. N., Prochazka, V., Kiefer, M. C., Travis, J., et al. (1995). Molecular cloning and structural characterization of the Arg-gingipain proteinase of *Porphyromonas gingivalis*. Biosynthesis as a proteinase-adhesin polyprotein. *J. Biol. Chem.* 270, 1007–1010. doi: 10.1074/jbc.270.3.1007

Pertea, M., Ayanbule, K., Smedinghoff, M., and Salzberg, S. L. (2009). OperonDB: a comprehensive database of predicted operons in microbial genomes. *Nucleic Acids Res.* 37, D479–D482. doi: 10.1093/nar/gkn784

Pike, R., McGraw, W., Potempa, J., and Travis, J. (1994). Lysine- and arginine-specific proteinases from *Porphyromonas gingivalis*. Isolation, characterization, and evidence for the existence of complexes with hemagglutinins. *J. Biol. Chem.* 269, 406–411.

Pomowski, A., Uson, I., Nowakowska, Z. M., Veillard, F., Sztukowska, M. N., Guevara, T., et al. (2017). Structural insights unravel the zymogenic mechanism of the virulence factor gingipain K from *Porphyromonas gingivalis*, a causative agent of gum disease from the human oral microbiome. *J. Biol. Chem.* 292, 5724–5735. doi: 10.1074/jbc.M117.776724

Posch, G., Andrukhov, O., Vinogradov, E., Lindner, B., Messner, P., Holst, O., et al. (2013). Structure and immunogenicity of the rough-type lipopolysaccharide from the periodontal pathogen *Tannerella forsythia*. *Clin. Vaccine Immunol.* 20, 945–953. doi: 10.1128/CVI.00139-13

Potempa, J., Banbula, A., and Travis, J. (2000). Role of bacterial proteinases in matrix destruction and modulation of host responses. *Periodontol. 2000* 24, 153–192. doi: 10.1034/j.1600-0757.2000.2240108.x

Potempa, J., Pike, R., and Travis, J. (1997). Titration and mapping of the active site of cysteine proteinases from *Porphyromonas gingivalis* (gingipains) using peptidyl chloromethanes. *Biol. Chem.* 378, 223–230. doi: 10.1515/bchm.1997.378.3-4.223

Potempa, J., Sroka, A., Imamura, T., and Travis, J. (2003). Gingipains, the major cysteine proteinases and virulence factors of *Porphyromonas gingivalis*: structure, function and assembly of multidomain protein complexes. *Curr. Protein Pept. Sci.* 4, 397–407. doi: 10.2174/1389203033487036

Quirke, A. M., Lundberg, K., Potempa, J., Mikuls, T. R., and Venables, P. J. (2015). PPAD remains a credible candidate for inducing autoimmunity in rheumatoid arthritis: comment on the article by Konig et al. *Ann. Rheum. Dis.* 74, e7. doi: 10.1136/annrheumdis-2014-206665

Rangarajan, M., Aduse-Opoku, J., Paramonov, N., Hashim, A., Bostanci, N., Fraser, O. P., et al. (2008). Identification of a second lipopolysaccharide in *Porphyromonas gingivalis* W50. *J. Bacteriol.* 190, 2920–2932. doi: 10.1128/JB.01868-07

Rangarajan, M., Smith, S. J., Sally, U., and Curtis, M. A. (1997). Biochemical characterization of the arginine-specific proteases of *Porphyromonas gingivalis* W50 suggests a common precursor. *Biochem. J.* 323(Pt 3), 701–709. doi: 10.1042/bj3230701

Remaut, H., Tang, C., Henderson, N. S., Pinkner, J. S., Wang, T., Hultgren, S. J., et al. (2008). Fiber formation across the bacterial outer membrane by the chaperone/usher pathway. *Cell* 133, 640–652. doi: 10.1016/j.cell.2008.03.033

Rhodes, R. G., Samarasam, M. N., Shrivastava, A., van Baaren, J. M., Pochiraju, S., Bollampalli, S., et al. (2010). *Flavobacterium johnsoniae* gldN and gldO are partially redundant genes required for gliding motility and surface localization of SprB. *J. Bacteriol.* 192, 1201–1211. doi: 10.1128/JB.01495-09

Rhodes, R. G., Samarasam, M. N., Van Groll, E. J., and McBride, M. J. (2011). Mutations in *Flavobacterium johnsoniae* sprE result in defects in gliding motility and protein secretion. *J. Bacteriol.* 193, 5322–5327. doi: 10.1128/JB.05480-11

Roman, S. J., Meyers, M., Volz, K., and Matsumura, P. (1992). A chemotactic signaling surface on CheY defined by suppressors of flagellar switch mutations. *J. Bacteriol.* 174, 6247–6255. doi: 10.1128/jb.174.19.6247-6255.1992

Rondelet, A., and Condemine, G. (2013). Type II secretion: the substrates that won't go away. *Res. Microbiol.* 164, 556–561. doi: 10.1016/j.resmic.2013.03.005

Russell, A. B., Wexler, A. G., Harding, B. N., Whitney, J. C., Bohn, A. J., Goo, Y. A., et al. (2014). A type VI secretion-related pathway in Bacteroidetes mediates interbacterial antagonism. *Cell Host Microbe* 16, 227–236. doi: 10.1016/j.chom.2014.07.007

Sagi, Y., Khan, S., and Eisenbach, M. (2003). Binding of the chemotaxis response regulator CheY to the isolated, intact switch complex of the bacterial flagellar motor: lack of cooperativity. *J. Biol. Chem.* 278, 25867–25871. doi: 10.1074/jbc.M303201200

Saier, M. H. Jr., and Reddy, B. L. (2015). Holins in bacteria, eukaryotes, and archaea: multifunctional xenologues with potential biotechnological and biomedical applications. *J. Bacteriol.* 197, 7–17. doi: 10.1128/JB.02046-14

Saiki, K., and Konishi, K. (2007). Identification of a *Porphyromonas gingivalis* novel protein sov required for the secretion of gingipains. *Microbiol. Immunol.* 51, 483–491. doi: 10.1111/j.1348-0421.2007.tb03936.x

Saiki, K., and Konishi, K. (2010a). Identification of a novel *Porphyromonas gingivalis* outer membrane protein, PG534, required for the production of active gingipains. *FEMS Microbiol. Lett.* 310, 168–174. doi: 10.1111/j.1574-6968.2010.02059.x

Saiki, K., and Konishi, K. (2010b). The role of Sov protein in the secretion of gingipain protease virulence factors of *Porphyromonas gingivalis*. *FEMS Microbiol. Lett.* 302, 166–174. doi: 10.1111/j.1574-6968.2009.01848.x

Saiki, K., and Konishi, K. (2014). *Porphyromonas gingivalis* C-terminal signal peptidase PG0026 and HagA interact with outer membrane protein PG27/LptO. *Mol. Oral Microbiol.* 29, 32–44. doi: 10.1111/omi.12043

Sakakibara, J., Nagano, K., Murakami, Y., Higuchi, N., Nakamura, H., Shimozato, K., et al. (2007). Loss of adherence ability to human gingival epithelial cells in S-layer protein-deficient mutants of *Tannerella forsythensis*. *Microbiology* 153(Pt 3), 866–876. doi: 10.1099/mic.0.29275-0

Sato, K., Naito, M., Yukitake, H., Hirakawa, H., Shoji, M., McBride, M. J., et al. (2010). A protein secretion system linked to bacteroidete gliding motility and pathogenesis. *Proc. Natl. Acad. Sci. U.S.A.* 107, 276–281. doi: 10.1073/pnas.0912010107

Sato, K., Sakai, E., Veith, P. D., Shoji, M., Kikuchi, Y., Yukitake, H., et al. (2005). Identification of a new membrane-associated protein that influences transport/maturation of gingipains and adhesins of *Porphyromonas gingivalis*. *J. Biol. Chem.* 280, 8668–8677. doi: 10.1074/jbc.M413544200

Sato, K., Yukitake, H., Narita, Y., Shoji, M., Naito, M., and Nakayama, K. (2013). Identification of *Porphyromonas gingivalis* proteins secreted by the Por secretion system. *FEMS Microbiol. Lett.* 338, 68–76. doi: 10.1111/1574-6968.12028

Schneewind, O., and Missiakas, D. M. (2012). Protein secretion and surface display in Gram-positive bacteria. *Philos. Trans. R. Soc. Lond. B Biol. Sci.* 367, 1123–1139. doi: 10.1098/rstb.2011.0210

Seers, C. A., Slakeski, N., Veith, P. D., Nikolof, T., Chen, Y. Y., Dashper, S. G., et al. (2006). The RgpB C-terminal domain has a role in attachment of RgpB to the outer membrane and belongs to a novel C-terminal-domain family found in *Porphyromonas gingivalis*. *J. Bacteriol.* 188, 6376–6386. doi: 10.1128/JB.00731-06

Sekot, G., Posch, G., Oh, Y. J., Zayni, S., Mayer, H. F., Pum, D., et al. (2012). Analysis of the cell surface layer ultrastructure of the oral pathogen *Tannerella forsythia*. *Arch. Microbiol.* 194, 525–539. doi: 10.1007/s00203-012-0792-3

Shah, H. N., Seddon, S. V., and Gharbia, S. E. (1989). Studies on the virulence properties and metabolism of pleiotropic mutants of *Porphyromonas gingivalis* (Bacteroides gingivalis) W50. *Oral Microbiol. Immunol.* 4, 19–23. doi: 10.1111/j.1399-302X.1989.tb00401.x

Shi, Y., Ratnayake, D. B., Okamoto, K., Abe, N., Yamamoto, K., and Nakayama, K. (1999). Genetic analyses of proteolysis, hemoglobin binding, and hemagglutination of *Porphyromonas gingivalis*. Construction of mutants with a combination of rgpA, rgpB, kgp, and hagA. *J. Biol. Chem.* 274, 17955–17960. doi: 10.1074/jbc.274.25.17955

Shoji, M., and Nakayama, K. (2016). Glycobiology of the oral pathogen *Porphyromonas gingivalis* and related species. *Microb. Pathog.* 94, 35–41. doi: 10.1016/j.micpath.2015.09.012

Shoji, M., Ratnayake, D. B., Shi, Y., Kadowaki, T., Yamamoto, K., Yoshimura, F., et al. (2002). Construction and characterization of a nonpigmented mutant of *Porphyromonas gingivalis*: cell surface polysaccharide as an anchorage for gingipains. *Microbiology* 148(Pt 4), 1183–1191. doi: 10.1099/00221287-148-4-1183

Shoji, M., Sato, K., Yukitake, H., Kondo, Y., Narita, Y., Kadowaki, T., et al. (2011). Por secretion system-dependent secretion and glycosylation of *Porphyromonas gingivalis* hemin-binding protein 35. *PLoS ONE* 6:e21372. doi: 10.1371/journal.pone.0021372

Shoji, M., Sato, K., Yukitake, H., Naito, M., and Nakayama, K. (2014). Involvement of the Wbp pathway in the biosynthesis of *Porphyromonas gingivalis* lipopolysaccharide with anionic polysaccharide. *Sci. Rep.* 4:5056. doi: 10.1038/srep05056

Shoji, M., Shibata, Y., Shiroza, T., Yukitake, H., Peng, B., Chen, Y. Y., et al. (2010). Characterization of hemin-binding protein 35 (HBP35) in *Porphyromonas gingivalis*: its cellular distribution, thioredoxin activity and role in heme utilization. *BMC Microbiol.* 10:152. doi: 10.1186/1471-2180-10-152

Shrivastava, A., Johnston, J. J., van Baaren, J. M., and McBride, M. J. (2013). *Flavobacterium johnsoniae* GldK, GldL, GldM, and SprA are required for secretion of the cell surface gliding motility adhesins SprB and RemA. *J. Bacteriol.* 195, 3201–3212. doi: 10.1128/JB.00333-13

Shrivastava, A., Lele, P. P., and Berg, H. C. (2015). A rotary motor drives Flavobacterium gliding. *Curr. Biol.* 25, 338–341. doi: 10.1016/j.cub.2014.11.045

Shrivastava, A., Rhodes, R. G., Pochiraju, S., Nakane, D., and McBride, M. J. (2012). *Flavobacterium johnsoniae* RemA is a mobile cell surface lectin involved in gliding. *J. Bacteriol.* 194, 3678–3688. doi: 10.1128/JB.00588-12

Siddiqui, H., Yoder-Himes, D. R., Mizgalska, D., Nguyen, K. A., Potempa, J., and Olsen, I. (2014). Genome sequence of *Porphyromonas gingivalis* strain HG66 (DSM 28984). *Genome Announc.* 2:e00947-14. doi: 10.1128/genomeA.00947-14

Simpson, W., Wang, C. Y., Mikolajczyk-Pawlinska, J., Potempa, J., Travis, J., Bond, V. C., et al. (1999). Transposition of the endogenous insertion sequence element IS1126 modulates gingipain expression in *Porphyromonas gingivalis*. *Infect. Immun.* 67, 5012–5020.

Slakeski, N., Seers, C. A., Ng, K., Moore, C., Cleal, S. M., Veith, P. D., et al. (2011). C-terminal domain residues important for secretion and attachment of RgpB in *Porphyromonas gingivalis*. *J. Bacteriol.* 193, 132–142. doi: 10.1128/JB.00773-10

Sleytr, U. B., and Beveridge, T. J. (1999). Bacterial S-layers. *Trends Microbiol.* 7, 253–260. doi: 10.1016/S0966-842X(99)01513-9

Smalley, J. W., Silver, J., Marsh, P. J., and Birss, A. J. (1998). The periodontopathogen *Porphyromonas gingivalis* binds iron protoporphyrin IX in the mu-oxo dimeric form: an oxidative buffer and possible pathogenic mechanism. *Biochem. J.* 331(Pt 3), 681–685. doi: 10.1042/bj3310681

Snel, B., Lehmann, G., Bork, P., and Huynen, M. A. (2000). STRING: a web-server to retrieve and display the repeatedly occurring neighbourhood of a gene. *Nucleic Acids Res.* 28, 3442–3444. doi: 10.1093/nar/28.18.3442

Sroka, A., Sztukowska, M., Potempa, J., Travis, J., and Genco, C. A. (2001). Degradation of host heme proteins by lysine- and arginine-specific cysteine proteinases (gingipains) of *Porphyromonas gingivalis*. *J. Bacteriol.* 183, 5609–5616. doi: 10.1128/JB.183.19.5609-5616.2001

Stanier, R. Y. (1942). The cytophaga group: a contribution to the biology of myxobacteria. *Bacteriol. Rev.* 6, 143–196.

Stanier, R. Y. (1947). Studies on nonfruiting myxobacteria; Cytophaga johnsonae, n. sp., a chitindecomposing myxobacterium. *J. Bacteriol.* 53, 297–315.

Stathopulos, J., Cambillau, C., Cascales, E., Roussel, A., and Leone, P. (2015). Crystallization and preliminary X-ray analysis of the C-terminal fragment of PorM, a subunit of the *Porphyromonas gingivalis* type IX secretion system. *Acta Crystallogr. F. Struct. Biol. Commun.* 71(Pt 1), 71–74. doi: 10.1107/S2053230X1402559X

Sztukowska, M., Veillard, F., Potempa, B., Bogyo, M., Enghild, J. J., Thogersen, I. B., et al. (2012). Disruption of gingipain oligomerization into non-covalent cell-surface attached complexes. *Biol. Chem.* 393, 971–977. doi: 10.1515/hsz-2012-0175

Taboada, B., Ciria, R., Martinez-Guerrero, C. E., and Merino, E. (2012). ProOpDB: prokaryotic operon database. *Nucleic Acids Res.* 40, D627–D631. doi: 10.1093/nar/gkr1020

Taguchi, Y., Sato, K., Yukitake, H., Inoue, T., Nakayama, M., Naito, M., et al. (2015). Involvement of an Skp-Like Protein, PGN_0300, in the type IX secretion system of *Porphyromonas gingivalis*. *Infect. Immun.* 84, 230–240. doi: 10.1128/IAI.01308-15

Takahara, H., Okamoto, H., and Sugawara, K. (1986). Calcium-dependent properties of peptidylarginine deiminase from rabbit skeletal muscle *Agric. Biol. Chem.* 50, 2899–2904.

Tomek, M. B., Neumann, L., Nimeth, I., Koerdt, A., Andesner, P., Messner, P., et al. (2014). The S-layer proteins of *Tannerella forsythia* are secreted via a type IX secretion system that is decoupled from protein O-glycosylation. *Mol. Oral Microbiol.* 29, 307–320. doi: 10.1111/omi.12062

Veith, P. D., Chen, Y. Y., Chen, D., O'Brien-Simpson, N. M., Cecil, J. D., Holden, J. A., et al. (2015). *Tannerella forsythia* outer membrane vesicles are enriched with substrates of the type IX secretion system and tonb-dependent receptors. *J. Proteome Res.* 14, 5355–5366. doi: 10.1021/acs.jproteome.5b00878

Veith, P. D., Chen, Y. Y., Gorasia, D. G., Chen, D., Glew, M. D., O'Brien-Simpson, N. M., et al. (2014). *Porphyromonas gingivalis* outer membrane vesicles exclusively contain outer membrane and periplasmic proteins and carry a cargo enriched with virulence factors. *J. Proteome Res.* 13, 2420–2432. doi: 10.1021/pr401227e

Veith, P. D., Chen, Y. Y., and Reynolds, E. C. (2004). *Porphyromonas gingivalis* RgpA and Kgp proteinases and adhesins are C terminally processed by the carboxypeptidase CPG70. *Infect. Immun.* 72, 3655–3657. doi: 10.1128/IAI.72.6.3655-3657.2004

Veith, P. D., Nor Muhammad, N. A., Dashper, S. G., Likic, V. A., Gorasia, D. G., Chen, D., et al. (2013). Protein substrates of a novel secretion system are numerous in the Bacteroidetes phylum and have in common a cleavable C-terminal secretion signal, extensive post-translational modification, and cell-surface attachment. *J. Proteome Res.* 12, 4449–4461. doi: 10.1021/pr400487b

Veith, P. D., O'Brien-Simpson, N. M., Tan, Y., Djatmiko, D. C., Dashper, S. G., and Reynolds, E. C. (2009). Outer membrane proteome and antigens of *Tannerella forsythia*. *J. Proteome Res.* 8, 4279–4292. doi: 10.1021/pr900372c

Veith, P. D., Talbo, G. H., Slakeski, N., Dashper, S. G., Moore, C., Paolini, R. A., et al. (2002). Major outer membrane proteins and proteolytic processing of RgpA and Kgp of *Porphyromonas gingivalis* W50. *Biochem. J.* 363(Pt 1), 105–115. doi: 10.1042/bj3630105

Vincent, M. S., Canestrari, M. J., Leone, P., Stathopoulos, J., Ize, B., Zoued, A., et al. (2017). Characterization of the *Porphyromonas gingivalis* type IX secretion trans-envelope PorKLMNP core complex. *J. Biol. Chem.* 292, 3252–3261. doi: 10.1074/jbc.M116.765081

Vincent, M. S., Durand, E., and Cascales, E. (2016). The PorX response regulator of the *Porphyromonas gingivalis* PorXY two-component system does not directly regulate the type IX secretion genes but binds the PorL subunit. *Front. Cell. Infect. Microbiol.* 6:96. doi: 10.3389/fcimb.2016.00096

Vossenaar, E. R., Zendman, A. J., van Venrooij, W. J., and Pruijn, G. J. (2003). PAD, a growing family of citrullinating enzymes: genes, features and involvement in disease. *Bioessays* 25, 1106–1118. doi: 10.1002/bies.10357

Wegner, N., Wait, R., Sroka, A., Eick, S., Nguyen, K. A., Lundberg, K., et al. (2010). Peptidylarginine deiminase from *Porphyromonas gingivalis* citrullinates human fibrinogen and alpha-enolase: implications for autoimmunity in rheumatoid arthritis. *Arthritis Rheum.* 62, 2662–2672. doi: 10.1002/art.27552

Wexler, A. G., Bao, Y., Whitney, J. C., Bobay, L. M., Xavier, J. B., Schofield, W. B., et al. (2016). Human symbionts inject and neutralize antibacterial toxins to persist in the gut. *Proc. Natl. Acad. Sci. U.S.A.* 113, 3639–3644. doi: 10.1073/pnas.1525637113

Whitmore, S. E., and Lamont, R. J. (2014). Oral bacteria and cancer. *PLoS Pathog.* 10:e1003933. doi: 10.1371/journal.ppat.1003933

Wilensky, A., Potempa, J., Houri-Haddad, Y., and Shapira, L. (2016). Vaccination with recombinant RgpA peptide protects against *Porphyromonas gingivalis*-induced bone loss. *J. Periodontal. Res.* 52, 285–291. doi: 10.1111/jre.12393

Wilson, M. M., Anderson, D. E., and Bernstein, H. D. (2015). Analysis of the outer membrane proteome and secretome of *Bacteroides fragilis* reveals a multiplicity of secretion mechanisms. *PLoS ONE* 10:e0117732. doi: 10.1371/journal.pone.0117732

Xu, Q., Shoji, M., Shibata, S., Naito, M., Sato, K., Elsliger, M. A., et al. (2016). A distinct type of pilus from the human microbiome. *Cell* 165, 690–703. doi: 10.1016/j.cell.2016.03.016

Yang, T., Bu, X., Han, Q., Wang, X., Zhou, H., Chen, G., et al. (2016). A small periplasmic protein essential for *Cytophaga hutchinsonii* cellulose digestion. *Appl. Microbiol. Biotechnol.* 100, 1935–1944. doi: 10.1007/s00253-015-7204-y

Yoshimura, M., Ohara, N., Kondo, Y., Shoji, M., Okano, S., Nakano, Y., et al. (2008). Proteome analysis of *Porphyromonas gingivalis* cells placed in a subcutaneous chamber of mice. *Oral Microbiol. Immunol.* 23, 413–418. doi: 10.1111/j.1399-302X.2008.00444.x

Zhang, Z., Liu, Q., and Hendrickson, W. A. (2014). Crystal structures of apparent saccharide sensors from histidine kinase receptors prevalent in a human gut symbiont. *FEBS J.* 281, 4263–4279. doi: 10.1111/febs.12904

Zhou, X. Y., Gao, J. L., Hunter, N., Potempa, J., and Nguyen, K. A. (2013). Sequence-independent processing site of the C-terminal domain (CTD) influences maturation of the RgpB protease from *Porphyromonas gingivalis. Mol. Microbiol.* 89, 903–917. doi: 10.1111/mmi.12319

Zhu, Y., and McBride, M. J. (2014). Deletion of the *Cytophaga hutchinsonii* type IX secretion system gene sprP results in defects in gliding motility and cellulose utilization. *Appl. Microbiol. Biotechnol.* 98, 763–775. doi: 10.1007/s00253-013-5355-2

13

Bacteria-Killing Type IV Secretion Systems

Germán G. Sgro[1†], Gabriel U. Oka[1†], Diorge P. Souza[1‡], William Cenens[1], Ethel Bayer-Santos[1‡], Bruno Y. Matsuyama[1], Natalia F. Bueno[1], Thiago Rodrigo dos Santos[1], Cristina E. Alvarez-Martinez[2], Roberto K. Salinas[1] and Chuck S. Farah[1]*

[1] Departamento de Bioquímica, Instituto de Química, Universidade de São Paulo, São Paulo, Brazil, [2] Departamento de Genética, Evolução, Microbiologia e Imunologia, Instituto de Biologia, University of Campinas (UNICAMP), Campinas, Brazil

***Correspondence:**
Chuck S. Farah
chsfarah@iq.usp.br

Bacteria have been constantly competing for nutrients and space for billions of years. During this time, they have evolved many different molecular mechanisms by which to secrete proteinaceous effectors in order to manipulate and often kill rival bacterial and eukaryotic cells. These processes often employ large multimeric transmembrane nanomachines that have been classified as types I–IX secretion systems. One of the most evolutionarily versatile are the Type IV secretion systems (T4SSs), which have been shown to be able to secrete macromolecules directly into both eukaryotic and prokaryotic cells. Until recently, examples of T4SS-mediated macromolecule transfer from one bacterium to another was restricted to protein-DNA complexes during bacterial conjugation. This view changed when it was shown by our group that many *Xanthomonas* species carry a T4SS that is specialized to transfer toxic bacterial effectors into rival bacterial cells, resulting in cell death. This review will focus on this special subtype of T4SS by describing its distinguishing features, similar systems in other proteobacterial genomes, and the nature of the effectors secreted by these systems and their cognate inhibitors.

Keywords: bacterial competition, Xanthomonadales, type IV immunity protein, type IV secretion effector, type IV secretion system, X-Tfe, X-Tfi, X-T4SS

INTRODUCTION

Type IV secretion systems (T4SSs) have been studied since the birth of modern molecular biology, starting with the description of bacterial conjugation over 70 years ago (Lederberg and Tatum, 1946). It quickly became evident that the T4SS-mediated horizontal transfer of genetic material is a major contributor to bacterial evolution, making it necessary to consider lateral connections between lineages for a complete description of the bacterial tree of life (de la Cruz and Davies, 2000). Horizontal gene transfer is also one of the principal mechanisms for the spread of genes conferring resistance to antibiotics (Cabezon et al., 2015). Moreover, many pathogenic bacteria use T4SSs to facilitate their proliferation and survival inside eukaryotic hosts, typically by the secretion of protein effectors or protein-DNA complexes (Gonzalez-Rivera et al., 2016). T4SSs are thus important virulence factors in a variety of human diseases, including whooping cough (*Bordetella pertussis*; Locht et al., 2011; Carbonetti, 2015), cat-scratch fever (*Bartonella henselae*; Siamer and Dehio, 2015), brucellosis (*Brucella* spp.; Ke et al., 2015), Legionnaire's pneumonia (*Legionella pneumophila*;

Finsel and Hilbi, 2015), Q fever (*Coxiella burnetii*; Moffatt et al., 2015) and peptic ulcer and gastric cancer (*Helicobacter pylori*; Naumann et al., 2017). One of the most well-characterized T4SSs is that of *Agrobacterium tumefaciens* which injects nucleoprotein complexes and protein factors into plant cells (Alvarez-Martinez and Christie, 2009; Li and Christie, 2018). Furthermore, specialized T4SSs from *Neisseria gonorrhoeae* or *H. pylori* secrete DNA to the extracellular milieu or uptake DNA from the environment to the bacterial cytoplasm, respectively (Hofreuter et al., 2001; Hamilton et al., 2005; Callaghan et al., 2017). Finally, the plant pathogen *Xanthomonas citri* (Oliveira et al., 2016; Sgro et al., 2018; Souza et al., 2015) and, more recently, the opportunistic human pathogen *Stenotrophomonas maltophilia* (preprint: Bayer-Santos et al., 2019), have been shown to use a T4SS to inject toxic effectors into target bacteria, thus inducing the death of rival cells (**Figure 1**).

T4SSs are structurally very diverse. For example, the related pKM101 and R388 plasmid-encoded conjugation systems (Chandran et al., 2009; Fronzes et al., 2009; Rivera-Calzada et al., 2013) and the pathogenic *Legionella* Dot/Icm (Ghosal et al., 2017; Chetrit et al., 2018) and *H. pylori* Cag (Frick-Cheng et al., 2016; Chang et al., 2018) effector-secreting systems, while all exhibiting an outer membrane-associated core complex with 14-fold or 13-fold symmetry, present significantly different features in terms of their overall size. These systems also display a varied set of both functional and structural subunits, and even the homologous subunits have very low sequence similarity and frequently present modified domain architectures (Alvarez-Martinez and Christie, 2009; Christie et al., 2014; Guglielmini et al., 2014; Christie, 2016; Grohmann et al., 2017). For these reasons, the T4SSs from Gram-negative bacteria have been divided into two major classes, denoted A and B (Christie and Vogel, 2000), and classification systems based on detailed phylogenetic analysis have divided Gram-negative and Gram-positive T4SSs into up to 8 classes (Guglielmini et al., 2014).

The canonical class A, best represented by the *A. tumefaciens vir* system and those coded by conjugative plasmids pKM101, R388, and RP4, have the basic set of 12 conserved subunits, named VirB1 to VirB11 plus VirD4 (Tzfira and Citovsky, 2006). The overall organization of the canonical class A T4SSs has been revealed in electron microscopy studies (Low et al., 2014; Redzej et al., 2017) and can be divided into two general (sub)complexes (**Figure 1**). The inner membrane complex is made up of subunits embedded in, or associated with, the inner membrane: VirB3, VirB4, VirB6, VirB8, VirB11, and VirD4. The outer membrane or "core" complex is comprised of the subunits VirB7, VirB9, and VirB10. These two complexes are connected by a flexible "stalk" of unknown composition, though it has been proposed to be made up, at least in part, by the disordered N-terminal domain of VirB10 (which also has an N-terminal transmembrane helix embedded in the inner membrane) and/or the C-terminal domain of VirB8 (Christie, 2016; Waksman, 2019). In addition to this transmembrane structure, there are extracellular pili made of subunits VirB2 and VirB5, that are presumably involved in making contact with the membrane of the target cell or organelle (Alvarez-Martinez and Christie, 2009). Even within the class A T4SSs, a large degree of sequence and size diversity has been observed for many of the subunits in different species. This is perhaps most starkly exemplified when considering the *H. pylori* Cag T4SS which, in addition to orthologs of the basic set of canonical class A subunits, possesses another five subunits that are required for proper function (Backert et al., 2015; Frick-Cheng et al., 2016).

The even more distantly related class B includes T4SSs found in the pathogens *L. pneumophila*, *C. burnetii*, and *Rickettsiella grylli* as well as in the IncI conjugative plasmids R64 and ColIb-P9 (Sexton and Vogel, 2002). *L. pneumophila* causes Legionnaire's disease in humans by infecting alveolar macrophages where it replicates within a specialized vacuole (Backert and Meyer, 2006; Ensminger and Isberg, 2009). Its Dot/Icm T4SS is made up of 27 components and secretes more than 300 effector proteins that manipulate signal transduction pathways in the host cell, primarily affecting organelle trafficking (Hilbi et al., 2017; Qiu and Luo, 2017). The bacteria-killing T4SSs, which is the topic of this review, belong to the canonical class A T4SSs, although they do have some structurally distinguishing features as described below.

The Xanthomonadales order of Gammaproteobacteria (Saddler and Bradbury, 2007), recently divided into two orders, Xanthomonadales (families *Xanthomonadaceae* and *Rhodanobacteraceae*) and Nevskiales (Naushad et al., 2015), include several hundred phytopathogenic species of the genera *Xanthomonas* and *Xylella* as well as important and ubiquitous soil, water and plant-associated bacteria of the genera *Stenotrophomonas*, *Lysobacter*, *Luteimonas*, *Pseudoxanthomonas*, *Rhodanobacter*, *Luteibacter*, *Dyella*, *Frateuria*, *Aquimonas*, and others (Van Sluys et al., 2002; Saddler and Bradbury, 2007; Looney et al., 2009; Mansfield et al., 2012). Some *Stenotrophomonas* strains are opportunistic pathogens of immunosuppressed human patients (Chang et al., 2015) and some *Stenotrophomonas* and *Lysobacter* strains have been recognized as potential biological control agents in combating plant diseases caused by fungi or other bacteria (Hayward et al., 2010; Mukherjee and Roy, 2016; Panthee et al., 2016). Other species from the genera *Lysobacter* and *Luteimonas* have been isolated from extreme environments (Brito et al., 2013; Zhang et al., 2015). Although the role of types II and III secretion systems in the virulence of species of the genus *Xanthomonas* is already well established (Buttner and Bonas, 2010), until a few years ago there was little information available on the functions of other secretion systems in these bacterial species. An accompanying article in this series deals with the recently discovered role of the *X. citri* Type VI secretion system (T6SS) in protection against predation by phagocytic amoebas (Bayer-Santos et al., 2018). In this review, we will focus on the special characteristics of the Xanthomonadales Type IV secretion systems, first described in *X. citri*, and their role in the contact-dependent killing of rival Gram-negative species. The review will focus on describing the distinguishing structural features of the T4SS components encoded by the chromosomal *virB* locus of *X. citri*, their conservation in homologous systems in the order Xanthomonadales and other proteobacterial genomes, the nature of the effectors secreted by these systems and the cognate inhibitors of these effectors.

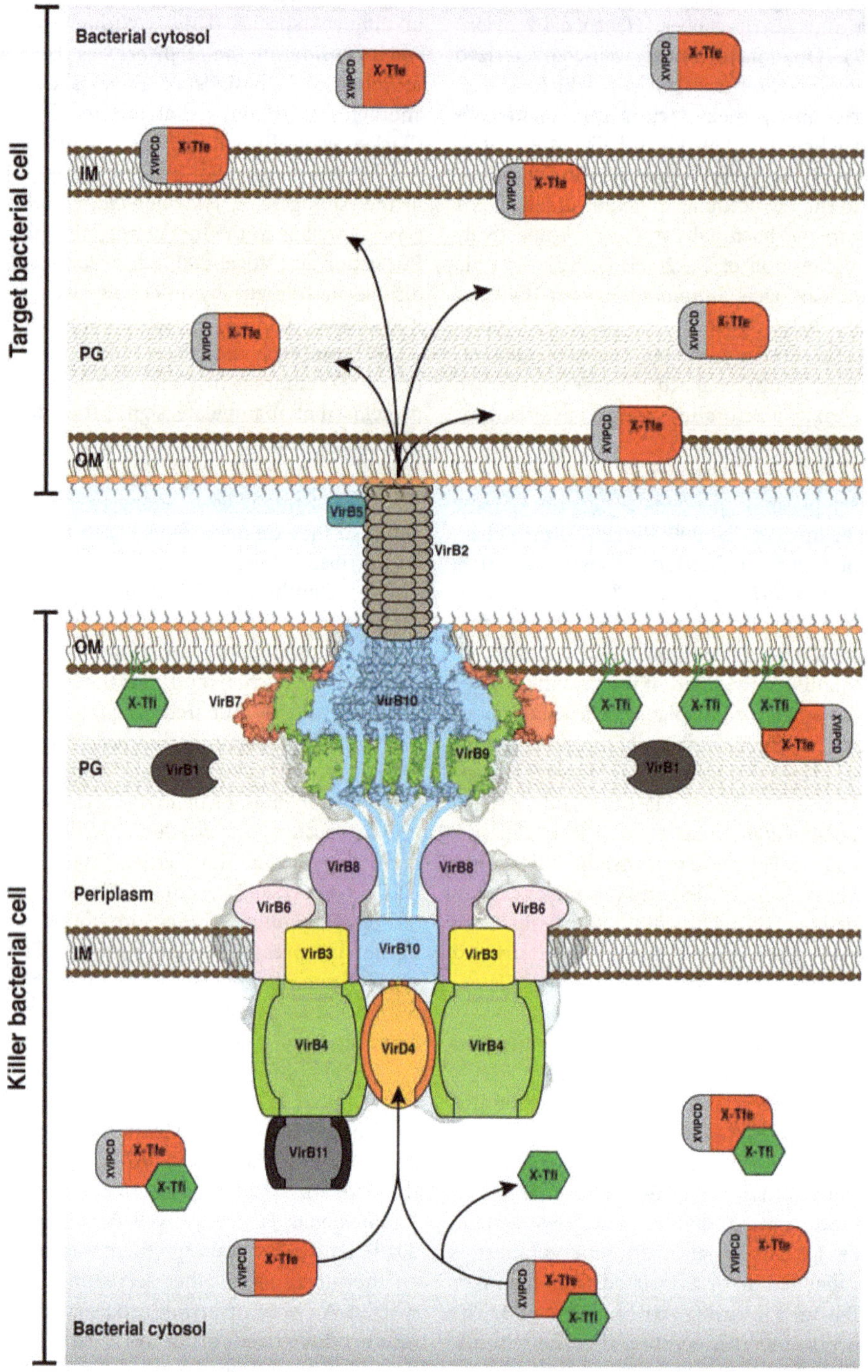

FIGURE 1 | Schematic model of the structure and function of the bacteria-killing Xanthomonadales-like Type IV secretion systems (X-T4SSs). The model shows the interface between two bacterial cells. The killer cell (below) is armed with an X-T4SS whose general architecture is based on the negative-stained electron microscope map of the R388 T4SS shown in the background (Low et al., 2014; Redzej et al., 2017) and the cryo-EM structure of the *X. citri* core complex (VirB7, VirB9, and VirB10; Sgro et al., 2018) associated with the outer membrane (OM). The disordered N-terminal domains of the VirB10 subunits extend down from the core complex and pass through the inner membrane. The inner membrane (IM) complex is made up of VirB3, VirB6, VirB8, the three ATPases VirB4, VirB11, and VirD4 as well as the aforementioned N-terminal segments of VirB10. Pili, made up of VirB2 and VirB5, mediate intercellular contacts. X-T4SS effectors (X-Tfes) interact, via their XVIPCD domains, with VirD4 and are subsequently transferred to the T4SS for translocation into the target cell where they will degrade target structures such as membrane phospholipids or carbohydrate and peptide linkages in the peptidoglycan (PG) layer. Prior to secretion, X-Tfes whose activities could target cytosolic substrates can be inhibited by cytosolic variants of their cognate immunity proteins (X-Tfis). If X-Tfes make their way into the periplasm, either by leakage from the secretion channel or by injection by neighboring cells of the same species, they will be inhibited by the periplasmic lipoprotein forms of the cognate X-Tfi. Portions of the Figure were adapted from Low et al. (2014) and Sgro et al. (2018) with permission from the publishers.

THE CHROMOSOMALLY CODED T4SS OF *Xanthomonas citri*

The T4SS encoded by the chromosomal *vir* locus of *X. citri* contains the canonical set of 12 structural components found in other class A T4SSs (**Figure 2**; Alegria et al., 2005; Souza et al., 2011). The presence of chromosomally encoded homologs in several other *Xanthomonas* species (see below) suggested an important function in *Xanthomonas* biology. A role in bacterial conjugation or nucleic acid transfer was deemed unlikely since the chromosomal *virB* locus does not contain genes coding for homologs of the DNA processing components of the relaxosome or characteristic palindromic *oriT* sites (Alegria et al., 2005). Furthermore, a knockout of the *virB7* gene in *X. citri* did not affect the development of canker symptoms in citrus plants (Souza et al., 2011) and the deletion of a large part of the homologous operon in *Xanthomonas campestris* pv. *campestris* 8004 did not modify the phenotype of infection in several plants of the *Brassicaceae* family (He et al., 2007), ruling out a direct involvement of the T4SS in *Xanthomonas* virulence (at least in these two species). Our group subsequently demonstrated that this secretion system confers to *X. citri* the capacity to kill other Gram-negative cells in a contact-dependent manner (Souza et al., 2015). The first bacterial killing experiments were performed by confronting *X. citri* with common laboratory strains of *Escherichia coli* as well as the Betaproteobacterium *Chromobacterium violaceum* (Souza et al., 2015) and subsequent experiments demonstrated similar T4SS-dependent killing of several other Gram-negative bacteria but not Gram-positive bacteria (DPS, GUO, WC, and CSF; unpublished). Recently, a CPRG-based colorimetric assay has been employed to monitor the real time kinetics of T4SS-dependent bacterial killing by both *X. citri* (Sgro et al., 2018) and *S. maltophilia* (Preprint: Bayer-Santos et al., 2019). Time-lapse microscopy clearly showed that bacterial killing by *X. citri* and *S. maltophilia* requires cell-cell contact and that the death of target cells is evidenced by the loss of cell turgor and contents over a very short period of time (Souza et al., 2015; Preprint: Bayer-Santos et al., 2019). These T4SSs share with some T6SSs the ability to transfer their toxic effectors directly into rival bacterial species of different orders and phyla and so are important factors for interspecies competition. In this sense, they differ from contact-dependent growth inhibition (CDI) systems (Hayes et al., 2014) and the *Staphylococcus aureus* Type VII secretion system (T7SS; Cao et al., 2016) that seem to be important for competition between cells of the same or closely related species (intraspecies competition).

IDENTIFICATION OF HOMOLOGOUS SYSTEMS IN THE ORDER XANTHOMONADALES AND OTHER PROTEOBACTERIAL GENOMES

Several of the *X. citri* T4SS components have some interesting features that distinguish them from their homologs in other more distantly related class A T4SSs involved in horizontal transfer of genetic material. For example, the VirB7 and VirB8 subunits have C-terminal extensions absent in most of their more distantly related homologs (see below). Genes coding for T4SSs with similar characteristics to that of *X. citri* can be identified in the chromosomes of many other *Xanthomonas* species (**Figure 2** and **Table 1**), for example *Xanthomonas campestris* pv. *campestris* B100 (Vorholter et al., 2008), *Xanthomonas albilineans* GPEPC73 (Pieretti et al., 2009), *X. campestris* pv. *vasculorum* NCPPB702 (Studholme et al., 2010) and *X. campestris* pv. *musacearum* NCPPB2005 (Wasukira et al., 2012). The corresponding locus is fragmented in *X. campestris* pv. *campestris* strains ATCC33913 (Da Silva et al., 2002) and 8004 (Qian et al., 2005), with the *virB5* and *virB6* genes found in other regions of the genomes. *X. campestris* pv. *vesicatoria* 85-10 (Thieme et al., 2005) lacks a significant part of the *vir* locus (all that remains is the 5′ region coding for VirD4, VirB7, VirB8, and VirB9). The system is also absent in *Xanthomonas oryzae* strains KACC10331 (Lee et al., 2005), MAFF311018 (Ochiai et al., 2005), PXO99A (Salzberg et al., 2008), and BLS256 (Salzberg et al., 2007), in *Xanthomonas fuscans* subsp. *aurantifolii* strains 10535 and 11122 (Moreira et al., 2010) and in all *Xylella* species sequenced to date. Homologous loci can be found in some Xanthomonadales species of the genera *Stenotrophomonas*, *Pseudoxanthomonas*, *Luteimonas*, *Lysobacter*, *Thermomonas*, *Rhodanobacter*, *Dyella*, *Frateuria*, and *Luteibacter* (**Table 1**). Interestingly, homologous systems are also found in some species of the Betaproteobacteria orders Burkholderiales (genera *Hydrogenophaga*, *Variovorax*) and Neisseriales (genera *Neisseria* and *Morococcus*) (**Table 1**). This is consistent with the observation that in some phylogenetic analyses, Xanthomonadales species are observed to branch anomalously with Betaproteobacteria, most probably due to horizontal gene transfer events (Martins-Pinheiro et al., 2004; Comas et al., 2006; Naushad and Gupta, 2013). We will therefore employ the term X-T4SS to designate all Xanthomonadales-like Type IV secretion systems.

Figure 2 presents the organization of genetic loci, homologous to the *X. citri* chromosomal *vir* locus, that are found in the genomes of a few bacterial species selected from genera of the *Xanthomonadaceae* family (*Xanthomonas*, *Stenotrophomonas*, and *Lysobacter*), and *Rhodanobacteraceae* family (*Dyella* and *Luteibacter*) within the order Xanthomonadales. Also shown are examples of genetic loci that code for X-T4SSs found in the more distant Betaproteobacteria genera of the *Comamonadaceae* family (*Hydrogenophaga*) and *Neisseriaceae* family (*Neisseria*). One interesting observation is that the loci in species from the Xanthomonadales order seem to have one operon coding for all 11 VirB components, beginning with the *virB7* gene. On the other hand, in *Hydrogenophaga crassostreae*, the operon has been divided into two segments (*virB7-11* and *virB1-6*) and in *Neisseria mucosa* and *N. flavescens* it has been divided into three or more segments (**Figure 2**). The positions of the *virD4* genes also vary: in most *Xanthomonas* and *Stenotrophomonas* species it is found immediately upstream of the *virB7* gene while in the more distantly related species it appears upstream, downstream or inserted between segments coding for the *virB* genes (**Figure 2**).

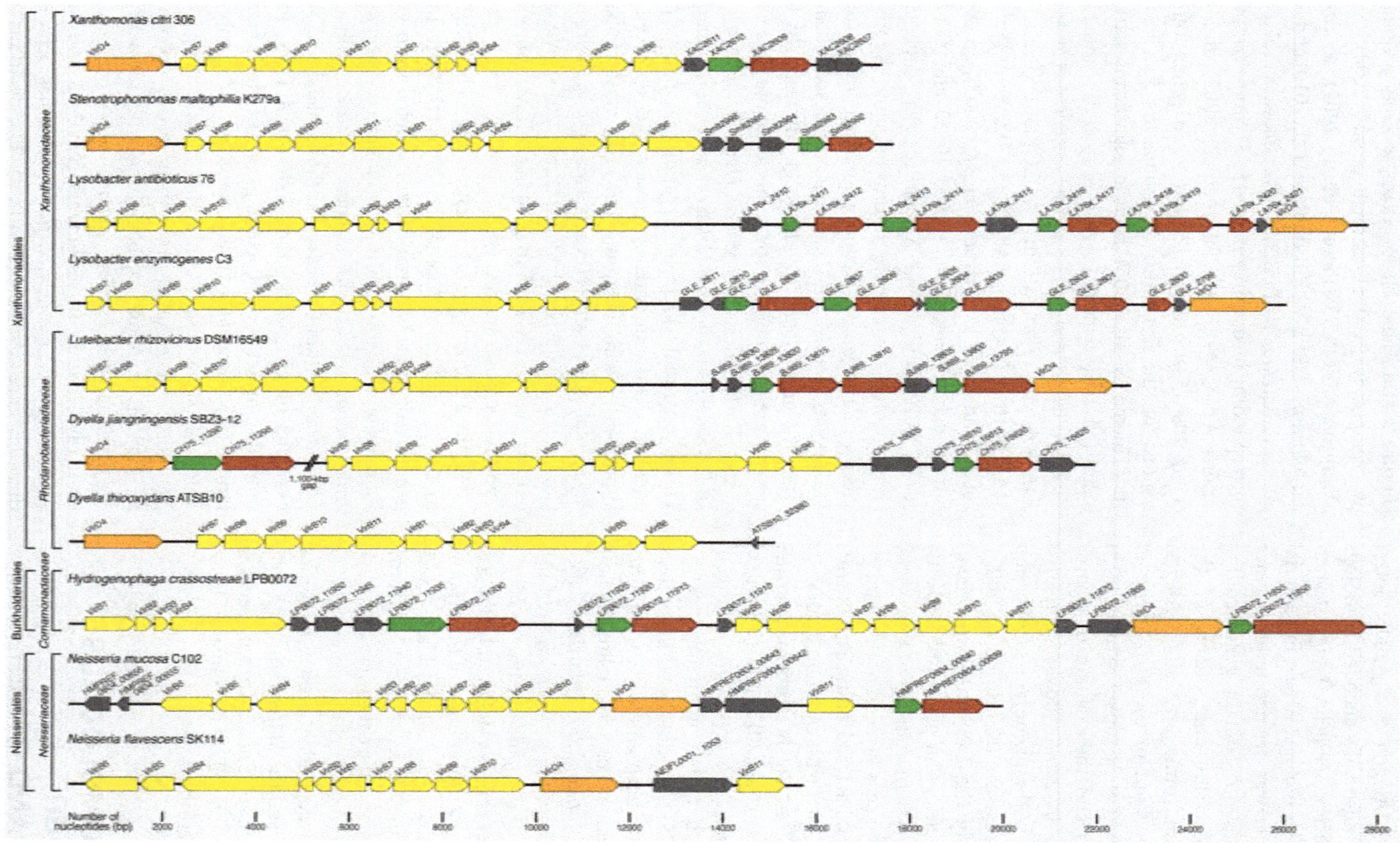

FIGURE 2 | *Xanthomonas citri* chromosomal *vir* locus and its homologs in other species. The top line presents the T4SS encoded by the chromosomal *vir* locus of *X. citri* 306 (Da Silva et al., 2002; Alegria et al., 2005). It contains the canonical set of 12 components found in other class A T4SSs. Genes coding for T4SSs with similar characteristics to that of *X. citri* can be identified in the chromosomes of many other species (see **Table 1** for an extensive list). Shown here are representative examples from *Stenotrophomonas maltophilia* K279a (Crossman et al., 2008), *Lysobacter antibioticus* 76 (de Bruijn et al., 2015), *Lysobacter enzymogenes* C3 (unpublished; GenBank accession CP013140), *Luteibacter rhizovicinus* DSM16549 (unpublished; GenBank accession CP017480), *Dyella jiangningensis* SBZ3-12 (Bao et al., 2014), *Dyella thiooxydans* ATSB10 (unpublished; GenBank accession CP014841), *Hydrogenophaga crassostreae* LPB0072 (unpublished; GenBank accession LVWD01000013), *Neisseria mucosa* C102 (unpublished, GenBank accession GCA_000186165) and *Neisseria flavescens* SK114 (unpublished; GenBank accession ACQV01000009). VirB and VirD4 genes are shown in yellow and orange, respectively. Xanthomonadales-like T4SS effectors (X-Tfes) and immunity proteins (X-Tfis) are colored red and green, respectively. Other open reading frames coding for proteins of unknown function are shown in gray.

DISTINGUISHING STRUCTURAL FEATURES OF THE BACTERIA-KILLING XANTHOMONADALES-LIKE T4SSs (X-T4SSs)

Supplementary Figures S1–S12 present multiple amino acid sequence alignments of VirB1–VirB11 and VirD4 (respectively) X-T4SS components coded by the homologous loci presented in **Figure 2**. What follows in this section is a brief description of some interesting structural features that can be identified from these alignments and, in some cases, their correlations with known structures and site-directed mutagenesis studies. The observations gleaned from these comparisons are likely to apply to most of the X-T4SSs listed in **Table 1**.

VirB7, VirB9, and VirB10: Components of the Core Complex

The 2.9 Å resolution crystal structure of the outer membrane layer of the pKM101 core complex (Chandran et al., 2009) and the recently published 3.3 Å resolution cryo-electron microscopy (cryo-EM) structure of the complete *X. citri* core complex (Sgro et al., 2018), along with the lower resolution EM maps of the complete pKM101 (Fronzes et al., 2009; Rivera-Calzada et al., 2013), R388 (Low et al., 2014) and *A. tumefaciens* (Gordon et al., 2017) core complexes have provided us with the greatest detail as yet of the periplasmic channel that connects the inner and outer membranes of class A T4SSs. These structures, are all made of 14 copies of VirB7–VirB9–VirB10 heterotrimers (named TraN-TraO-TraF in pKM101 and TrwH-TrwF-TrwE in R388) and can be divided into two layers: the O-layer associated with the outer membrane, consisting of VirB7 and the C-terminal domains of VirB9 and VirB10, and the I-layer made up of the N-terminal domains of VirB9 and VirB10 (**Figures 3, 4**; Fronzes et al., 2009).

The VirB7 lipoprotein component of X-T4SSs is much larger (ranging from 130 to 185 amino acids; **Supplementary Figure S7**) than that found in other class A T4SSs (normally ~40 amino acids). This large size is due to an extra globular C-terminal domain called N0 (Souza et al., 2011). Interestingly, similar N0 domains are also found in a myriad of transport systems located in Gram-negative bacterial outer membranes, ranging from secretins of T2SSs, Type IV pilus biogenesis machineries (Korotkov et al., 2009), T3SSs (Spreter et al., 2009), filamentous phages (Spagnuolo et al., 2010), long-tailed bacteriophages (Kanamaru et al., 2002; Kondou et al., 2005), signal-transduction domains in TonB-dependent receptors (Garcia-Herrero and Vogel, 2005; Ferguson et al., 2007) and membrane-penetrating devices in T6SSs (Leiman et al., 2009). The N0 domain is also the C-terminal domain of the outer membrane lipoprotein DotD of the class B T4SSs found in the human pathogens *L. pneumophila* and *C. burnetii* (Nakano et al., 2010). The presence of this domain in many outer membrane transport systems could reflect an unexplored evolutionary relationship between them (Souza et al., 2011). The function of the VirB7 N0 domain is possibly related to the observation that it mediates VirB7 oligomerization and, as the VirB7 subunits are highly concentrated in the context of the core complex, it was predicted that the VirB7 domain could assemble an extra peripheral ring in the O-layer of the X-T4SS (Souza et al., 2011), subsequently confirmed by the resolution of the *X. citri* core complex structure (Sgro et al., 2018). This external ring of N0 domains give the *X. citri* core complex its characteristic profile that resembles a flying saucer (**Figure 3**; Sgro et al., 2018). The motifs that mediate VirB7 oligomerization (specific residues in the N0 domain and a [T/S]EIPL) motif that immediately precedes it, contribute to T4SS assembly in the *X. citri* periplasm and are essential for its antibacterial activity (Souza et al., 2011; Oliveira et al., 2016; Sgro et al., 2018). The multiple sequence alignment in **Supplementary Figure S7** shows that these motifs, as well as the region involved in interaction with VirB9, are conserved among X-T4SS VirB7 proteins.

Like their homologs in other class A T4SSs, the X-T4SS VirB9 proteins have two domains connected by a central linker. They all possess an N-terminal signal peptide with a cleavage site immediately after a highly conserved alanine residue (**Supplementary Figure S9**). The cryo-EM structure of the *X. citri* core complex (Sgro et al., 2018) and the NMR solution structure of the *X. citri* VirB7–VirB9 binary complex (Oliveira et al., 2016) showed that the *X. citri* VirB9 C-terminal domain interacts with VirB7 and with the VirB10 C-terminal domain in the O-layer of the core complex in a manner similar to that observed for pKM101 (**Figure 4**). The *X. citri* core complex structure provided us with the first high resolution structure of the I-layer, composed of 14 VirB9 N-terminal β-sandwich domains that pack against each other side-by-side, forming a ring with an internal diameter of 80 Å (**Figure 3**; Sgro et al., 2018). At the base of the I-layer, small 12-residue helices from the N-terminal domains of VirB10 fit into grooves at the interfaces between VirB9 subunits (Sgro et al., 2018). The multiple sequence alignment of X-T4SS VirB9 proteins shows that the N- and C-terminal domains are quite well conserved but the central linker is variable in both sequence and length (**Supplementary Figure S9**). This is consistent with the observation that deletion of six residues in the linker region did not affect the stability or function of the T4SS in *X. citri* (Sgro et al., 2018).

VirB10 subunits in class A T4SSs can be divided into three substructures: the N-terminal cytosolic portion with its contiguous transmembrane helix that spans the bacterial inner membrane, the periplasmic portion of the N-terminal domain that is largely unstructured in the NMR analysis of the isolated domain and the cryo-EM structure of the *X. citri* core complex (Sgro et al., 2018) and the C-terminal domain localized in the O-layer of the core complex. The alignments shown in **Supplementary Figure S10** reveal that the C-terminal domains of X-T4SS VirB10 subunits are very well conserved. The sequences are also very similar to their counterparts in pKM101, R388 and *A. tumefaciens* (Sgro et al., 2018). One region in this domain that presents a relatively high degree of variability is the "antenna" (Chandran et al., 2009), made up of two alpha helices (α1 and α2) that form the actual pore through the outer membrane. **Figure 4** presents a comparison of the relative orientations of the VirB10 antennae when the *X. citri* core complex and pKM101 O-layer structures are superposed. In the *X. citri* core complex

TABLE 1 | Bacterial strains that code for a putative X-T4SS and X-Tfes substrates.

Organism	Accession#	Organism	Accession#
Xanthomonadaceae			
Luteimonas sp. 83-4	NZ_CP029556.1	*Xanthomonas axonopodis* pv. *citrumelo* F1	CP002914.1
***Lysobacter antibioticus* 76**	NZ_CP011129.1	*Xanthomonas axonopodis* pv. *melhusii* LMG9050	LOJW01000012.1
Lysobacter capsici AZ78	JAJA02000001.1	*Xanthomonas axonopodis* pv. *vasculorum* NCPPB900	KN173625.1
***Lysobacter enzymogenes* C3**	CP013140.1	*Xanthomonas axonopodis* Xac29-1	CP004399.1
Lysobacter gummosus 3.2.11	CP011131.1	*Xanthomonas campestris* pv. *campestris* B100	NC_010688.1
Lysobacter maris HZ9B	CP029843.1	*Xanthomonas campestris* pv. *campestris* str. 8004	CP000050.1
Lysobacter silvestris AM20-91	NZ_NPZB01000002.1	*Xanthomonas campestris* pv. *campestris* str. ATCC33913	NC_003902.1
Lysobacter sp. 4284/11	NZ_RFLY01000011.1	*Xanthomonas campestris* pv. *musacearum* NCPPB2005	AKBE01000043.1
Lysobacter sp. cf310	FOSS01000003.1	*Xanthomonas campestris* pv. *raphani* 756C	CP002789.1
Lysobacter sp. Root494	NZ_LMFH01000005.1	*Xanthomonas campestris* pv. *vitiscarnosae* LMG939	LOKI01000031.1
Lysobacter sp. Root604	LMGS01000001.1	*Xanthomonas campestris* pv. *durantae* LMG696	LOKP01000030.1
Lysobacter sp. TY2-98	NZ_CP031413.1	*Xanthomonas cannabis* pv. *cannabis* NCPPB3753	JSZF01000027.1
Lysobacter sp. yr284	FNPT01000001.1	***Xanthomonas citri* 306**	AE008923.1
Lysobacter sp. zong2l5	NZ_QTSU01000001.1	*Xanthomonas citri* pv. *fuscans* str. 4834-R	FO681494.1
[Pseudomonas] geniculata N1	AJLO02000016.1	*Xanthomonas citri* pv. *glycines* str. 8ra	JDSU01000002.1
Pseudoxanthomonas sp. CF125	NZ_FNLD01000002.1	*Xanthomonas citri* pv. *malvacearum* MSCT	CP017020.1
Pseudoxanthomonas sp. GM95	FOAX01000001.1	*Xanthomonas citri* pv. *phaseoli* var. *fuscans*	CP020979.1
Pseudoxanthomonas sp. KAs_5_3	PKSO01000004.1	*Xanthomonas citri* pv. *vignicola* CFBP7113	CP022270.1
Pseudoxanthomonas spadix DSM18855	NZ_RDQN01000004.1	*Xanthomonas codiaei* CFBP4690	NZ_MDEC01000025.1
Pseudoxanthomonas suwonensis S2	QFNC01000012.1	*Xanthomonas cynarae* CFBP4188	NZ_MDFM01000055.1
Pseudoxanthomonas wuyuanensis CGMCC1.10978	NZ_OCND01000011.1	*Xanthomonas dyei* CFBP7245	NZ_MDEE01000016.1
Stenotrophomonas chelatiphaga DSM21508	NZ_LDJK01000096.1	*Xanthomonas euvesicatoria* 66b	JSZG01000018.1
Stenotrophomonas daejeonensis JCM16244	NZ_LDJP01000037.1	*Xanthomonas euvesicatoria* pv. *citrumelonis* CFBP3371	MDCC01000019.1
Stenotrophomonas ginsengisoli DSM24757	NZ_LDJM01000025.1	*Xanthomonas floridensis* WHRI8848	NZ_LXNG01000007.1
Stenotrophomonas indicatrix WS40	NZ_PEJS01000001.1	*Xanthomonas fragariae* PD5205	LT853885.1
Stenotrophomonas koreensis DSM17805	NZ_LDJH01000013.1	*Xanthomonas gardneri* ATCC19865	AEQX01000084.1
Stenotrophomonas lactitubi M15	NZ_PHQX01000001.1	*Xanthomonas hortorum* pv. *hederae* CFBP4925	MDEF01000040.1
Stenotrophomonas maltophilia Ab55555	JH791780.1	*Xanthomonas hyacinthi* CFBP1156	NZ_MDEG01000039.1
***Stenotrophomonas maltophilia* K279a**	NC_010943.1	*Xanthomonas hyacinthi* DSM19077	JPLD01000728.1
Stenotrophomonas maltophilia MF89	ATAP01000112.1	*Xanthomonas melonis* CFBP4644	MDEH01000006.1
Stenotrophomonas maltophilia R551-3	CP001111.1	*Xanthomonas nasturtii* WHRI8853	NZ_LYMI01000032.1
Stenotrophomonas maltophilia RA8	CALM01000806.1	*Xanthomonas perforans* Xp4-20	JZUZ01000033.1
Stenotrophomonas maltophilia WJ66	KN849114.1	*Xanthomonas phaseoli* pv. *dieffenbachiae* LMG25940	JPYI02000041.1
Stenotrophomonas pavanii DSM25135	LDJN01000042.1	*Xanthomonas phaseoli* pv. *manihotis* LMG784	LKKP01000141.1
Stenotrophomonas rhizophila OG2	NZ_NCWX01000002.1	*Xanthomonas phaseoli* pv. *phaseoli* NCPPB1158	JSBS02000062.1
Stenotrophomonas sp. 92mfcol6.1	FWEU01000001.1	*Xanthomonas pisi* CFBP4643	NZ_MDEI01000004.1
Stenotrophomonas sp. AG209	QXDB01000001.1	*Xanthomonas prunicola* CFBP8355	NZ_PHKX01000001.1
Stenotrophomonas sp. CC120222-04	FZQI01000004.1	*Xanthomonas sacchari* R1	NZ_CP010409.1
Stenotrophomonas sp. BIIR7	NZ_MKCZ01000002.1	*Xanthomonas* sp. CFBP7698	PRDN01000001.1
Thermomonas fusca DSM15424	NZ_AUIV01000008.1	*Xanthomonas* sp. CFBP7912	MDSN01000006.1
Xanthomonas albilineans GPEPC73	FP565176.1	*Xanthomonas* sp. Leaf131	LMOG01000019.1
Xanthomonas alfalfae GEV-Rose-07	MIKD01000086.1	*Xanthomonas* sp. Leaf148	LMOP01000008.1
Xanthomonas arboricola pv. *arracaciae* CFBP7407	MIGU01000001.1	*Xanthomonas* sp. NCPPB1128	NZ_LFME01000006.1
Xanthomonas arboricola pv. *corylina* CFBP2565	MDSJ01000034.1	*Xanthomonas theicola* CFBP4691	NZ_MIGX01000080.1
Xanthomonas arboricola pv. *fragariae* CFBP6773	OEQD01000019.1	*Xanthomonas translucens* pv. *arrhenatheri* LMG727	CXOI01000012.1
Xanthomonas arboricola pv. *guizotiae* CFBP7408	MDSK01000048.1	*Xanthomonas translucens* pv. *phlei* LMG730	CXOJ01000010.1
Xanthomonas arboricola pv. *juglandis* Xaj417	CP012251.1	*Xanthomonas translucens* pv. *poae* B99	LWSU01000053.1
Xanthomonas arboricola pv. *populi* CFBP 3122	MIGV01000035.1	*Xanthomonas translucens* pv. *translucens* DSM18974	CAPJ01000354.1
Xanthomonas arboricola pv. *pruni* MAFF301420	BAVC01000014.1	*Xanthomonas vasicola* NCPPB1060	CP034649.1
Xanthomonas arboricola pv. *pruni* str. MAFF311562	BAVB01000420.1	*Xanthomonas vasicola* pv. *vasculorum* NCPPB702	NZ_GG699328.2
Xanthomonas axonopodis pv. *begoniae* CFBP2524	MPSX01000020.1	*Xanthomonas vesicatoria* ATCC35937	AEQV01000175.1

(Continued)

TABLE 1 | Continued

Organism	Accession#	Organism	Accession#
Rhodanobacteraceae			
***Dyella jiangningensis* SBZ3-12**	CP007444.1	*Luteibacter* sp. 329MFSha	NZ_FOJE01000001.1
Dyella marensis UNC178MFTsu3.1	FONH01000012.1	*Luteibacter* sp. OK325	QAOX01000004.1
Dyella sp. 333MFSha	FNBR01000009.1	*Luteibacter* sp. UNCMF331Sha3.1	FOBU01000002.1
Dyella sp. 4MSK11	NZ_QRBF01000004.1	*Luteibacter* sp. UNCMF366Tsu5.1	FPIS01000002.1
Dyella sp. AD56	NRDP01000015.1	*Luteibacter yeojuensis* SU11	JZRB01000062.1
Dyella sp. AtDHG13	NZ_QICJ01000003.1	*Rhodanobacter fulvus* Jip2	NZ_AJXU01000014.1
Dyella sp. OK004	FOZI01000001.1	*Rhodanobacter* sp. 67-28	MKTU01000080.1
***Dyella thiooxydans* ATSB10**	CP014841.1	*Rhodanobacter* sp. C01	NZ_MUNR01000011.1
Frateuria terrea CGMCC1.7053	FOXL01000004.1	*Rhodanobacter* sp. C06	NZ_MUNP01000039.1
***Luteibacter rhizovicinus* DSM16549**	CP017480.1	*Rhodanobacter* sp. OK091	FRCH01000001.1
Luteibacter sp. 22Crub2.1	FUYT01000025.1	*Rhodanobacter* sp. Root627	NZ_LMGW01000002.1
Neisseriaceae			
Morococcus cerebrosus CIP81.93	NZ_JUFZ01000115.1	*Neisseria* sp. HMSC069H12	NZ_KV810249.1
Neisseria dentiae NCTC13012	NZ_UGQR01000001.1	*Neisseria* sp. HMSC06F02	KQ001448.1
***Neisseria flavescens* SK114**	ACQV01000009.1	*Neisseria* sp. HMSC070A01	LTII01000031.1
***Neisseria mucosa* C102**	GL635793.1	*Neisseria* sp. HMSC071C03	KV836738.1
Neisseria sp. HMSC056A03	KV821597.1	*Neisseria* sp. oral taxon 014 str. F0314	GL349413.1
Neisseria sp. HMSC064D07	KV831649.1	*Neisseria subflava* C2012011976	NZ_POXP01000001.1
Comamonadaceae			
***Hydrogenophaga crassostreae* LPB0072**	LVWD01000013.1	*Hydrogenophaga* sp. H7	MCIC01000014.1
Hydrogenophaga sp. A37	MUNZ01000181.1	*Variovorax* sp. Root318D1	NZ_LMCQ01000008.1
Others			
Acinetobacter baumannii 4300STDY7045681	UFGS01000006.1	*Burkholderiales* bacterium GWF1_66_17	MERT01000006.1
Bacillus sp. SRB_336	NZ_NADW01000001.1	*Xanthomonadales* bacterium RIFOXYA1FULL_69_10	MIDV01000097.1
Bacterium AM6	MUYX01000125.1	*Xanthomonadales* bacterium 14-68-21	NCKH01000003.1
Betaproteobacteria bacterium HGW	PHCC01000002.1		

X-T4SSs were identified according to the following criteria: (i) located in chromosomal DNA, (ii) VirB7 subunits have C-terminal N0 domains, (iii) genes for all twelve class A T4SS subunits are present, and (iv) the genomes carry genes for putative effectors (X-Tfes) with C-terminal XVIPCD required for recognition by X-T4SS VirD4. Species names are organized in alphabetical order within each bacterial family. Species discussed in more detail in the main text are shown in bold. #NCBI Reference Sequences or GenBank accession number.

structure, the antenna helices are twisted clockwise (~50°) and tilted vertically (~20°) with respect to the corresponding helices in pKM101, producing a more open outer membrane pore in the *X. citri* structure (45 Å versus 35 Å; **Figure 4**; Sgro et al., 2018). We also observe variability in sequence and length of the linker between the alpha helices that is expected to form a loop on the extracellular side of the outer membrane. This loop is particularly rich in threonine, serine and glycine residues and is longer in the Xanthomonadales VirB10 proteins than in their counterparts in *A. tumefaciens* and pKM101 (**Supplementary Figure S10**; Sgro et al., 2018). In both *X. citri* core complex and pKM101 O-layer structures, these loops are disordered with no significant density in the corresponding maps. Since 14 such loops are expected to be in close proximity at the extracellular face of the outer membrane, they could interact to facilitate closing and opening of the pore. However, an *X. citri* VirB10-msfGFP chimera with an 11 residue deletion in this loop is still partially functional (Sgro et al., 2018).

In contrast to the VirB10 C-terminal domain, its N-terminal domain is known to be highly variable in size and sequence. Xanthomonadales VirB10 proteins have relatively long N-terminal cytosolic segments that precede the transmembrane helix that passes through the inner membrane. While this cytosolic peptide is only 38 or 22 residues long and lacks proline residues in pKM101 and *A. tumefaciens*, it is 57–68 residues long and is rich in proline residues (around 15%) in most X-T4SS VirB10 subunits (**Supplementary Figure S10**). The N-terminal region of VirB10 has been observed to interact with VirD4 of the T4SSs from *A. tumefaciens* (Garza and Christie, 2013) and plasmids R388 (Llosa et al., 2003; Segura et al., 2013) and R27 (Gilmour et al., 2003). Whether similar interactions occur in the X-T4SS remains to be investigated.

The periplasmic portions of the N-terminal domains (NTDs) of VirB10 subunits in many T4SSs are particularly rich in prolines (Jakubowski et al., 2009) and this is also the case for the X-T4SSs (**Supplementary Figure S10**; Sgro et al., 2018). NMR studies of the periplasmic VirB10 NTD revealed it to be intrinsically disordered but with a 12 residue segment that samples a helical conformation and suffers conformational perturbations when mixed with a near 2:1 excess of isolated N-terminal domain of VirB9 at sub-millimolar concentrations (Sgro et al., 2018). This VirB10 N-terminal helix (residues 151–162 in *X. citri*; **Supplementary Figure S10**) fits into the groove between two VirB9 N-terminal domains in the

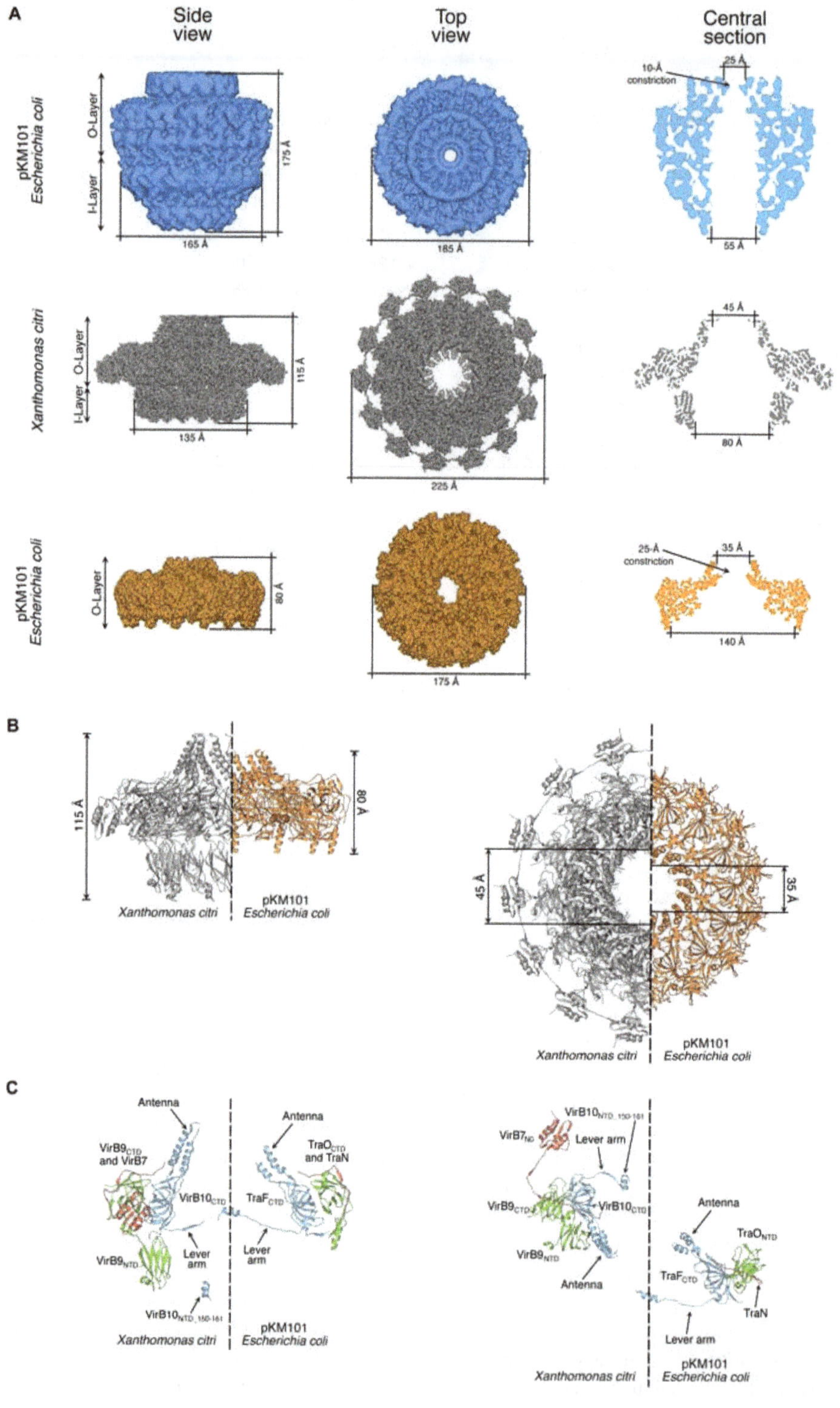

FIGURE 3 | Comparison of core complex structures. **(A)** Comparison of the electron microscopy maps of the full-length core complexes from pKM101 (12.4 Å resolution; top row; Rivera-Calzada et al., 2013) and *X. citri* T4SSs (3.3 Å resolution; middle row; Sgro et al., 2018). Also shown is the electron density map of the O-layer of the pKM101 core complex obtained by X-ray crystallography (2.9 Å resolution; lower row; Chandran et al., 2009). General features and dimensions are shown for side and top views, and for a central section. **(B)** Side-by-side comparison of the atomic models of the *X. citri* core complex (gray) and pKM101 (orange) O-layers. General features and dimensions are shown for side and top views. **(C)** Side-by-side comparison of the atomic models of the VirB7–VirB9–VirB10 trimer and TraN-TraO-TraF trimer in the *X. citri* core complex and pKM101 O-layer, respectively. Colors: VirB10 and TraF (blue), VirB9 and TraO (green), VirB7 and TraN (red). Side (left) and top (right) views are shown of diametrically opposed trimers taken from the side-by-side comparisons shown in **B**. NTD, N-terminal domain; CTD, C-terminal domain. Portions of the Figure were adapted from Rivera-Calzada et al. (2013) and Sgro et al. (2018) with permission from the publishers.

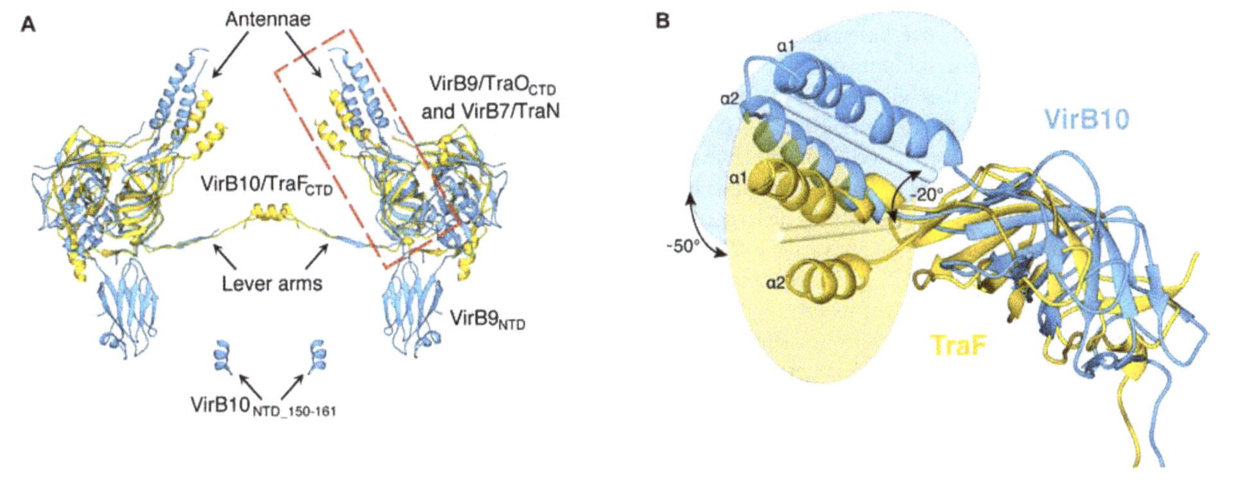

FIGURE 4 | Relative orientations of the antennae that form the outer membrane pore in the *X. citri* and pKM101 core complexes. **(A)** Superposition of the atomic models of diametrically opposed VirB7–VirB9–VirB10 trimers of the *X. citri* core complex (blue) and TraN-TraO-TraF trimers of the pKM101 O-layer (yellow). **(B)** Details of the relative orientations of the VirB10 and TraF C-terminal domains. The structures shown correspond to the red rectangle in **(A)**. The blue and yellow circles represent the planes that contain the central axes of the two antenna helices (α1 and α2). The blue and yellow rods represent the average vector between the two helices in each protein. The angles between the planes (~50°) and between the rods (~20°) are shown. Figure derived from Sgro et al. (2018) with modifications. NTD, N-terminal domain; CTD, C-terminal domain. This Figure was adapted from and Sgro et al. (2018) with permission from the publishers.

X. citri core complex structure (Sgro et al., 2018). The $VirB9_{NTD}$-$VirB10_{NTD}$ interaction, in addition to the VirB7–VirB7 interactions mentioned above (Souza et al., 2011) are two examples of interactions that are relatively weak when measured in isolation but reveal themselves to be physiologically relevant in the context of a large multi-subunit complex whose assembly is expected to be highly cooperative. The helical region is in fact the only well-conserved sequence in the N-terminal domains of the Xanthomonadales and *H. crassostreae* X-T4SS VirB10 subunits and can be described as a P[S/T]Lh[E/D/Q]RRh motif where h is a hydrophobic residue (**Supplementary Figure S10**). The VirB10 subunits from the two *Neisseria* species shown in **Supplementary Figure S10** do not seem to carry this motif.

One interesting observation is the very small number of stereospecific contacts between the I- and O-layers in the *X. citri* core complex. This immediately brings up the question as to what maintains the relative orientations between the two layers. The answer may be that individually weak interactions, multiplied fourteen times in the mature complex, could together be strong enough to favor specific conformational states between the two layers. Another interesting observation is that the long flexible N-terminal linkers that emerge from the VirB9 and VirB10 C-terminal domains in the direction of the I-layer point in opposite directions and pass by each other with their main chain atoms coming within 7 Å of each other (**Figure 3C**; Sgro et al., 2018). Therefore, the covalent linkages between the VirB9 and VirB10 N- and C-domains can be looked upon as forming an intricate cross-weave pattern at the interface of the I- and O-layers. This detail could have a role in maintaining the two layers in a preferential orientation by restricting the excessive relative rotations in both clockwise and counter-clockwise directions. Enigmatically, however, small (6 or 8 residue) deletions in these linkers had only moderate effects on T4SS-dependent bacterial killing by *X. citri* (Sgro et al., 2018).

VirB1

In *A. tumefaciens*, VirB1 undergoes cleavage of its N-terminal signal peptide upon transport to the periplasm and a second cleavage reaction that produces two fragments: (i) an N-terminal SLT (soluble lytic transglycosylase) domain predicted to be involved in peptidoglycan remodeling during T4SS biogenesis and (ii) a 76 residue C-terminal fragment (named VirB1*) that is subsequently transported to the extracellular milieu (Baron et al., 1997; Llosa et al., 2000). The VirB1 proteins in the X-T4SSs all have a well-conserved 150 residue N-terminal domain with predicted SLT activity (**Supplementary Figure S1**). These proteins lack an N-terminal signal sequence, however, and so their mechanism of transport into the periplasm is not yet known. The X-T4SSs VirB1 C-terminal domains vary in length from 130 to over 200 residues and are highly variable in sequence (**Supplementary Figure S1**). Whether X-T4SS VirB1 proteins undergo C-terminal processing in a manner analogous to that observed in *A. tumefaciens* remains to be investigated.

VirB2 and VirB5: The Components of the T4SS Pilus

The VirB2 pilin subunits in the Xanthomonadales species and more distant *H. crassostreae*, *N. flavescens*, and *N. mucosa* all have similar sizes and a very well conserved central hydrophobic region as well as a predicted cleavable 31–39 residue long N-terminal signal peptide (**Supplementary Figure S2**). After removal of the signal peptide, these pilins are predicted to have lengths between 80 and 104 residues. This is significantly greater than the 70 and 64 residue long mature F-pilin and its close homolog from plasmid pED208 (respectively) whose cryo-EM structures have been determined in the context of the assembled sex pilus (Costa et al., 2016). Sequence-based secondary structure predictions for the X-T4SS VirB2 subunits correspond well with the two pilin structures and this allowed us to predict the positions of the two major helices (α2 and α3) in X-T4SS VirB2 as well as the intervening positively charged loop which interacts with the head groups of bound phospholipids in the pilus lumen (**Supplementary Figure S2**; Costa et al., 2016). The larger size of the X-T4SS VirB2 subunits is due to highly variable C-terminal extensions (**Supplementary Figure S2**). It is not clear whether these C-terminal extensions decorate the external pilus surface in X-T4SSs, perhaps providing binding sites for species-specific targets, or whether they are processed as has been observed for some P-pili (Eisenbrandt et al., 1999).

VirB5 is thought to be associated with the T4SS pilus, perhaps as a minor pilin at the pilus tip (Schmidt-Eisenlohr et al., 1999; Aly and Baron, 2007; Alvarez-Martinez and Christie, 2009). Due to the very high sequence variability in VirB5 proteins, its annotation as a bona-fide T4SS component in deposited genomic sequences is often ambiguous. In the bacteria-killing T4SSs under consideration here, these proteins have between 200 and 280 residues and are highly variable in sequence. They all have a predicted N-terminal cleavable signal peptide as well as a pair of cysteine residues found in the central portion of the amino acid sequence that are separated by 11 to 33 residues (**Supplementary Figure S5**). Interestingly, the genetic loci coding for X-T4SSs in the two *Lysobacter* species shown in **Figure 2** each carry two *virB5* genes in tandem. These protein pairs are 73% and 43% identical in *Lysobacter antibioticus* and *Lysobacter enzymogenes*, respectively. The predicted involvement of VirB5 in mediating the binding of the pilus to specific structures on the target cell (Alvarez-Martinez and Christie, 2009), could be a causative factor in this subunit's accelerated evolution.

VirB8, VirB6, and VirB3: Integral Membrane Proteins of the Inner Membrane Complex

VirB8 is an integral membrane protein with an N-terminal cytosolic peptide, a transmembrane helix and a globular C-terminal domain localized in the periplasm, the latter of which has been shown to interact with several other T4SS components, including VirB6, VirB9, and VirB10 (Alvarez-Martinez and Christie, 2009; Sivanesan et al., 2010; Villamil Giraldo et al., 2012). High resolution structures of the soluble C-terminal region of VirB8 proteins and homologs from diverse T4SSs have been determined: *A. tumefaciens* (Bailey et al., 2006), pKM101 (Casu et al., 2016), *H. pylori* (ComB10) and *Brucella suis* (Terradot et al., 2005), *Clostridium perfringens*, *Rickettsia typhi* and several *Bartonella* species (Gillespie et al., 2015), *L. pneumophila* and plasmid R64 (Kuroda et al., 2015). All these structures present the same fold, a β-sheet juxtaposed against a group of α-helices, and in most cases have been shown to oligomerize to different degrees (see references above). Since there are an estimated 12 copies of VirB8 in each class A T4SS (Low et al., 2014), these domains could associate to form an as-yet unknown structure in the bacterial periplasm. Interestingly, the bacteria-killing X-T4SSs have highly distinctive VirB8 components that are significantly longer (between 290 and 370 residues in length) than the canonical VirB8 components observed in the species listed above (all less than 250 residues). This greater size is, in large part, due to a C-terminal extension enriched in Ala, Gln, Gly, and Pro (AQGP) residues (**Table 2** and **Supplementary Figure S8**). The length of this extension and its enrichment in these residues are particularly evident in the Xanthomonadales order (53–73%) and *H. crassostreae* (45%) and less so in the X-T4SS VirB8 proteins of *Neisseria* species (**Table 2**). The role, if any, of the AQGP-rich extensions in these proteins is not yet known.

VirB6 is predicted to be a polytopic integral protein. In both *A. tumefaciens* and *B. suis*, the VirB6 N-terminus is located in the periplasm and the C-terminus is located in the cytosol, implying an odd number of transmembrane helices, estimated to be five in *A. tumefaciens* (Jakubowski et al., 2004) and seven in *B. suis* (Villamil Giraldo et al., 2015). **Supplementary Figure S6** presents the multiple sequence alignment of X-T4SS VirB6 proteins that also align well with their homologs in *A. tumefaciens* and *B. suis* (data not shown). The precise number and positions of the transmembrane helices is again ambiguous since transmembrane helix pairs 3/4 and 5/6 could alternatively be longer single helices (**Supplementary Figure S6**). Another common feature of these proteins is a large loop between transmembrane helices 2 and 3, predicted to be localized in the periplasm for both *A. tumefaciens*

TABLE 2 | Characteristics of C-terminal extensions in VirB8 proteins from X-T4SSs.

Organism	Extension size (aa)	% Ala	% Gln	% Gly	% Pro	% AQGP
Xanthomonas citri 306	98	21	25	11	15	72
Stenotrophomonas maltophilia K279a	104	19	19	12	15	65
Lysobacter antibioticus 76	97	26	4	10	32	72
Lysobacter enzymogenes C3	100	25	7	10	31	73
Luteibacter rhizovicinus DSM16549	129	26	11	12	22	71
Dyella jiangningensis SBZ3-12	70	16	9	11	17	53
Dyella thiooxydans ATSB10	48	33	2	8	27	70
Hydrogenophaga crassostreae LPB0072	53	13	6	11	15	45
Neisseria mucosa C102	55	6	16	4	13	39
Neisseria flavescens SK114	52	6	14	6	6	32

Analysis is based on the alignment shown in ***Supplementary Figure S8****.*

and *B. suis*. The periplasmic loops of the estimated 24 copies of VirB6 per T4SS (Low et al., 2014) are expected to interact with other periplasmic components of the inner membrane complex (**Figure 1**; Ding et al., 2003; Alvarez-Martinez and Christie, 2009; Villamil Giraldo et al., 2012, 2015; Christie, 2016).

X-T4SS VirB3 proteins are predicted to be bitopic or polytopic membrane proteins with one or two transmembrane helices located within the region encompassed by residues 15 and 57 (see **Supplementary Figure S3** for details). This is consistent with the difficulty in defining VirB3 topology in other T4SSs (Alvarez-Martinez and Christie, 2009). In some organisms, gene fusions have been observed between VirB3 and VirB4 (Batchelor et al., 2004) but this does not seem to be the case in the X-T4SSs. These gene fusions and the highly conserved synteny of *virB3* and *virB4* genes in most organisms suggests that these two proteins could interact with each other at or within the inner membrane (Peña et al., 2012). This hypothesis is supported by the observation that *A. tumefaciens* VirB4 is required to maintain normal levels of VirB3 (Jones et al., 1994) and that recombinant R388 VirB4 and VirB3 can be co-purified as a 1:1 complex (Low et al., 2014).

VirB4, VirB11, and VirD4: The ATPases of the Inner Membrane Complex

VirB4, VirB11, and VirD4 are P-loop ATPases with conserved Walker A and Walker B motifs and, in most T4SSs characterized to date, all three proteins are required for biogenesis and/or function (Alvarez-Martinez and Christie, 2009; Christie et al., 2014; Christie, 2016). These proteins use the hydrolysis of ATP to carry out mechanical work, expected to manifest itself in substrate unfolding, transfer and/or extrusion through the T4SS channel (Atmakuri et al., 2004).

VirB4 is the most well conserved T4SS subunit and has been used in phylogenetic analyses to trace evolutionary relationships and propose models for the emergence of T4SS subclasses (Guglielmini et al., 2014). Studies on different T4SSs have reported evidence that VirB4 interacts, at least transiently, with all of the other inner membrane complex components (Jones et al., 1994; Atmakuri et al., 2004; Cascales and Christie, 2004; Jakubowski et al., 2004; Paschos et al., 2006; Ripoll-Rozada et al., 2013; Low et al., 2014; Christie, 2016).

VirB4 has been localized to two 3-tiered barrel-like pedestals at the base of the inner membrane complex in EM reconstructions of the complete R388 T4SS, with each barrel corresponding to a VirB4 hexamer (Low et al., 2014; Redzej et al., 2017). VirB4 proteins can be divided into N- and C-terminal domains. The C-terminal domain carries all the conserved motifs required for nucleotide binding and hydrolysis (Walker A and Walker B boxes and motifs C, D, and E) and these motifs are present in X-T4SS VirB4 proteins (**Supplementary Figure S4**). The N-terminal domain, known to mediate interactions with the inner membrane, is expected to correspond to the upper tier in the R388 T4SS structure (Low et al., 2014; Redzej et al., 2017). One variable in the family of VirB4 proteins is the presence or absence of one or more predicted N-terminal transmembrane helices and the question as to their requirement for VirB4 function has proven to be controversial (Rabel et al., 2003), with the additional caveat that VirB4/TraB from pKM101 can be purified in soluble and membrane-bound forms (Durand et al., 2010). Therefore, it is not clear whether VirB4 should be considered an integral or peripheral membrane protein, or both (Arechaga et al., 2008; Christie, 2016; Waksman, 2019). The X-T4SS VirB4 proteins do not have predicted transmembrane helices using the TMHMM v2.0 (Krogh et al., 2001) and PSort (Nakai and Horton, 1999) prediction algorithms.

VirB11 is a soluble membrane-associated AAA+ ATPase that has been shown to interact with both VirD4 and VirB4 (Ripoll-Rozada et al., 2013). The crystal structures of VirB11 homologs from *B. suis* (Hare et al., 2006) and *H. pylori* (Yeo et al., 2000) are both two-tiered hexameric rings in which each ring layer consists of six N- or C-terminal domains from the constituent monomers. Within VirB11 monomers, the domains are connected by a central linker of varying length, short in *H. pylori* and 17 residues longer (linker B and α2C) in *B. suis*, resulting in a domain-swapped architecture in the latter (Hare et al., 2006). As a consequence, the nucleotide binding site in *H. pylori* VirB11 is located at the interface between the two domains of the same monomer while in *B. suis* the nucleotide binds at the interface between the N-terminal domain of one monomer and the C-terminal domain of the neighboring monomer (Hare et al., 2006). VirB11 proteins from X-T4SSs show a high degree of sequence similarity and all have the long version of the linker, which aligns well with the *B. suis* linker B and α2C sequences (**Supplementary Figure S11**). We can therefore expect that the X-T4SS VirB11 proteins exhibit a domain-swapped structure similar to that of *B. suis* (Hare et al., 2006).

The VirD4 ATPase and its homologs are often called coupling proteins due to their role in selecting substrates for export by the T4SS. Analysis of the X-T4SS VirD4 proteins suggests that they have a canonical VirD4-like architecture (Llosa and Alkorta, 2017) with two N-terminal transmembrane helices with a predicted intervening ~30 amino acid periplasmic loop and a cytosolic C-terminal domain. The cytosolic domain can be separated into a nucleotide binding domain (NBD), with conserved Walker A and Walker B motifs, and a so-called all alpha domain (AAD) (**Supplementary Figure S12**; Gomis-Ruth et al., 2002). The VirD4 N-terminal transmembrane domain helices have been implicated in interacting with the VirB10 N-terminal region that includes its transmembrane helix (Segura et al., 2013) and the VirD4 all alpha domain is involved in substrate recognition (Gomis-Ruth et al., 2002; Whitaker et al., 2015). TrwB, the VirD4 homolog of the conjugative plasmid R388, has been crystallized as a hexameric ring (Gomis-Ruth et al., 2002). It has been proposed that VirB4 and VirD4 could form transient heterohexameric complexes during substrate transport (Peña et al., 2012; Waksman, 2019) and low resolution electron microscopy studies of the intact VirB3-B10/D4 T4SS from R388 observed VirD4 dimers sandwiched between the two hexameric VirB4 barrels (Redzej et al., 2017). Therefore, the oligomeric structure of VirD4 in a fully assembled and functioning T4SS is still not clear (Redzej et al., 2017; Chetrit et al., 2018; Waksman, 2019).

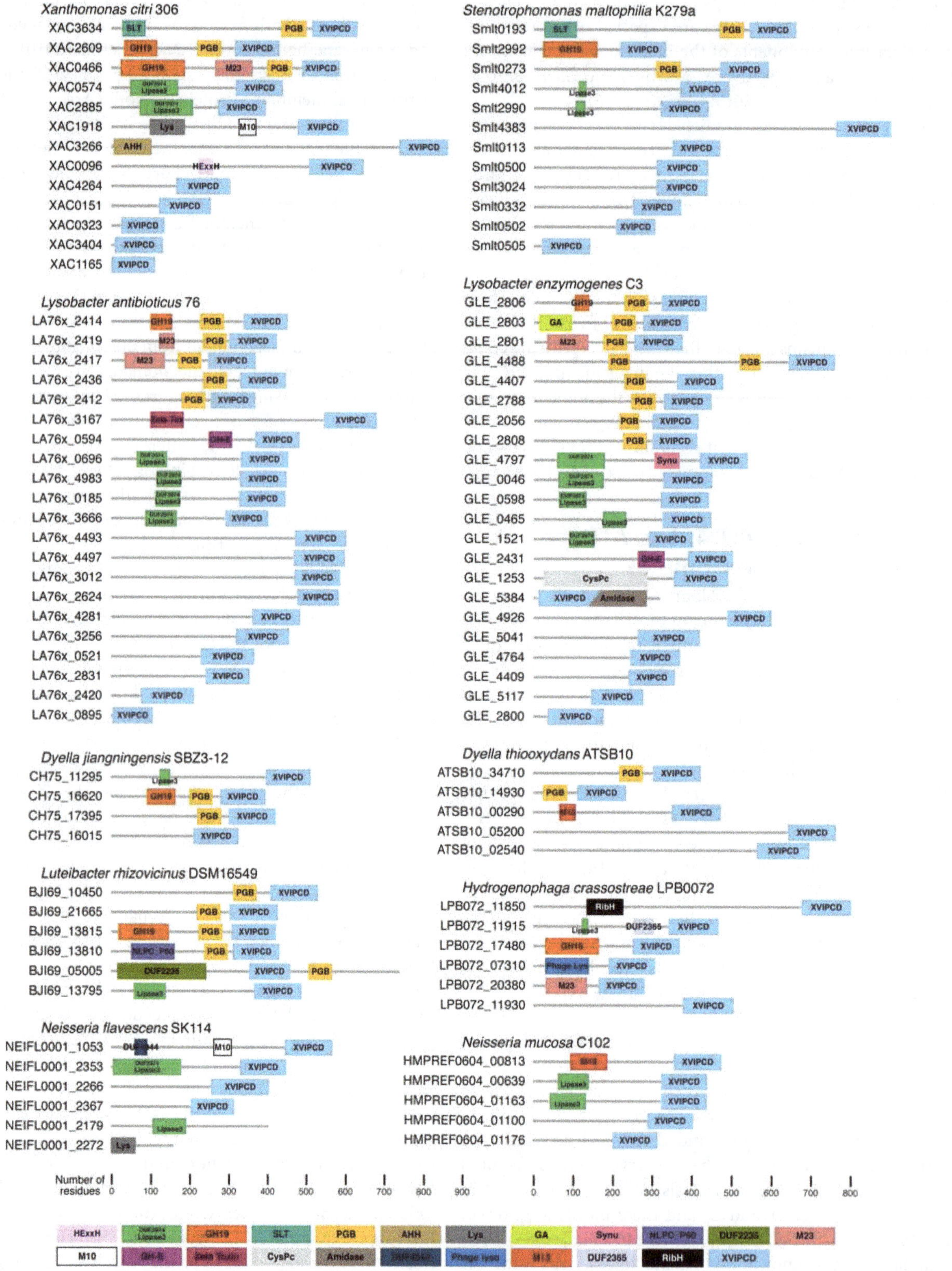

FIGURE 5 | Putative Xanthomonadales-like T4SS effectors (X-Tfes) found in selected species that carry an X-T4SS. Shown here are representative examples from *Xanthomonas citri* 306 (Da Silva et al., 2002), *Stenotrophomonas maltophilia* K279a (Crossman et al., 2008), *Lysobacter antibioticus* 76 (de Bruijn et al., 2015), *Lysobacter enzymogenes* C3 (unpublished; GenBank accession CP013140), *Luteibacter rhizovicinus* DSM16549 (unpublished; GenBank accession CP017480),

(Continued)

FIGURE 5 | Continued
Dyella jiangningensis SBZ3-12 (Bao et al., 2014), *Dyella thiooxydans* strain ATSB10 (unpublished; GenBank accession CP014841), *Hydrogenophaga crassostreae* LPB0072 (unpublished; GenBank accession LVWD01000013), *Neisseria mucosa* C102 (unpublished, GenBank accession GCA_000186165) and *Neisseria flavescens* SK114 (unpublished; GenBank accession ACQV01000009). Protein domains were identified by sequence comparison with the Pfam (El-Gebali et al., 2019) and/or CDD databases (Marchler-Bauer et al., 2015) and are colored according to the scheme presented at the bottom of the Figure. Domain abbreviations: M10 (Pfam accession PF08548), M13 (Pfam accession PF01431), M23 (Pfam accession PF01551), Lipase3 (Pfam accession PF01764), DUF2974 (Pfam accession PF11187), GH-E (Pfam accession PF14410), GH19 (Pfam accession PF00182), Zeta Toxin (Pfam accession PF06414), SLT (CDD accession cd00254), CysPc (CDD accession cd00044), PGB (Pfam accession PF01471), Amidase (Pfam accession PF01510), AHH (Pfam accession PF14412), DUF4344 (Pfam accession PF14247), Lys (CDD accession cl00222), Phage lyso (Pfam accession PF00959), GA (Pfam accession PF01832), Synu (CDD accession cl03193), DUF2365 (Pfam accession PF10157), NLPC_P60 (Pfam accession PF00877), RibH (Pfam accession PF02267), DUF2235 (Pfam accession PF09994), HExxH (HExxH motif in putative metalloprotease domain; Firczuk and Bochtler, 2007).

XANTHOMONADALES-LIKE T4SS EFFECTORS (X-Tfes) AND THEIR COGNATE INHIBITORS (X-Tfis)

X-Tfes

The first clues regarding the physiological role of the *X. citri* T4SS came from the identification of T4SS substrates using the VirD4 coupling protein as a bait in yeast two-hybrid assays against a *Xanthomonas* genomic library (Alegria et al., 2005). The strategy was based on the reasoning that in other well-characterized T4SSs, the VirD4 component is known to interact with the macromolecular substrates prior to transport (Llosa and Alkorta, 2017). This screening originally identified 12 so-called "*Xanthomonas* VirD4 interacting proteins," or XVIPs (Alegria et al., 2005), later called *Xanthomonadaceae* T4SS effectors (Souza et al., 2015) and from here on Xanthomonadales-like T4SS effectors (X-Tfes, **Figure 5**). In *X. citri*, the gene for one X-Tfe (XAC2609) is found in the *vir* locus while the remaining X-Tfe genes are dispersed throughout the genome. Interestingly, all of these proteins have a common C-terminal domain entitled "XVIP conserved domain" or XVIPCD (**Figures 1, 5**), typically around 120 residues long, required for interaction with VirD4 (Alegria et al., 2005) and for secretion in a T4SS-dependent manner (Souza et al., 2015). The XVIPCD is characterized by a few conserved motifs in its N-terminal region and a glutamine-rich C-terminal region (Alegria et al., 2005).

The discovery of the XVIPCD as the secretion signal for the *X. citri* X-Tfes allowed for a large-scale bioinformatics identification of X-Tfe genes present in other bacterial genomes (Souza et al., 2015). **Figure 5** shows the domain architectures of the X-Tfes identified by bioinformatics analysis of bacterial genomes whose X-T4SSs are described in **Figure 2**. The N-terminal portions of the *X. citri* X-Tfes are highly variable in size and architecture and most are predicted to function within the periplasm as peptidoglycan (PG) glycohydrolases, lytic transglycosylases, PG peptidases or lipases (**Figure 5**). Therefore, these bacterial species probably use their X-T4SSs to inject not one, but a diverse cocktail of X-Tfes that will simultaneously attack multiple structures in the target cell (**Figure 1**). Two purified *X. citri* X-Tfes (XAC2609 and XAC0466) with predicted PG hydrolase activities have been shown to lyse PG and induce the lysis of Gram-positive cells, which have exposed bacterial cell walls (Souza et al., 2015). It is interesting that a considerable fraction of X-Tfes have N-terminal sequences with no identifiable domains, opening the possibility that new domain families with antibacterial activities could be characterized in the future. One such X-Tfe, Smlt3024 from *S. maltophilia* K279a (**Figure 5**), has been shown to inhibit *E. coli* growth when heterologously expressed and directed to the periplasm (preprint: Bayer-Santos et al., 2019).

It is worth noting that we often encounter several open reading frames that code for small proteins, sometimes possessing little more than an intact XVIPCD; for example XAC0323, XAC1165, and XAC3404 in *X. citri* (respectively 136, 127, and 132 residues in length; **Figure 5**; Souza et al., 2015). In some cases, these open reading frames appear to be fragments of ancestral X-Tfes genes that suffered frameshift mutations. One example of this phenomenon is provided by the XAC1165 gene whose first 37 nucleotides overlap with the 3′ end of the upstream XAC1164 gene which codes for a 437 protein of unknown function. The amino acid sequences of XAC1164 and XAC1165 align very well with the N-terminal and XVIPCD regions, respectively, of the Smlt0113 X-Tfe protein from *S. maltophilia* (**Figure 5**). Thus *X. citri* XAC1164 and XAC1165 proteins are homologous, and probably the non-functional, fragments of a functional X-Tfe (Smlt0113) in *S. maltophilia*.

X-Tfis

To protect against the toxicity of endogenous or exogenous X-Tfes, *X. citri* and *S. maltophilia* produce specific immunity proteins that bind to their cognate toxins (Alegria et al., 2005; Souza et al., 2015; preprint: Bayer-Santos et al., 2019). These inhibitors have been termed *Xanthomonadaceae* T4SS immunity proteins (Souza et al., 2015) and from here on Xanthomonadales-like T4SS immunity proteins (X-Tfis). The genes coding for X-Tfis are usually found upstream and are probably co-transcribed with their cognate X-Tfe (Souza et al., 2015; preprint: Bayer-Santos et al., 2019). All bacterial species identified so far that carry an X-T4SS also code for multiple X-Tfe/X-Tfi pairs and, in most cases, the genes for at least one pair is found within, or in close proximity to, the locus that codes for the structural components of the X-T4SS (see **Figure 2**). Furthermore, in almost all cases where the X-Tfe is predicted to act upon periplasmic structures (glycosidic and peptide bonds in peptidoglycan or ester linkages in phospholipids), the cognate X-Tfi carries an N-terminal signal peptide and lipobox for periplasmic localization and anchoring in the outer membrane (Souza et al., 2015; preprint: Bayer-Santos et al., 2019). On the other hand, some X-Tfes with N-terminal

X-Tfe	X-Tfi	N-terminal amino acid sequence of X-Tfi	Putative alternative X-Tfi initiation codon and RBS
XAC3634	XAC3633	MLVRKISLVLALATIAACTQATPDATAPKTAAAAAGTPTKPSEKDASPM...	agaaaaggatgcatctcccatg
XAC2609	XAC2610	MLTRELARAVAGVIYLICVVSITACSPSNAPSAEADGEKSPAKNQASKKPEYELQKDLKM...	aaaaggatttgaaaatg
XAC0466	XAC0467	MPPFRLLIPILAVALVACNGPQAADAPETPANAPAAAAQPPSPAASPPATPTQGTVPM...	aagggactgtacccatg
XAC0096	XAC0097	MRFPRAALLFLTALCAPALSACAHGPLKPLPKEHADM...	gaaggagcacgctgacatg
XAC0574	XAC0573	MAAHLPRRPALRQMLTPSLLALLLTACHSPETSM...	cggagaccagcatg
XAC2885	XAC2884	MQPRFPALLVLATSFFAVSCTASPGAKEQTTM...	aaggagcaaaccaccatg
XAC1918	XAC1917	MKIKSVGCVALALFFITGCTVVSAGADM...	gcgggcgcggacatg

FIGURE 6 | Possible alternative translation start codons that could lead to the production of soluble cytosolic X-Tfis in *Xanthomonas citri*. The first two columns list the names of *X. citri* X-Tfe/X-Tfi pairs in which the X-Tfi is predicted to be a lipoprotein (Souza et al., 2015). The third column presents the N-terminal amino acid sequence of the X-Tfi in which the signal sequence and Lipobox are shown in bold. The basic nucleotides at the N-terminus of the signal sequence are shown in blue. The four Lipobox residues are shown in red. Underlined residues are those from the absolutely conserved Cys residue at the site of cleavage in the Lipobox to the next Met residue (green) in the protein sequence. The last column presents the nucleotide sequence (lowercase letters) immediately upstream of the putative alternative start codon (green). The putative Shine–Dalgarno sequence (ribosome binding site) for this alternative start codon is shown in red.

TABLE 3 | List of proteins in the KEGG database with greatest similarity[a] to the N-terminal domain (residues 1–240) of Smlt0332 from *S. maltophilia* K279a.

Organism	Accession[b]	*E*-value	Description
Xanthomonas campestris pv. *campestris* B100	xcc-b100_0624	3 E-88	X-T4SS X-Tfe
Xanthomonas campestris pv. *campestris* 8004	XC_3909	2 E-83	X-T4SS X-Tfe
Xanthomonas campestris pv. *campestris* ATCC33913	XCC3567	2 E-83	X-T4SS X-Tfe
Xanthomonas vasicola pv. *vasculorum* SAM119	C7V42_12340	2 E-79	X-T4SS X-Tfe
Xanthomonas vesicatoria ATCC35937	BJD12_15640	2 E-76	X-T4SS X-Tfe
Metakosakonia sp. MRY16-398	MRY16398_33930	2 E-26	Type VI secretion system secreted protein VgrG
Pantoea ananatis LMG20103	PANA_2352	9 E-26	Type VI secretion system secreted protein VgrG
Pantoea vagans FDAARGOS_160	AL522_12495	4 E-25	Type VI secretion system secreted protein VgrG
Kosakonia radicincitans GXGL-4A	A3780_13240	4 E-22	Type VI secretion system secreted protein VgrG/Rhs
Enterobacter hormaechei subsp. *xiangfangensis* LMG27195	BFV63_12735	4 E-21	Type VI secretion system secreted protein VgrG/Rhs
Enterobacter hormaechei subsp. *xiangfangensis* 34399	LI66_12735	9 E-21	Type VI secretion system secreted protein VgrG/Rhs
Enterobacter hormaechei subsp. *hoffmannii* ECR091	ECR091_12370	9 E-21	Type VI secretion system secreted protein VgrG
Enterobacter hormaechei subsp. *hoffmannii* ECNIH3	ECNIH3_12435	2 E-20	Type VI secretion system secreted protein VgrG
Enterobacter cloacae ECNIH5	ECNIH5_12380	3 E-20	Type VI secretion system secreted protein VgrG/Rhs
Burkholderia stabilis ATCCBAA-67	BBJ41_25130	2 E-20	Type VI secretion system secreted protein VgrG
Enterobacter hormaechei subsp. *hormaechei* 34983	LI64_12500	2 E-20	Type VI secretion system secreted protein VgrG/Rhs
Methylocaldum marinum S8	sS8_3556	6 E-20	Type VI secretion system secreted protein VgrG
Ralstonia solanacearum FQY_4	F504_2863	2 E-19	Type VI secretion system secreted protein VgrG
Ralstonia solanacearum Po82	RSPO_c00015	2 E-19	Type VI secretion system secreted protein VgrG
Burkholderia territorii RF8-non-BP5	WS51_08400	4 E-19	Type VI secretion system secreted protein VgrG
Cronobacter turicensis z3032	CTU_00910	3 E-19	Type VI secretion system secreted protein VgrG
Ralstonia pseudosolanacearum RS 476	CDC45_17535	5 E-19	Type VI secretion system secreted protein VgrG
Ralstonia solanacearum GMI1000	RSc3430	5 E-19	Type VI secretion system secreted protein VgrG
Ralstonia solanacearum PSI07	RPSI07_0016	1 E-17	Type VI secretion system secreted protein VgrG
Burkholderia stagnalis MSMB735WGS	WT74_22275	3 E-17	Type VI secretion system secreted protein VgrG
Xanthomonas fragariae Fap21	BER92_04245	2 E-17	Type VI secretion system secreted protein VgrG
Ralstonia solanacearum FQY_4	F504_3476	4 E-17	Type VI secretion system secreted protein VgrG
Xanthomonas campestris pv. *raphani* 756C	XCR_2915	4 E-17	Hypothetical protein
Mycolicibacterium hassiacum DSM44199	MHAS_03665	1 E-16	Hypothetical protein
Burkholderia ubonensis MSMB22	BW23_4367	3 E-16	Type VI secretion system secreted protein VgrG/Rhs
Enterobacter sp. R4-368	H650_00935	2 E-12	Type VI secretion system secreted protein VgrG
Kosakonia cowanii 888-76	BWI95_18245	7 E-09	Type VI secretion system secreted protein VgrG/Rhs

[a] *only proteins with significant coverage in the alignment are shown.*
[b] *KEGG (Kyoto Encyclopedia of Genes and Genomes) accession number.*

domains predicted to act in the cytosol of the target cell (for example the *X. citri* X-Tfe XAC3266 with an N-terminal AHH domain with predicted nuclease activity; **Figure 5**) have a cognate X-Tfi (for example XAC3267) lacking a lipoprotein signal (Souza et al., 2015). Finally, some X-Tfes are expected to be active in both the cytosol and periplasm, as are the cases of the X-Tfes with predicted lipase domains with phospholipase activities (NFB, DPS, BM, and CSF, manuscript in preparation; **Figure 5**). This brings up the question regarding the cellular localization of the X-Tfis. An analysis of the *X. citri* X-Tfis with putative N-terminal signal peptide and Lipobox sites indicates that their coding genes have potential alternative downstream start (ATG) codons with associated ribosome binding sites (**Figure 6**). This raises the possibility that many X-Tfes can be produced in two versions: (i) a membrane-associated periplasmic lipoprotein and (ii) a soluble cytosolic protein (**Figure 1**). Thus, if X-Tfes make their way into the periplasm, either by leakage from the secretion channel or by injection by neighboring cells of the same species, they will be inhibited by the periplasmic lipoprotein forms of the cognate X-Tfi. On the other hand, X-Tfes whose activities could target cytosolic substrates can be inhibited by cytosolic variants of their cognate X-Tfis. If this is in fact the case, for at least this latter subset of X-Tfes, transport will necessarily involve previous dissociation of the X-Tfe/X-Tfi cytosolic pair.

Parallels Between X-T4SS X-Tfe/X-Tfi, T6SS Effector/Immunity Protein and Plasmid-Encoded Toxin/ Antitoxin (TA) Pairs

X-Tfe/X-Tfi pairs share many of the characteristics observed for T6SS effectors and their inhibitors (Russell et al., 2011, 2013). For example, one immunity protein from *X. citri* (X-$Tfi^{XAC2610}$) inhibits the GH19 family PG hydrolase X-$Tfe^{XAC2609}$ and has a very similar topology, though very little sequence similarity, to the PG hydrolase inhibitors PliI and Tsi1 (Van Herreweghe et al., 2010; Russell et al., 2011) the latter of which is an inhibitor of the T6SS effector Tse1 from *Pseudomonas aeruginosa* (Souza et al., 2015). Another example is provided by the X-Tfe Smlt0332 from *S. maltophilia* K279a, which has many X-Tfe homologs in other Xanthomonadales species (data not shown) but whose N-terminal region has no similarity with annotated domains in the Pfam or CCD databases. Interestingly, Blast searches against the curated KEGG database (Kanehisa et al., 2017) using this domain identified a large number of homologous sequences fused to VgrG domains in effectors predicted to be secreted by T6SSs of *Metakosakonia*, *Pantoea*, *Kosakonia*, *Enterobacter*, *Burkholderia*, *Methylocaldum*, *Ralstonia*, *Cronobacter*, and *Xanthomonas* species (**Table 3**). Searches against the non-redundant protein sequence database (Altschul et al., 1990) identified many more such homologs in other bacterial species (data not shown). These findings raise interesting questions regarding the evolution, distribution and exchange of T4SS and T6SS effectors in the biosphere. In fact, we can make a general observation that anti-bacterial Type IV and Type VI secretion systems share many enzymatic effector and cognate inhibitory modules and differ only in the specific sequences recognized for transport. It also raises the possibility that the acquisition of immunity proteins could be advantageous even in the absence of the cognate effector by offering a defense against the toxic activity of substrates launched by both T4SS and T6SSs during encounters with rival bacteria. We have in fact recently observed the reciprocal T4SS-dependent dueling between *S. maltophilia* and *X. citri* cells which could mimic similar encounters between soil- and/or plant-associated bacteria in the environment (preprint: Bayer-Santos et al., 2019). The differences in X-Tfe and X-Tfi repertoires between rival species will contribute to the outcome of these encounters.

Effector/immunity protein pairs associated with T4SS and T6SSs show intriguing parallels with toxin/anti-toxin modules that function to guarantee vertical transmission of mobile elements (Jensen and Gerdes, 1995). For example, Harms et al. (2017) have shown that the pVbh plasmid of *Bartonella schoenbuchensis*, codes for a toxin/antitoxin module in which the toxin component, VbhT, acquired a C-terminal BID (Bep Intracellular Delivery) domain that confers its transfer to recipient cells during conjugation. They propose that its function may be to support intercellular DNA transfer by pre-emptively addicting the recipient cell to the plasmid, which also carries the gene for the antitoxin antidote. It is not difficult to imagine a scenario in which the T4SS coded by such a plasmid could lose its capacity to transfer DNA but retain its capacity to transfer the toxin, and in this way evolve into a single-purpose bacteria-killing T4SS. Therefore, we can expect bactericidal T4SSs, perhaps with very different recognition signals, to have arisen on multiple occasions in distantly related bacterial species.

CLOSING REMARKS

These are early days in the characterization of antibacterial T4SSs. The structure of the *X. citri* core complex has provided a good reference for comparison with other T4SSs, and has illustrated the structural variability that we can expect to encounter even within the class A T4SSs. While X-T4SS activities have only been experimentally verified for *X. citri* and *S. maltophilia*, bioinformatics analysis allowed us to confidently expand the list of bacterial families both within the Gammaproteobacteria class as well as to other families within the Betaproteobacteria (**Table 1**) that carry proteins with many of the characteristic X-T4SSs features, including VirB7 proteins with N0 domains, VirB8 proteins with AQGP-rich extensions as well as recognizable X-Tfe/X-Tfi pairs in which the effector carries a C-terminal XVIPCD. The list of X-T4SSs will most surely expand significantly in the future. However, it is unlikely that bactericidal T4SSs are restricted to the X-T4SSs described here. It is more probable that many other bacterial species carry as yet uncharacterized and perhaps unrecognized T4SSs that recruit effectors with recognition signals significantly different from the XVIPCDs associated with X-T4SSs as predicted (Souza et al., 2015) and as illustrated by the results obtained for the T4SS encoded by the *B. schoenbuchensis* pVbh plasmid (Harms et al., 2017).

AUTHOR CONTRIBUTIONS

GS, GO, EB-S, and CF produced the figures and tables. CF wrote the manuscript. All authors contributed with critical discussions and revisions that led to the final version of the manuscript.

FUNDING

This work was supported by grants from the Fundação de Amparo à Pesquisa do Estado de São Paulo (FAPESP) to CF (Grant # 2017/17303-7), CA-M (Grant # 2018/01852-4), and EB-S (Grant # 2017/02178-2).

ACKNOWLEDGMENTS

GS, GO, DS, WC, BM, and EB-S acknowledge scholarships from FAPESP. DS, TdS, and NB acknowledge fellowships from Coordenação de Aperfeiçoamento de Pessoal de Nível Superior (CAPES).

REFERENCES

Alegria, M. C., Souza, D. P., Andrade, M. O., Docena, C., Khater, L., Ramos, C. H. I., et al. (2005). Identification of new protein-protein interactions involving the products of the chromosome- and plasmid-encoded type IV secretion loci of the phytopathogen *Xanthomonas axonopodis* pv. *citri*. *J. Bacteriol.* 187, 2315–2325. doi: 10.1128/JB.187.7.2315-2325.2005

Altschul, S. F., Gish, W., Miller, W., Myers, E. W., and Lipman, D. J. (1990). Basic local alignment search tool. *J. Mol. Biol.* 215, 403–410. doi: 10.1016/S0022-2836(05)80360-2

Alvarez-Martinez, C. E., and Christie, P. J. (2009). Biological diversity of prokaryotic type IV secretion systems. *Microbiol. Mol. Biol. Rev.* 73, 775–808. doi: 10.1128/MMBR.00023-09

Aly, K. A., and Baron, C. (2007). The VirB5 protein localizes to the T-pilus tips in *Agrobacterium tumefaciens*. *Microbiology* 153, 3766–3775. doi: 10.1099/mic.0.2007/010462-0

Arechaga, I., Pena, A., Zunzunegui, S., del Carmen Fernandez-Alonso, M., Rivas, G., and de la Cruz, F. (2008). ATPase activity and oligomeric state of TrwK, the VirB4 homologue of the plasmid R388 type IV secretion system. *J. Bacteriol.* 190, 5472–5479. doi: 10.1128/JB.00321-08

Atmakuri, K., Cascales, E., and Christie, P. J. (2004). Energetic components VirD4, VirB11 and VirB4 mediate early DNA transfer reactions required for bacterial type IV secretion. *Mol. Microbiol.* 54, 1199–1211. doi: 10.1111/j.1365-2958.2004.04345.x

Backert, S., and Meyer, T. F. (2006). Type IV secretion systems and their effectors in bacterial pathogenesis. *Curr. Opin. Microbiol.* 9, 207–217. doi: 10.1016/j.mib.2006.02.008

Backert, S., Tegtmeyer, N., and Fischer, W. (2015). Composition, structure and function of the *Helicobacter pylori* cag pathogenicity island encoded type IV secretion system. *Future Microbiol.* 10, 955–965. doi: 10.2217/fmb.15.32

Bailey, S., Ward, D., Middleton, R., Grossmann, J. G., and Zambryski, P. C. (2006). *Agrobacterium tumefaciens* VirB8 structure reveals potential protein-protein interaction sites. *Proc. Natl. Acad. Sci. U.S.A.* 103, 2582–2587. doi: 10.1073/pnas.0511216103

Bao, Y., Kwok, A. H. Y., He, L., Jiang, J., Huang, Z., Leung, F. C. C., et al. (2014). Complete genome sequence of *Dyella jiangningensis* strain SBZ3-12, isolated from the surfaces of weathered rock. *Genome Announc.* 2:e00416-14. doi: 10.1128/genomeA.00416-14

Baron, C., Llosa, M., Zhou, S., and Zambryski, P. C. (1997). VirB1, a component of the T-complex transfer machinery of *Agrobacterium tumefaciens*, is processed to a C-terminal secreted product, VirB1. *J. Bacteriol.* 179, 1203–1210. doi: 10.1128/jb.179.4.1203-1210.1997

Batchelor, R. A., Pearson, B. M., Friis, L. M., Guerry, P., and Wells, J. M. (2004). Nucleotide sequences and comparison of two large conjugative plasmids from different *Campylobacter* species. *Microbiology* 150(Pt 10), 3507–3517. doi: 10.1099/mic.0.27112-0

Bayer-Santos, E., Cenens, W., Matsuyama, B. Y., Di Sessa, G., Mininel, I. D. V., and Farah, C. S. (2019). The opportunistic pathogen *Stenotrophomonas maltophilia* utilizes a type IV secretion system for interbacterial killing. *bioRxiv* [Preprint]. doi: 10.1101/557322

Bayer-Santos, E., Lima, L., dos, P., Ceseti, L., de, M., Ratagami, C. Y., et al. (2018). *Xanthomonas citri* T6SS mediates resistance to *Dictyostelium* predation and is regulated by an ECF σ factor and cognate Ser/Thr kinase. *Environ. Microbiol.* 20, 1562–1575. doi: 10.1111/1462-2920.14085

Brito, E. M., Pinon-Castillo, H. A., Guyoneaud, R., Caretta, C. A., Gutierrez-Corona, J. F., Duran, R., et al. (2013). Bacterial biodiversity from anthropogenic extreme environments: a hyper-alkaline and hyper-saline industrial residue contaminated by chromium and iron. *Appl. Microbiol. Biotechnol.* 97, 369–378. doi: 10.1007/s00253-012-3923-5

Buttner, D., and Bonas, U. (2010). Regulation and secretion of *Xanthomonas* virulence factors. *FEMS Microbiol. Rev.* 34, 107–133. doi: 10.1111/j.1574-6976.2009.00192.x

Cabezon, E., Ripoll-Rozada, J., Pena, A., de la Cruz, F., and Arechaga, I. (2015). Towards an integrated model of bacterial conjugation. *FEMS Microbiol. Rev.* 39, 81–95. doi: 10.1111/1574-6976.12085

Callaghan, M. M., Heilers, J. H., van der Does, C., and Dillard, J. P. (2017). Secretion of chromosomal DNA by the *Neisseria gonorrhoeae* type IV secretion system. *Curr. Top. Microbiol. Immunol.* 413, 323–345. doi: 10.1007/978-3-319-75241-9_13

Cao, Z., Casabona, M. G., Kneuper, H., Chalmers, J. D., and Palmer, T. (2016). The type VII secretion system of *Staphylococcus aureus* secretes a nuclease toxin that targets competitor bacteria. *Nat. Microbiol.* 2:16183. doi: 10.1038/nmicrobiol.2016.183

Carbonetti, N. H. (2015). Contribution of pertussis toxin to the pathogenesis of pertussis disease. *Pathog. Dis.* 73:ftv073. doi: 10.1093/femspd/ftv073

Cascales, E., and Christie, P. J. (2004). Definition of a bacterial type IV secretion pathway for a DNA substrate. *Science* 304, 1170–1173. doi: 10.1126/science.1095211

Casu, B., Smart, J., Hancock, M. A., Smith, M., Sygusch, J., and Baron, C. (2016). Structural analysis and inhibition of TraE from the pKM101 type IV secretion system. *J. Biol. Chem.* 291, 23817–23829. doi: 10.1074/jbc.M116.753327

Chandran, V., Fronzes, R., Duquerroy, S., Cronin, N., Navaza, J., and Waksman, G. (2009). Structure of the outer membrane complex of a type IV secretion system. *Nature* 462, 1011–1015. doi: 10.1038/nature08588

Chang, Y. T., Lin, C. Y., Chen, Y. H., and Hsueh, P. R. (2015). Update on infections caused by *Stenotrophomonas maltophilia* with particular attention to resistance mechanisms and therapeutic options. *Front. Microbiol.* 6:893. doi: 10.3389/fmicb.2015.00893

Chang, Y. W., Shaffer, C. L., Rettberg, L. A., Ghosal, D., and Jensen, G. J. (2018). In vivo structures of the *Helicobacter pylori* cag type IV secretion system. *Cell Rep.* 23, 673–681. doi: 10.1016/j.celrep.2018.03.085

Chetrit, D., Hu, B., Christie, P. J., Roy, C. R., and Liu, J. (2018). A unique cytoplasmic ATPase complex defines the *Legionella pneumophila* type IV secretion channel. *Nat. Microbiol.* 3, 678–686. doi: 10.1038/s41564-018-0165-z

Christie, P. J. (2016). The mosaic type IV secretion systems. *EcoSal Plus* 7:ecosalplus.ESP-0020-2015. doi: 10.1128/ecosalplus.ESP-0020-2015

Christie, P. J., and Vogel, J. P. (2000). Bacterial type IV secretion: conjugation systems adapted to deliver effector molecules to host cells. *Trends Microbiol.* 8, 354–360. doi: 10.1016/s0966-842x(00)01792-3

Christie, P. J., Whitaker, N., and González-Rivera, C. (2014). Mechanism and structure of the bacterial type IV secretion systems. *Biochim. Biophys. Acta* 1843, 1578–1591. doi: 10.1016/j.bbamcr.2013.12.019

Comas, I., Moya, A., Azad, R. K., Lawrence, J. G., and Gonzalez-Candelas, F. (2006). The evolutionary origin of Xanthomonadales genomes and the nature of the horizontal gene transfer process. *Mol. Biol. Evol.* 23, 2049–2057. doi: 10.1093/molbev/msl075

Costa, T. R. D., Ilangovan, A., Ukleja, M., Redzej, A., Santini, J. M., Smith, T. K., et al. (2016). Structure of the bacterial sex F pilus reveals an assembly of a stoichiometric protein-phospholipid complex. *Cell* 166, 1436–1444.e10. doi: 10.1016/j.cell.2016.08.025

Crossman, L. C., Gould, V. C., Dow, J. M., Vernikos, G. S., Okazaki, A., Sebaihia, M., et al. (2008). The complete genome, comparative and functional analysis of *Stenotrophomonas maltophilia* reveals an organism heavily shielded by drug resistance determinants. *Genome Biol.* 9:R74. doi: 10.1186/gb-2008-9-4-r74

Da Silva, A. C. R., Ferro, J. A., Reinach, F. C., Farah, C. S., Furlan, L. R., Quaggio, R. B., et al. (2002). Comparison of the genomes of two *Xanthomonas* pathogens with differing host specificities. *Nature* 417, 459–463. doi: 10.1038/417459a

de Bruijn, I., Cheng, X., de Jager, V., Expósito, R. G., Watrous, J., Patel, N., et al. (2015). Comparative genomics and metabolic profiling of the genus *Lysobacter*. *BMC Genomics* 16:991. doi: 10.1186/s12864-015-2191-z

de la Cruz, F., and Davies, J. (2000). Horizontal gene transfer and the origin of species: lessons from bacteria. *Trends Microbiol.* 8, 128–133. doi: 10.1016/s0966-842x(00)01703-0

Ding, Z., Atmakuri, K., and Christie, P. J. (2003). The outs and ins of bacterial type IV secretion substrates. *Trends Microbiol.* 11, 527–535. doi: 10.1016/j.tim.2003.09.004

Durand, E., Oomen, C., and Waksman, G. (2010). Biochemical dissection of the ATPase TraB, the VirB4 homologue of the *Escherichia coli* pKM101 conjugation machinery. *J. Bacteriol.* 192, 2315–2323. doi: 10.1128/JB.01384-09

Eisenbrandt, R., Kalkum, M., Lai, E. M., Lurz, R., Kado, C. I., and Lanka, E. (1999). Conjugative pili of IncP plasmids, and the Ti plasmid T pilus are composed of cyclic subunits. *J. Biol. Chem.* 274, 22548–22555. doi: 10.1074/jbc.274.32.22548

El-Gebali, S., Mistry, J., Bateman, A., Eddy, S. R., Luciani, A., Potter, S. C., et al. (2019). The Pfam protein families database in 2019. *Nucleic Acids Res.* 47, D427–D432. doi: 10.1093/nar/gky995

Ensminger, A. W., and Isberg, R. R. (2009). *Legionella pneumophila* Dot/Icm translocated substrates: a sum of parts. *Curr. Opin. Microbiol.* 12, 67–73. doi: 10.1016/j.mib.2008.12.004

Ferguson, A. D., Amezcua, C. A., Halabi, N. M., Chelliah, Y., Rosen, M. K., Ranganathan, R., et al. (2007). Signal transduction pathway of TonB-dependent transporters. *Proc. Natl. Acad. Sci. U.S.A.* 104, 513–518. doi: 10.1073/pnas.0609887104

Finsel, I., and Hilbi, H. (2015). Formation of a pathogen vacuole according to *Legionella pneumophila*: how to kill one bird with many stones. *Cell. Microbiol.* 17, 935–950. doi: 10.1111/cmi.12450

Firczuk, M., and Bochtler, M. (2007). Folds and activities of peptidoglycan amidases. *FEMS Microbiol. Rev.* 31, 676–691. doi: 10.1111/j.1574-6976.2007.00084.x

Frick-Cheng, A. E., Pyburn, T. M., Voss, B. J., McDonald, W. H., Ohi, M. D., and Cover, T. L. (2016). Molecular and structural analysis of the *Helicobacter pylori* cag type IV secretion system core complex. *mBio* 7:e02001-15. doi: 10.1128/mBio.02001-15

Fronzes, R., Schafer, E., Wang, L., Saibil, H. R., Orlova, E. V., and Waksman, G. (2009). Structure of a type IV secretion system core complex. *Science* 323, 266–268. doi: 10.1126/science.1166101

Garcia-Herrero, A., and Vogel, H. J. (2005). Nuclear magnetic resonance solution structure of the periplasmic signalling domain of the TonB-dependent outer membrane transporter FecA from *Escherichia coli*. *Mol. Microbiol.* 58, 1226–1237. doi: 10.1111/j.1365-2958.2005.04889.x

Garza, I., and Christie, P. J. (2013). A putative transmembrane leucine zipper of *Agrobacterium* VirB10 is essential for T-Pilus biogenesis but not type IV secretion. *J. Bacteriol.* 195, 3022–3034. doi: 10.1128/JB.00287-13

Ghosal, D., Chang, Y. W., Jeong, K. C., Vogel, J. P., and Jensen, G. J. (2017). *In situ* structure of the *Legionella* Dot/Icm type IV secretion system by electron cryotomography. *EMBO Rep.* 18, 726–732. doi: 10.15252/embr.201643598

Gillespie, J. J., Phan, I. Q. H., Scheib, H., Subramanian, S., Edwards, T. E., Lehman, S. S., et al. (2015). Structural insight into how bacteria prevent interference between multiple divergent type IV secretion systems. *mBio* 6:e01867-15. doi: 10.1128/mBio.01867-15

Gilmour, M. W., Gunton, J. E., Lawley, T. D., and Taylor, D. E. (2003). Interaction between the IncHI1 plasmid R27 coupling protein and type IV secretion system: TraG associates with the coiled-coil mating pair formation protein TrhB. *Mol. Microbiol.* 49, 105–116. doi: 10.1046/j.1365-2958.2003.03551.x

Gomis-Ruth, F. X., Moncalian, G., de la Cruz, F., and Coll, M. (2002). Conjugative plasmid protein TrwB, an integral membrane type IV secretion system coupling protein. Detailed structural features and mapping of the active site cleft. *J. Biol. Chem.* 277, 7556–7566. doi: 10.1074/jbc.m110462200

Gonzalez-Rivera, C., Bhatty, M., and Christie, P. J. (2016). Mechanism and function of type IV secretion during infection of the human host. *Microbiol. Spectr.* 4:VMBF-0024-2015. doi: 10.1128/microbiolspec.VMBF-0024-2015

Gordon, J. E., Costa, T. R. D., Patel, R. S., Gonzalez-Rivera, C., Sarkar, M. K., Orlova, E. V., et al. (2017). Use of chimeric type IV secretion systems to define contributions of outer membrane subassemblies for contact-dependent translocation. *Mol. Microbiol.* 105, 273–293. doi: 10.1111/mmi.13700

Grohmann, E., Christie, P. J., Waksman, G., and Backert, S. (2017). Type IV secretion in Gram-negative and Gram-positive bacteria. *Mol. Microbiol.* 107, 455–471. doi: 10.1111/mmi.13896

Guglielmini, J., Neron, B., Abby, S. S., Garcillan-Barcia, M. P., de la Cruz, F., and Rocha, E. P. (2014). Key components of the eight classes of type IV secretion systems involved in bacterial conjugation or protein secretion. *Nucleic Acids Res.* 42, 5715–5727. doi: 10.1093/nar/gku194

Hamilton, H. L., Dominguez, N. M., Schwartz, K. J., Hackett, K. T., and Dillard, J. P. (2005). *Neisseria gonorrhoeae* secretes chromosomal DNA via a novel type IV secretion system. *Mol. Microbiol.* 55, 1704–1721. doi: 10.1111/j.1365-2958.2005.04521.x

Hare, S., Bayliss, R., Baron, C., and Waksman, G. (2006). A large domain swap in the VirB11 ATPase of *Brucella suis* leaves the hexameric assembly intact. *J. Mol. Biol.* 360, 56–66. doi: 10.1016/j.jmb.2006.04.060

Harms, A., Liesch, M., Körner, J., Québatte, M., Engel, P., and Dehio, C. (2017). A bacterial toxin-antitoxin module is the origin of inter-bacterial and inter-kingdom effectors of *Bartonella*. *PLoS Genet.* 13:e1007077. doi: 10.1371/journal.pgen.1007077

Hayes, C. S., Koskiniemi, S., Ruhe, Z. C., Poole, S. J., and Low, D. A. (2014). Mechanisms and biological roles of contact-dependent growth inhibition systems. *Cold Spring Harb. Perspect. Med.* 4:a010025. doi: 10.1101/cshperspect.a010025

Hayward, A. C., Fegan, N., Fegan, M., and Stirling, G. R. (2010). *Stenotrophomonas* and Lysobacter: ubiquitous plant-associated gamma-proteobacteria of developing significance in applied microbiology. *J. Appl. Microbiol.* 108, 756–770. doi: 10.1111/j.1365-2672.2009.04471.x

He, Y. Q., Zhang, L., Jiang, B. L., Zhang, Z. C., Xu, R. Q., Tang, D. J., et al. (2007). Comparative and functional genomics reveals genetic diversity and determinants of host specificity among reference strains and a large collection of Chinese isolates of the phytopathogen *Xanthomonas campestris* pv. *campestris*. *Genome Biol.* 8:R218.

Hilbi, H., Nagai, H., Kubori, T., and Roy, C. R. (2017). Subversion of host membrane dynamics by the legionella Dot/Icm type IV secretion system. *Curr. Top. Microbiol. Immunol.* 413, 221–242. doi: 10.1007/978-3-319-75241-9_9

Hofreuter, D., Odenbreit, S., and Haas, R. (2001). Natural transformation competence in *Helicobacter pylori* is mediated by the basic components of a type IV secretion system. *Mol. Microbiol.* 41, 379–391. doi: 10.1046/j.1365-2958.2001.02502.x

Jakubowski, S. J., Kerr, J. E., Garza, I., Krishnamoorthy, V., Bayliss, R., Waksman, G., et al. (2009). *Agrobacterium* VirB10 domain requirements for type IV secretion and T pilus biogenesis. *Mol. Microbiol.* 71, 779–794. doi: 10.1111/j.1365-2958.2008.06565.x

Jakubowski, S. J., Krishnamoorthy, V., Cascales, E., and Christie, P. J. (2004). *Agrobacterium tumefaciens* VirB6 domains direct the ordered export of a DNA substrate through a type IV secretion system. *J. Mol. Biol.* 341, 961–977. doi: 10.1016/j.jmb.2004.06.052

Jensen, R. B., and Gerdes, K. (1995). Programmed cell death in bacteria: proteic plasmid stabilization systems. *Mol. Microbiol.* 17, 205–210. doi: 10.1111/j.1365-2958.1995.mmi_17020205.x

Jones, A. L., Shirasu, K., and Kado, C. I. (1994). The product of the VirB4 gene of *Agrobacterium tumefaciens* promotes accumulation of VirB3 protein. *J. Bacteriol.* 176, 5255–5261. doi: 10.1128/jb.176.17.5255-5261.1994

Kanamaru, S., Leiman, P. G., Kostyuchenko, V. A., Chipman, P. R., Mesyanzhinov, V. V., Arisaka, F., et al. (2002). Structure of the cell-puncturing device of bacteriophage T4. *Nature* 415, 553–557. doi: 10.1038/415553a

Kanehisa, M., Furumichi, M., Tanabe, M., Sato, Y., and Morishima, K. (2017). KEGG: new perspectives on genomes, pathways, diseases and drugs. *Nucleic Acids Res.* 45, D353–D361. doi: 10.1093/nar/gkw1092

Ke, Y., Wang, Y., Li, W., and Chen, Z. (2015). Type IV secretion system of *Brucella* spp. and its effectors. *Front. Cell. Infect. Microbiol.* 5:72. doi: 10.3389/fcimb.2015.00072

Kondou, Y., Kitazawa, D., Takeda, S., Tsuchiya, Y., Yamashita, E., Mizuguchi, M., et al. (2005). Structure of the central hub of bacteriophage Mu baseplate determined by X-ray crystallography of gp44. *J. Mol. Biol.* 352, 976–985. doi: 10.1016/j.jmb.2005.07.044

Korotkov, K. V., Pardon, E., Steyaert, J., and Hol, W. G. (2009). Crystal structure of the N-terminal domain of the secretin GspD from ETEC determined with the assistance of a nanobody. *Structure* 17, 255–265. doi: 10.1016/j.str.2008.11.011

Krogh, A., Larsson, B., von Heijne, G., and Sonnhammer, E. L. (2001). Predicting transmembrane protein topology with a hidden Markov model: application to complete genomes. *J. Mol. Biol.* 305, 567–580. doi: 10.1006/jmbi.2000.4315

Kuroda, T., Kubori, T., Thanh Bui, X., Hyakutake, A., Uchida, Y., Imada, K., et al. (2015). Molecular and structural analysis of *Legionella* DotI gives insights into an inner membrane complex essential for type IV secretion. *Sci. Rep.* 5:10912. doi: 10.1038/srep10912

Lederberg, J., and Tatum, E. L. (1946). Gene recombination in *Escherichia coli*. *Nature* 158:558. doi: 10.1038/158558a0

Lee, B. M., Park, Y. J., Park, D. S., Kang, H. W., Kim, J. G., Song, E. S., et al. (2005). The genome sequence of *Xanthomonas oryzae* pathovar oryzae KACC10331, the bacterial blight pathogen of rice. *Nucleic Acids Res.* 33, 577–586. doi: 10.1093/nar/gki206

Leiman, P. G., Basler, M., Ramagopal, U. A., Bonanno, J. B., Sauder, J. M., Pukatzki, S., et al. (2009). Type VI secretion apparatus and phage tail-associated protein complexes share a common evolutionary origin. *Proc. Natl. Acad. Sci. U.S.A.* 106, 4154–4159. doi: 10.1073/pnas.0813360106

Li, Y. G., and Christie, P. J. (2018). The *Agrobacterium* VirB/VirD4 T4SS: mechanism and architecture defined through in vivo mutagenesis and chimeric systems. *Curr. Top. Microbiol. Immunol.* 418, 233–260. doi: 10.1007/82_2018_94

Llosa, M., and Alkorta, I. (2017). Coupling proteins in type IV secretion. *Curr. Top. Microbiol. Immunol.* 413, 143–168. doi: 10.1007/978-3-319-75241-9_6

Llosa, M., Zunzunegui, S., and de la Cruz, F. (2003). Conjugative coupling proteins interact with cognate and heterologous VirB10-like proteins while exhibiting specificity for cognate relaxosomes. *Proc. Natl. Acad. Sci. U.S.A.* 100, 10465–10470. doi: 10.1073/pnas.1830264100

Llosa, M., Zupan, J., Baron, C., and Zambryski, P. (2000). The N- and C-terminal portions of the *Agrobacterium* VirB1 protein independently enhance tumorigenesis. *J. Bacteriol.* 182, 3437–3445. doi: 10.1128/jb.182.12.3437-3445.2000

Locht, C., Coutte, L., and Mielcarek, N. (2011). The ins and outs of pertussis toxin. *FEBS J.* 278, 4668–4682. doi: 10.1111/j.1742-4658.2011.08237.x

Looney, W. J., Narita, M., and Mühlemann, K. (2009). *Stenotrophomonas maltophilia*: an emerging opportunist human pathogen. *Lancet Infect. Dis.* 9, 312–323. doi: 10.1016/S1473-3099(09)70083-0

Low, H. H., Gubellini, F., Rivera-Calzada, A., Braun, N., Connery, S., Dujeancourt, A., et al. (2014). Structure of a type IV secretion system. *Nature* 508, 550–553. doi: 10.1038/nature13081

Mansfield, J., Genin, S., Magori, S., Citovsky, V., Sriariyanum, M., Ronald, P., et al. (2012). Top 10 plant pathogenic bacteria in molecular plant pathology. *Mol. Plant Pathol.* 13, 614–629. doi: 10.1111/j.1364-3703.2012.00804.x

Marchler-Bauer, A., Derbyshire, M. K., Gonzales, N. R., Lu, S., Chitsaz, F., Geer, L. Y., et al. (2015). CDD: NCBI's conserved domain database. *Nucleic Acids Res.* 43, D222–D226. doi: 10.1093/nar/gku1221

Martins-Pinheiro, M., Galhardo, R. S., Lage, C., Lima-Bessa, K. M., Aires, K. A., and Menck, C. F. M. (2004). Different patterns of evolution for duplicated DNA repair genes in bacteria of the Xanthomonadales group. *BMC Evol. Biol.* 4:29. doi: 10.1186/1471-2148-4-29

Moffatt, J. H., Newton, P., and Newton, H. J. (2015). *Coxiella burnetii*: turning hostility into a home. *Cell. Microbiol.* 17, 621–631. doi: 10.1111/cmi.12432

Moreira, L. M., Almeida, N. F. Jr., Potnis, N., Digiampietri, L. A., Adi, S. S., Bortolossi, J. C., et al. (2010). Novel insights into the genomic basis of citrus canker based on the genome sequences of two strains of *Xanthomonas fuscans* subsp. *aurantifolii*. *BMC Genomics* 11:238. doi: 10.1186/1471-2164-11-238

Mukherjee, P., and Roy, P. (2016). Genomic potential of *Stenotrophomonas maltophilia* in bioremediation with an assessment of its multifaceted role in our environment. *Front. Microbiol.* 7:967. doi: 10.3389/fmicb.2016.00967

Nakai, K., and Horton, P. (1999). PSORT: a program for detecting sorting signals in proteins and predicting their subcellular localization. *Trends Biochem. Sci.* 24, 34–35. doi: 10.1016/S0968-0004(98)01336-X

Nakano, N., Kubori, T., Kinoshita, M., Imada, K., and Nagai, H. (2010). Crystal structure of *Legionella* DotD: insights into the relationship between type IVB and type II/III secretion systems. *PLoS Pathog.* 6:e1001129. doi: 10.1371/journal.ppat.1001129

Naumann, M., Sokolova, O., Tegtmeyer, N., and Backert, S. (2017). *Helicobacter pylori*: a paradigm pathogen for subverting host cell signal transmission. *Trends Microbiol.* 25, 316–328. doi: 10.1016/j.tim.2016.12.004

Naushad, H. S., and Gupta, R. S. (2013). Phylogenomics and molecular signatures for species from the plant pathogen-containing order Xanthomonadales. *PLoS One* 8:e55216. doi: 10.1371/journal.pone.0055216

Naushad, S., Adeolu, M., Wong, S., Sohail, M., Schellhorn, H. E., and Gupta, R. S. (2015). A phylogenomic and molecular marker based taxonomic framework for the order *Xanthomonadales*: proposal to transfer the families *Algiphilaceae* and *Solimonadaceae* to the order *Nevskiales* ord. nov. and to create a new family within the order *Xanthomonadales*, the family *Rhodanobacteraceae* fam. nov., containing the genus *Rhodanobacter* and its closest relatives. *Antonie Van Leeuwenhoek* 107, 467–485. doi: 10.1007/s10482-014-0344-8

Ochiai, H., Inoue, V., Takeya, M., Sasaki, A., and Kaku, H. (2005). Genome sequence of *Xanthomonas oryzae* pv. *oryzae* suggests contribution of large numbers of effector genes and insertion sequences to its race diversity. *Jpn. Agric. Res. Q.* 39, 275–287. doi: 10.6090/jarq.39.275

Oliveira, L. C., Souza, D. P., Oka, G. U., Lima, F., da, S., Oliveira, R. J., et al. (2016). VirB7 and VirB9 interactions are required for the assembly and antibacterial activity of a type IV secretion system. *Structure* 24, 1707–1718. doi: 10.1016/j.str.2016.07.015

Panthee, S., Hamamoto, H., Paudel, A., and Sekimizu, K. (2016). *Lysobacter* species: a potential source of novel antibiotics. *Arch. Microbiol.* 198, 839–845. doi: 10.1007/s00203-016-1278-5

Paschos, A., Patey, G., Sivanesan, D., Gao, C., Bayliss, R., Waksman, G., et al. (2006). Dimerization and interactions of *Brucella suis* VirB8 with VirB4 and VirB10 are required for its biological activity. *Proc. Natl. Acad. Sci. U.S.A.* 103, 7252–7257. doi: 10.1073/pnas.0600862103

Peña, A., Matilla, I., Martín-Benito, J., Valpuesta, J. M., Carrascosa, J. L., De La Cruz, F., et al. (2012). The hexameric structure of a conjugative VirB4 protein ATPase provides new insights for a functional and phylogenetic relationship with DNA translocases. *J. Biol. Chem.* 287, 39925–39932. doi: 10.1074/jbc.M112.413849

Pieretti, I., Royer, M., Barbe, V., Carrere, S., Koebnik, R., Cociancich, S., et al. (2009). The complete genome sequence of *Xanthomonas albilineans* provides new insights into the reductive genome evolution of the xylem-limited *Xanthomonadaceae*. *BMC Genomics* 10:616. doi: 10.1186/1471-2164-10-616

Qian, W., Jia, Y., Ren, S. X., He, Y. Q., Feng, J. X., Lu, L. F., et al. (2005). Comparative and functional genomic analyses of the pathogenicity of phytopathogen *Xanthomonas campestris* pv. *campestris*. *Genome Res.* 15, 757–767. doi: 10.1101/gr.3378705

Qiu, J., and Luo, Z. Q. (2017). *Legionella* and *Coxiella* effectors: strength in diversity and activity. *Nat. Rev. Microbiol.* 15, 591–605. doi: 10.1038/nrmicro.2017.67

Rabel, C., Grahn, A. M., Lurz, R., and Lanka, E. (2003). The VirB4 family of proposed traffic nucleoside triphosphatases: common motifs in plasmid RP4 TrbE are essential for conjugation and phage adsorption. *J. Bacteriol.* 185, 1045–1058. doi: 10.1128/JB.185.3.1045-1058.2003

Redzej, A., Ukleja, M., Connery, S., Trokter, M., Felisberto-Rodrigues, C., Cryar, A., et al. (2017). Structure of a VirD4 coupling protein bound to a VirB type IV secretion machinery. *EMBO J.* 36, 3080–3095. doi: 10.15252/embj.201796629

Ripoll-Rozada, J., Zunzunegui, S., de la Cruz, F., Arechaga, I., and Cabezón, E. (2013). Functional interactions of VirB11 traffic ATPases with VirB4 and VirD4 molecular motors in type IV secretion systems. *J. Bacteriol.* 195, 4195–4201. doi: 10.1128/JB.00437-13

Rivera-Calzada, A., Fronzes, R., Savva, C. G., Chandran, V., Lian, P. W., Laeremans, T., et al. (2013). Structure of a bacterial type IV secretion core complex at subnanometre resolution. *EMBO J.* 32, 1195–1204. doi: 10.1038/emboj.2013.58

Russell, A. B., Hood, R. D., Bui, N. K., LeRoux, M., Vollmer, W., and Mougous, J. D. (2011). Type VI secretion delivers bacteriolytic effectors to target cells. *Nature* 475, 343–347. doi: 10.1038/nature10244

Russell, A. B., LeRoux, M., Hathazi, K., Agnello, D. M., Ishikawa, T., Wiggins, P. A., et al. (2013). Diverse type VI secretion phospholipases are functionally plastic antibacterial effectors. *Nature* 496, 508–512. doi: 10.1038/nature12074

Saddler, G. S., and Bradbury, J. F. (2007). "Xanthomonadales ord. nov," in *Bergey's Manual of Systematic Bacteriology*, eds D. J. Brenner, N. R. Krieg, J. T. Staley, G. M. Garrity, D. R. Boone, P. Vos, et al. (Boston, MA: Springer). doi: 10.1007/0-387-28022-7_3

Salzberg, S., Schatz, M., Delcher, A., Roberts, M., Rabinowicz, P., Inman, J., et al. (2007). *Xanthomonas oryzae* pv. oryzicola BLS256, whole genome shotgun sequencing project. Submitt. to GenBank database (AAQN00000000.1).

Salzberg, S. L., Sommer, D. D., Schatz, M. C., Phillippy, A. M., Rabinowicz, P. D., Tsuge, S., et al. (2008). Genome sequence and rapid evolution of the rice pathogen *Xanthomonas oryzae* pv. *oryzae* PXO99A. *BMC Genomics* 9:204. doi: 10.1186/1471-2164-9-204

Schmidt-Eisenlohr, H., Domke, N., Angerer, C., Wanner, G., Zambryski, P. C., and Baron, C. (1999). Vir proteins stabilize VirB5 and mediate its association with the T pilus of *Agrobacterium tumefaciens*. *J. Bacteriol.* 181, 7485–7492.

Segura, R. L., Águila-Arcos, S., Ugarte-Uribe, B., Vecino, A. J., De La Cruz, F., Goñi, F. M., et al. (2013). The transmembrane domain of the T4SS coupling protein TrwB and its role in protein-protein interactions. *Biochim. Biophys. Acta* 1828, 2015–2025. doi: 10.1016/j.bbamem.2013.05.022

Sexton, J. A., and Vogel, J. P. (2002). Type IVB secretion by intracellular pathogens. *Traffic* 3, 178–185. doi: 10.1034/j.1600-0854.2002.030303.x

Sgro, G. G., Costa, T. R. D., Cenens, W., Souza, D. P., Cassago, A., Coutinho de Oliveira, L., et al. (2018). Cryo-EM structure of the bacteria-killing type IV secretion system core complex from *Xanthomonas citri*. *Nat. Microbiol.* 3, 1429–1440. doi: 10.1038/s41564-018-0262-z

Siamer, S., and Dehio, C. (2015). New insights into the role of *Bartonella* effector proteins in pathogenesis. *Curr. Opin. Microbiol.* 23, 80–85. doi: 10.1016/j.mib.2014.11.007

Sivanesan, D., Hancock, M. A., Villamil Giraldo, A. M., and Baron, C. (2010). Quantitative analysis of VirB8-VirB9-VirB10 interactions provides a dynamic model of type IV secretion system core complex assembly. *Biochemistry* 49, 4483–4493. doi: 10.1021/bi902201y

Souza, D. P., Andrade, M. O., Alvarez-Martinez, C. E., Arantes, G. M., Farah, C. S., and Salinas, R. K. (2011). A component of the Xanthomonadaceae type IV secretion system combines a VirB7 motif with a N0 domain found in outer membrane transport proteins. *PLoS Pathog.* 7:e1002031. doi: 10.1371/journal.ppat.1002031

Souza, D. P., Oka, G. U., Alvarez-Martinez, C. E., Bisson-Filho, A. W., Dunger, G., Hobeika, L., et al. (2015). Bacterial killing via a type IV secretion system. *Nat. Commun.* 6:6453. doi: 10.1038/ncomms7453

Spagnuolo, J., Opalka, N., Wen, W. X., Gagic, D., Chabaud, E., Bellini, P., et al. (2010). Identification of the gate regions in the primary structure of the secretin pIV. *Mol. Microbiol.* 76, 133–150. doi: 10.1111/j.1365-2958.2010.07085.x

Spreter, T., Yip, C. K., Sanowar, S., Andre, I., Kimbrough, T. G., Vuckovic, M., et al. (2009). A conserved structural motif mediates formation of the periplasmic rings in the type III secretion system. *Nat. Struct. Mol. Biol.* 16, 468–476. doi: 10.1038/nsmb.1603

Studholme, D. J., Kemen, E., Maclean, D., Schornack, S., Aritua, V., Thwaites, R., et al. (2010). Genome-wide sequencing data reveals virulence factors implicated in banana *Xanthomonas* wilt. *FEMS Microbiol. Lett.* 310, 182–192. doi: 10.1111/j.1574-6968.2010.02065.x

Terradot, L., Bayliss, R., Oomen, C., Leonard, G. A., Baron, C., and Waksman, G. (2005). Structures of two core subunits of the bacterial type IV secretion system, VirB8 from *Brucella suis* and ComB10 from *Helicobacter pylori*. *Proc. Natl. Acad. Sci. U.S.A.* 102, 4596–4601. doi: 10.1073/pnas.0408927102

Thieme, F., Koebnik, R., Bekel, T., Berger, C., Boch, J., Buttner, D., et al. (2005). Insights into genome plasticity and pathogenicity of the plant pathogenic bacterium *Xanthomonas campestris* pv. vesicatoria revealed by the complete genome sequence. *J. Bacteriol.* 187, 7254–7266. doi: 10.1128/JB.187.21.7254-7266.2005

Tzfira, T., and Citovsky, V. (2006). Agrobacterium-mediated genetic transformation of plants: biology and biotechnology. *Curr. Opin. Biotechnol.* 17, 147–154. doi: 10.1016/j.copbio.2006.01.009

Van Herreweghe, J. M., Vanderkelen, L., Callewaert, L., Aertsen, A., Compernolle, G., Declerck, P. J., et al. (2010). Lysozyme inhibitor conferring bacterial tolerance to invertebrate type lysozyme. *Cell. Mol. Life Sci.* 67, 1177–1188. doi: 10.1007/s00018-009-0241-x

Van Sluys, M. A., Monteiro-Vitorello, C. B., Camargo, L. E. A., Menck, C. F. M., da Silva, A. C., Ferro, J. A., et al. (2002). Comparative genomic analysis of plant-associated bacteria. *Annu. Rev. Phytopathol.* 40, 169–189. doi: 10.1146/annurev.phyto.40.030402.090559

Villamil Giraldo, A. M., Mary, C., Sivanesan, D., and Baron, C. (2015). VirB6 and VirB10 from the *Brucella* type IV secretion system interact via the N-terminal periplasmic domain of VirB6. *FEBS Lett.* 589, 1883–1889. doi: 10.1016/j.febslet.2015.05.051

Villamil Giraldo, A. M., Sivanesan, D., Carle, A., Paschos, A., Smith, M. A., Plesa, M., et al. (2012). Type IV secretion system core component VirB8 from *Brucella* binds to the globular domain of VirB5 and to a periplasmic domain of VirB6. *Biochemistry* 51, 3881–3890. doi: 10.1021/bi300298v

Vorholter, F. J., Schneiker, S., Goesmann, A., Krause, L., Bekel, T., Kaiser, O., et al. (2008). The genome of *Xanthomonas campestris* pv. campestris B100 and its use for the reconstruction of metabolic pathways involved in xanthan biosynthesis. *J. Biotechnol.* 134, 33–45. doi: 10.1016/j.jbiotec.2007.12.013

Waksman, G. (2019). From conjugation to T4S systems in Gram-negative bacteria: a mechanistic biology perspective. *EMBO Rep.* 20:e47012. doi: 10.15252/embr.201847012

Wasukira, A., Tayebwa, J., Thwaites, R., Paszkiewicz, K., Aritua, V., Kubiriba, J., et al. (2012). Genome-wide sequencing reveals two major sub-lineages in the genetically monomorphic pathogen *Xanthomonas campestris* pathovar musacearum. *Genes* 3, 361–377. doi: 10.3390/genes3030361

Whitaker, N., Chen, Y., Jakubowski, S. J., Sarkar, M. K., Li, F., and Christie, P. J. (2015). The all-alpha domains of coupling proteins from the *Agrobacterium tumefaciens* VirB/VirD4 and *Enterococcus faecalis* pCF10-encoded type IV secretion systems confer specificity to binding of cognate DNA substrates. *J. Bacteriol.* 197, 2335–2349. doi: 10.1128/JB.00189-15

Yeo, H. J., Savvides, S. N., Herr, A. B., Lanka, E., and Waksman, G. (2000). Crystal structure of the hexameric traffic ATPase of the *Helicobacter pylori* type IV secretion system. *Mol. Cell* 6, 1461–1472. doi: 10.1016/s1097-2765(00)00142-8

Zhang, L., Wang, X., Yu, M., Qiao, Y., and Zhang, X. H. (2015). Genomic analysis of *Luteimonas abyssi* XH031(T): insights into its adaption to the subseafloor environment of South Pacific Gyre and ecological role in biogeochemical cycle. *BMC Genomics* 16:1092. doi: 10.1186/s12864-015-2326-2

14

Expression of the Gene for Autotransporter AutB of *Neisseria meningitidis* Affects Biofilm Formation and Epithelial Transmigration

Jesús Arenas [1], Fernanda L. Paganelli [2], Patricia Rodríguez-Castaño [1], Sara Cano-Crespo [1], Arie van der Ende [3], Jos P. M. van Putten [4] and Jan Tommassen [1]*

[1] Department of Molecular Microbiology and Institute of Biomembranes, Utrecht University, Utrecht, Netherlands, [2] Department of Medical Microbiology, University Medical Center Utrecht, Utrecht, Netherlands, [3] Department of Medical Microbiology, Academic Medical Center, Amsterdam, Netherlands, [4] Department of Infectious Diseases and Immunology, Faculty of Veterinary Medicine, Utrecht University, Utrecht, Netherlands

***Correspondence:**
Jesús Arenas
j.a.arenasbusto@uu.nl;
jesusarenasbust@yahoo.es

Neisseria meningitidis is a Gram-negative bacterium that resides as a commensal in the upper respiratory tract of humans, but occasionally, it invades the host and causes sepsis and/or meningitis. The bacterium can produce eight autotransporters, seven of which have been studied to some detail. The remaining one, AutB, has not been characterized yet. Here, we show that the *autB* gene is broadly distributed among pathogenic *Neisseria* spp. The gene is intact in most meningococcal strains. However, its expression is prone to phase variation due to slipped-strand mispairing at AAGC repeats located within the DNA encoding the signal sequence and is switched off in the vast majority of these strains. Moreover, various genetic disruptions prevent *autB* expression in most of the strains in which the gene is in phase indicating a strong selection against AutB synthesis. We observed that *autB* is expressed in two of the strains examined and that AutB is secreted and exposed at the cell surface. Functionality assays revealed that AutB synthesis promotes biofilm formation and delays the passage of epithelial cell layers in *vitro*. We hypothesize that this autotransporter is produced during the colonization process only in specific niches to facilitate microcolony formation, but its synthesis is switched off probably to evade the immune system and facilitate human tissue invasion.

Keywords: autotransporters, protein secretion, biofilms, infection, *Neisseria meningitidis*, *Haemophilus influenzae*, pathogenesis

INTRODUCTION

The Gram-negative diplococcus *Neisseria meningitidis* is a common inhabitant of the human nasopharynx, but it is also the causative agent of meningococcal disease, a life-threatening infection characterized by fast development of septicemia and/or meningitis. The colonization and its persistence in the host involve the formation of microcolonies in the nasopharynx (Sim et al., 2000). Microcolonies are biofilm-like structures, which are defined as multicellular microbial communities often encased within a self-produced extracellular matrix (Costerton et al., 1995) and presumably help the bacteria to survive adverse circumstances, such as host defense mechanisms.

Amongst others, several autotransporters (ATs) have been demonstrated to play a role in biofilm formation in *N. meningitidis* (Arenas and Tommassen, 2016).

ATs are a class of proteins secreted by Gram-negative bacteria (Grijpstra et al., 2013). They contain an N-terminal signal sequence for transport across the inner membrane via the Sec machinery and a C-terminal translocator domain that inserts as a β-barrel in the outer membrane via the Bam complex and that assists in the translocation of an associated passenger domain across the outer membrane. Based on the structure of the translocator domain, two main types of ATs can be discriminated, the classical monomeric ATs and the trimeric ATs. In classical monomeric ATs, the C-terminal translocator domain forms a 12-stranded β-barrel, whilst in trimeric ATs, the translocator domain of each subunit contributes four β-strands to form a similar 12-stranded β-barrel as in the monomeric ATs. The passenger of classical ATs usually forms an extended β-helix on which smaller globular domains are displayed. The C-terminal part of these passengers often harbors a linker domain that, in some cases, has been demonstrated to contain autochaperone activity, i.e., it helps in the folding of the passenger after its secretion to the cell surface (Oliver et al., 2003; Peterson et al., 2010). After secretion, the passenger can remain attached to the cell surface or it can be released into the external medium by one of a variety of possible proteolytic mechanisms. Their functions can be very diverse, but they are often involved in virulence (Grijpstra et al., 2013).

Based on the analysis of genome sequences, it appears that *N. meningitidis* can produce up to eight different ATs, i.e., IgA1 protease, App, AusI, NalP, NhhA, NadA, AutA, and AutB (van Ulsen and Tommassen, 2006). Seven of them have been characterized to at least some extent. The passenger of IgA1 protease consists of two domains, the protease domain, which cleaves, amongst others, human immunoglobulin A1, the IgA subclass that predominates in the nasopharynx, and an α-peptide that can be released from the cell surface together with the protease domain, or it can remain attached to the cell surface where it is implicated in biofilm formation by binding extracellular DNA (eDNA) (Arenas et al., 2013a). Like IgA1 protease, App and AusI (a.k.a. MspA) are monomeric ATs with a protease domain, and both have been implicated in adhesion to epithelial cells (Serruto et al., 2003; Turner et al., 2006). Also NalP has protease activity; amongst others, it releases proteins from the bacterial cell surface, including the α-peptide of IgA1 protease and the neisserial heparin-binding antigen NHBA, a surface-exposed lipoprotein, which, like the α-peptide, is involved in biofilm formation by binding eDNA (van Ulsen et al., 2003; Serruto et al., 2010; Arenas et al., 2013a). Thus, NalP regulates biofilm formation. NhhA and NadA are cell-associated trimeric ATs with a role in adhesion to eukaryotic cells (Capecchi et al., 2005; Scarselli et al., 2006), whilst AutA is a monomeric AT involved in bacterial autoaggregation, a function that affects biofilm structure (Arenas et al., 2015). The remaining AT, AutB, has not been characterized yet. It is evolutionary related to a poorly characterized AT designated Lav, present in some strains of *Haemophilus influenzae*, another inhabitant of the nasopharynx, from which it was suggested to be acquired by horizontal gene transfer. Expression of its gene and its function remain enigmatic.

The expression of the genes for most ATs in *N. meningitidis* is prone to phase variation by slipped-strand mispairing at short nucleotide repeats (Turner et al., 2002; van Ulsen et al., 2006; Arenas et al., 2015). Besides, expression of several AT genes, e.g., *ausI* and *autA*, can be prevented in certain lineages by genetic disruptions, such as deletions or frame-shift mutations, possibly evolved by selection pressure imposed by the immune system (van Ulsen et al., 2006; Arenas et al., 2015). The expression of *autB* also seems to be prone to phase variation. The gene contains a variable number of AAGC nucleotide repeats immediately downstream of the start codon (Peak et al., 1999). These repeats are also present in the *autA* gene, where they were shown to be implicated in phase variation (Arenas et al., 2015). However, expression of *autB* has not been demonstrated so far. In fact, early studies suggested that *autB* is a pseudogene (Ait-Tahar et al., 2000). This conclusion was based on the lack of reactivity of two anti-AutB antisera against nine meningococcal and one gonococcal strains. However, the number of AAGC repeats and the presence of genetic disruptions in the *autB* genes of those strains were not evaluated. Therefore, the conclusion that *autB* is a pseudogene may be premature. The objective of the present work was to determine whether AutB can be produced in *N. meningitidis* and to elucidate its possible function.

MATERIALS AND METHODS

Bioinformatics Analysis

Amino-acid sequences encoded by the *autB* genes were predicted after alteration of the number of AAGC repeat units to create the correct reading frame and, in some cases, by removal of frameshift mutations and premature stop codons. The cleavage site of the N-terminal signal sequence was predicted using publicly available web tools (http://www.cbs.dtu.dk/services/SignalP/). The mature protein was then used for phylogenetic analysis using the neighbor-joining with bootstrap analysis (100 replications) considering distances based on p-distance with the available MEGA software version 6.0 (http://www.megasoftware.net/) (Tamura et al., 2013). For secondary and tertiary structure predictions, the public web-based programs PsiPred (Buchan et al., 2013) and PHYRE2 (http://www.sbg.bio.ic.ac.uk/phyre2/html/page.cgi?id=index), respectively, were used. Alignment of protein sequences was performed in MAFFT version 7 (http://mafft.cbrc.jp/alignment/server/). AutB variants were defined based on phylogeny of the N-terminal part of the passenger. Each variant was considered when the bootstrap value of the precedent node was 100, the distance within the group was lower than the overall distance for AutB, and the distance from other groups higher than the overall distance for AutB.

Bacterial Strains and Growth Conditions

Meningococcal strains used in this study include reference strains MC58 (Tettelin et al., 2000), FAM18 (Bentley et al., 2007), α14

(Schoen et al., 2008), and α153 (Schoen et al., 2008). HB-1 (Bos and Tommassen, 2005) and BB-1 (Arenas et al., 2013a) are unencapsulated derivatives of H44/76 and B16B6, respectively. A panel of 102 meningococcal strains isolated from patients suffering from meningococcal disease in the Netherlands was already described (Arenas et al., 2015). All meningococcal strains were grown at 37°C on GC medium base (Difco) supplemented with IsovitaleX (Becton Dickinson) at 37°C in a candle jar overnight. To grow the bacteria in liquid cultures, bacteria were collected from GC plates and diluted in tryptic soy broth (TSB) (Beckton Dickinson) to an OD_{550} of 0.1 and incubated in 25-cm^2 polystyrene cell culture flasks or 125-ml square media bottles with constant shaking at 110 rpm. *Escherichia coli* strains used in this study were DH5α and BL21(DE3) (Invitrogen), which were grown in Lysogeny broth (LB) or LB agar at 37°C.

For all strains, media were supplemented with the antibiotics kanamycin (100 μg ml^{-1}), chloramphenicol (25 μg ml^{-1}) or ampicillin (100 μg ml^{-1}) when required and with 0.1 mM of isopropyl-β-D-1-thiogalactopyranoside (IPTG) to induce gene expression.

PCR Analysis and Sequencing of the *autB* Gene

Segments of *autB* were amplified by PCR from bacteria grown on plates with primers listed in Table S1 using High Fidelity Polymerase (Roche Diagnostics GmbH, Germany) or DreamTaq-DNA Polymerase (Fermentas, UK). PCR products were visualized in agarose gels stained with ethidium bromide. When required, they were purified with the PCR Clean-Up System (Promega Corporation) and sequenced at the Macrogen sequencing service (Amsterdam). Large sequences were assembled using the SeqMan II software (DNAstart) using at least two independent PCR reactions.

Cloning and Transformation

For cloning, PCR fragments were obtained from DNA of strain HB-1 using primers described in Table S1. PCR fragments were purified and digested with restriction enzymes (Fermentas, UK) for which sites were included in the primers, to be subsequently cloned in appropriate vectors. To generate an *autB* knockout construct, PCR fragments from immediately upstream and downstream of the *autB* gene were cloned into pKO*nhbA-kan* (Arenas et al., 2013a). In the resulting plasmid, called pKO*autB-kan*, these segments flank a kanamycin-resistance cassette.

To generate a plasmid for the production of a part of the passenger domain of AutB of strain HB-1 in *E. coli*, the corresponding PCR product was cloned into pET16b (Invitrogen) resulting in plasmid pET16b-AutBp. To generate plasmids for expression of AutB variants in *N. meningitidis*, the entire *autB* genes from isolates 2081107 and α153 were amplified and cloned into plasmid $pFPIORF_1$ (Arenas et al., 2013b), resulting in $pENAutB_1$ and $pENAutB_2$, respectively. *N. meningitidis* and *E. coli* were transformed with intact or linearized plasmids following standard protocols (Arenas et al., 2015) and transformants were selected on solid medium supplemented with appropriate antibiotics. The proper generation of knockout mutants or the presence of the plasmid was verified by PCR. In addition, protein synthesis was confirmed by Western blotting or gene expression was confirmed by RT-PCR as described below.

Purification of Recombinant AutB and Antiserum Production

A fragment of the AutB passenger domain of strain HB-1 was purified as described (Arenas et al., 2015). Briefly, the recombinant polypeptide, corresponding to amino-acid residues 151–278 of the mature AutB protein, with an N-terminal His-tag was produced in *E. coli* BL21(DE3) carrying pET16b-AutBp after induction with IPTG and purified as inclusion bodies. The protein band corresponding to the recombinant protein was excised from SDS-polyacrylamide gel electrophoresis (SDS-PAGE) gels and used for the production of rabbit antiserum at Eurogentec (Liège, Belgium). The concentration of the purified protein was determined with the BCA assay kit (Thermo Fisher Scientific, Rockford, IL, USA) and its purity was estimated in SDS-PAGE gels.

RNA Purification and RT-PCR Assays

To obtain RNA, cells from exponentially growing cultures were collected by centrifugation for 10 min at 5000 rpm in an Eppendorf Centrifuge 5424, adjusted to an OD_{550} of 4, and resuspended in trizol (Invitrogen, U.K.). Then, 200 μl of chloroform were added per ml of trizol, followed by centrifugation at 5000 rpm for 30 min. The resulting upper layer was mixed with an equal amount of ice-cold 75% ethanol. Next, RNA was isolated using the Nucleospin RNA II kit (Macherey-Nagel, U.S.A.) according to the manufacturer's instructions. The resulting solution was treated with Turbo DNA free (Ambion, Germany) for 1 h at 37°C to remove genomic DNA followed by inactivation of the DNase according to the recommendations of the manufacturer. The resulting pure RNA was used immediately to generate cDNA using the Transcriptor High Fidelity cDNA Synthesis Kit (Roche, The Netherlands). RNA, cDNA, and chromosomal DNA were used as templates in PCRs to determine the generation of specific transcripts with primers listed in Table S1. PCRs started with an incubation for 5 min at 95°C, followed by 30 cycles of 30 s at 95°C, 30 s at 65°C and 10 s at 72°C. Reactions ended with 10 min of incubation at 72°C.

SDS-PAGE and Western Blotting

Whole cell lysates, supernatants and cell envelopes were prepared and adjusted as previously described (Arenas et al., 2015). Protein concentrations were determined with the BCA assay kit. Before SDS-PAGE, samples were diluted 1:1 in double-strength sample buffer and heated for 10 min at 100°C. Proteins separated on gels were stained with Coomassie brilliant blue G250 or transferred to nitrocellulose membranes. These membranes were next blocked with phosphate-buffered saline (PBS) containing 0.1% (v/v) Tween 20 and 0.5% (w/v) non-fat dried milk (PBS-T-M), and then incubated with primary antibodies and subsequently with horseradish peroxidase-conjugated goat anti-rabbit IgG or anti-mouse IgG antibodies (Biosource International), as previously described (Arenas et al., 2006). All incubations were performed for 1 h and followed by three washes for 15 min with PBS-T-M. Blots were developed with the Pierce ECL Western Blotting Substrate. The monoclonal antibody MN2D6D directed against RmpM and the antiserum directed against fHbp were generously provided by the Netherlands Vaccine Institute (Bilthoven, The Netherlands) and by GlaxoSmithKline (Rixensart, Belgium), respectively. The antisera directed against the α-peptide and the translocator domain of IgA protease were from our laboratory collection (Roussel-Jazédé et al., 2014).

Proteinase K Accessibility Assays

Proteinase K accessibility assays were performed as described (Arenas et al., 2015) with few modifications. Briefly, bacteria recovered from a culture grown for 4 h in TSB were adjusted to an optical density at 550 nm (OD_{550}) of 1 and incubated with 2 μg ml^{-1} of proteinase K (Fermentas) for 1 h at 37°C, after which the protease was inactivated with 2 mM phenylmethylsulfonyl fluoride Sigma-Aldrich). Cells were harvested by centrifugation and protein degradation was examined by SDS-PAGE and Western blotting.

Settling Experiments and Biofilm Formation

For biofilm formation and settling experiments, bacteria were initially grown in TSB with or without IPTG and adjusted to a similar OD_{550}. Settling experiments were performed as described (Arenas et al., 2015). Biofilm formation was analyzed under static conditions in polystyrene plates and in a flow-cell model as described before (Arenas et al., 2013a, 2015), with some modifications. Where indicated, 100 μg ml^{-1} of DNase I was added to the cultures during biofilm formation. For the flow-cell model, pictures were taken at different time intervals during biofilm formation. After 16 h, biofilms were stained with LIVE/DEAD stain (Life Technologies Europe BV, the Netherlands) dissolved in Dulbecco's PBS (DPBS) (Lonza, USA) as suggested by the manufacturer. Structural parameters of the biofilms were analyzed using COMSTAT (Heydorn et al., 2000)/MATLAB R2010b software (The MathWorks) program, using eight image stacks randomly generated of each sample. For statistical analysis, data from at least three independent experiments performed in duplicate were used. Statistical comparisons of all biofilm parameters were calculated using an unpaired *t*-test with GRAPH PAD v 6.0 (Graph Pad Software, Inc).

Infection Assays

The epithelial cell line NCI-H292 (ATCC CRL 1848) was cultured in RPMI 1640 medium supplemented with 5% fetal calf serum, which was heat inactivated before use (1 h at 56°C). All cell-culture medium components were purchased from Laboratories PAA. The cells were cultured at 37°C in a humidified atmosphere containing 5% CO_2 and maintained in 25-cm^2 tissue-culture flasks (Nunc) until ~80% confluence was reached.

Bacterial adherence was determined as previously described (van Putten and Paul, 1995). In short, 2 days before the assays, NCI-H292 cells from 4 to 25 passages were seeded in 24-well plates. Bacteria grown overnight on plate were suspended in HEPES buffer (10 mM HEPES, 145 mM NaCl, 5 mM KCl, 5 mM glucose, 1 mM $CaCl_2$ and 1 mM $MgCl_2$, pH 7.2), washed by centrifugation (1500 *g*, 10 min) and incubated with cultured cells at a multiplicity of infection of 100 for 3 h. Non-adherent bacteria were removed by sequential washings with DPBS, and the viable adhering bacteria were counted by determining the colony-forming units (CFU) after disruption of the cell layer with 1% saponin diluted in DPBS for 15 min and subsequent mechanic homogenization.

Passage of cell layers was assayed as described previously (van Schilfgaarde et al., 1995) with modifications. In short, cells were grown on transparent tissue culture inserts with 1-μm pores (model no. 353104; Falcon) placed in 24-well plates (Falcon) containing 0.5 ml of medium. The culture medium was refreshed every 2 days. After 6 days, the transepithelial resistance of the cellular layers was measured with the Millicell-ERS Resistance system (Millipore, Bedford, Mass.), and the insert was moved to a new well containing 300 μl of RPMI in the basal compartment with 100 μg/ml of DNase I for avoid biofilm formation. Before starting the infection, the culture medium above the insert was replaced, and the cellular layers were then infected with $\sim 10^7$ CFU for in total 12 h. After 3 h, the medium in the upper compartment was replaced to avoid medium acidification, and the number of CFU in the basal compartment was determined at regular time intervals.

Nucleic Acid Accession Numbers

The nucleotide sequences of the *autB* genes of disease isolates 2081107, 2061551, and 2070077 were deposited in GenBank ID (KT367782, KT367783, and KT367784, respectively).

RESULTS

Characterization and Distribution of the *autB* Gene

BLASTn searches identified the *autB* gene in available genome sequences of the pathogenic Neisseria spp. *N. meningitidis* and *N. gonorrhoeae* but not in those of non-pathogenic species, such as *N. lactamica* (**Table 1** and Table S2). The gene was also identified in some strains of Haemophilus spp. (**Table 1** and Table S2). **Figure 1** illustrates the position of the *autB* gene in representative genomes. The *autB* gene is ubiquitous in both pathogenic Neisseria spp. with the exception of one meningococcal strain, i.e., strain 053442. In this strain, as well as in *N. lactamica*, the flanking genes are preserved, but the *autB* gene is substituted by a 1415-bp sequence. Interestingly, the sequences flanking the *autB* gene in *H. influenzae* strains, including the 5′ end of the *holB* gene and the 3′ end of the *tmk* gene are also present as intergenic regions flanking *autB* in *N. meningitidis* and *N. gonorrhoeae* (**Figure 1**). This indicates that *autB* and the flanking regions may have been transferred en bloc from Haemophilus to Neisseria as suggested previously (Davis et al., 2001). However, many Haemophilus strains do neither contain the *autB* gene (**Table 1**), nor the alternative region found in *N. lactamica* (**Figure 1** and data not shown). Interestingly, a sequence containing the 3′ ends of the *autB* and *tmk* genes is

TABLE 1 | Distribution of *autB* within available genome sequences of *Neisseria* and *Haemophilus* species.

Species	Strains analyzed	Presence *autB*	Intact[a]	In frame[b]
N. meningitidis	118	117	104	2
N. gonorrhoeae	16	16	0	0
N. lactamica	4	0		
N. flavescens	2	0		
N. polysaccharea	2	0		
N. sicca	4	0		
H. influenzae	15	7	7	2
H. haemolyticus	9	2	2	2
H. parainfluenzae	2	1	1	?
H. aegyptius	3	3	3	0

[a]*Strains having an intact autB gene that is either in or out of frame at the AAGC repeats.*
[b]*Strains having an intact autB gene that is in frame because of an appropriate number of AAGC repeats. In the case of the H. parainfluenzae strain, it cannot be determined whether the gene is in frame because the sequence upstream of the AAGC repeats is not available.*

tandem repeated in *H. haemolyticus* (**Figure 1**), indicating that this region is prone to genetic recombination.

The genetic characteristics of the *autB* gene in a panel of Neisseria and Haemophilus strains are listed in Table S2. **Table 1** summarizes the numbers of strains in which the gene can be expressed. The number of AAGC nucleotide repeats is considerably lower in Neisseria spp. (3–19) than in Haemophilus spp. (17–30 repeats). In the meningococcal *autA* gene, the same repeat is present, but the range of copies is considerably larger (6–40) (Arenas et al., 2015) than in meningococcal *autB*. In 12 of the 117 meningococcal strains examined (10.3%), the *autB* gene is in frame at these repeats, but in 10 of them the gene is disrupted further downstream of the repeats by frame-shift mutations, premature stop codons or insertion of a transposase element (Table S2). Thus, only two strains (1.7%), i.e., α153 and LNP27256, putatively express *autB* (**Table 1**). In stark contrast, in the 105 meningococcal strains, in which the *autB* gene is out of phase at the AAGC repeats, the gene is further intact with only three exceptions (Table S2). Hence, all these strains can potentially express the gene after phase variation occurs, but, apparently, this is prevented by a very strong selection pressure. Due to downstream disruptions, none of the gonococcal strains can express *autB*, independent of number or repeats. Such disruptions are not present in the *autB* genes of the Haemophilus strains examined, and the gene is in frame in 28% of them (Table S2), but all strains can potentially express *autB* after slipped-strand mispairing. To summarize, *autB* can be expressed, but expression seems to be prone to phase variation at the AAGC repeats and to different genetic disruptions. In addition, these data indicate a strong selection against *autB* expression in Neisseria, but not in Haemophilus spp.

Structure and Variability of AutB

The *autB* gene from *N. meningitidis* reference strain MC58 is not expressed because the number of AAGC repeats renders the gene out of frame (Table S2). Deletion of two repeats results in an N-terminally extended ORF coding for a hypothetical protein of 674 amino-acid residues (aa). The signal peptide cleavage site in this protein was predicted between aa residues A_{30} and V_{31} resulting in a mature protein of 644 aa, which is similar to that of AutA (660 aa), and with a calculated molecular mass of 73.2 kDa. The passenger of AutB is constituted of two parts, a C-terminal linker domain (aa 231–338), which shows homology to the autochaperone domain of other ATs and could accordingly be modeled as a right-handed β-helix (data not shown), and an N-terminal domain. Secondary structure predictions indicate that this N-terminal part of the passenger contains two conserved α-helices (with approximate positions between aa 1–20 and 90–110 of the mature aa sequences) separated by a largely unstructured region of ~80 aa and followed by a segment that is rich in β-sheet but occasionally also contains some α-helix prediction (Figure S1). Rather similar secondary structure was predicted for the corresponding fragment of AutA (Figure S1). The passengers of AutB proteins each contain one or two pairs of cysteines, which probably form a disulfide bond, but they are located at different positions in the sequence (Figure S2). The translocator domain of AutB (aa 360–644) is predicted to form a 12-stranded β-barrel that is connected via an α-helix (aa 337–354) to the passenger.

To determine sequence conservation, the predicted mature AutB proteins from several *Neisseria* and *Haemophilus* strains were aligned. The alignments (see Figure S2 for representatives) revealed that the sequence of the translocator domain was better conserved than that of the passenger. The translocator domain also showed considerable similarity to that of AutA of MC58 (not included in the alignments, but see below). However, the passenger domain showed high sequence diversity (see Figure S2 for examples). To investigate this variability in more detail, we performed independent phylogenetic analysis for the N-terminal part of the passenger, the linker and the translocator domain of representative AutB proteins and AutA of MC58 (**Figure 2**). Indeed, the translocator domain showed limited variability as compared with the other two domains (compare overall mean distances of the separate domains of the AutB proteins). Although similar to the translocator domain of the AutB proteins, the translocator domain of AutA clustered in a different branch, demonstrating that AutA is a different AT, which is consistent with its distinct genomic location. When the N-terminal domain of the passengers was analyzed, three major branches were identified, here designated AutB1, AutB2, and AutB3. The assignment of the AutB proteins in the different strains to these clusters is shown in Table S2. AutA again formed a separate branch. Interestingly, the phylogenic relationships of the AutB proteins do not parallel the boundaries of the species in which these proteins are found, suggesting that specific variants did not evolve in one specific organism, but that there is regular exchange of the genes between these species. AutB1 is the predominant variant in three species, i.e., *N. meningitidis*, *N. gonorrhoeae*, and *H. influenzae*. The AutB3 variant was found in three *Haemophilus* spp. and the AutB2 variant is present in all species except in *N. gonorrhoeae* and *H. parainfluenzae*. Variant AutB3 showed a larger diversity in the N-terminal domain of the passenger than the other variants and, interestingly, clustered with the passenger of AutA, suggesting the exchange of sequences

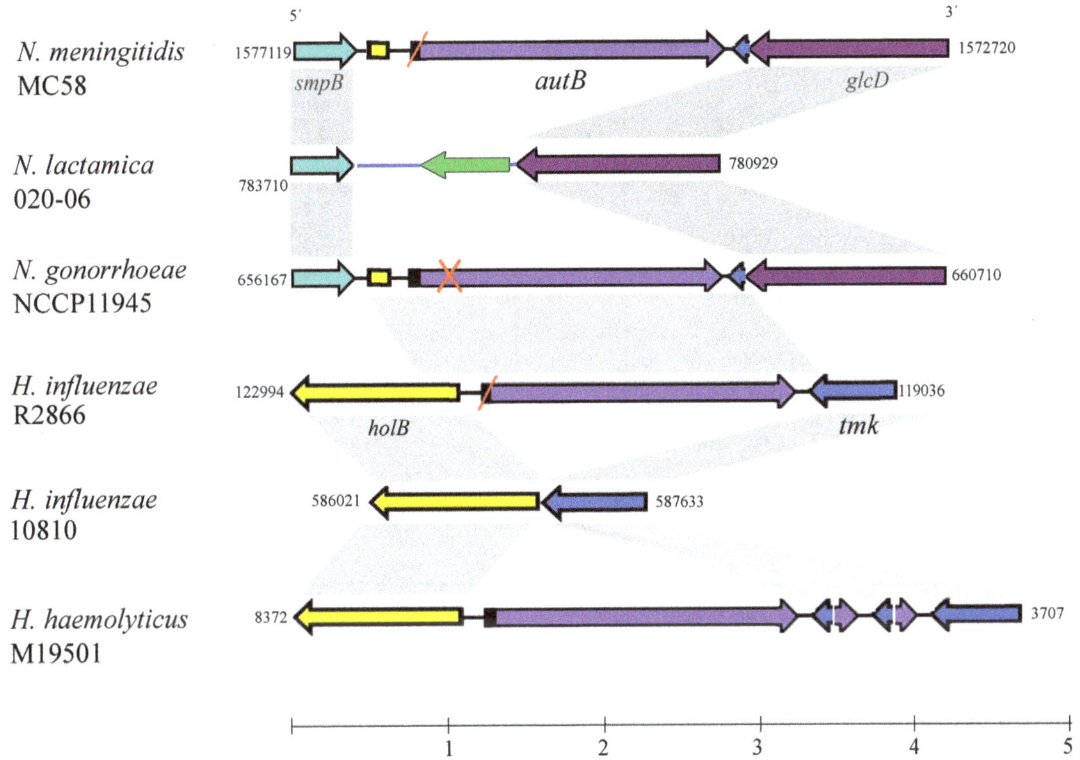

FIGURE 1 | Genomic context of the *autB* gene. The relevant part of the genome sequences of *N. meningitidis* strain MC58, *N. lactamica* strain 020-06, *N. gonorrhoeae* strain NCCP11945, *H. influenzae* strains R2866 and 10810, and *H. haemolyticus* strain M19501 are schematically depicted. Numbers at the side of each map indicate the first and last nucleotide position of the DNA fragment shown in accordance with genome annotations. The genes (arrows) and intergenic regions (lines) with high sequence similarity between different genome sequences are colored identically. Gray shadowing indicates regions with >85% of sequence identity. Red slashes indicate that the gene is out of phase at the AAGC repeats but can potentially be expressed after phase variation. A red cross indicates that the gene is disrupted and cannot be expressed even if it is in phase at the AAGC repeat region. The genes flanking *autB* are conserved in the *Neisseria* genomes. The upstream gene, *smpB*, encodes a protein of 148 amino-acid residues (aa), which is a component of the *trans*-translation system for releasing stalled ribosomes from damaged messenger RNAs. The downstream gene is a homolog of *glcD* of *E. coli*, which encodes the D subunit of glycolate oxidase. *N. lactamica* misses the *autB* gene and its flanking sequences; instead, it contains an alternative intergenic sequence (colored blue) and a gene encoding a hypothetical protein of 168 aa with a conserved DUF1877 domain (colored green). BLAST searches using this gene as query indicated that it is present in the genomes of other *Neisseria* spp. that lack *autB* as well as in many other bacteria. The *autB* gene is also present in some strains of *Haemophilus* spp. but in a different genomic context. In these species, the gene is located between the *holB* gene, which encodes the δ′ subunit of DNA polymerase III, and the *tmk* gene, which encodes thymidylate kinase. It is noteworthy that the intergenic region upstream of *autB* in the *Neisseria* genomes contains part of the 5′ end of the *holB* gene of *Haemophilus*; also downstream of *autB*, a part of the intergenic region and the 3′ end of the *tmk* gene is shared between *N. meningitidis* and *Haemophilus*, suggesting that a DNA segment containing *autB*, the flanking intergenic regions and parts of the *holB* and *tmk* genes from *Haemophilus* was inserted en bloc into a common ancestor of *N. meningitidis* and *N. gonorrhoeae*. Interestingly, a DNA fragment containing the 5′ ends of *autB* and *tmk* and their intergenic region is repeated several times downstream of *autB* in *H. haemolyticus* strain M19501.

between both AT, but limited to this domain. Cluster analysis of the linker domain also indicated the presence of the three main branches with AutA being a separate cluster. The groups were constituted of the same *autB* genes as for the N-terminal domain of the passenger; therefore, the same nomenclature is maintained. However, the relation between the groups varied notably. In this part of the protein, AutB1 was closely related to AutB3 and only distantly related to AutB2. This analysis confirmed that the passenger is rather variable as compared with the translocator domain, which is in agreement with its expected surface exposure and accessibility to the immune system. In addition, this analysis reflects shuffling of different domains within the passenger as suggested before (Davis et al., 2001).

To gain more insight in the evolution of *autB*, we calculated the GC content in the three regions in several *autB* genes. The GC content was similar in the regions encoding the N-terminal part of the passenger and the linker domain (35 ± 2%), but remarkably different for that encoding the translocator domain (44 ± 2%), which suggests that the passenger and the translocator domains have different evolutionary origins that are both different from the pathogenic *Neisseria* spp. with a GC content of 52% in their genome sequences. No differences were found in this respect between the three *autB* variants, suggesting that they evolved in the same species. In the *autA* gene, the GC content of the three regions was remarkably different, i.e., 40 ± 3, 52 ± 3, and 56 ± 1% for the N-terminal part of the passenger, the linker and the translocator domain, respectively. The two latter regions are closer to the average GC content in *Neisseria* genomes. Together, this analysis supports the hypothesis that both ATs have a different origin and suggests the exchange of

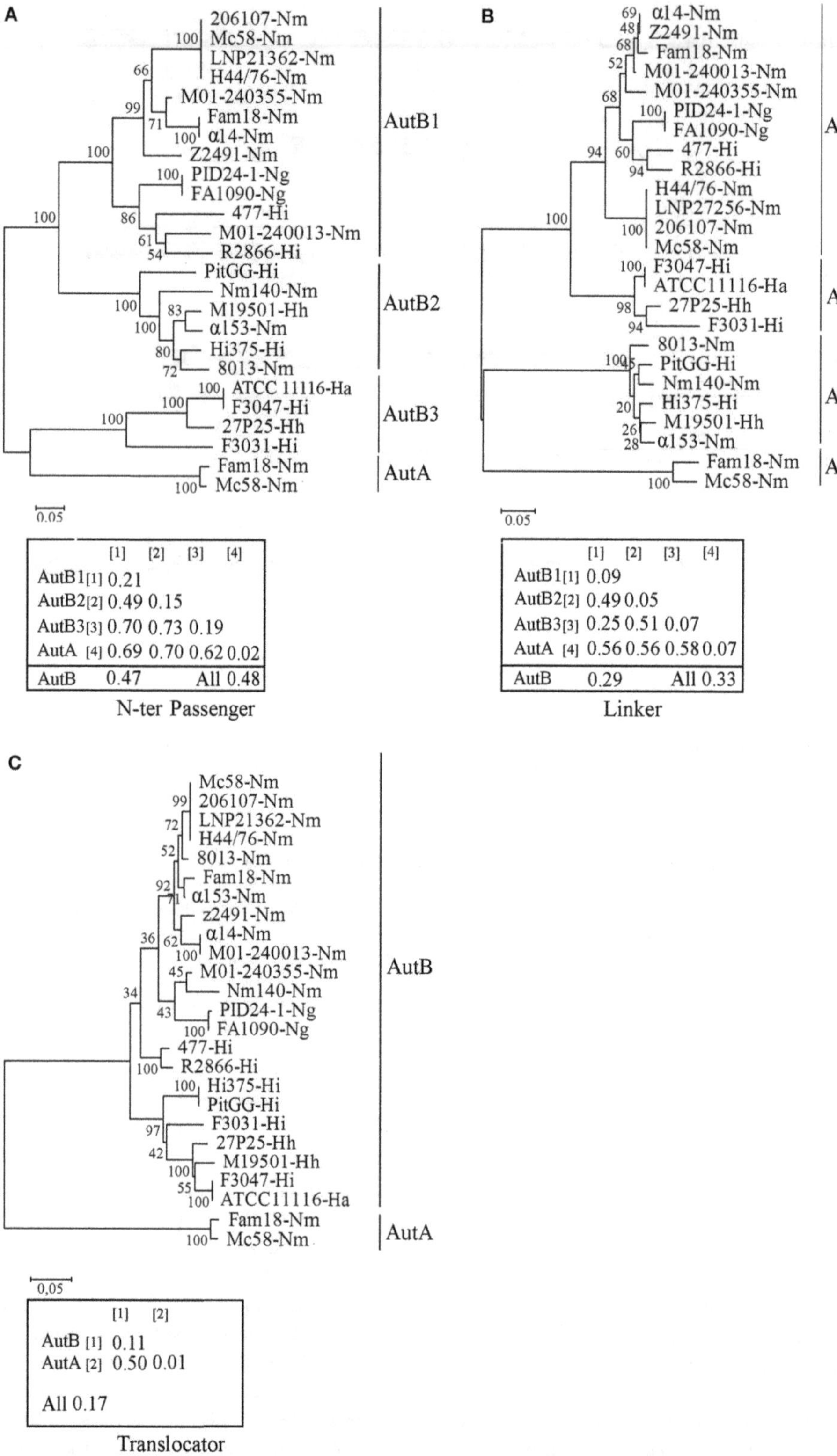

FIGURE 2 | Phylogenetic trees of *autB* gene sequences. Cluster analysis was performed on the N-terminal part of the passenger **(A)**, the linker **(B)**, and the translocator domain **(C)** of mature AutB and AutA proteins derived from representative genomes of *N. meningitidis* (*Nm*), *N. gonorrhoeae* (*Ng*), *H. influenzae* (*Hi*), *H. aegyptius* (*Ha*), and *H. haemolyticus* (*Hh*) strains. The *autB* genes from *H. influenzae* strain R2866 and *H. aegyptius* ATCC11116 were previously called *lav* and *las*, respectively (Davis et al., 2001). The bootstraps values are shown on the branches. Genetic distances within and between groups and overall mean distances for AutBs are included in the insets.

genetic material between genes of different ATs in the region encoding the passenger.

Phase Variation of *autB* in Clinical Meningococcal Isolates

To study phase variation of *autB*, we analyzed large sets of meningococcal disease isolates from the same genetic origin. If phase variation indeed occurs frequently, different isolates of the same cc should contain different numbers of repeats and, in the absence of selection pressure, ~33% should have the gene in the proper reading frame. We analyzed collections of cc213 and cc32 isolates, two hyper-invasive clonal complexes. The number of repeat units in the *autA* gene of these isolates was previously analyzed (Arenas et al., 2015) allowing us to compare phase variation in these two AT genes. In cc213 strain M01-240355, *autB* is in phase at the AAGC repeat but it is disrupted by a downstream frameshift mutation (Table S2). In the cc32 strains listed in Table S2 ($n = 17$), the *autB* gene is out of phase but it does not contain additional disruptions. All these genomes harbor an AutB1 variant (Table S2).

The repeat region of the *autB* gene was amplified by PCR and sequenced in a panel of 53 isolates of cc213 and 49 isolates of cc32 collected in The Netherlands between 2000 and 2010 from patients with meningococcal disease. The number of repeat units varied and ranged from 2 to 10 in *autB* and from 5 to 32 in *autA* (Table S3 and **Figure 3**). These results illustrate that slipped-strand mispairing at the AAGC repeats occurs in both genes and in both clonal complexes. However, in only 1 of the 49 cc32 isolates (2%), i.e., strain 2081107, and none of the 53 cc213 isolates the *autB* gene was in phase. This low frequency contrasts drastically with that observed for *autA*, where the gene was found to be in phase in 28% and 45% for cc213 and cc32 isolates, respectively (**Figure 3**), i.e., close to the 33% that would be expected in the absence of any selection pressure (Arenas et al., 2015). Thus, the results support the hypothesis that, although slipped-strand mispairing resulting in frameshifts does occur at the AAGC repeats in *autB*, there is a strong selection pressure against the occurrence of a number of repeats that would render the gene in frame in both clonal complexes. Further sequence examination revealed that cc213 isolates do not contain the same additional frameshift that disrupts the *autB* gene downstream of the AAGC repeats in strain M01-240355, suggesting that this feature is not conserved in cc213 strains. Therefore, the gene could potentially be expressed in this cc after slipped-strand mispairing. Interestingly, examination of the sequence after the repeats revealed that isolate 2041085 harbors an AutB2 variant, whilst all other cc213 isolates harbor an AutB1 variant, evidencing horizontal genetic transfer. The full-length *autB* gene was sequenced in three isolates of cc32, i.e., 2081107, which is in frame at the AAGC repeats, and 2061551 and 2070077, which are out of phase. All these isolates revealed only variation in the number of repeat units and no other genetic disruptions or amino-acid substitutions relative to that of strain MC58. Thus,

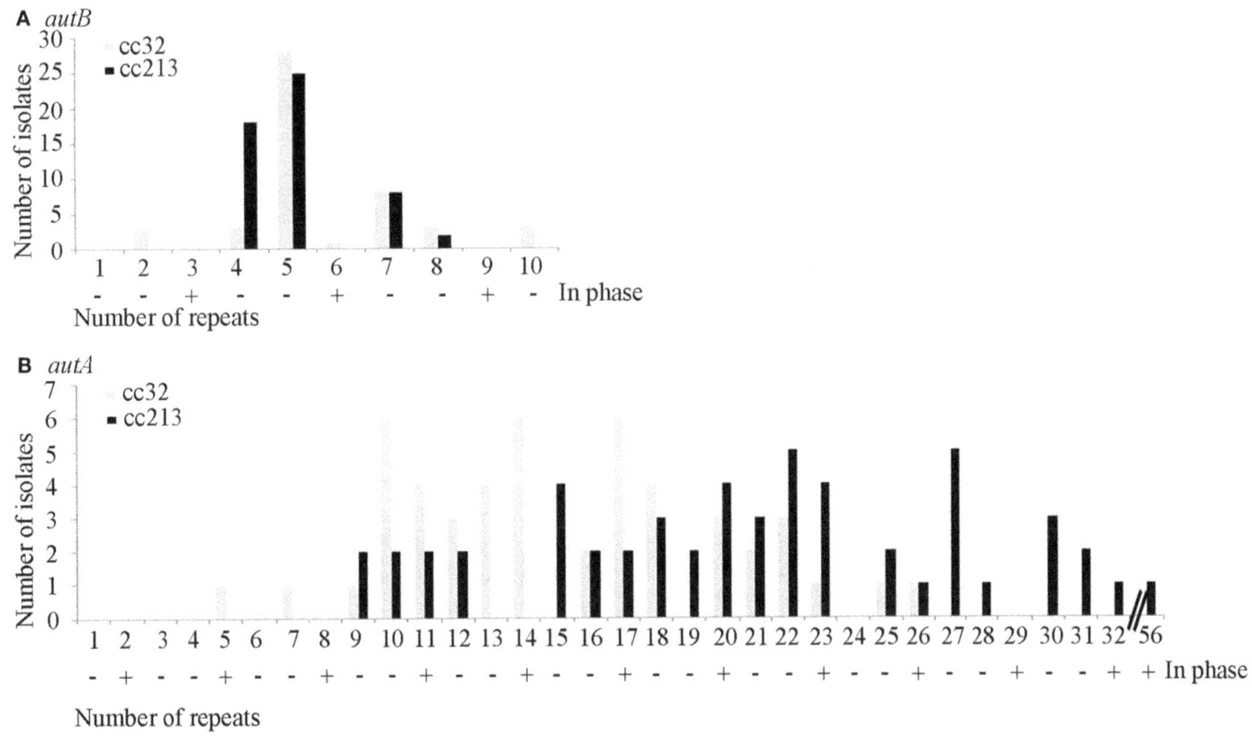

FIGURE 3 | Variable numbers of AAGC repeats. The numbers of AAGC repeats were determined in the *autB* **(A)** and *autA* **(B)** genes of 49 cc32 and 53 cc213 meningococcal strains isolated from patients with meningococcal disease. Data for AutA were taken from Arenas et al. (2015). The numbers of repeats that would render the gene in phase are indicated by a plus sign.

the *autB* gene of isolate 2081107 is intact and, therefore, probably expressed.

Phase Variation of *autB* in Carriage Isolates

Since the vast majority of isolates analyzed in Tables S2, S3 are from patients with invasive meningococcal disease, our selection of strains may not be representative for those residing in the nasopharynx. Thus, we analyzed the *autB* gene in the genome sequences of a collection of carriage isolates available in a public data base (http://pubmlst.org/software/database/bigsdb/). A total of 207 strains was analyzed. The number of repeat units in the *autB* gene ranged from 2 to 22. In total, 10.6% of these isolates had 3, 6, or 12 repeats that render *autB* in frame. However, in the majority of these strains, the gene is disrupted by downstream-located single-nucleotide insertions and only 2.4% of isolates (28871, 28881, 28942, 28955, 28959) had an undisrupted *autB* gene in frame. Hence, these data do not show obvious differences in possible *autB* expression between carrier and disease isolates.

Expression of Meningococcal AutB

We next analyzed whether AutB is indeed synthesized in strains where the gene is in phase at the AAGC repeats and has no other genetic disruptions. Plasmids encoding the *autB1* and *autB2* genes from strains 2081107 and α153, respectively, were introduced in HB-1Δ*autB*. Although the *autB* gene is phase off in HB-1 (Table S2), we deleted the chromosomal copy of the gene to avoid genetic exchange with the *autB* gene on the plasmids. Western blot analysis showed a band with an apparent molecular weight of ~73 kDa in strain HB-1Δ*autB* carrying pENAutB$_1$ only when the strain was grown in the presence of IPTG (**Figure 4A**), thus identifying this band AutB$_1$. A band of similar size was detected in isolate 2081107, which contains an intact in-frame *autB* gene on the chromosome, but not in preparations of other strains where the *autB1* gene is out of phase (**Figure 4A**). This result demonstrates that AutB is synthesized in isolate 2081107. Unfortunately, an *autB* mutant of this strain could not be created, because the strain was not transformable. No reaction was observed in strains HB-1Δ*autB* carrying pENAutB$_2$ (data not shown) or α153, which is expected to express AutB2 from the chromosome (**Figure 4A**), presumably due to lack of cross-reactivity of the antiserum, which was raised against a part of AutB1 that shows little sequence similarity to AutB2 (Figure S2). The antiserum did also not react with a preparation of strain α14 (**Figure 4A**), which expresses AutA, confirming the specificity of the antiserum.

To investigate if *autB2* is expressed in α153, RT-PCR assays were done using primers targeting internal DNA fragments of *autB1* and *autB2*. With chromosomal DNA from HB-1 and α153 as templates, the amplicons for *autB1* and *autB2* were according the expected size, i.e., 100 and 150 bp, respectively (**Figure 4B**). No amplicons were obtained from RNA preparations as templates (data not shown), but they were obtained from cDNA preparations of strains HB-1Δ*autB* containing pENAutB$_1$ and grown in presence of IPTG and α153, but not of strains HB-1 and the α153Δ*autB* mutant (**Figure 4B**). Primers for *rmpM* yielded an amplicon in all preparations, evidencing that all contained similar amounts of cDNA. The lack of detection of *autB* transcripts in strain HB-1 could be due to degradation of the mRNA by the presence of a premature stop codon resulting from the frameshift at the AAGC repeat region. Together, these data show that *autB* is expressed in at least some meningococcal strains and confirm that its expression is determined by phase variation at the AAGC repeat units.

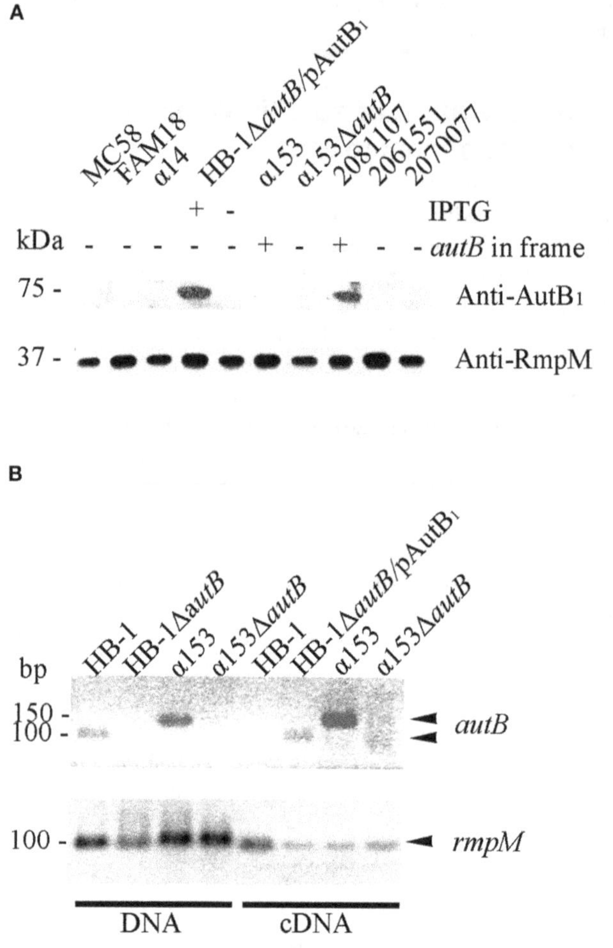

FIGURE 4 | Expression of AutB. (A) Western blots of cell envelope preparations of various *N. meningitidis* strains were probed with antisera directed against AutB1 and, as a loading control, against RmpM. HB-1Δ*autB* containing pENAutB$_1$ (pAutB$_1$) was grown in the presence or absence of IPTG as indicated. Also indicated is whether the chromosomal *autB* gene is in frame or not. Positions of molecular mass standards are shown at the left. Only the relevant parts of the blot are shown. **(B)** Agarose gels showing PCR products obtained with either chromosomal DNA or cDNA as templates as indicated at the bottom. The cDNA was generated from RNA, which was extracted from the *N. meningitidis* strains, using primers for *autB* or *rmpM* as indicated. HB-1Δ*autB* containing pENAutB$_1$ was grown in the presence of IPTG. Size standards are shown at the left. Only the relevant parts of the gels are shown.

Exposure of AutB at the Cell Surface

Our Western blotting analysis detected the full-length AutB in cell envelope preparations (**Figure 4A**). To determine whether the passenger domain may be released from a proportion of the AutB molecules into the extracellular medium, whole cell lysates, cell envelopes and supernatants of strain HB-1Δ*autB* expressing AutB1 from pENAutB$_1$ were analyzed by SDS-PAGE and Western blotting. The expected 73-kDa band was detected in cell-envelope preparations but no band reacting with the antiserum was detected in supernatant preparations (**Figure 5A**). As a control, the secretion of IgA protease was also analyzed using specific antibodies against its translocator domain and the α-peptide, which is released into the milieu after cleavage by NalP (Roussel-Jazédé et al., 2014). As expected, the translocator domain and the α-peptide were detected in the cell envelope fraction and the culture supernatant, respectively (**Figure 5A**). Hence, the passenger of AutB is not released into the extracellular medium. To confirm its cell-surface exposition, we used proteinase K accessibility assays in intact bacteria (**Figure 5B**). The protease degraded AutB and fHbp, a surface-exposed lipoprotein that was analyzed as a positive control (Bos et al., 2014). In contrast, the periplasmically exposed outer membrane-associated protein RmpM remained unaffected, confirming the integrity of the outer membrane. Thus, the passenger of AutB is secreted but remains attached via the translocator domain to the cell surface.

AutB Expression Impacts Biofilm Formation

Previously, we demonstrated that AutA has a role in autoaggregation and biofilm formation (Arenas et al., 2015). To investigate whether AutB also has a role in autoaggregation, settling assays were performed. These assays showed a clear effect of the of AutA production on bacterial autoaggregation (Figure S3A); however, such an effect was not observed when *autB1* was expressed from plasmid in HB-1Δ*autB*, and also no difference between α153 and its *autB* mutant derivative was observed (Figure S3A). Thus, in contrast to AutA, synthesis of AutB does not induce strong autoaggregation.

A possible role of AutB in biofilm formation was first studied under static conditions on polystyrene plates. The presence of a capsule is known to inhibit biofilm formation (Yi et al., 2004; Lappann et al., 2006), but α153 is a natural capsule null mutant. We also included the capsule-deficient reference strains HB-1 and BB-1, which were previously used in biofilm assays (Arenas et al., 2013a). After 1 h of incubation, α153 generated a biofilm mass intermediate between that of BB-1 and HB-1 (**Figure 6A**). Interestingly, deletion of *autB* drastically impaired biofilm formation to a level comparable with that of strain BB-1 (**Figure 6A**). This phenotype was complemented when either AutB1 or AutB2 was expressed *in trans* from plasmid (**Figure 6A**), demonstrating that both variants have a similar role.

N. meningitidis has two different strategies of biofilm formation, either dependent or independent of eDNA (Lappann et al., 2010). HB-1 and BB-1 follow the eDNA-dependent and -independent routes of biofilm formation, respectively (Arenas et al., 2013a). To investigate whether AutB-mediated biofilm formation is dependent on eDNA, biofilm formation of strain α153 and its *autB* mutant derivative was assessed in the presence of DNase I. This treatment considerably reduced biofilm mass in α153 to the level of the Δ*autB* mutant, but it did not impact on the residual biofilm formation of the mutant (**Figure 6A**, right panel). This data indicates that AutB-mediated biofilm formation is dependent on eDNA and suggests that the remaining biofilm formation in the *autB* mutant of α153 is eDNA independent. Presumably, AutB at the cell surface binds eDNA that acts as a glue facilitating interbacterial and bacterium-substratum interactions. Previously, the α-peptide of IgA protease and NHBA were reported to represent the main surface-exposed DNA-binding proteins involved in biofilm formation in strain HB-1 (Arenas et al., 2013a). Western blot analysis, however, revealed that the α-peptide of IgA protease is released into the medium in strain α153 (**Figure 5A**), whilst examination of the α153 genome sequence revealed that the *nhbA* gene is disrupted. Thus, probably, AutB is the main DNA-binding protein in α153 and, therefore, its inactivation has a drastic impact on biofilm formation. To investigate the DNA-binding capacities of AutB, we produced the entire passenger of AutB of strain HB-1 in *E. coli*. The protein formed inclusion bodies, which were purified, but we could not establish proper conditions to fold the protein *in vitro*.

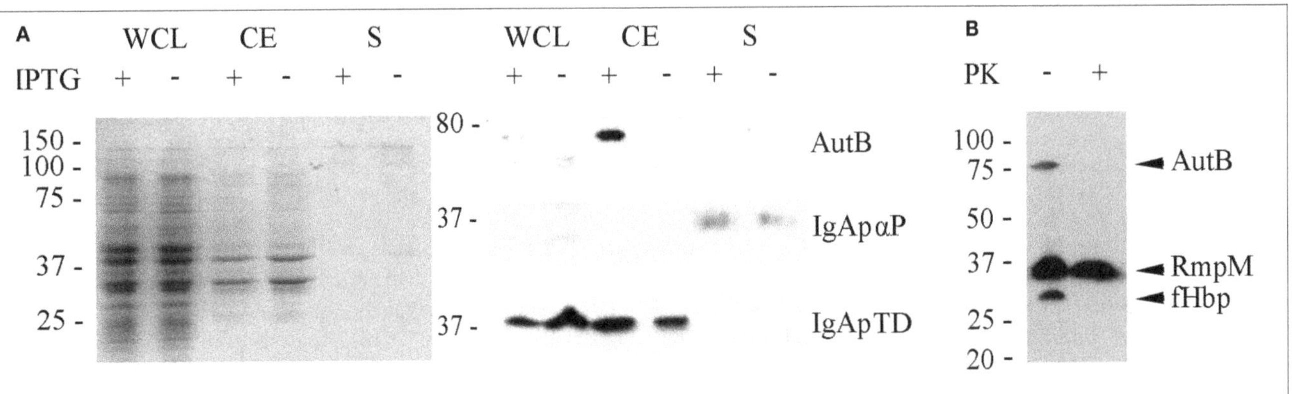

FIGURE 5 | Localization of AutB. (A) Strain HB-1Δ*autB* containing pENAutB1 was grown in the presence or absence of IPTG and whole cell lysates (WCL), cell envelopes (CE) and culture supernatants (S) were prepared and separated by SDS-PAGE. The left panel shows a Coomassie-stained gel, and corresponding Western blots with antisera directed against AutB1, and the α-peptide (αP) and the translocator domain (TD) of IgA protease (IgAp) are shown in the right panel. Only the relevant parts of the blots are shown. **(B)** Protease-accessibility assay. Cells of HB-1Δ*autB* containing pENAutB1 were grown in the presence of 0.1 mM IPTG and treated or not with 2 μg/ml of proteinase K (PK). The degradation of AutB, RmpM, and fHbp was analyzed by Western blotting using specific antibodies.

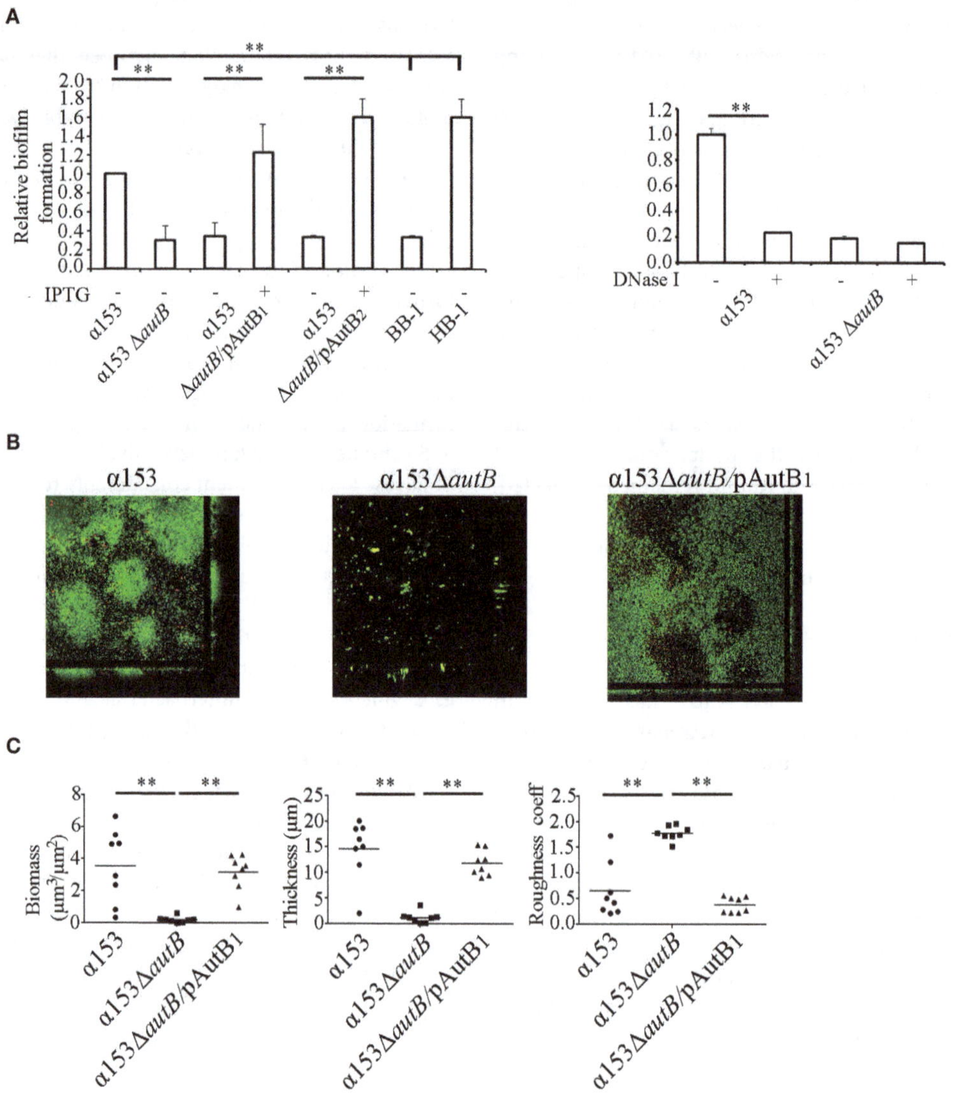

FIGURE 6 | AutB mediates biofilm formation. (A) Biofilm formation under static conditions. Bacteria were pre-cultured in TSB with or without 0.1 mM of IPTG and adjusted to an OD_{550} of 1.0. Aliquots were then transferred into 24-well plates and incubated under static conditions for 1 h (left panel). The impact of DNase I on biofilm formation in α153 and its Δ*autB* mutant derivative is shown in the right panel. 100 μg/ml of DNase I was added to the cultures, which were subsequently incubated for 1 h under static conditions. Biofilms formed were quantified after staining with crystal violet by measuring the OD_{630}. The data represent means and standard deviations of at least three independent experiments, and values are given as relative to α153, which was set at 1.0. Statistically significant differences between groups are marked with two asterisks (unpaired *t*-test of $P < 0.01$). **(B)** Biofilm formation under flow conditions. Representative pictures are shown of structures of 16 h-old biofilms of α153, α153Δ*autB*, and α153Δ*autB* carrying pENAutB1 cultured in presence of 0.1 mM IPTG (α153Δ*autB*/pAutB$_1$). Bacteria were stained with Dead/Live staining for visualization. Green and red bacteria are live and dead cells, respectively. **(C)** Quantification of biomass, thickness, and roughness of 16 h-old biofilms under flow conditions. The biofilm parameters were determined with COMSTAT/MATLAB software. Asterisks indicate statistically significant differences ($P < 0.0005$) between groups calculated by unpaired *t*-test using GraphPad software.

To investigate the influence of AutB synthesis on biofilm formation in more detail, we used a flow-cell model. With this method, the flow in the nasopharynx or the bloodstream is mimicked, and biofilm development can continuously be monitored by microscopy. Biofilms formed by α153 were constituted of round aggregates of different sizes, which were surrounded by single cells (see representative pictures in **Figure 6B** and the development of the biofilm in Figure S3B). These aggregates fused into larger aggregates, which constituted the biomass of the biofilm (Figure S3B). These biofilm structures had a clearly different appearance than those reported previously for strains HB-1, BB-1, and α14 (Arenas et al., 2013a, 2015). Analysis of the α153Δ*autB* mutant did not reveal structured biofilms; instead, only few single cells or very small aggregates were randomly attached to the substratum (**Figure 6B**). COMSTAT analysis revealed a biomass and thickness significantly reduced as compared with the wild type (**Figure 6C**) in accordance with the results of the biofilm assays under static conditions (**Figure 6A**). Furthermore, biofilm roughness, also determined by COMSTAT, increased significantly. All phenotypic differences were complemented when $AutB_1$ was expressed *in trans* from plasmid (**Figures 6B,C**). These data confirm that AutB is required for biofilm formation and architecture and demonstrate its biological relevance.

AutB Synthesis Interferes with Meningococcal Translocation across Epithelial Cell Layers

To investigate whether the synthesis of AutB also affects the interaction of the bacteria with eukaryotic cells, we first determined the adherence of α153 and its *autB* mutant derivative to NCI-H292 cells by counting the number of cell-associated CFU 3 h after initiating infection. Although adherence of the mutant appeared slightly reduced (~25%), a defect that was complemented when AutB was expressed *in trans* (**Figure 7A**), this difference was not statistically significant.

Next, we studied the ability of the strains to cross epithelial cell layers, a process necessary for host invasion. NCI-H292 cells were grown for 6 days on a permeable support to generate cellular junctions, as verified by a trans-epithelial resistance of 30 ± 2 $\Omega \times cm^2$, in accordance with values previously reported (van Schilfgaarde et al., 1995). The cell layers were then infected with bacteria and the numbers of bacteria that reached the basal compartment after passage of the cell layers were determined between 6 and 12 h post infection by counting CFU. Cells of the *autB* mutant reached the basal compartment faster than those of the parental strain as demonstrated, for example, by the significantly higher numbers of *autB* mutant bacteria than of wild-type bacteria in the basal compartment 10 h after infection (**Figure 7B**), a phenotype that was complemented by expression of a functional copy of *autB* from $pENAutB_1$. Clones of cells derived from the wild type that reached the trans-epithelial compartment early after infection were collected from different experiments and further analyzed. To investigate whether AutB synthesis and, consequently, their biofilm-formation capacity was altered, we tested biofilm formation under static conditions. Interestingly, all clones had a reduced biofilm-forming capacity like the *autB* mutant (see **Figure 7C** for representatives). Sequencing of the AAGC region in all clones did not show alterations, suggesting that phase variation was not the origin of such defect. To test whether *autB* expression was lost we analyzed one clone by RT-PCR assays and found no detectable *autB* expression (**Figure 7C**). Sequencing of the complete *autB* gene and flanking regions, however, did not reveal an obvious reason for this down-regulation, suggesting these clones had acquired a mutation in a regulatory gene. Together, these data demonstrate that *autB* expression negatively affects bacterial epithelial transmigration and suggests that biofilm formation is inversely correlated with invasion.

DISCUSSION

The *autB* gene is present in bacteria colonizing the human mucosa and is restricted to certain species of the genera *Neisseria* and *Haemophilus*. This distribution was earlier explained by the transfer of the gene from an unidentified microorganism to *H. influenzae* and then to a recent ancestor of both *N. meningitidis* and *N. gonorrhoeae* (Davis et al., 2001). This hypothesis was mainly based on the observation that the gene is placed in *H. influenzae* between the *tmk* and *holB* genes, two genes that are contiguous in many gram-negative bacteria, whilst it is placed in a different context in *N. meningitidis* and *N. gonorrhoeae* but flanked by fragments of the *tmk* and *holB* genes from *H. influenzae* (**Figure 1**). These observations were made by the examination of the few genome sequences of *Neisseria* and *Haemophilus* strains that were available at that time (Davis et al., 2001). Now, many more genome sequences of both genera are available, and this allowed us to extend the earlier analysis. Indeed, our analysis confirms initial observations and adds new evidence about the evolution and expression of the gene.

First, the *autB* gene is not present in all *H. influenzae* isolates, indicating that the gene does not originate from this species. We found the gene in three other *Haemophilus* spp., i.e., *H. haemolytica, H. parainfluenzae,* and *H. aegyptius*, which are closely related to *H. influenzae.* Also in these species, the gene is found only in a limited number of isolates, indicating that they did not evolve from *autB*-containing *H. influenzae* strains but also acquired the gene by horizontal gene transfer. Second, the gene was ubiquitously present in *N. meningitidis* and *N. gonorrhoeae* genomes, but not in other *Neisseria* spp., consistent with the proposed acquisition of the gene by a recent ancestor of both pathogenic *Neisseria* spp. In agreement with its acquisition by horizontal gene transfer, the GC content of *autB* is substantially lower than that of *Neisseria* genomes. Third, our phylogenetic analysis revealed the existence of three main allelic variants of *autB*. Each variant was not restricted to one single species, but *N. meningitidis, H. influenzae, H. haemolyticus,* and *H. aegyptius* each contained several of these variants, a clear indication that they share a common pool of *autB* genes. In contrast, only *autB1* was detected in *N. gonorrhoeae*, indicating that this species does not participate in the exchange of *autB* variants which is consistent with its different niche. In the evolutionary context, it is also interesting to consider the origin of AutA, which is structurally related to AutB. In contrast to *autB*, *autA* is present in both pathogenic and commensal *Neisseria* species (Arenas et al., 2015). Therefore, it did not arise by gene duplication after introduction of *autB* into a common ancestor of the pathogenic *Neisseria* spp. Because it is ubiquitous among *Neisseria* spp., it may originate from a common ancestor of *Neisseria* spp. Its subsequent transfer to and evolution in other microorganisms may eventually have resulted in its return as *autB* in *Neisseria.* In agreement with the neisserial origin of *autA* is the GC content of the segments encoding the linker and translocator domains of the protein, which, in contrast to the corresponding domains of *autB*, are in accordance with those of neisserial genomes. However, the GC content of the segment encoding the N-terminal part of the AutA passenger is substantially lower indicating a different evolutionary origin of this part of the gene. Shuffling of domains is also suggested from the phylogenetic analysis of the *autB* genes. The translocator domain of AutB is well conserved, whilst the linker is more conserved than the N-terminal part of the

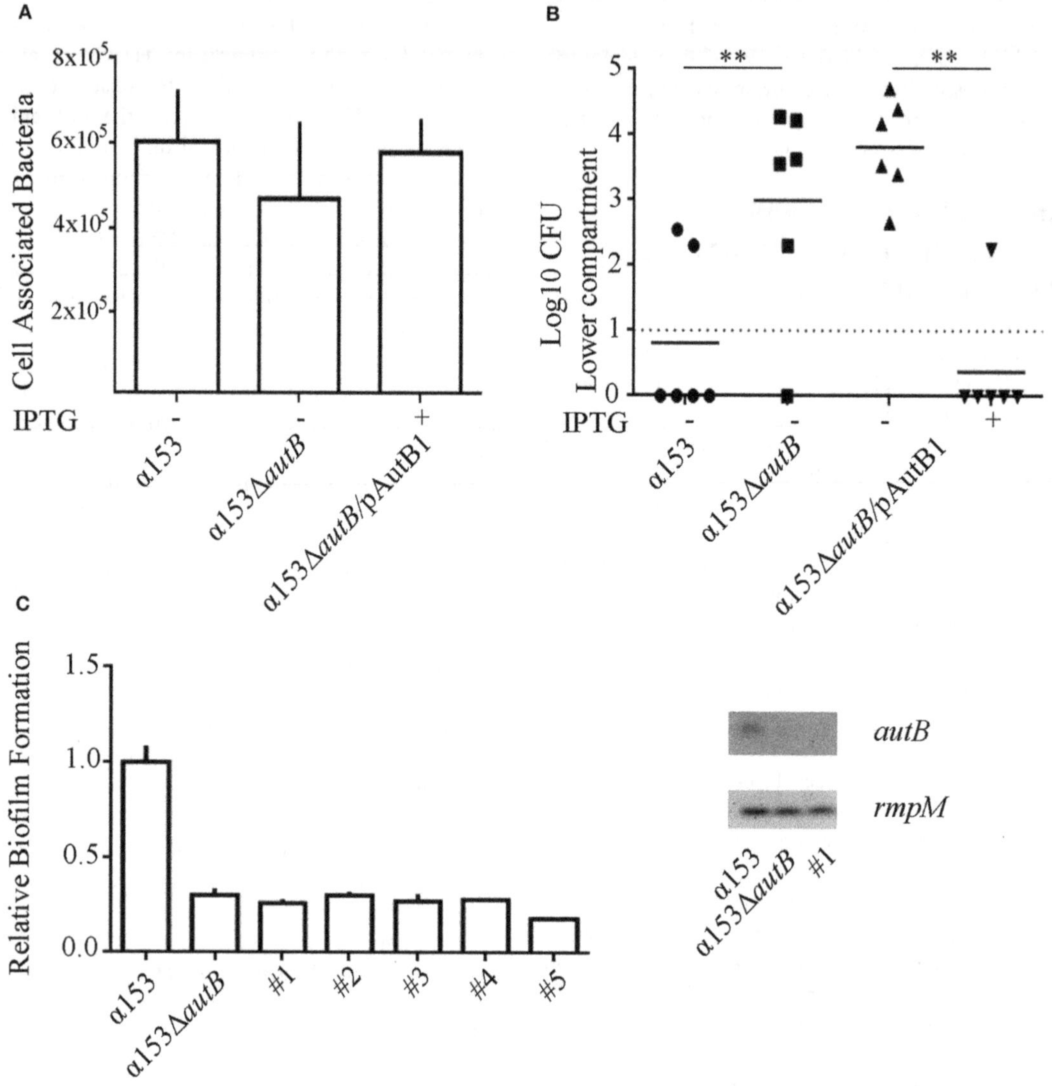

FIGURE 7 | Inactivation of *autB* affects passage of NCI-H292 cell layers. (A) Adherence of *N. meningitidis* strains α153, α153Δ*autB*, and α153Δ*autB* carrying pENAutB$_1$ to NCI-H292 cell layers. The complemented strain was grown in the presence of IPTG. The NCI-H292 cells were incubated with the bacteria for 3 h, washed, and cell-associated CFU were determined after lysing the cells with saponin. Means and standard deviations of three independent experiments performed in duplicate are shown. Differences observed were not statistically significant. **(B)** Passage of cells of strain α153, its Δ*autB* mutant derivative and the complemented mutant through NCI-H292 cell layers. The complemented mutant was grown with or without IPTG as indicated. The passage of bacteria through the cell layers was determined by counting CFUs from the basal compartment 10 h after inoculation. Results of three independent experiments performed in duplicate are shown. Asterisks show statistically significant differences between groups ($P < 0.001$, unpaired t-test). Before statistical analysis, CFUs were log10 converted. **(C)** Analysis of clones of cells of strain α153 that reached the trans-epithelial compartment. Several clones were recovered in independent infection experiments (#1–5). Their biofilm-forming capacity was determined as described for **Figure 6A** and is shown in the graft at the left. Expression of *autB* was determined by RT-PCR as described for **Figure 4B**, and agarose gels with PCR products obtained with cDNA as templates are shown in the right panel.

passenger. The N-terminal domain of AutB3 is only distantly related to the corresponding domains of AutB1 and AutB2. In contrast, its linker domain is closely related to that of AutB1, from which it probably evolved after having been linked to a different N-terminal domain.

In all *N. gonorrhoeae* strains examined, the *autB* gene cannot be expressed because of genetic disruptions downstream of the AAGC repeat region, indicating that AutB synthesis is not relevant in the particular niche of this species. In contrast, although phase off in most cases, an intact *autB* gene is preserved in the vast majority of *N. meningitidis* isolates, indicating that it is advantageous for this species to be able to synthesize AutB at some stage in the colonization process. However, it is also evident that it is important for the bacteria to be able to shut off the synthesis of AutB. With only very few exceptions, the number of AAGC repeats renders the gene phase off in meningococci with an intact *autB* gene (Tables S2, S3, **Figure 3**). Such an extreme preference for the off-phase of a phase-variable gene has, to the best of our knowledge, not been reported before. As compared with *Haemophilus autB*, the number of AAGC repeats in *N. meningitidis autB* is generally lower. A lower number of repeats is expected to result in a reduced frequency of phase variation. However, the variable number of repeats observed in the *autB* gene of isolates of the same clonal complex demonstrates that loss and gain of these repeats through slipped-strand mispairing is still occurring in the meningococcus. When the number of these repeats is reduced to three, the gene is in the on phase and the frequency of phase variation is expected to be very low. In this case, the majority of the isolates have lost the possibility to express the *autB* gene through mutations further downstream in the gene, which accentuates the importance for the bacteria to switch off the expression of the gene.

Why is an intact *autB* gene retained in *N. meningitidis*, while its expression is shut off in the vast majority of the isolates? Like AutB, many other surface-exposed proteins of *N. meningitidis* show phase-variable expression (Saunders et al., 2000), most likely to escape from the immune system. As these proteins have important functions for colonization and persistence in the host, the functions of some of these proteins may be taken over by others when their expression is turned off. The *autB* gene has been considered to be a pseudogene because its expression could not be demonstrated in a limited set of meningococcal strains (Ait-Tahar et al., 2000). We demonstrate here that AutB is synthesized in at least some isolates and that it has a role in biofilm formation presumably by binding eDNA. This role would be equivalent to those of NHBA and the α-peptide of IgA protease (Arenas et al., 2013a). Although the expression of the genes for NHBA and IgA protease has not been reported to be phase variable, these proteins are cleaved from the cell surface by the AT protease NalP (Serruto et al., 2003; van Ulsen et al., 2003; Roussel-Jazédé et al., 2014), the expression of which is phase variable (Saunders et al., 2000). Thus, AutB may serve as a backup mechanism that enables biofilm formation if the amount of cell-surface-exposed NHBA and α-peptide is low.

Then, why is *autB* expression switched off in most isolates? Phase variation by slipped-strand mispairing is a random process and, with the AAGC repeats being located within the coding region, one would expect that 33% of the isolates are in phase on. Such a frequency was indeed found for the *autA* gene (Arenas et al., 2015), but *autB* was found to be in phase on in only ~1% of the same set of isolates, indicating the existence of a strong selection pressure against expression of the gene. Possibly, AutB elicits a strong immune response. Consistent with this hypothesis is the high sequence variability we observed in the passenger domain of AutB, which may reflect antigenic variability due to immune pressure. However, another explanation for selection against *autB* expression in disease isolates is that biofilm formation, whilst presumably important in the colonization of the mucosal surfaces, may be hindering the passage of the epithelial layers to cause invasive disease. Indeed, we observed that AutB synthesis delays the passage of epithelial cell layers *in vitro*. It is noteworthy in this respect that no evidence for selection pressure against *autB* expression was observed in the limited number of *Haemophilus* genomes analyzed. The *H. influenzae* strains in which *autB* (*lav*) was found are nontypeable strains, which seldom cause invasive disease (Davis et al., 2001). Furthermore, *H. haemolyticus* is generally considered as a commensal in the nasopharynx, although also few cases of invasive disease by this bacterium have been reported (Jordan et al., 2011). Thus, these observations suggest a role for AutB during colonization of the nasopharynx and a negative effect of AutB synthesis on bacterial invasion. However, also the vast majority of strains isolated from carriers did not express *autB*. A possible explanation is that the isolation methods for carriage isolates selectively fail to collect AutB-expressing strains. Carriage strains are often isolated from healthy people using swabs. This method underestimates the number of carriers as was demonstrated by Sim et al. (2000), who reported that swabs allowed for the isolation of meningococci from 10% of the people examined whilst meningococci were detected in 45% of these people by immunohistochemistry. In addition, microcolonies were found with the latter technique below the epithelial surface, which could explain the observed underestimation of meningococcal carriage through swab isolation. Thus, it is possible that AutB facilitates microcolony formation in this specific niche.

In summary, we showed here for the first time the synthesis of AutB in some meningococcal isolates and the existence of strong selection pressure against *autB* expression. We also demonstrated the localization of AutB at the bacterial cell surface, its function in biofilm formation, and the negative consequences of its expression on the transit of the bacteria through epithelial cell layers. This work completes the initial characterization of the eight ATs identified so far in available meningococcal genome sequences and provides new insights in the commensal/virulence relationship of pathogenic *Neisseria* and *Haemophilus* species.

AUTHOR CONTRIBUTIONS

JA, FP, JP, and JT conceived and designed the experiments; JA, SC, AE, and JT performed bioinformatics analysis; JA, FP, PR, and SC performed the experiments; JA, JT analyzed the data and wrote the paper. All authors have read and approved the manuscript.

FUNDING

This work was partially supported by Utrecht University. PR, SC were supported by personal fellowships for student mobility (Spanish government) and by an Erasmus fellowship, respectively.

ACKNOWLEDGMENTS

We would like to thank Tom van den Hoeven and Donia Tajouri for technical assistance and fruitful discussions.

REFERENCES

Ait-Tahar, K., Wooldridge, K. G., Turner, D. P. J., Atta, M., Todd, I., and Ala'Aldeen, D. A. A. (2000). Auto-transporter A protein of *Neisseria meningitidis*: a potent CD4+ T-cell and B-cell stimulating antigen detected by expression cloning. *Mol. Microbiol.* 37, 1094–1105. doi: 10.1046/j.1365-2958.2000.02061.x

Arenas, J., Abel, A., Sánchez, S., Alcalá B., Criado, M. T., and Ferreirós, C. M. (2006). Locus NMB0035 codes for a 47-kDa surface-accessible conserved antigen in Neisseria. *Int. Microbiol.* 9, 273–280.

Arenas, J., Cano, S., Nijland, R., van Dongen, V., Rutten, L., van der Ende, A., et al. (2015). The meningococcal autotransporter AutA is implicated in autoaggregation and biofilm formation. *Environ. Microbiol.* 17, 1321–1337. doi: 10.1111/1462-2920.12581

Arenas, J., Nijland, R., Rodriguez, F. J., Bosma, T. N. P., and Tommassen, J. (2013a). Involvement of three meningococcal surface-exposed proteins, the heparin-binding protein NhbA, the α-peptide of IgA protease and the autotransporter protease NalP, in initiation of biofilm formation. *Mol. Microbiol.* 87, 254–268. doi: 10.1111/mmi.12097

Arenas, J., Schipper, K., van Ulsen, P., van der Ende, A., and Tommassen, J. (2013b). Domain exchange at the 3' end of the gene encoding the fratricide meningococcal two-partner secretion protein A. *BMC Genomics* 14:622. doi: 10.1186/1471-2164-14-622

Arenas, J., and Tommassen, J. (2016). Meningococcal biofilm formation: let's stick together. *Trends Microbiol.* doi: 10.1016/j.tim.2016.09.005. [Epub ahead of print].

Bentley, S. D., Vernikos, G. S., Snyder, L. A., Churcher, C., Arrowsmith, C., Chillingworth, T., et al. (2007). Meningococcal genetic variation mechanisms viewed through comparative analysis of serogroup C strain FAM18. *PLoS Genet.* 3:e23. doi: 10.1371/journal.pgen.0030023

Bos, M. P., Grijpstra, J., Tommassen-van Boxtel, R., and Tommassen, J. (2014). Involvement of *Neisseria meningitidis* lipoprotein GNA2091 in the assembly of a subset of outer membrane proteins. *J. Biol. Chem.* 289, 15602–15610. doi: 10.1074/jbc.M113.539510

Bos, M. P., and Tommassen, J. (2005). Viability of a capsule- and lipopolysaccharide-deficient mutant of *Neisseria meningitidis*. *Infect. Immun.* 73, 6194–6197. doi: 10.1128/IAI.73.9.6194-6197.2005

Buchan, D. W., Minneci, F., Nugent, T. C., Bryson, K., and Jones, D. T. (2013). Scalable web services for the PSIPRED protein analysis workbench. *Nucleic Acids Res.* 41, W349–W357. doi: 10.1093/nar/gkt381

Capecchi, B., Adu-Bobie, J., Di Marcello, F., Ciucchi, L., Masignani, V., Taddei, A., et al. (2005). *Neisseria meningitidis* NadA is a new invasin which promotes bacterial adhesion to and penetration into human epithelial cells. *Mol. Microbiol.* 55, 687–698. doi: 10.1111/j.1365-2958.2004.04423.x

Costerton, J. W., Lewandowski, Z., Caldwell, D. E., Korber, D. R., and Lappin-Scott, H. M. (1995). Microbial biofilms. *Annu. Rev. Microbiol.* 49, 711–745. doi: 10.1146/annurev.mi.49.100195.003431

Davis, J., Smith, A. L., Hughes, W. R., and Golomb, M. (2001). Evolution of an autotransporter: domain shuffling and lateral transfer from pathogenic *Haemophilus* to *Neisseria*. *J. Bacteriol.* 183, 4626–4635. doi: 10.1128/JB.183.15.000-000.2001

Grijpstra, J., Arenas, J., Rutten, L., and Tommassen, J. (2013). Autotransporter secretion: varying on a theme. *Res. Microbiol.* 164, 562–582. doi: 10.1016/j.resmic.2013.03.010

Heydorn, A., Nielsen, A. T., Hentzer, M., Sternberg, C., Givskov, M., Ersbøll, B. K., et al. (2000). Quantification of biofilm structures by the novel computer program COMSTAT. *Microbiology* 146, 2395–2407. doi: 10.1099/00221287-146-10-2395

Jordan, I. K., Conley, A. B., Antonov, I. V., Arthur, R. A., Cook, E. D., Cooper, G. P., et al. (2011). Genome sequences for five strains of the emerging pathogen *Haemophilus haemolyticus*. *J. Bacteriol.* 193, 5879–5880. doi: 10.1128/JB.05863-11

Lappann, M., Claus, H., van Alen, T., Harmsen, M., Elias, J., Molin, S., et al. (2010). A dual role of extracellular DNA during biofilm formation of *Neisseria meningitidis*. *Mol. Microbiol.* 75, 1355–1371. doi: 10.1111/j.1365-2958.2010.07054.x

Lappann, M., Haagensen, J. A., Claus, H., Vogel, U., and Molin, S. (2006). Meningococcal biofilm formation: structure, development and phenotypes in a standardized continuous flow system. *Mol. Microbiol.* 62, 1292–1309. doi: 10.1111/j.1365-2958.2006.05448.x

Oliver, D. C., Huang, G., Nodel, E., Pleasance, S., and Fernandez, R. C. (2003). A conserved region within the *Bordetella pertussis* autotransporter BrkA is necessary for folding of its passenger domain. *Mol. Microbiol* 47, 1367–1383. doi: 10.1046/j.1365-2958.2003.03377.x

Peak, I. R., Jennings, M. P., Hood, D. W., and Moxon, E. R. (1999). Tetranucleotide repeats identify novel virulence determinant homologues in *Neisseria meningitidis*. *Microb. Pathog.* 26, 13–23. doi: 10.1006/mpat.1998.0243

Peterson, J. H., Tian, P., Ieva, R., Dautin, N., and Bernstein, H. D. (2010). Secretion of a bacterial virulence factor is driven by the folding of a C-terminal segment. *Proc. Natl. Acad. Sci. U.S.A.* 107, 17739–17744. doi: 10.1073/pnas.1009491107

Roussel-Jazédé, V., Arenas, J., Langereis, J. D., Tommassen, J., and van Ulsen, P. (2014). Variable processing of the IgA protease autotransporter at the cell surface of *Neisseria meningitidis*. *Microbiology* 160, 2421–2431. doi: 10.1099/mic.0.082511-0

Saunders, N. J., Jeffries, A. C., Peden, J. F., Hood, D. W., Tettelin, H., Rappuoli, R., et al. (2000). Repeat-associated phase variable genes in the complete genome sequence of *Neisseria meningitidis* strain MC58. *Mol. Microbiol.* 37, 207–215. doi: 10.1046/j.1365-2958.2000.02000.x

Scarselli, M., Serruto, D., Montanari, P., Capecchi, B., Adu-Bobie, J., Veggi, D., et al. (2006). *Neisseria meningitidis* NhhA is a multifunctional trimeric autotransporter adhesin. *Mol. Microbiol.* 61, 631–644. doi: 10.1111/j.1365-2958.2006.05261.x

Schoen, C., Blom, J., Claus, H., Schramm-Glück, A., Brandt, P., Müller, T., et al. (2008). Whole-genome comparison of disease and carriage strains provides insights into virulence evolution in *Neisseria meningitidis*. *Proc. Natl. Acad. Sci. U.S.A.* 105, 3473–3478. doi: 10.1073/pnas.0800151105

Serruto, D., Adu-Bobie, J., Scarselli, M., Veggi, D., Pizza, M., Rappuoli, R., et al. (2003). *Neisseria meningitidis* App, a new adhesin with autocatalytic serine protease activity. *Mol. Microbiol.* 48, 323–334. doi: 10.1046/j.1365-2958.2003.03420.x

Serruto, D., Spadafina, T., Ciucchi, L., Lewis, L. A., Ram, S., Tontini, M., et al. (2010). *Neisseria meningitidis* GNA2132, a heparin-binding protein that induces protective immunity in humans. *Proc. Natl. Acad. Sci. U.S.A.* 23, 3770–3775. doi: 10.1073/pnas.0915162107

Sim, R. J., Harrison, M. M., Moxon, E. R., and Tang, C. M. (2000). Underestimation of meningococci in tonsillar tissue by nasopharyngeal swabbing. *Lancet* 356, 1653–1654. doi: 10.1016/S0140-6736(00)03162-7

Tamura, K., Stecher, G., Peterson, D., Filipski, A., and Kumar, S. (2013). MEGA6: molecular evolutionary genetics analysis version 6.0. *Mol. Biol. Evol.* 30, 2725–2729. doi: 10.1093/molbev/mst197

Tettelin, H., Saunders, N. J., Heidelberg, J., Jeffries, A. C., Nelson, K. E., Eisen, J. A., et al. (2000). Complete genome sequence of *Neisseria meningitidis* serogroup B strain MC58. *Science* 287, 1809–1815. doi: 10.1126/science.287.5459.1809

Turner, D. P. J., Marietou, A. G., Johnston, L., Ho, K. K. L., Rogers, A. J., Wooldridge, K. G., et al. (2006). Characterization of MspA, an immunogenic autotransporter protein that mediates adhesion to epithelial and endothelial cells in *Neisseria meningitidis*. *Infect. Immun.* 74, 2957–2964. doi: 10.1128/IAI.74.5.2957-2964.2006

Turner, D. P. J., Wooldridge, K. G., and Ala'Aldeen, D. A. A. (2002). Autotransported serine protease A of *Neisseria meningitidis*: an immunogenic, surface-exposed outer membrane, and secreted protein. *Infect. Immun.* 70, 4447–4461. doi: 10.1128/IAI.70.8.4447-4461.2002

van Putten, J. P. M., and Paul, S. M. (1995). Binding of syndecan-like cell surface proteoglycan receptors is required for *Neisseria gonorrhoeae* entry into human mucosal cells. *EMBO J.* 14, 2144–2154.

van Schilfgaarde, M., van Alphen, L., Eijk, P., Everts, V., and Dankert, J. (1995). Paracytosis of *Haemophilus influenzae* through cell layers of NCI-H292 lung epithelial cells. *Infect. Immun.* 63, 4729–4737.

van Ulsen, P., Adler, B., Fassler, P., Gilbert, M., van Schilfgaarde, M., van der Ley, P., et al. (2006). A novel phase-variable autotransporter serine protease, AusI, of *Neisseria meningitidis*. *Microbes Infect.* 8, 2088–2097. doi: 10.1016/j.micinf.2006.03.007

van Ulsen, P., and Tommassen, J. (2006). Protein secretion and secreted proteins in pathogenic *Neisseriaceae. FEMS Microbiol. Rev.* 30, 292–319. doi: 10.1111/j.1574-6976.2006.00013.x

van Ulsen, P., van Alphen, L., ten Hove, J., Fransen, F., van der Ley, P., and Tommassen, J. (2003). A *Neisserial* autotransporter NalP modulating the processing of other autotransporters. *Mol. Microbiol.* 50, 1017–1030. doi: 10.1046/j.1365-2958.2003.03773.x

Yi, K., Rasmussen, A. W., Gudlavalleti, S. K., Stephens, D. S., and Stojiljkovic, I. (2004). Biofilm formation by *Neisseria meningitidis. Infect. Immun.* 72, 6132–6138. doi: 10.1128/IAI.72.10.6132-6138.2004

15

Structural and Functional Characterization of the Type Three Secretion System (T3SS) Needle of *Pseudomonas aeruginosa*

Charlotte Lombardi[1†], James Tolchard[2†], Stephanie Bouillot[3], Luca Signor[1], Caroline Gebus[3], David Liebl[3‡], Daphna Fenel[1], Jean-Marie Teulon[1], Juliane Brock[1], Birgit Habenstein[2], Jean-Luc Pellequer[1], Eric Faudry[3], Antoine Loquet[2], Ina Attrée[3], Andréa Dessen[1,4] and Viviana Job[1,3]*

[1] Univ. Grenoble Alpes, CEA, CNRS, Institut de Biologie Structurale (IBS), Grenoble, France, [2] Institute of Chemistry and Biology of Membranes and Nanoobjects, Institut Européen de Chimie et Biologie (CBMN), UMR5248 CNRS, University of Bordeaux, Pessac, France, [3] Univ. Grenoble Alpes, Bacterial Pathogenesis and Cellular Responses Group, U1036 INSERM, ERL5261 CNRS, CEA, Grenoble, France, [4] Brazilian Biosciences National Laboratory (LNBio), Centro Nacional de Pesquisa em Energia e Materiais (CNPEM), Campinas, Brazil

***Correspondence:**
Viviana Job
viviana.job@cea.fr

The type three secretion system (T3SS) is a macromolecular protein nano-syringe used by different bacterial pathogens to inject effectors into host cells. The extracellular part of the syringe is a needle-like filament formed by the polymerization of a 9-kDa protein whose structure and proper localization on the bacterial surface are key determinants for efficient toxin injection. Here, we combined *in vivo*, *in vitro,* and *in silico* approaches to characterize the *Pseudomonas aeruginosa* T3SS needle and its major component PscF. Using a combination of mutagenesis, phenotypic analyses, immunofluorescence, proteolysis, mass spectrometry, atomic force microscopy, electron microscopy, and molecular modeling, we propose a model of the *P. aeruginosa* needle that exposes the N-terminal region of each PscF monomer toward the outside of the filament, while the core of the fiber is formed by the C-terminal helix. Among mutations introduced into the needle protein PscF, D76A, and P47A/Q54A caused a defect in the assembly of the needle on the bacterial surface, although the double mutant was still cytotoxic on macrophages in a T3SS-dependent manner and formed filamentous structures in *vitro*. These results suggest that the T3SS needle of *P. aeruginosa* displays an architecture that is similar to that of other bacterial needles studied to date and highlight the fact that small, targeted perturbations in needle assembly can inhibit T3SS function. Therefore, the T3SS needle represents an excellent drug target for small molecules acting as virulence blockers that could disrupt pathogenesis of a broad range of bacteria.

Keywords: type III secretion system, *Pseudomonas aeruginosa*, T3SS needle, structure, virulence, immunofluorescence microscopy, mutagenesis

INTRODUCTION

Bacterial pathogens have developed different strategies to colonize, invade and kill eukaryotic cells. One of the most successful mechanisms involves the use of the type III secretion system (T3SS), a macromolecular complex present on the surface of numerous pathogenic and colonizing species such as *Salmonella, Shigella, enteropathogenic Escherichia coli* (EPEC), *Yersinia,* and

Pseudomonas spp. (Galán and Collmer, 1999; Galán et al., 2014; Wagner et al., 2018). The T3SS can be described as a multicomponent protein structure consisting of four major constituents: (i) a basal body that anchors the system to the bacterial membranes; (ii) an export apparatus which includes a cytoplasmic sorting platform that selects substrates and provides energy for the secretion process; (iii) a needle filament which protrudes toward the outside of the bacterial surface and serves as a passage for translocator proteins and effectors; and (iv) a translocation pore formed in the eukaryotic cell membrane that allows the entry of virulence effectors into the host cytoplasm.

The basal body and the needle form the so-called needle complex (NC), which represents the core structure of the T3SS. The number of NCs per bacterial cell varies between species. For instance, *Salmonella typhimurium*, assembles between 10 and 100 NCs per cell (Kubori et al., 1998), while only a few NCs were detected on the surface of *Pseudomonas aeruginosa* (Perdu et al., 2015). Notably, the T3SS needle is formed by a single polymerized protein that has been studied in the context of vaccine development against several pathogens (Charro and Mota, 2015; Jneid et al., 2016; Koroleva et al., 2017). It has been shown that immunization with needle proteins induces specific humoral and T cell responses and abrogates bacterial pathogenicity in animal models (Koroleva et al., 2017). In addition, small molecules such as phenoxyacetamide, that are directed against specific residues of the needle protein PscF can inhibit *P. aeruginosa* T3SS secretion (Bowlin et al., 2014) and the same compound also inhibits abscess formation in mice by directly blocking the T3SS (Berube et al., 2017). These results highlight the need for further characterization of molecular aspects and structures of NC assemblies to develop more specific anti-microbial molecules (Izoré et al., 2011).

Formation of the T3SS needle is a spatio-temporally regulated process. Protein monomers of the T3SS needle from different bacterial species have an approximate molecular weight of 9-kDa and display 13% sequence identity and 42% sequence similarity (considering the main human pathogens: *Salmonella, Shigella, P. aeruginosa,* and *Yersinia* sp.) (Kubori et al., 2000; Hoiczyk and Blobel, 2001; Pastor et al., 2005). Prior to secretion and assembly on the bacterial surface the spontaneous assembly of needle monomers in the bacteria cytosol is prevented by binding to two distinct chaperones concomitantly (Quinaud et al., 2005; Sun et al., 2008; Sal-Man et al., 2013), as is also the case for translocator proteins (Job et al., 2010; Discola et al., 2014; Nguyen et al., 2015). High resolution structures of T3SS needle proteins from different bacteria that have been solved to date (Deane et al., 2006; Quinaud et al., 2007; Wang et al., 2007; Sun et al., 2008; Poyraz et al., 2010) by crystallography and solution NMR reveal a similar protein fold composed of a helix-turn-helix motif with two long helices. Furthermore, one notable feature of T3SS needle proteins is an amphipathic C-terminal helix, which is 'trapped' within a hydrophobic concave region of the dual chaperone interface, presumably in order to block self-association (and early polymerization) (Quinaud et al., 2007; Sun et al., 2008). Upon T3SS activation, the needle protein dissociates from its chaperones, binding to the inner rod protein within the basal body (Kuhlen et al., 2018). Polymerization then occurs through addition of 100s of monomers to the distal end of growing needle. Interestingly, some bacteria possess accessory proteins that aid in assembly of the needle filament and accelerate the polymerization process *in vitro,* such as recently reported for *Salmonella typhimurium* (Kato et al., 2018). The final assembled needle in all bacteria is then capped by a tip protein (or soluble translocator), which is absolutely necessary to allow the formation of the translocation pore for the injection of effectors (Matteï et al., 2011; Harmon et al., 2013). During cell contact the specific needle length is essential for proper function yet the exact mechanism of length control still remains controversial (Cornelis, 2006). It has been suggested that a molecular ruler is involved (Kubori et al., 2000; Journet et al., 2003; Wagner et al., 2010; Bergeron et al., 2016), or that needle length is regulated by a precise timing of substrate switching, as suggested by recent mathematical models (Nariya et al., 2016).

The length of a fully assembled T3SS needle varies between bacterial species from 45 to 80 nm (Kubori et al., 1998; Tamano et al., 2000; Pastor et al., 2005; Radics et al., 2014; Park et al., 2018) while the outer and inner diameter range from 5–13 and 2–2.5 nm, respectively (Kubori et al., 2000; Pastor et al., 2005; Poyraz et al., 2010; Fujii et al., 2012; Loquet et al., 2012; Demers et al., 2013; Radics et al., 2014; Hu et al., 2018). Solid-state NMR structures of the T3SS needles of PrgI from *Salmonella* (Loquet et al., 2012) and MxiH from *Shigella* (Demers et al., 2014) indicated a super helical multimeric structure with 5.7 subunits per turn (Loquet et al., 2012) composed of three intermolecular subunit–subunit interfaces, one of which is axial (subunit i to i+11) and two are lateral (subunit i to i+5/6). Interestingly, the orientation of the two aforementioned helices within the needle structure has been the subject of debate (Fujii et al., 2012; Demers et al., 2013, 2014; Verasdonck et al., 2015). The first cryo-electron microscopy studies performed on the *Shigella* T3SS suggested that the C-terminus of each protomer points toward the outside (Deane et al., 2006; Fujii et al., 2012), while studies involving a combination of cryo-EM and solid state NMR indicated that at least in *Salmonella* and *Shigella* T3SS needles have the N-terminus that points toward the outside of the super-helical structure (Demers et al., 2013, 2014; Verasdonck et al., 2015).

In this work we address the architecture of the T3SS needle of *P. aeruginosa* using a combination of mutagenesis followed by phenotypic studies, proteolysis, mass spectrometry (MS), electron and atomic force microscopies (EM and AFM) and molecular modeling. We show that the *P. aeruginosa* T3SS needle monomer PscF has an N-terminal region oriented toward the outside of the filament, while the C-terminal helix of PscF forms the needle core. Using mutagenesis, we found that D76 is essential for needle polymerization as well as its assembly on the bacterial surface, while residues P47 and Q54 are concomitantly dispensable for polymerization but affect needle stability and effector secretion. Our results, analyzed in the context of other published studies, suggest that a common architecture exists between T3SS needles of different bacterial species, which could facilitate the rational design of

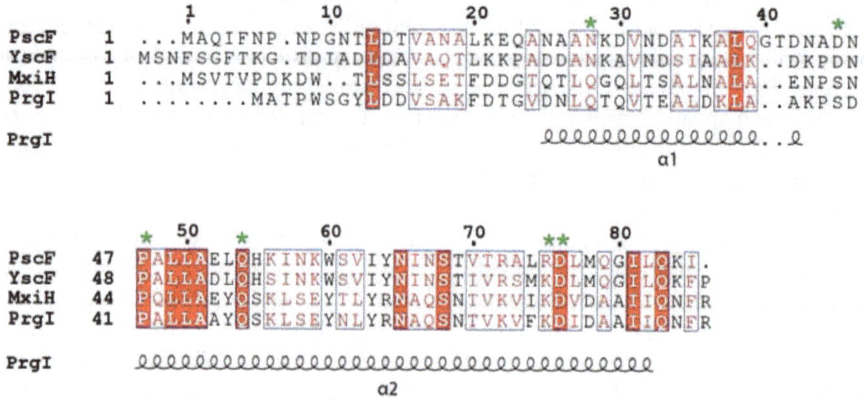

FIGURE 1 | Sequence alignment of needle proteins from different bacteria. PscF from *Pseudomonas aeruginosa*, YscF from *Yersinia* sp., MxiH from *Shigella* sp., PrgI from *Salmonella* sp. The residues mutated in this study are indicated with a green asterisk. Numbers refer to the PscF sequence. Secondary structure elements from the PrgI structure are indicated underneath the sequence alignment. The figure was generated with ESPript, using the new ENDscript server (Robert and Gouet, 2014). Conserved and similar residues are shown in red and blue boxes, respectively.

needle-specific anti-virulence molecules that block or destabilize the T3SS machinery.

RESULTS AND DISCUSSION

Identification of Key Functional Residues of PscF

To uncover the structural elements that are important for the functionality of the T3SS needle in *P. aeruginosa*, we first used a mutagenesis approach coupled to phenotypic studies. We designed seven different PscF point mutants on several bases: conservation of residues between different bacterial species, results obtained in *Shigella flexneri* (Kenjale et al., 2005; Veenendaal et al., 2007), *Yersinia pestis* (Davis and Mecsas, 2007), and *Yersinia pseudotuberculosis* (Torruellas et al., 2005) and predictions/models of PscF fold (**Figure 1**). We generated six single mutants: N28S, D45A, P47A, Q54A, R75A, D76A, and an additional double mutant (P47A/Q54A) whose homologous residues in the *Shigella* needle protein (MxiH-P44A/Q51A) had been shown to be critical for wild-type function (Kenjale et al., 2005; Veenendaal et al., 2007). The D76A mutant had already been studied by our groups and others (Kenjale et al., 2005; Quinaud et al., 2007) and it was further characterized in this study. All mutations were introduced into the pIApG-*pscF* plasmid and transformed into a *P. aeruginosa* clinical isolate CHA strain deleted for the PscF-encoding gene (Δ*pscF*) (Pastor et al., 2005). The cytotoxicity toward macrophages of the Δ*pscF*/*pscF*wt complemented strain had already been reported to be the same as the original CHA strain (Quinaud et al., 2007). We then tested the ability of all complemented strains to infect macrophages measuring the release of the host cytoplasmic enzyme lactate dehydrogenase (LDH) into the supernatant. Most mutant strains killed macrophages with comparable kinetics as the wild-type strain suggesting the existence of a robust core in the protein that can accept local perturbation. However, the two strains carrying PscF-D76A or the double mutant PscF-P47A/Q54A showed significantly attenuated cytotoxicity (with $P < 0.001$) toward macrophages. The *P. aeruginosa* PscF-D76A strain killed only 7.0 ± 1.8% of all cells present in the assay while *P. aeruginosa* PscF-P47A/Q54A strain killed 43.3 ± 6.2% of cells during 3 h of infection. As a comparison, the wild-type *P. aeruginosa* strain killed 87.5 ± 2.8% of all cells during the same period (**Figure 2A**). Both mutations P47A and Q54A alone had no effect on cytotoxicity after 3 h of infection, in agreement with previous observations of hemolysis and invasion in *Shigella* (Kenjale et al., 2005).

To understand the cause of decreased virulence observed with the selected mutants, we first analyzed the expression of the PscF mutants and the secretion profiles of translocator proteins PopB and PcrV in those strains (**Figure 2B**). The T3SS was induced *in vitro* by Ca^{2+} depletion in bacterial cultures, the pellet (containing the entire cell content) and supernatant (containing secreted proteins) were separated by centrifugation and analyzed by Western blotting. All *P. aeruginosa* mutants expressed the different PscF variants (**Figure 2B**), demonstrating that the mutations did not affect the expression of PscF. Analysis of PopB and PcrV in secreted fractions showed reduced levels for the P47A/Q54A strain and a thin band of PopB and no PcrV for the D76A strain, results that are consistent with the decreased cytotoxicity of these two mutants in our macrophage killing assay.

Our results point out that among the conserved residues of the needle protein PscF, D76, P47 and Q54 play essential roles in T3SS functionality, in agreement with other reports on *Shigella flexneri* and *Yersinia pestis* (Kenjale et al., 2005; Torruellas et al., 2005). Interestingly in *Shigella*, the corresponding mutants (MxiH-D73A and P44A/Q51A) secrete Ipa/Ipg proteins constitutively, and are unable to invade epithelial cells and to cause hemolysis (Kenjale et al., 2005; Veenendaal et al., 2007). Other mutations like PscF-R75A in *P. aeruginosa* have no effect on cytotoxicity toward macrophages, while the homologous mutation (MxiH-K72A) in *Shigella* has a significant impact in hemolysis, suggesting a potential different mode of regulation/activation

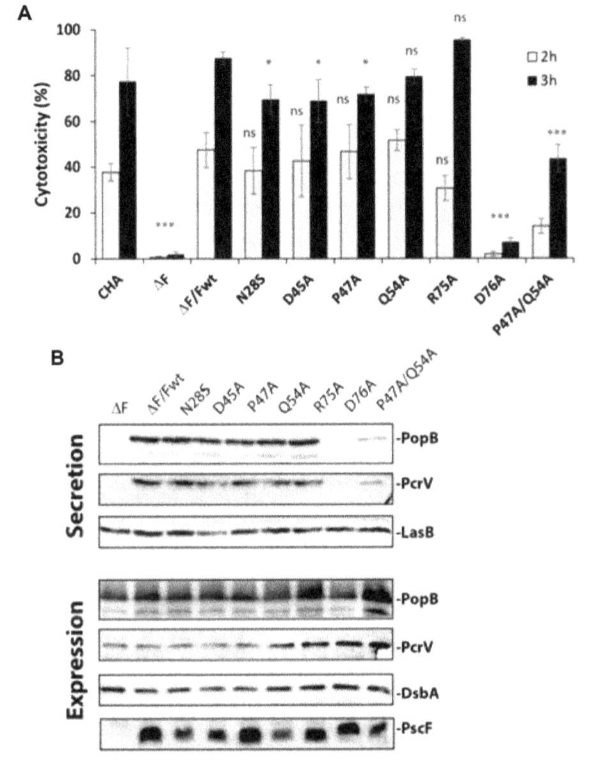

FIGURE 2 | T3SS activity in *Pseudomonas* PscF mutants. **(A)** The cytotoxicity of *P. aeruginosa* strains toward macrophage cells was measured by monitoring LDH release after 2 and 3 h of infection using a multiplicity of infection (MOI) of 5. The PscF deletion mutant (ΔF), D76A, and P47A/Q54A strains show a higher statistical difference at both 2 and 3 h of infection compared to wild-type complemented strain (ΔF/Fwt). LDH measurements were corrected with values corresponding to cells that were not infected; we considered as 100% of cytotoxicity a 1% Triton X-100 treated well. Pairwise differences relative to ΔF/Fwt based on the Tukey test are indicated: ns, non-significant, $^{***}P < 0.001$, $^{*}P < 0.05$. Cytotoxicity of original CHA strain is also reported. **(B)** Western blot of the supernatant (secreted proteins) and total bacteria (expression) fractions after centrifugation were developed with anti-PopB and anti-PcrV antibodies. The expression of PscF variants was confirmed by loading total bacterial extracts on SDS- 15% PAGE. The Western blot was developed using anti-PscF antibodies obtained using a monomeric 6His-PscF (see section "Materials and Methods"). The D76A strain secretes almost no PopB or PcrV while P47A/Q54A secretes less of both translocators as compared to other mutants and the wild-type strain. LasB was used as loading control for the secreted protein, and DsbA as loading control for bacterial expression and as a lysis control for the supernatant (data not shown).

of needle protein polymerization. We thus set out to further understand the specific role of these residues in regards to: (i) proper folding of PscF, (ii) PscF's ability to polymerize and form the needle, (iii) interaction of PscF with the tip translocator protein PcrV, (iv) secretion, localization and abundance of the PscF needle on the bacterial surface.

In vitro Characterization of PscF Needle Mutants

In order to investigate the first two possibilities, i.e., that D76A and P47A/Q54A mutations could affect PscF folding and needle polymerization, we expressed and purified the two PscF mutants in *E. coli* in the absence of their two chaperones PscE and PscG. This allowed the *in vitro* production of filaments, as it was shown in the case of wild-type PscF (Quinaud et al., 2005). Purified PscF wild-type, PscF-D76A and PscF-P47A/Q54A filaments were then analyzed by negative staining electron microscopy (EM) and atomic force microscopy (AFM) (**Figure 3A** and **Supplementary Figure S1**). Both the wild-type and the P47A/Q54A PscF variants formed elongated fibers with outer diameters ranging from 2 to 10 nm indicating that the P47A/Q54A mutation does not prevent the needle polymerization process. The measurement of the diameters of both filaments on EM images suggested a tendency of P47A/Q54A PscF filaments to be slightly thinner than the wild-type ones with a statistically significant difference on diameter size distribution (*t*-test, $P < 0.001$) (**Figure 3B**). The diameter measurements by both EM and AFM thus indicated smaller values than the 8 nm-diameter determined by high resolution methods. This is probably due to a difficulty in identifying the borders of thin needles by EM, and the strong adsorption of the filaments on mica in the AFM experiments, as already found for cylindrical viruses (Godon et al., 2017). The D76A mutant protein could not form filaments suggesting a loss of capacity to polymerize (**Figure 3A**), thus explaining the lack of cytotoxicity of *P. aeruginosa* strains expressing PscF-D76A. On the other hand, in the PscF-P47A/Q54A mutant the 50% decrease in cytotoxicity could be linked to the formation of thinner fibers or could be correlated to a more subtle folding defect of the needle filament.

In order to investigate this last hypothesis we incubated both wild-type and P47A/Q54A PscF needle filaments with trypsin at room temperature and monitored protease digestion for up to 23 h. Samples were taken at different times and analyzed by SDS-PAGE and by liquid chromatography coupled to electrospray ionization mass spectrometry (LC/ESI-MS) (**Figure 3C** and **Table 1**). In our experiments, PscF filaments are a result of the polymerization of a 93-residue monomeric protein that carries a 6His-tag at the C-terminus with an expected mass of 10,218 Da (for the wild-type) and 10,135 Da (for the P47A/Q54A mutant). The SDS-PAGE patterns were apparently similar: both wild-type and P47A/Q54A proteins were surprisingly stable to trypsin digestion, and the full-length protein was also still apparent after 23 h. A major fragment at 6,500 Da (corresponding to fragment Ala37-His93) appeared on SDS-PAGE after 10 min (one asterisk in **Figure 3C**). The kinetics of trypsin cleavage were followed by LC/ESI-MS analysis at different time points (10, 30 min and 6 h of digestion) which allowed precise identification and relative quantification of proteolytic fragments (**Table 1**). All expected trypsin cleavage sites and the fragments identified by LC/ESI-MS are reported in **Figure 3C**. The first trypsin cleavage occurred after Lys21 and Lys36, generating the following three fragments: (Ala2-Lys21), (Ala2-Lys36) and (Ala37-His93). Subsequently, cleavage occurred after Lys56, leading to fragments (Lys37-Lys56) and (Ile57-His93). Moreover, LC/ESI-MS analyses of digested fragments highlighted interesting differences between PscF wild-type and PscF P47A/Q54A needle filaments. Indeed, an additional digested band at a lower molecular mass was visible on SDS-PAGE after 90 min for the wild-type filaments

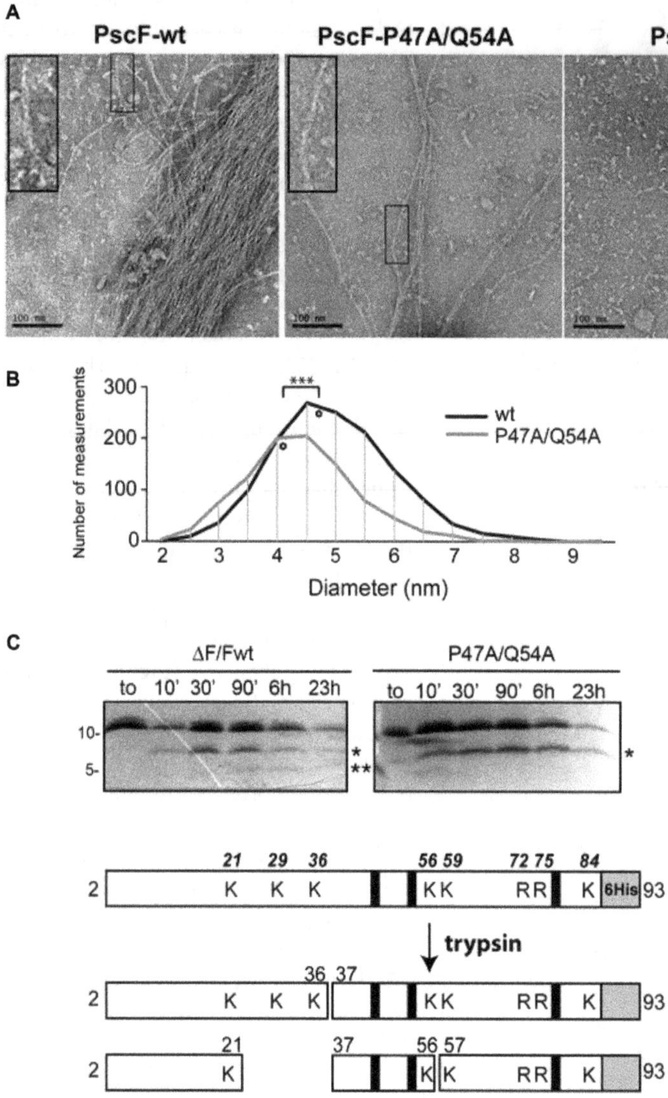

FIGURE 3 | Characterization of PscF wild-type and mutant filaments. **(A)** Negative-staining electron microscopy images of purified PscF wild-type (left panel), PscF P47A/Q54A (middle panel) and PscF D76A (right panel) visualized at the same protein concentration (0.1 mg/ml). Scale bar: 100 nm. **(B)** Diameter distribution of PscF filaments measured on EM images shown in **(A)**. The diamonds represent the average diameter. Wild-type PscF has an average diameter of 4.72 ± 1.02 nm (n = 1390) while PscF P47A/Q54A filaments are thinner with average diameters of 4.15 ± 0.97 nm (n = 986). Statistical analysis: ***$P < 0.001$. **(C)** Trypsin digestion profiles of purified wild-type PscF and P47A/Q54A filaments were analyzed by 16.5% Tris-Tricine and LC/ESI Mass spectrometry. Both proteins are stable with a major cleavage-band at 6.5 kDa (one asterisk) corresponding to fragments 37–93. Only for the wild-type protein is visible a second lower band of 4.5 kDa (residues 57–93) (two asterisks). A scheme of trypsin digestion kinetics determined by MS analysis is reported below, with the corresponding identified fragments. The gray box represents the 6His tag, black lines show the position of D76, P47, and Q54 residues mutated in this study. All trypsin-cleavable sites (lysines, K and arginines, R) are shown with their relative position on the top scheme.

only, corresponding to specific cleavage after Lys56 (two asterisks in **Figure 3C**). This fragment of 4,454 Da (residues Ile57-His93) for the PscF-P47A/Q54A mutant was not visible on SDS-PAGE and detectable only by MS analysis after 6 h in the proteolysis experiment representing 1.1% of the fragment population versus 10.5% in the wild-type PscF at the same time point (**Table 1**). These results suggest that Lys56 is less accessible to proteolysis by trypsin in the PscF-P47A/Q54A filament compared to the PscF wild-type filament. An opposite effect was observed for Lys36, that is more accessible to trypsin cleavage in the PscF-P47A/Q54A filament (with 10.7% of fragment population corresponding to Ala37-His93 with a mass of 6,472 Da) compared to the PscF wild-type filament (with 2.5% of fragment population) (**Table 1** and one asterisk in **Figure 3C**). Therefore, the two filaments are structurally different at least in the region around Lys36 and Lys56.

These results indicate that the P47A/Q54A and wild-type filaments only present a small difference on the outer surface structure (see below). Along with the fact that P47A/Q54A filaments could be slightly thinner, this could explain the decreased capacities of secretion and cytotoxicity of the strains carrying these mutations. However, one must also consider that the filaments purified form *E. coli* could be structurally distinct from needles assembled within the T3SS apparatus in *P. aeruginosa*.

Needle Visualization on the Surface of *P. aeruginosa* PscF Mutants

In order to further characterize the aforementioned mutations on PscF in a more physiological context, we looked at the localization and/or abundance of the needle on the *P. aeruginosa* surface as well as its interaction with the PcrV tip protein using fluorescence microscopy. We performed immune detection of PscF on fixed cells, using antibodies generated against the PscF native needles (produced during this study) (**Figure 4**). Fixed cells were prepared as described in Section "Materials and Methods" and then separated into two samples: one was incubated with anti-PcrV antibodies (shown in cyan), while the other one was incubated with anti-PscF antibodies (shown in green). In both samples, DNA was stained with SYTO24 (shown in red). The Δ*pscF* and Δ*pcrV* samples were used as negative controls and presented no unspecific labeling with the anti-PcrV antibodies and just weak background with the anti-PscF used at higher concentrations. ΔPscF/PscF-wt and ΔPcrV/PcrV-wt were used as positive controls and showed clearly distinct cell surface-associated fluorescent spots for both proteins all around the bacteria (**Figures 4A,B**). Of note, PcrV could not be detected on the surface of the ΔPscF strain because it only assembles at the tip of the PscF needle. All PscF mutants showed similar patterns of labeling as the positive controls except for the PscF D76A- and P47A/Q54A-expressing strains that showed markedly smaller amounts of PscF and PcrV spots all around their surface (**Figure 4B** and **Supplementary Figure S2**). To eliminate the possibility that the absence of PscF on the *P. aeruginosa* surface was due to a defect in expression of PscF D76A and P47A/Q54A, we repeated the experiment with cells made permeable with Triton X-100 in order to allow the entry of the antibody into the cell. The antibodies directed toward PscF detected the protein in both permeabilized mutant strains (**Supplementary Figure S3**). These data are in agreement with the Western blot results and indicate that PscF mutant proteins were produced within *P. aeruginosa*. Moreover, this experiment showed that D76A and P47A/Q54A mutants have a defect in PscF export and/or assembly onto the bacterial surface.

We then quantified the PscF and PcrV spots per cell using the MicrobeJ plugin (Ducret et al., 2016) of the ImageJ program (Schneider et al., 2012), considering that one spot corresponded to one needle. Between 30 and 40% of wild-type bacterial cells showed one or more PscF spots (up to 6) per cell, with a majority of cells with 1 or 2 spots/cell (**Figure 5B**). Immunolabeling of bacteria expressing PscF D76A showed that only 6.9 $\pm$ 1.6% of the counted cells (n = 1713) presented a single visible spot and the P47A/Q54A mutant displayed 8.9 $\pm$ 2.4% of the population with 1 or 2 spots per cell (n = 2307). For comparison, the complemented ΔPscF/PscF-wt stain presented 32.8 $\pm$ 4.0% of cells with at least one needle (n = 1829) (**Figures 5A,B**) while the negative control ΔPscF strain presented 2.3 $\pm$ 1.4% of spots near the bacteria. In all samples, except in D76A and P47A/Q54A, the percentage of cells with PscF and PcrV spots was very similar, indicating that the mutations do not affect binding between the tip protein and the needle. In the case of D76A and P47A/Q54A only 3.2 $\pm$ 1.2% (n = 2126) and 5.6 $\pm$ 2.5% (n = 2128) of cells presented PcrV spots, respectively, suggesting that the tip/needle interaction is present, but we could not exclude that some D76A and P47A/Q54A needles do not present PcrV at their tip.

These observations explain the absence of cytotoxicity toward macrophages in the case of D76A. Interestingly, although P47A/Q54A mutations affected the number of needles detected,

TABLE 1 | Identification and relative quantifation of PscF (*wt/mutant*) proteolytic fragments by LC/ESI MS.

Proteolysis time	10 min		30 min		6 h	
Theoretical mass (Da) for tryptic fragments of PscF (wt/mutant)	**PscF-WT**	**PscF-P47A/Q54A**	**PscF-WT**	**PscF- P47A/Q54A**	**PscF-WT**	**PscF- P47A/Q54A**
	Measured mass (Da) (*% Area of EIC peaks*)					
2097.09 [(1)] (2-21)	2097.08 (*9.4%*)	2097.09 (*5.6%*)	2097.09 (*18.1%*)	2097.09 (*10.8%*)	2097.08 (*28.1%*)	2097.09 (*30.8%*)
2118.07/2035.03 [(1)] (37-56)	2118.07 (*1.6%*)	2035.02 (*0.2%*)	2118.07 (*3.7%*)	2035.03 (*0.3%*)	2118.07 (*17.6%*)	2035.03 (*3.5%*)
3678.86 [(1)] (2-36)	3678.87 (*7.7%*)	3678.86 (*13.2%*)	3678.85 (*11.4%*)	3678.85 (*12.6%*)	3678.85 (*2.9%*)	3678.85 (*3.9%*)
4454.15 [(2)] (57-93)	4454.36 (*2.6%*)	n.d.	4454.52 (*3.4%*)	n.d.	4454.88 (*10.5%*)	4454.18 (*1.1%*)
6555.45/6472.36 [(2)] (37-93)	6555.63 (*9.4%*)	6472.50 (*9.1%*)	6555.72 (*9.4%*)	6472.55 (*8.5%*)	6555.60 (*2.5%*)	6472.55 (*10.7%*)
10218.47/10135.38 [(3)] (2-93)	10218.67 (*69.3%*)	10135.59 (*71.9%*)	10218.68 (*54.0%*)	10135.46 (*67.8%*)	10218.80 (*38.5%*)	10135.46 (*49.8%*)

Theoretical mass values for tryptic fragments of PscF (wild-type and P47A/Q54A mutant) are reported in the first column. Both PscFwt and P47A/Q54A mutant were digested with trypsin (trypsin:protein ratio 1:500 w/w) at room temperature. After 10 min, 30 min and 6 h of incubation the samples were analyzed by LC/ESI-MS. The area of the extracted ion chromatogram (EIC) peaks for each fragment were calculated and reported as a percentage of the sum of all fragment (total area of all the peaks). [(1)] *monoisotopic mass,* [(2)] *average mass,* [(3)] *mass value for the intact undigested protein, missing the methionine at N-termini; n.d., not detected.*

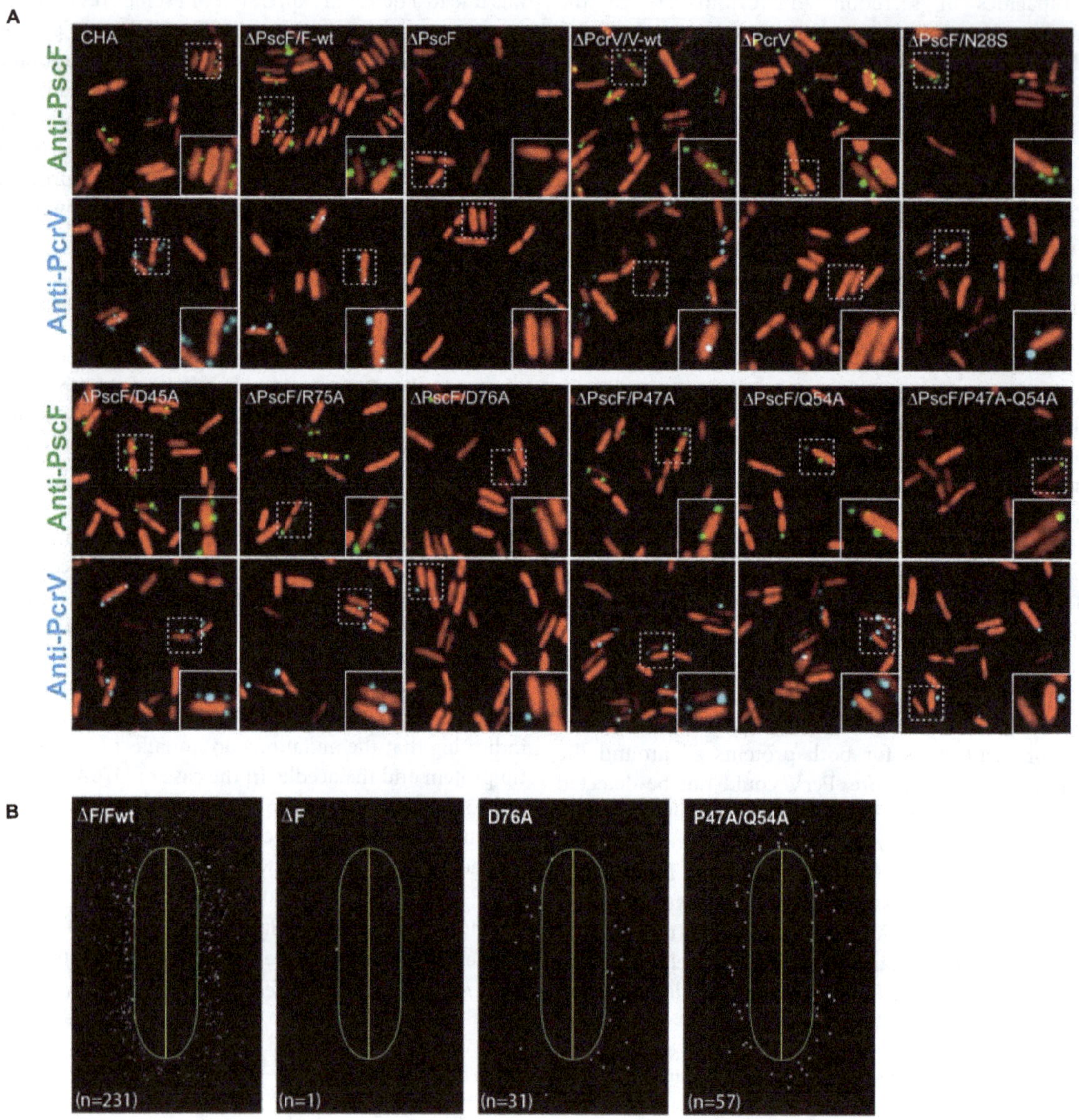

FIGURE 4 | Localization of PscF-needles on the surface of *Pseudomonas aeruginosa*. **(A)** *P. aeruginosa* CHA strain isolated on cystic fibrosis patient depleted for the *pscF* gene (Δ*pscF*) and complemented with pIApG-*pscF* constructs were grown in T3SS-inducing conditions. PscF needles were visualized by immuno fluorescence on fixed bacteria using anti-PscF (in green) or anti-PcrV (in cyan). SYTO24 was used to visualize bacteria (in red). As a negative controls we used *P. aeruginosa* ΔF and ΔV, while ΔF/Fwt and ΔV/Vwt were used as a positive control. Only few PscF and PcrV spots were visible on *P. aeruginosa* strains carrying a PscF-D76A or a PscF-P47A/Q54A. **(B)** MicrobeJ reconstitution of PscF distribution around the bacteria. n = number of spots in the image.

the synthesized needles still allowed injection of toxins, suggesting that the number of needles on the bacterial surface is less crucial than the structure of the needle *per se*. All these data strongly suggest that in *P. aeruginosa* D76A and P47A/Q54A mutants are defective in the *in vivo* needle assembly process while a concomitant instability or defect in the export of PscF through the basal body could not be excluded.

In *Yersinia pestis*, the YscF-D77A variant also shows a defect in the surface exposure of the needle whilst maintaining normal protein expression levels (Torruellas et al., 2005). In contrast, the MxiH-D73A and P44A/Q51A mutants in *Shigella flexneri* were both able to export the needle protein and assemble a NC almost normally (Kenjale et al., 2005; Veenendaal et al., 2007). Furthermore, MxiH-D73A was able to polymerize (Fujii et al., 2012) (unlike PscF-D76A) with no significant structural changes but it lacks the tip complex. Once again, this suggests that the same mutation will cause different effects on the assembly of *Shigella*, *Yersinia*, and *Pseudomonas* T3SS needles.

Modeling of the *P. aeruginosa* PscF Needle

In order to understand at the molecular level the impact of the D76A and P47A/Q54A mutations, we performed molecular modeling of the *P. aeruginosa* PscF needle, taking advantage of the solid-state NMR structure of the *Salmonella* PrgI needle

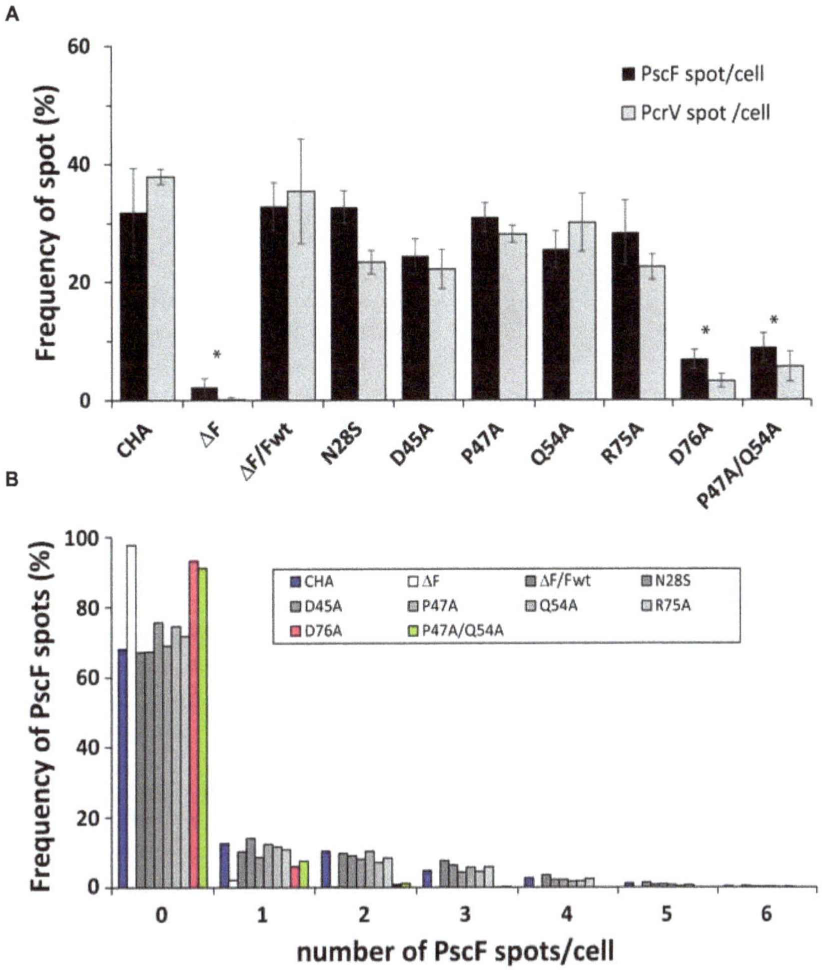

FIGURE 5 | Presence of PscF and PcrV on *Pseudomonas aeruginosa* PscF-mutant strains. **(A)** Images of immunolabeled fixed bacteria in **Figure 4** were analyzed with MicrobeJ to detect and associate each PscF or PcrV spot to only one bacterium. Frequency was considered as the percentage of bacteria with at least one PscF and PcrV spot on the total counted bacteria. About 30–40% of cells had needles with the PcrV tip protein on their surface, with the exception of the D76A strain with only 6.9 ± 1.6% (PscF) and 3.2 ± 1.2% (PcrV), and the P47A/Q54A strain with 8.9 ± 2.4% (PscF) and 5.6 ± 2.5% (PcrV) of cells with spots. **(B)** Distribution of the number of PscF spots/needles per bacterial cell. Between 630 and 2300 individual bacteria were counted. *P. aeruginosa* wild-type and mutant strains had between 1 to 3 PscF spots per cell, except for D76A (in pink) and P47A/Q54A (in green) that presented only one or two spots per cell. Overall comparisons using the Kruskal–Wallis' test indicates significant differences between classes ($P < 0.001$). Pairwise differences relative to wild-type based on Dunn's *post hoc* test are shown: $^*P<0.05$.

(Loquet et al., 2012). We constructed two different models for the PscF needle: one using the protein in the same orientation as PrgI in the filament (i.e., with the C-termini inside and the N-termini outside the needle; that model will be named PscF-forward); and the other one supposing that the PscF protomer is inverted with the N-termini residue inside and the C-termini residue outside the needle structure (PscF-reverse) (**Figure 6**). Optimal models were subjected to a brief structural minimization protocol using the Chimera molecular modeling/visualization package (Pettersen et al., 2004) (default parameters) to remove atomic clashes (VDW overlap). Pre- and post-minimization structures were analyzed using the PSVS webserver (Bhattacharya et al., 2007) to evaluate the structural improvements in the monomeric models. After minimization, all homology models showed significant improvements in both clash scores and favorable Ramachandran angles. The energetically minimized structures were then used to reconstruct PrgI-like T3SS needles, and were built up from 29 monomers to form the needle filaments. To compare the two models of PscF to the needle architecture in *Salmonella* we also constructed a PrgI-inverted needle (PrgI-reverse).

The three resulting needle architectures: PscF-reverse, PscF-forward and PrgI-reverse are shown in **Figure 6**. We then tried to understand if one of the two PscF needle models (PscF-reverse or PscF-forward) was more favorable. To do so, we computed several parameters related to the global architecture: surface electrostatic potential (**Figure 6A**), position of conserved residues (**Figure 6B**) and hydrophobicity (**Figure 6C**) and compared them to the experimental solid-state NMR *Salmonella* PrgI needle structure. Surprisingly none of the PscF needle models showed

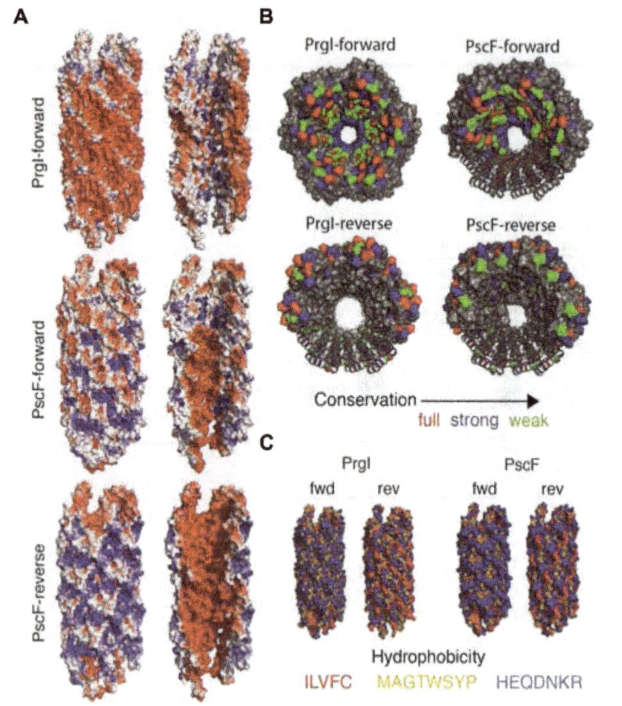

FIGURE 6 | Needle reconstruction for PscF wild-type and mutants. **(A)** The PrgI Solid-state NMR structure was used as a model for the construction of PscF in the Forward and Reverse orientations. Mutants D76A and P74A/Q54A were constructed on the PscF-forward model. The exterior view (left) and lumen view (right) of the T3SS needle models are colored by surface electrostatic potentials, at pH 7, using the APBS plugin for PyMol. **(B)** Distribution of conserved residues distribution on PrgI and PscF needle models in Forward and Reverse orientations. **(C)** Hydrophobicity distribution of the different models shown in **(B)**.

the same electrostatic distribution as the experimental PrgI needle structure (top in **Figure 6A**), displaying an astonishing pattern of circular succession of negative/positive charges at the lumen surface, while the external surface was predominantly negatively charged. Both PscF needle models showed a strong negative charge distribution at the inner surface, while the external surfaces were much more positively charged compared to PrgI needles. In addition, no particular succession of positively/negatively charged patterns could be seen for either PscF model. In PrgI needles, this lumen pattern arises mostly from D70 and Q77 (negative) and K66 and R80 (positive). Equivalent amino acid positions in PscF D76, Q83, and R72 are conserved (**Figures 1, 6B**); however, R80, the last residue in PrgI, is absent from PscF, leading to a pronounced change in the electrostatic charge distribution at the lumen surface.

Next, we investigated the hydrophobic surface of the models (**Figure 6C**) considering that the PrgI needle is characterized by a strong network of hydrophobic interactions at the lateral interfaces between subunit i and i+5/6 (Loquet et al., 2012). PscF-reverse and PrgI-reverse models both exhibit an unfavorable hydrophobic external surface while the PscF-forward model shows a favorable hydrophilic surface, strengthening the energetic relevance of the PscF-forward model. Finally, we examined the distribution of the conserved residues on the different needle models (**Figure 6B**). The PrgI needle structure has been defined by a typical distribution of conserved residues among the T3SS needle subunits, with almost all conserved residues pointing inside the needle pore while the external surface is made of non-conserved amino acids. Visualization of these conserved needle residues on the PscF models lead to two distinct situations: PscF-forward presents many conserved residues at the lumen surface, while this lumen surface in the PscF-reverse model is mostly composed of non-conserved residues. It has been suggested that the presence of non-conserved residues exposed to the external surface of PrgI could provide a way to evade immune response of the host cell (Loquet et al., 2012). The same distribution is observed for the PscF-forward model, and together with our observations on the hydrophobic and electrostatic surfaces it provides a substantial hint toward the relevance of the PscF-forward model compared to the PscF-reverse model.

Subsequently, we constructed PscF needle models for the two mutants: D76A and P47A/Q54A (**Figure 7B**), adopting the forward model orientation. In the D76A model, the distribution of the charges is drastically affected by the point mutation; D76 is located in the central hollow section of the needle and the mutation into alanine modifies the overall negative charge distribution, which could be an explanation to the lack of polymerization *in vitro* of this mutant. The P47A/Q54A model, however, suggests that the mutated residues are buried in the subunit–subunit interfaces and the overall charges are more similar to the wild-type PscF-forward model. According to the atomic depth measurements (Chen and Pellequer, 2013), the regions 45–47 is the deepest, farthest away from the solvent, in the whole needle. Any change in deeply buried residues is expected to impact proteins stability (Chakravarty and Varadarajan, 1999), that could explain the significant difference in the number of needle on bacteria surface. Considering the equivalent amino acids in PrgI (i.e., P41 and Q48), we examined the residues involved in the subunit–subunit interfaces by taking into account the solid-state NMR restraints used for the PrgI needle structure determination (see **Figure 2** in Loquet et al., 2012). P41 in PrgI is involved in strong contacts between subunit i to i+11 forming the so-called axial interface, while Q48 is weakly involved in the intramolecular fold. This suggests that the double P47A/Q54A mutation in PscF could lead just to a moderate perturbation of the needle arrangement that could explain why this mutant still polymerizes *in vitro*.

We then used the data obtained from trypsin proteolysis and MS analysis to explore the structural differences between wild-type and mutant P47A/Q54A filaments and to validate our model. As mentioned above, we monitored trypsin digestion of both fibers by LC/ESI-MS (**Figure 3C** and **Table 1**). This experiment allowed us to conclude that the residues that were the most accessible to trypsin digestion, and thus were solvent exposed are: Lys36, Lys21, and Lys56 (and probably Lys29, absent in MS digested-fragments). Interestingly, these experimental results are only in agreement with the PscF-forward wild-type model (with the N-termini exposed toward the outside), where Lys36, Lys29, and Lys21 are expected to be the most exposed

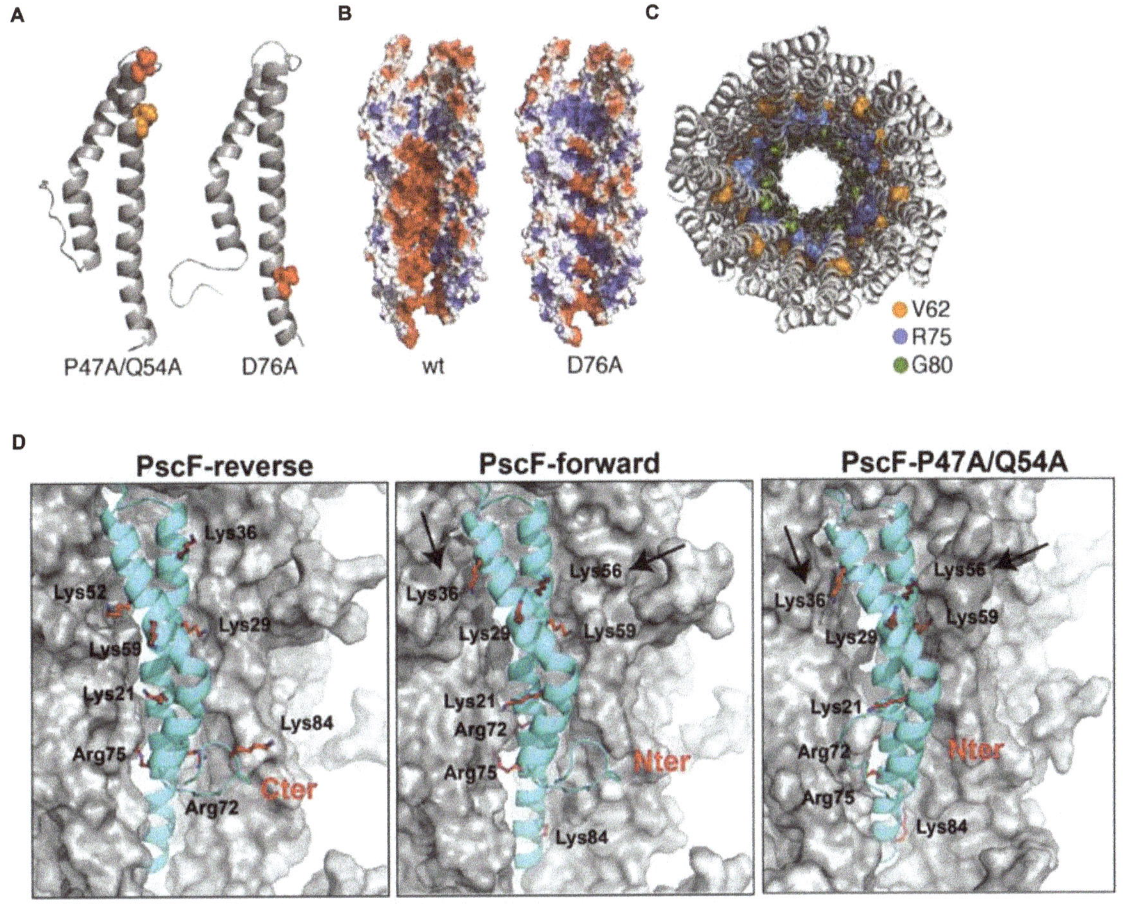

FIGURE 7 | Model of the PscF P47A/Q54A and PscF D76 assembled filament. **(A)** Ribbon representation of PscF monomer carrying the two mutations: D76A and P47A/Q54A. **(B)** Electrostatic surface representation of the two mutant reconstituted filaments with a channel view. **(C)** Top view of a PscF-forward wild-type model, colors show residues implicated in binding of the T3SS-inhibitor phenoxyacetamide (Bowlin et al., 2014). **(D)** Comparison between reverse and forward PscF and PscF-P47A/Q54A filaments. PscF-forward model (with the N-termini exposed toward the outside), with Lys36, Lys29, and Lys21 solvent-exposed, Lys56 and Lys59 less accessible, and Lys84, Arg72, and Arg75 completely buried. PscF-reverse model (with the C-termini exposed toward the outside), with solvent accessible residues: Lys84, Arg75, Lys59, and Lys36. The PscF-P47A/Q54A forward model showing accessibility of the same residues as compared to the PscF-forward wild-type model except for the Lys56 and Lys36 that are slightly less or more trypsin-accessible, respectively (indicated by two arrows). All needle models are represented as surfaces with one monomer of PscF represented as a cyan ribbon. All trypsin-cleavable sites are shown as sticks.

to the solvent, Lys56 and Lys59 are less accessible, and Lys84, Arg72 and Arg75 are completely buried (middle in **Figure 7D**). On the other hand, in the PscF-reverse wild-type model (with the C-termini exposed toward the outside), the residues that would be solvent accessible are: Lys84, Arg75, Lys59, and Lys36 (left in **Figure 7D**). Lys84, in particular, is located just before the C-terminus. In this configuration, the C-terminal 6His-tag would have been expected to be quickly cleaved by trypsin, but no fragment corresponding to this cleavage was observed for any of the peptides analyzed by LC/ESI-MS (**Table 1**). Moreover, the PscF-forward P47A/Q54A model with Lys56 less solvent-exposed and Lys36 more solvent-exposed (right in **Figure 7D**) is also in agreement with our trypsin digestion results. The digestion-fragment at 4,454 Da (corresponding to a cleavage after Lys56) was less abundant in the mutant compared to the wild-type (1.1 vs. 10.5%), while the digestion fragment corresponding to a cleavage after Lys36 was more abundant in the mutant compared to the wild-type (10.7 vs. 2.5%) as discussed above (**Figure 3C** and **Table 1**).

Thus, based on our biochemical, structural and molecular modeling data, we hypothesize that the T3SS needle of *P. aeruginosa* follows the PscF-forward model with the N-terminus pointing toward the outside of the fiber and the C-terminus consequently hidden inside the needle's hollow cavity. Our results imply that the overall architecture of the needle is therefore conserved between *Pseudomonas*, *Salmonella*, and *Shigella* spp., highlighting the importance of the orientation of the small 9-kDa protein inside the oligomeric structure. D76A and P47A/Q54A mutations are located at the C-terminal helix, which is well-conserved in the sequence among bacterial species. Their effects on needle polymerization and stability as well as their importance for functional regulation of needle assembly as shown by our analyses of electrostatic charges present at the lumen surface point to an important role of the C-terminal helix in the assembly mechanism. The impact of the mutations D76A and P47A/Q54A, and their homologs in T3SS needles of other bacteria, suggests that regions facing the inner cavity or deeply buried within the needle play a significant role in needle stability and/or function. It also suggests that local changes of the sequence of the subunit protein in crucial regions, as exemplified here for the two mutants and in previous studies, might lead to important perturbations on different aspects of the needle structure-function interplay, on both a structural (e.g., structural instability, surface electrostatic distribution) and functional basis. Moreover, the charge distribution in the lumen may be critical in needle assembly as suggest by the defect in polymerization in the D76A variant and the previous observation that the PscF-D76A protein overexpressed in *P. aeruginosa* CHA strain has a dominant-negative effect on assembly of the wild-type PscF needle (Quinaud et al., 2007).

Understanding the Mode of Action of T3SS Inhibitors

To go further we used our proposed *P. aeruginosa* T3SS needle model to understand the mode of action of T3SS-inhibitors, such as the phenoxyacetamide family, that was hypothesized to act inside the cavity of PscF (Bowlin et al., 2014). In this work, the authors suggested that PscF residues V62, R75 and G80 were involved in direct binding of phenoxyacetamide. In our model, only G80 is exposed to the lumen surface (**Figure 7C** in green), while V62 (in orange) and R75 (in blue) are located at subunit interfaces. These observations suggest that the three amino acid positions, upon binding with phenoxyacetamide, may decrease needle stability (for V62 and R75); in addition, it is also possible that binding could change the surface of the lumen (G80). These three residues appear to be close enough in our PscF needle model to speculate the presence of a single binding site, as suggested by the Moir group (Bowlin et al., 2014). We therefore suggest that it is possible to design other molecules that interact with multiple residues starting from the lumen structure model in order to block T3SS action.

The T3SS needle represents an excellent and promising molecular target in the fight against Gram-negative pathogens, since it is easily accessible to small molecules that do not need to cross bacterial membranes, and is non-essential for survival. Thus, small molecules affecting its function could block virulence without eliciting high levels of antibiotic resistance.

Our work provides a new model for the *P. aeruginosa* PscF-needle, that was validated *in vitro* by experimental data combining mutagenesis, proteolysis, and Mass Spectrometry experiments. Moreover, the phenotypic characterization of PscF mutants *in vivo* showed that the majority of the single mutations introduced in the needle have no effect on T3SS-toxicity and are not sufficient to disrupt needle polymerization, with the exception of D76A. This underlines the importance of the charge in the face of the lumen for assembly of a functional needle.

A detailed molecular comprehension of the structure–function relationship of the T3SS needle should advance future developments of anti-virulence molecules.

MATERIALS AND METHODS

Bacterial Strains and Culture Conditions for T3SS Expression

Strains and plasmids used in this study are presented in **Supplementary Table S2.** Cytotoxic *P. aeruginosa* cystic fibrosis isolate CHA carrying appropriate chromosomal deletions of *pscF* gene (Δ*pscF)* was transformed with plasmid pIApG-*pscF* wild-type or mutants that expressed *pscF* with a T3SS inducible promoter. Cultures were grown overnight in Luria-Bertani (LB) at 37°C at 300 rpm in the presence of 300 μg/ml of carbenicillin. Then next day, they were diluted to an optical density measured at 600 nm (OD_{600}) of 0.1 A.U. in LB in T3SS-inducing conditions by adding 5 mM EGTA and 20 mM $MgCl_2$ (Pastor et al., 2005; Dasgupta et al., 2006). When the OD_{600} reached 1.0 A.U., cells were centrifuged, and then the pellet (entire bacterial protein content) and the supernatant (the secreted protein fraction) was analyzed by Western blotting. Anti-PopB and anti-PcrV antibodies (Goure et al., 2004) were diluted to 1:10,000 and 1:3,000, respectively. Anti-PscF antibodies were raised in rabbits (Covalab, France) using monomeric 6His-PscF (Quinaud et al., 2005). The antibodies were further purified on Protein-A column and diluted 1:500 for Western blot analysis. As a loading control we used LasB (a secreted protein) and DsbA (a periplasmic protein) diluted to 1:2,000 and 1:10,000, respectively. Lysis control was done on secreted protein fractions using DsbA antibodies. All mutants were produced using the Quick-Change site-directed mutagenesis II kit (Stragatene). Primers are listed in **Supplementary Table S2.**

Cytotoxicity Assay

Lactate dehydrogenase release into the supernatant was measured using the Cytotoxicity Detection Kit by Roche Applied Science, following the recommended protocol. Briefly, J774 cells were seeded at 2 × 10^5 in 48-well plates the day prior to the experiment, and infected in DMEM medium at MOI of 5 with *P. aeruginosa*Δ*pscF*-pIApG-*pscF* constructs at OD_{600} = 1 A.U. After 2 and 3 h, 30 μL of cell supernatants were mixed with 100 μl of reaction mix and the OD was read at 490 nm. OD values were subtracted from that of uninfected cells. The 100% cell death value was quantified after addition of 1% Triton X-100, in duplicates. The experiment was performed in triplicate wells (except for the P47A/Q54A mutant for which six replicates were performed). Results represent the means and standard deviations of the triplicates. Statistics were calculated using SigmaPlot software. For multiple comparisons, a one-way analysis of variance (ANOVA) test was performed, followed by Tukey's test for pairwise comparisons.

Immunofluorescence

Two different *P. aeruginosa* genetic backgrounds were used: CHAΔ*pcrV* complemented or not with pIApG-*pcrV*-wt, and CHAΔ*pscF* complemented with all pIApG-*pscF* constructs or with the wild-type *pscF*. Cells were grown under T3SS-inducing conditions up to an optical density measured at 600 nm (OD_{600}) of 1 A.U. and then culture was fixed with 4% PFA in 25 mM

HEPES pH 7.4 overnight at 4°C. After centrifugation at 6,000 rpm for 15 min the pellet was washed three times with 1 ml PBS, then incubated for 30 min at RT in 1 ml PBS with 0.5% BSA (BS, Blocking Solution). Then cells were divided into two Eppendorf tubes and spin down, each pellet was resuspended and incubated for 30 min at room temperature in 50 μl of BS containing of anti-PcrV (1:200) (Goure et al., 2004) or 50 μl BS with anti-PscF (1:50). Anti-PscF antibodies were produced in rabbits (Biotem) from the PscF fibers purified under native conditions from *E. coli* BL21 (DE3). After three washing steps with 1 ml PBS, the pellet was resuspended into 50 μl of BS containing anti-rabbit coupled to Cy3 (Jackson ImmunoResearch Laboratories) with a final dilution of (1:500) and SYTO24-Green (Life Technologies) with a final dilution of (1:2000) and further incubated 30 min at RT. After three final washes, the cells were resuspended into BS. One drop of each sample was deposited on a 8-chambered labteck (Thermo Fisher Scientific) and liquid 1.5% low-melting agarose at 37°C or 1.5% agar pad was added on the top of the drop and visualized on a IX71 Olympus microscope controlled by the CellR Olympus system and driven by Xcellence software (Olympus). Images were captured with a Hammamatsu Orca-ER camera using a 100x (N.A. 1,30) oil objective.

To investigate for the presence of PscF inside the cells in PscF-mutants, cells were fixed with 4% PFA, washed as previously described, then permeabilized with 0.25% Triton X-100 for 5 min at room temperature to allow the anti-PscF to enter cells (method adapted from Cimino et al., 2006). Triton X-100 was then washed out three times with 1 ml PBS before continuing the protocol as described above from BS incubation.

Quantification of Fluorescent Spots Associated With Bacteria

Quantification was done using the MicrobeJ plugin of ImageJ (Ducret et al., 2016)[1] and [2]. Briefly, for bacterial identification we used the same setting (area, length, width, curvature of bacteria) for all images. For PcrV and PscF spot analyses a Tolerance of 100 was used, and only in the case of PscF a filter of intensity between 250-max was added in order to eliminate background noise and unrelated spots. For the final step of analyses by MicrobeJ, namely the association between each identified bacterium and the spots, we used two filters: inside and outside with "exclusive" settings, in order to associate each spot (that could be inside or outside the bacteria) with just one bacterium. Averages were calculated from the results of 5 to 11 independent images taken for each mutant. The frequency was considered as being the percentage of cells with at least one spot.

Statistics were calculated using SigmaPlot. For multiple comparisons, a one-way analysis of variance (ANOVA) test was performed, followed by Dunn's test.

PscF Expression and Purification and Mutant Construction

Escherichia coli BL21 (DE3) cells were transformed with pET22b-PscF (wild-type, D76A and P47A/Q54A) that generated a protein with a 6His-tag at the C terminus (Quinaud et al., 2005). Cells were grown in LB media supplemented with 100 μg/ml ampicillin at 37°C, under agitation (200 rpm) until they reached an OD_{600} = 0.7–0.8 A.U. Protein expression was induced by addition of 1 mM IPTG and growth was continued for up to 3 h, then cells were centrifuged for 30 min at 5,500 rpm at 4°C. Pellets were resuspended at 4°C in 25 ml of lysis buffer (25 mM Tris-HCl pH 8.0, 200 mM NaCl, 25 mM Imidazole) containing benzonase. Cells were lysed at 18 kPsi in a cell disrupter and centrifuged for 30 min at 15,000 rpm at 4°C. The soluble fraction was applied on a 1 ml resin Ni-NTA superflow (QIAGEN) in a batch column. The column was washed with lysis buffer and eluted the same buffer containing 200 mM imidazole. Sample purity was checked by SDS-PAGE and Mass Spectrometry. Mutants were produced using the Quick-Change site-directed mutagenesis II kit (Stragatene) and verified by DNA sequencing. Primers are listed in the **Supplementary Table S2**.

Trypsin Digestion

PscF-wt and PscF-P47A/Q54A proteins were purified as described above. Trypsin digestion was carried out according to the following procedure: trypsin was dissolved into a buffer containing 25 mM Tris-HCl pH 8.0, 200 mM NaCl and digestion was performed using a (trypsin:protein) ratio of 1:500 (w/w). The reaction was performed at RT and samples were collected at different time points (10 min, 30 min, 1 h 30 min, 6 h, ON) and analyzed by 16.5% Tris-Tricine gel and by LC/ESI-MS.

Electron Microscopy

Four μl of the protein samples were absorbed to the clean side of a carbon film on mica, stained with sodium silico tungstate and transferred to a 400-mesh copper grid. The images were taken under low dose conditions ($<10\ e^-/Å^2$) at a magnification of 23,000 and 49,000 times with defocus values between 1.2 and 2.5 μm on a Tecnai 12 LaB6 electron microscope at 120 kV accelerating voltage using a CCD Camera Gatan Orius 1000. Size determination of the PscF filaments was performed in Gwyddion (Nečas and Klapetek, 2012) using the raw.dm3 EM files, measurements were done at different positions along the filaments using the "Measure distance" tool. Additional measurements were performed in ImageJ (Schneider et al., 2012). Statistics were calculated using SigmaPlot. For single comparisons, a Mann–Whitney Rank Sum Test was used.

Atomic Force Microscopy

A 2.5 μl drop of reconstituted filaments in deionized water (dilution 1/5000) was deposited on freshly cleaved mica, incubated for 3 min, washed with 1 ml of water with 80 μl drop steps to remove excessive salt crystals, and finally dried with nitrogen gas. Imaging was performed on a Multimode 8, Nanoscope V (Bruker) equipped with NanoScope software (Bruker, Santa Barbara, CA, United States). Imaging was done with peak force imaging mode at ~1 Hz rate, with 512 or 1024 pixel sampling and other parameters were adjusted automatically with ScanAsyst mode in air. A ScanAsyst-air (Bruker) cantilever with nominal 2 nm tip radius, 70 kHz frequency and 0.4 N/m spring constant was used. Images

[1] https://imagej.nih.gov/ij/

[2] http://www.microbej.com/

were processed with Gwyddion (Nečas and Klapetek, 2012), and if needed stripe noise was removed using DeStripe (Chen and Pellequer, 2011). Size determination of the filaments was performed in Gwyddion by using manual cross-sections (3px thick) and by measuring their maximum heights. Average values and standard deviations are reported. The computation of atomic depth was performed using the Adepth server (Chen and Pellequer, 2013).

LC/ESI Mass Spectrometry

Liquid Chromatography Electrospray Ionization Mass Spectrometry (LC/ESI-MS) was performed using a 6210 LC/ESI-TOF mass spectrometer interfaced with an HPLC binary pump system (Agilent Technologies). The mass spectrometer was calibrated in the mass-to-charge (*m/z*) 300–3200 range with standard calibrants (ESI-L, Low concentration tuning mix, Agilent Technologies) before measurements and mass spectra were recorded in the 300–3200 *m/z* range. MS acquisition was carried out in the positive ion mode with spectra in the profile mode. The MS instrument was operated with the following experimental settings: the ESI source temperature was set at 300°C; nitrogen was used as drying gas (7 l/min) and as nebulizer gas (10 psi); the capillary needle voltage was set at 4000 V. Spectra acquisition rate was of 1.03 spectra/s. All solvents used were HPLC grade (Chromasolv, Sigma-Aldrich), trifluoroacetic acid (TFA) was from Acros Organics (puriss., p.a.). Solvent A was 0.03% TFA in water, solvent B was 95% acetonitrile-5% water-0.03% TFA. The MS spectra were acquired and the data processed with MassHunter workstation software (*v.* B.02.00, Agilent Technologies) and with GPMAW software (v. 7.00b2, Lighthouse Data, Denmark).

Just before analysis each trypsin digested protein was diluted with solvent A to a final concentration of 5 μM and thermostatted at 10°C in the autosampler; 8 μl of each sample were injected. Samples were first trapped and desalted on a reverse phase-C8 cartridge (Zorbax 300SB-C8, 5 μm, 300 μm ID × 5 mm, Agilent Technologies) for 3 min at a flow rate of 50 μl/min with 100% solvent A and then eluted and separated onto a RP-C8 column (Jupiter, 5 μm, 300 Å, 1 mm ID × 50 mm, Phenomenex) at a flow rate of 50 μl/min using the following linear gradient: from 5 to 95% solvent B in 15 min, then remaining 2 min at 100% solvent B and finally re-equilibrating the column at 5% solvent B for 10 min.

Modeling

Optimal models of PscF-forward, PscF-reverse and PrgI-reverse protomers were built based on the PrgI protomer structure of the *Salmonella* needle structure by extracting chain A from the 2LPZ pdb file. MODELLER (Eswar et al., 2007), version 9.16, was used to individually align the forward (N-C:N-C) and reverse (N-C:C-N) PscF sequences to PrgI as well as a reverse (N-C:C-N) variant of PrgI for comparison (align2d.py). Initial single-chain models for the D76A and P47A/Q54A were prepared in the same way. The resulting alignment files and the PrgI subunit model were used as additional input to MODELLER to construct subunit models with secondary structure corresponding to that of PrgI (model-single.py). Ten models were calculated in each case and an overall assessment was manually carried out, judging energetic qualities and alignment to PrgI, to derive single optimal models for all cases. In the case of both forward and reverse PscF models, C-terminal helices were additionally enforced by alteration of the Phi and Psi backbone angles with PyMOL. Optimal models were subjected to a brief structural minimization protocol using the Chimera molecular modeling/visualization package (Pettersen et al., 2004) (default parameters) to remove atomic clashes (VDW overlap). PrgI-like T3SS needles were reconstructed in PyMol by aligning the constructed subunit models, by secondary structure, to the 29 chains of the PrgI (PDB code: 2LPZ) needle model.

The complete 29-chain needle structures, for wild-type (forward and reverse) and mutated subunits, were refined using a cluster-based installation of Rosetta (Das and Baker, 2008) (relax.mpi.linuxgccrelease – relax:fast), wherein the backbone heavy atoms were fixed in space but the positions of side-chains were allowed to evolve with respect to energetic minimization. The best resulting structures (as determined by overall Rosetta energy), calculated from a pool of 3 were then submitted to the MolProbity webserver (Davis et al., 2007) in a protonated form for validation (**Supplementary Table S1**).

AUTHOR CONTRIBUTIONS

VJ, IA, and AL designed the study and assembled the results. CL performed protein purifications and sample preparations for biochemical, EM and AFM experiments. DF and J-MT performed the EM and AFM experiments, respectively. J-LP analyzed and interpreted both images. All model building, computer minimizations and structure interpretations were performed by JT, with the supervision of AL and BH. CG constructed plasmids and mutants and perform initial cytotoxicity assays under the supervision of IA and EF. Macrophages cultures were prepared by SB. VJ performed cytotoxicity, florescence microscopy and biochemical experiments, with data analysis and interpretation. SB and DL contributed to the microscopy experiments and ImageJ/MicrobeJ analysis, while JB helped with Western blots. LS performed mass spectrometry experiments, data analysis, and interpretation. VJ, AD, and AL wrote the paper, with input from all authors.

FUNDING

This work used the platforms of the Grenoble Instruct-ERIC Center (ISBG: UMS 3518 CNRS-CEA-UGA-EMBL) with support from FRISBI (ANR-10 INBS-05-02) and GRAL (ANR-10-LABX-49-01) within the Grenoble Partnership for Structural Biology (PSB). The electron microscope facility is supported by the Rhône-Alpes Region, the Fondation Recherche Médicale (FRM), the fonds FEDER, the Centre National de la Recherche Scientifique (CNRS), the CEA, the University of Grenoble, EMBL, and the GIS-Infrastrutures en Biologie Santé et Agronomie (IBISA). The authors wish to acknowledge ERC Starting Grant No. 639020, ANR-14-CE09-

0020-01 and the Fondation pour la Recherche Médicale (FRM)—AJE20140630090 to AL, as well as grant VLM (RF20150501349) to EF, Fondation pour la Recherche Médicale (DEQ20170336705) to IA, and VLM (RIF20150501457) to AD.

ACKNOWLEDGMENTS

The authors thank Michel Ragno for antibody purification. This work acknowledges the AFM platform at the IBS.

REFERENCES

Bergeron, J. R. C., Fernández, L., Wasney, G. A., Vuckovic, M., Reffuveille, F., Hancock, R. E. W., et al. (2016). The structure of a type 3 secretion system (T3SS) ruler protein suggests a molecular mechanism for needle length sensing. *J. Biol. Chem.* 291, 1676–1691. doi: 10.1074/jbc.M115.684423

Berube, B. J., Murphy, K. R., Torhan, M. C., Bowlin, N. O., Williams, J. D., Bowlin, T. L., et al. (2017). Impact of type III secretion effectors and of phenoxyacetamide inhibitors of type III secretion on abscess formation in a mouse model of *Pseudomonas aeruginosa* infection. *Antimicrob. Agents Chemother.* 61, e1202–e1217. doi: 10.1128/AAC.01202-17

Bhattacharya, A., Tejero, R., and Montelione, G. T. (2007). Evaluating protein structures determined by structural genomics consortia. *Proteins* 66, 778–795. doi: 10.1002/prot.21165

Bowlin, N. O., Williams, J. D., Knoten, C. A., Torhan, M. C., Tashjian, T. F., Li, B., et al. (2014). Mutations in the *Pseudomonas aeruginosa* needle protein gene pscF confer resistance to phenoxyacetamide inhibitors of the type III secretion system. *Antimicrob. Agents Chemother.* 58, 2211–2220. doi: 10.1128/AAC.02795-13

Chakravarty, S., and Varadarajan, R. (1999). Residue depth: a novel parameter for the analysis of protein structure and stability. *Struct. Lond. Engl.* 7, 723–732. doi: 10.1016/S0969-2126(99)80097-5

Charro, N., and Mota, L. J. (2015). Approaches targeting the type III secretion system to treat or prevent bacterial infections. *Expert Opin. Drug Discov.* 10, 373–387. doi: 10.1517/17460441.2015.1019860

Chen, S. W., and Pellequer, J.-L. (2011). DeStripe: frequency-based algorithm for removing stripe noises from AFM images. *BMC Struct. Biol.* 11:7. doi: 10.1186/1472-6807-11-7

Chen, S. W., and Pellequer, J.-L. (2013). Adepth: New Representation and its implications for atomic depths of macromolecules. *Nucleic Acids Res.* 41, W412–W416. doi: 10.1093/nar/gkt299

Cimino, M., Alamo, L., and Salazar, L. (2006). Permeabilization of the mycobacterial envelope for protein cytolocalization studies by immunofluorescence microscopy. *BMC Microbiol.* 6:35. doi: 10.1186/1471-2180-6-35

Cornelis, G. R. (2006). The type III secretion injectisome. *Nat. Rev. Microbiol.* 4, 811–825. doi: 10.1038/nrmicro1526

Das, R., and Baker, D. (2008). Macromolecular modeling with rosetta. *Annu. Rev. Biochem.* 77, 363–382. doi: 10.1146/annurev.biochem.77.062906.171838

Dasgupta, N., Ashare, A., Hunninghake, G. W., and Yahr, T. L. (2006). Transcriptional induction of the *Pseudomonas aeruginosa* type III secretion system by low Ca2+ and host cell contact proceeds through two distinct signaling pathways. *Infect. Immun.* 74, 3334–3341. doi: 10.1128/IAI.00090-06

Davis, A. J., and Mecsas, J. (2007). Mutations in the *Yersinia pseudotuberculosis* type III secretion system needle protein, YscF, that specifically abrogate effector translocation into host cells. *J. Bacteriol.* 189, 83–97. doi: 10.1128/JB.01396-06

Davis, I. W., Leaver-Fay, A., Chen, V. B., Block, J. N., Kapral, G. J., Wang, X., et al. (2007). MolProbity: all-atom contacts and structure validation for proteins and nucleic acids. *Nucleic Acids Res.* 35, W375–W383. doi: 10.1093/nar/gkm216

Deane, J. E., Roversi, P., Cordes, F. S., Johnson, S., Kenjale, R., Daniell, S., et al. (2006). Molecular model of a type III secretion system needle: implications for host-cell sensing. *Proc. Natl. Acad. Sci. U.S.A.* 103, 12529–12533. doi: 10.1073/pnas.0602689103

Demers, J.-P., Habenstein, B., Loquet, A., Kumar Vasa, S., Giller, K., Becker, S., et al. (2014). High-resolution structure of the *Shigella* type-III secretion needle by solid-state NMR and cryo-electron microscopy. *Nat. Commun.* 5:4976. doi: 10.1038/ncomms5976

Demers, J.-P., Sgourakis, N. G., Gupta, R., Loquet, A., Giller, K., Riedel, D., et al. (2013). The common structural architecture of *Shigella flexneri* and *Salmonella typhimurium* type three secretion needles. *PLoS Pathog.* 9:e1003245. doi: 10.1371/journal.ppat.1003245

Discola, K. F., Förster, A., Boulay, F., Simorre, J.-P., Attree, I., Dessen, A., et al. (2014). Membrane and chaperone recognition by the major translocator protein PopB of the type III secretion system of *Pseudomonas aeruginosa*. *J. Biol. Chem.* 289, 3591–3601. doi: 10.1074/jbc.M113.517920

Ducret, A., Quardokus, E. M., and Brun, Y. V. (2016). MicrobeJ, a tool for high throughput bacterial cell detection and quantitative analysis. *Nat. Microbiol.* 1:16077. doi: 10.1038/nmicrobiol.2016.77

Eswar, N., Webb, B., Marti-Renom, M. A., Madhusudhan, M. S., Eramian, D., Shen, M.-Y., et al. (2007). Comparative protein structure modeling using MODELLER. *Curr. Protoc. Protein Sci.* 50, 2.9.1–2.9.31. doi: 10.1002/0471140864.ps0209s50 Unit 2.9,

Fujii, T., Cheung, M., Blanco, A., Kato, T., Blocker, A. J., and Namba, K. (2012). Structure of a type III secretion needle at 7-Å resolution provides insights into its assembly and signaling mechanisms. *Proc. Natl. Acad. Sci. U.S.A.* 109, 4461–4466. doi: 10.1073/pnas.1116126109

Galán, J. E., and Collmer, A. (1999). Type III secretion machines: bacterial devices for protein delivery into host cells. *Science* 284, 1322–1328. doi: 10.1126/science.284.5418.1322

Galán, J. E., Lara-Tejero, M., Marlovits, T. C., and Wagner, S. (2014). Bacterial type III secretion systems: specialized nanomachines for protein delivery into target cells. *Annu. Rev. Microbiol.* 68, 415–438. doi: 10.1146/annurev-micro-092412-155725

Godon, C., Teulon, J.-M., Odorico, M., Basset, C., Meillan, M., Vellutini, L., et al. (2017). Conditions to minimize soft single biomolecule deformation when imaging with atomic force microscopy. *J. Struct. Biol.* 197, 322–329. doi: 10.1016/j.jsb.2016.12.011

Goure, J., Pastor, A., Faudry, E., Chabert, J., Dessen, A., and Attree, I. (2004). The V antigen of *Pseudomonas aeruginosa* is required for assembly of the functional PopB/PopD translocation pore in host cell membranes. *Infect. Immun.* 72, 4741–4750. doi: 10.1128/IAI.72.8.4741-4750.2004

Harmon, D. E., Murphy, J. L., Davis, A. J., and Mecsas, J. (2013). A mutant with aberrant extracellular LcrV-YscF interactions fails to form pores and translocate Yop effector proteins but retains the ability to trigger Yop secretion in response to host cell contact. *J. Bacteriol.* 195, 2244–2254. doi: 10.1128/JB.02011-12

Hoiczyk, E., and Blobel, G. (2001). Polymerization of a single protein of the pathogen *Yersinia enterocolitica* into needles punctures eukaryotic cells. *Proc. Natl. Acad. Sci. U.S.A.* 98, 4669–4674. doi: 10.1073/pnas.071065798

Hu, J., Worrall, L. J., Hong, C., Vuckovic, M., Atkinson, C. E., Caveney, N., et al. (2018). Cryo-EM analysis of the T3S injectisome reveals the structure of the needle and open secretin. *Nat. Commun.* 9:3840. doi: 10.1038/s41467-018-06298-8

Izoré, T., Job, V., and Dessen, A. (2011). Biogenesis, regulation, and targeting of the type III secretion system. *Struct. Lond. Engl.* 1993, 603–612. doi: 10.1016/j.str.2011.03.015

Jneid, B., Moreau, K., Plaisance, M., Rouaix, A., Dano, J., and Simon, S. (2016). Role of T3SS-1 SipD protein in protecting mice against Non-typhoidal *Salmonella* typhimurium. *PLoS Negl. Trop. Dis.* 10:e0005207. doi: 10.1371/journal.pntd.0005207

Job, V., Matteï, P.-J., Lemaire, D., Attree, I., and Dessen, A. (2010). Structural basis of chaperone recognition of type III secretion system minor translocator proteins. *J. Biol. Chem.* 285, 23224–23232. doi: 10.1074/jbc.M110.111278

Journet, L., Agrain, C., Broz, P., and Cornelis, G. R. (2003). The needle length of bacterial injectisomes is determined by a molecular ruler. *Science* 302, 1757–1760. doi: 10.1126/science.1091422

Kato, J., Dey, S., Soto, J. E., Butan, C., Wilkinson, M. C., De Guzman, R. N., et al. (2018). A protein secreted by the *Salmonella* type III secretion system controls needle filament assembly. *eLife* 7:e35886. doi: 10.7554/eLife.35886

Kenjale, R., Wilson, J., Zenk, S. F., Saurya, S., Picking, W. L., Picking, W. D., et al. (2005). The needle component of the type III secreton of *Shigella* regulates the activity of the secretion apparatus. *J. Biol. Chem.* 280, 42929–42937. doi: 10.1074/jbc.M508377200

Koroleva, E. A., Kobets, N. V., Shcherbinin, D. N., Zigangirova, N. A., Shmarov, M. M., Tukhvatulin, A. I., et al. (2017). Chlamydial type III secretion system needle protein induces protective immunity against *Chlamydia muridarum* intravaginal infection. *Biomed Res. Int.* 2017:3865802. doi: 10.1155/2017/3865802

Kubori, T., Matsushima, Y., Nakamura, D., Uralil, J., Lara-Tejero, M., Sukhan, A., et al. (1998). Supramolecular structure of the *Salmonella* typhimurium type III protein secretion system. *Science* 280, 602–605. doi: 10.1126/science.280.5363.602

Kubori, T., Sukhan, A., Aizawa, S. I., and Galán, J. E. (2000). Molecular characterization and assembly of the needle complex of the *Salmonella* typhimurium type III protein secretion system. *Proc. Natl. Acad. Sci. U.S.A.* 97, 10225–10230. doi: 10.1073/pnas.170128997

Kuhlen, L., Abrusci, P., Johnson, S., Gault, J., Deme, J., Caesar, J., et al. (2018). Structure of the core of the type III secretion system export apparatus. *Nat. Struct. Mol. Biol.* 25, 583–590. doi: 10.1038/s41594-018-0086-9

Loquet, A., Sgourakis, N. G., Gupta, R., Giller, K., Riedel, D., Goosmann, C., et al. (2012). Atomic model of the type III secretion system needle. *Nature* 486, 276–279. doi: 10.1038/nature11079

Matteï, P.-J., Faudry, E., Job, V., Izoré, T., Attree, I., and Dessen, A. (2011). Membrane targeting and pore formation by the type III secretion system translocon. *FEBS J.* 278, 414–426. doi: 10.1111/j.1742-4658.2010.07974.x

Nariya, M. K., Israeli, J., Shi, J. J., and Deeds, E. J. (2016). Mathematical model for length control by the timing of substrate switching in the type III secretion system. *PLoS Comput. Biol.* 12:e1004851. doi: 10.1371/journal.pcbi.1004851

Nečas, D., and Klapetek, P. (2012). Gwyddion: an open-source software for SPM data analysis. *Open Phys.* 10, 181–188. doi: 10.2478/s11534-011-0096-2

Nguyen, V. S., Jobichen, C., Tan, K. W., Tan, Y. W., Chan, S. L., Ramesh, K., et al. (2015). Structure of AcrH-AopB chaperone-translocator complex reveals a role for membrane hairpins in type III secretion system translocon assembly. *Struct. Lond. Engl.* 23, 2022–2031. doi: 10.1016/j.str.2015.08.014

Park, D., Lara-Tejero, M., Waxham, M. N., Li, W., Hu, B., Galán, J. E., et al. (2018). Visualization of the type III secretion mediated *Salmonella*-host cell interface using cryo-electron tomography. *eLife* 7:e39514. doi: 10.7554/eLife.39514

Pastor, A., Chabert, J., Louwagie, M., Garin, J., and Attree, I. (2005). PscF is a major component of the *Pseudomonas aeruginosa* type III secretion needle. *FEMS Microbiol. Lett.* 253, 95–101. doi: 10.1016/j.femsle.2005.09.028

Perdu, C., Huber, P., Bouillot, S., Blocker, A., Elsen, S., Attrée, I., et al. (2015). ExsB is required for correct assembly of the *Pseudomonas aeruginosa* type III secretion apparatus in the bacterial membrane and full virulence in vivo. *Infect. Immun.* 83, 1789–1798. doi: 10.1128/IAI.00048-15

Pettersen, E. F., Goddard, T. D., Huang, C. C., Couch, G. S., Greenblatt, D. M., Meng, E. C., et al. (2004). UCSF Chimera–a visualization system for exploratory research and analysis. *J. Comput. Chem.* 25, 1605–1612. doi: 10.1002/jcc.20084

Poyraz, O., Schmidt, H., Seidel, K., Delissen, F., Ader, C., Tenenboim, H., et al. (2010). Protein refolding is required for assembly of the type three secretion needle. *Nat. Struct. Mol. Biol.* 17, 788–792. doi: 10.1038/nsmb.1822

Quinaud, M., Chabert, J., Faudry, E., Neumann, E., Lemaire, D., Pastor, A., et al. (2005). The PscE-PscF-PscG complex controls type III secretion needle biogenesis in *Pseudomonas aeruginosa*. *J. Biol. Chem.* 280, 36293–36300. doi: 10.1074/jbc.M508089200

Quinaud, M., Plé, S., Job, V., Contreras-Martel, C., Simorre, J.-P., Attree, I., et al. (2007). Structure of the heterotrimeric complex that regulates type III secretion needle formation. *Proc. Natl. Acad. Sci. U.S.A.* 104, 7803–7808. doi: 10.1073/pnas.0610098104

Radics, J., Königsmaier, L., and Marlovits, T. C. (2014). Structure of a pathogenic type 3 secretion system in action. *Nat. Struct. Mol. Biol.* 21, 82–87. doi: 10.1038/nsmb.2722

Robert, X., and Gouet, P. (2014). Deciphering key features in protein structures with the new ENDscript server. *Nucleic Acids Res.* 42, W320–W324. doi: 10.1093/nar/gku316

Sal-Man, N., Setiaputra, D., Scholz, R., Deng, W., Yu, A. C. Y., Strynadka, N. C. J., et al. (2013). EscE and EscG are cochaperones for the type III needle protein EscF of enteropathogenic *Escherichia coli*. *J. Bacteriol.* 195, 2481–2489. doi: 10.1128/JB.00118-13

Schneider, C. A., Rasband, W. S., and Eliceiri, K. W. (2012). NIH Image to ImageJ: 25 years of image analysis. *Nat. Methods* 9, 671–675. doi: 10.1038/nmeth.2089

Sun, P., Tropea, J. E., Austin, B. P., Cherry, S., and Waugh, D. S. (2008). Structural characterization of the *Yersinia pestis* type III secretion system needle protein YscF in complex with its heterodimeric chaperone YscE/YscG. *J. Mol. Biol.* 377, 819–830. doi: 10.1016/j.jmb.2007.12.067

Tamano, K., Aizawa, S., Katayama, E., Nonaka, T., Imajoh-Ohmi, S., Kuwae, A., et al. (2000). Supramolecular structure of the *Shigella* type III secretion machinery: the needle part is changeable in length and essential for delivery of effectors. *EMBO J.* 19, 3876–3887. doi: 10.1093/emboj/19.15.3876

Torruellas, J., Jackson, M. W., Pennock, J. W., and Plano, G. V. (2005). The *Yersinia pestis* type III secretion needle plays a role in the regulation of Yop secretion. *Mol. Microbiol.* 57, 1719–1733. doi: 10.1111/j.1365-2958.2005.04790.x

Veenendaal, A. K. J., Hodgkinson, J. L., Schwarzer, L., Stabat, D., Zenk, S. F., and Blocker, A. J. (2007). The type III secretion system needle tip complex mediates host cell sensing and translocon insertion. *Mol. Microbiol.* 63, 1719–1730. doi: 10.1111/j.1365-2958.2007.05620.x

Verasdonck, J., Shen, D.-K., Treadgold, A., Arthur, C., Böckmann, A., Meier, B. H., et al. (2015). Reassessment of MxiH subunit orientation and fold within native *Shigella* T3SS needles using surface labelling and solid-state NMR. *J. Struct. Biol.* 192, 441–448. doi: 10.1016/j.jsb.2015.10.005

Wagner, S., Grin, I., Malmsheimer, S., Singh, N., Torres-Vargas, C. E., and Westerhausen, S. (2018). Bacterial type III secretion systems: a complex device for the delivery of bacterial effector proteins into eukaryotic host cells. *FEMS Microbiol. Lett.* 365:fny201. doi: 10.1093/femsle/fny201

Wagner, S., Stenta, M., Metzger, L. C., Dal Peraro, M., and Cornelis, G. R. (2010). Length control of the injectisome needle requires only one molecule of Yop secretion protein P (YscP). *Proc. Natl. Acad. Sci. U.S.A.* 107, 13860–13865. doi: 10.1073/pnas.1006985107

Wang, Y., Ouellette, A. N., Egan, C. W., Rathinavelan, T., Im, W., and De Guzman, R. N. (2007). Differences in the electrostatic surfaces of the type III secretion needle proteins PrgI, BsaL, and MxiH. *J. Mol. Biol.* 371, 1304–1314. doi: 10.1016/j.jmb.2007.06.034

16

Tools and Approaches for Dissecting Protein Bacteriocin Import in Gram-Negative Bacteria

*Iva Atanaskovic and Colin Kleanthous**

Department of Biochemistry, University of Oxford, Oxford, United Kingdom

Bacteriocins of Gram-negative bacteria are typically multi-domain proteins that target and kill bacteria of the same or closely related species. There is increasing interest in protein bacteriocin import; from a fundamental perspective to understand how folded proteins are imported into bacteria and from an applications perspective as species-specific antibiotics to combat multidrug resistant bacteria. In order to translocate across the cell envelope and cause cell death, protein bacteriocins hijack nutrient uptake pathways. Their import is energized by parasitizing intermembrane protein complexes coupled to the proton motive force, which delivers a toxic domain into the cell. A plethora of genetic, structural, biochemical, and biophysical methods have been applied to find cell envelope components involved in bacteriocin import since their discovery almost a century ago. Here, we review the various approaches that now exist for investigating how protein bacteriocins translocate into Gram-negative bacteria and highlight areas of research that will need methodological innovations to fully understand this process. We also highlight recent studies demonstrating how bacteriocins can be used to probe organization and architecture of the Gram-negative cell envelope itself.

Keywords: bacteriocin, import, Gram-negative bacteria, cell envelope, methods

***Correspondence:**
Colin Kleanthous
colin.kleanthous@bioch.ox.ac.uk

INTRODUCTION

When exposed to environmental or competition stress bacteria often release proteinaceous toxins called bacteriocins that target and kill neighboring bacteria (Cascales et al., 2007; Cornforth and Foster, 2013). Bacteriocins of Gram-positive bacteria are mostly post-translationally modified peptides with a broad species target range, the best known example being the widely used food preservative nisin. Peptidic bacteriocins have been reviewed extensively (Héchard and Sahl, 2002; Cotter, 2014). The focus of the present review is on protein bacteriocins from Gram-negative bacteria. These are large folded proteins (40–80 kDa) that are composed of multiple domains and tend to have a narrow killing spectrum because of the numerous specific interactions at the cell surface involved in their import. A bacteriocin producer cell is protected from its own bacteriocin by an immunity protein, while sensitive strains lack such protection. These toxins can form pores in the inner membrane, act as nucleases to degrade DNA or RNA in the target cell, or interfere with cell

---

Abbreviations: CCCP, carbonyl cyanide 3-chlorophenylhydrazone; ColE9, colicin E9; CPA, common polysaccharide antigen; EK, enterokinase; FRAP, Forster recovery after photobleaching; FRET, Forster resonance energy transfer; Im9, ColE9 immunity protein; IM, inner membrane; ITC, isothermal titration calorimetry; LPS, lipopolysaccharide; MMBL, monocot mannose-binding lectin; NMR, nuclear magnetic resonance; NTD, N-terminal domain; OBS, OmpF-binding site; OM, outer membrane; OMP, outer membrane protein; PMF, proton motive force; PPI, protein–protein interactions; SAXS, small-angle X-ray scattering; TIRF, total internal reflection fluorescence.

wall biosynthesis. To do so, protein bacteriocins (hereafter referred to merely as bacteriocins) have to cross a multi-layered cell envelope which is accomplished by parasitizing host proteins involved in nutrient and metabolite trafficking (**Figure 1**).

Bacteriocins have the potential to be developed as much-needed therapeutics to treat multidrug resistant bacterial infections (Cotter, 2014; Behrens et al., 2017). A prerequisite for successfully applying bacteriocins as antimicrobials, however, is to understand how they are imported. Moreover, these import pathways might reveal further processes that could be exploited for newly designed drugs or chimeric bacteriocins with more potent toxicity (Lukacik et al., 2012).

The discovery of new bacteriocins has been accelerated by whole-genome sequencing technologies and implementation of gene mining tools (Jamet and Nassif, 2015; Sharp et al., 2017). While peptide Gram-negative bacteriocins, such as microcins, have been reviewed elsewhere (Duquesne et al., 2007), here we focus on methods used for the study of multidomain protein bacteriocins. The two most explored groups of protein bacteriocins are colicins produced by *Escherichia coli* (Cascales et al., 2007) and pyocins produced by *Pseudomonas aeruginosa* (Ghequire and De Mot, 2014). Nuclease colicins contain an N-terminal translocation domain, a central receptor binding domain, and a C-terminal cytotoxic domain that binds a cognate immunity protein, while in pyocins the location of the translocation and receptor binding domains appears reversed (Michel-Briand and Baysse, 2002). Bacteriocins can be divided into two groups based on the periplasmic energy transducing system they exploit for import. Group A use the Tol–Pal system, which is composed of periplasmic and IM proteins, Pal, TolA, TolB, TolR, TolQ. All but the outer membrane lipoprotein Pal have been documented to be involved in bacteriocin import.

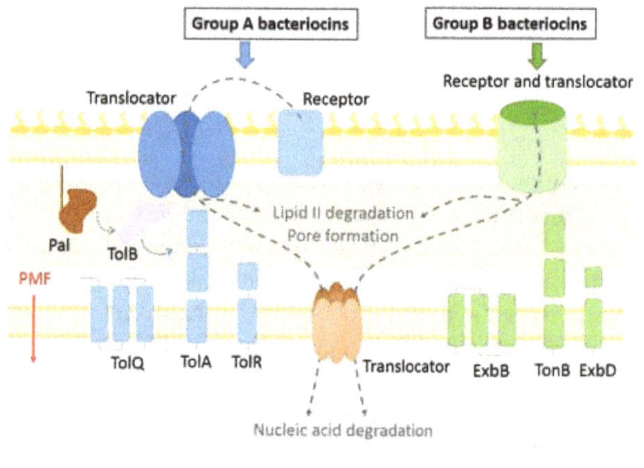

FIGURE 1 | Bacteriocin import pathways. Bacteriocins bind to outer membrane receptors to get imported into the cell. Some bacteriocins (group B) use the receptor protein also as a translocator to cross the outer membrane, while exploiting the TonB system and PMF as an energy source. In case of group A bacteriocins the translocator differs from the receptor protein and the Tol system is used to enter the periplasm. Bacteriocins that degrade lipid II and prevent peptidoglycan recycling remain in the periplasm, while pore forming bacteriocins are inserted in the inner membrane. Nuclease bacteriocins use a distinct protein translocator to cross the inner membrane.

Group B use the Ton system, composed of TonB, ExbB, and ExbD proteins (**Figure 1**). It is likely that all protein bacteriocins fall into these two such groups (Kleanthous, 2010).

Colicin E9 is one of the best understood of the Group A bacteriocins in terms of its translocation mechanism. Import of ColE9 involves assembly of a translocon complex. The OM portion of the translocon includes BtuB, its receptor, its porin translocator OmpF or OmpC, TolB, its periplasmic target, and Im9, its immunity protein. In order to form this OM translocon, ColE9 uses its intrinsically unstructured N-terminus to pass through a porin channel to engage the PMF-coupled Tol–Pal system in the periplasm (Housden et al., 2005). How ColE9 translocates across the OM is not understood, but it is known that the colicin exploits FtsH, the AAA$^+$ ATPase/protease, to cross the IM. Once inside the cell, the ColE9 DNase causes nonspecific cleavage of double-stranded DNA which results in cell death (Walker et al., 2007). Group B colicins and pyocins pass through Ton-dependent receptors without the involvement of porins. For instance, pyocin S2 binds to a TonB-coupled siderophore receptor FpvAI, and passes through the FpvAI lumen mimicking its cognate ligand (White et al., 2017).

Gram-negative bacteriocins use a variety of pathways and distinct combinations of cell envelope proteins to kill cells, making it challenging to dissect their import mechanisms. Since their discovery, genetic, structural, biochemical, and biophysical approaches have all been deployed to define these pathways often in combination (**Figure 2**). Here, we give an overview of these approaches, pointing out the most recent advancements in the toolkit used for dissecting bacteriocin translocation in Gram-negative bacteria.

PAIRING UP BACTERIOCINS WITH THEIR RECEPTORS

Every bacteriocin begins its journey through the cell envelope by binding to a specific receptor on the bacterial surface. While most bacteriocins bind OM proteins, some use LPS as their primary receptor (Kim et al., 2014; McCaughey et al., 2014, 2016). The specificity of a bacteriocin–receptor interaction narrows down the target range of these toxins. Therefore, pairing up bacteriocins with their receptors is an important first step in applying them as therapeutics (Cotter, 2014). If a sufficient number of bacteriocin receptors are known, a screen for receptor genes in a genome of a pathogen isolated from the site of infection could guide the design of bacteriocin cocktails to specifically eradicate the cause of infection. Additionally, linking a bacteriocin to a receptor of known biological function is the starting point for understanding which import pathway is being hijacked by the toxin.

When searching for a bacteriocin receptor, the first issue to address is its chemical nature. Bacteriocin *neutralization experiments* have often been used to determine if the receptor is within the protein or LPS fraction of the outer membrane (Weltzien and Jesaitis, 1971). If a certain cell fraction contains the receptor, it will bind to a bacteriocin and inhibit its toxic activity, which can be assessed by a plate killing assay (**Figure 2**). Neutralization experiments can also be used to test if a specific

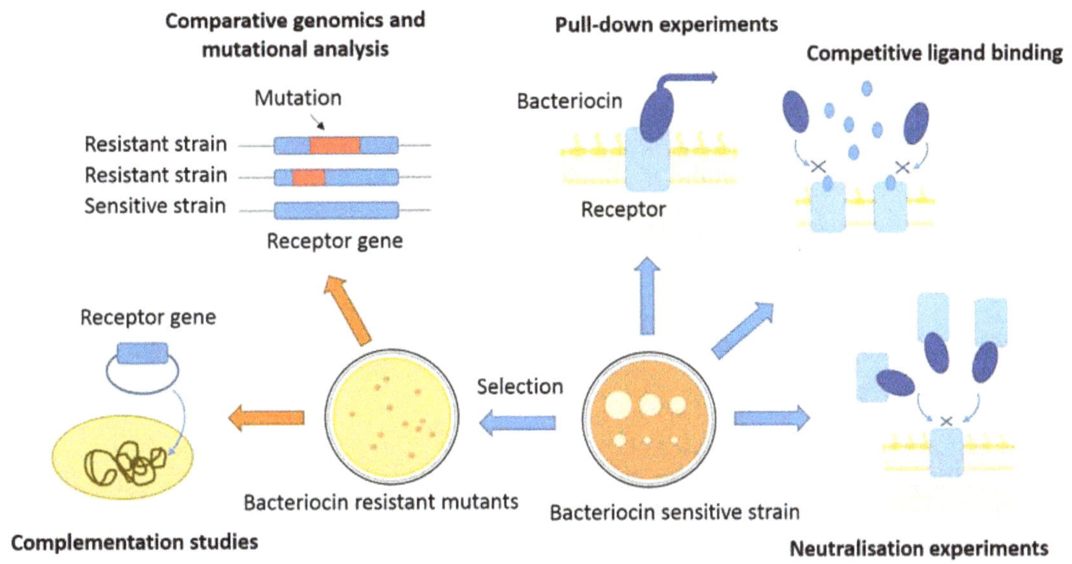

FIGURE 2 | Approaches to finding bacteriocin translocon components. Translocon components can be isolated from membranes of sensitive strains by use of affinity tagged bacteriocins as bait. Competitive ligand binding or bacteriocin binding to a purified translocon component can inhibit bacteriocin activity and give indications about proteins engaged in bacteriocin entry. Bacteriocin-resistant mutants can be selected by use of high bacteriocin concentrations, or generated by transposon mutagenesis. Genomes of resistant mutants can further be analyzed for mutations underlying the resistance phenotype, which can give gene candidates for translocon components. A component of bacteriocin entry has to be further confirmed by complementation studies, where bacteriocin sensitivity is re-established once a resistant mutant is transformed with a gene of interest.

nutrient import pathway is being hijacked by a bacteriocin. If cells are exposed to a bacteriocin in the presence of a nutrient with which it shares its import pathway, competitive binding of the ligand should either inhibit bacteriocin activity or nutrient import. Such experiments were successful in early attempts at receptor discovery. For instance, competitive binding of cyanocobalamin and E-type colicins gave early indications that they all share BtuB as a receptor (Masi et al., 1973). Similarly, such experiments suggested that pyocin S3 and pyoverdine both bind to the ferripyoverdine type II receptor in *P. aeruginosa* (Baysse et al., 1999), and ferredoxin and pectocin M bind to the same ferredoxin receptor in *Pectobacterium artrosepticum* (Grinter et al., 2012).

An alternative approach is one that combines *neutralization assays with cell wall fractionation and protein purification.* OM fractions can be tested for bacteriocin neutralization activity. After singling out the OM fraction with neutralization activity, further analysis by mass spectrometry can identify the receptor. Use of protease inhibitors is important for preventing OM proteases from degrading the bacteriocin, which can be misinterpreted as bacteriocin neutralization. Misinterpretations can also be avoided by co-fractionating OM proteins isolated from a bacteriocin resistant and a bacteriocin sensitive strain, where all OM proteins from each strain have been labeled with two different fluorescent or radioactive labels. Since the resistant mutants should lack the receptor, a fraction with receptor activity should contain only proteins that originate from the sensitive strain (Sabet and Schnaitman, 1973). A limitation of this approach is that receptor concentrations obtained by OM fractionation can often be insufficient to achieve neutralization. This approach is therefore limited to cases where bacteriocin receptors are expressed to high levels or bind the bacteriocin with high affinity.

Instead of testing for neutralization activity, bacteriocin OM receptors can be identified directly by *pull-down experiments*, using a bacteriocin of interest as a bait (**Figure 2**). A bacteriocin should co-elute from the chromatography column with its receptor, where further analysis of the co-eluent by proteolysis and peptide fingerprinting by mass spectrometry can give a receptor candidate. For example, Housden et al. (2005) used a hexahistidine-tagged immunity protein complexed to ColE9 and immobilized on a nickel affinity column to purify components of the ColE9 translocon from OM extracts. These pull-down experiments can be challenging in cases of low-abundance receptors. One way to circumvent this problem is to find receptor overproducers, marked by an increased sensitivity to a bacteriocin of interest (Bowles et al., 1983). Another option is to cultivate cells in conditions that increase bacteriocin sensitivity by inducing receptor expression (Bindereif et al., 1982). Defining growth conditions where a bacteriocin receptor is overexpressed can also give valuable hints about the nature of the receptor. This was the case for several S-type pyocin receptors where it was observed that killing of *P. aeruginosa* was more effective if cultivated in iron-limited conditions (Smith et al., 1992; Sano et al., 1993). This observation indicated that siderophore receptors, which are overexpressed when cells are starved of iron, are involved in import of S-type pyocins. Receptors for pyocins S3, S2, S4, and S5 (Baysse et al., 1999; Denayer et al., 2007; Elfarash et al., 2012, 2014) were all discovered by this route.

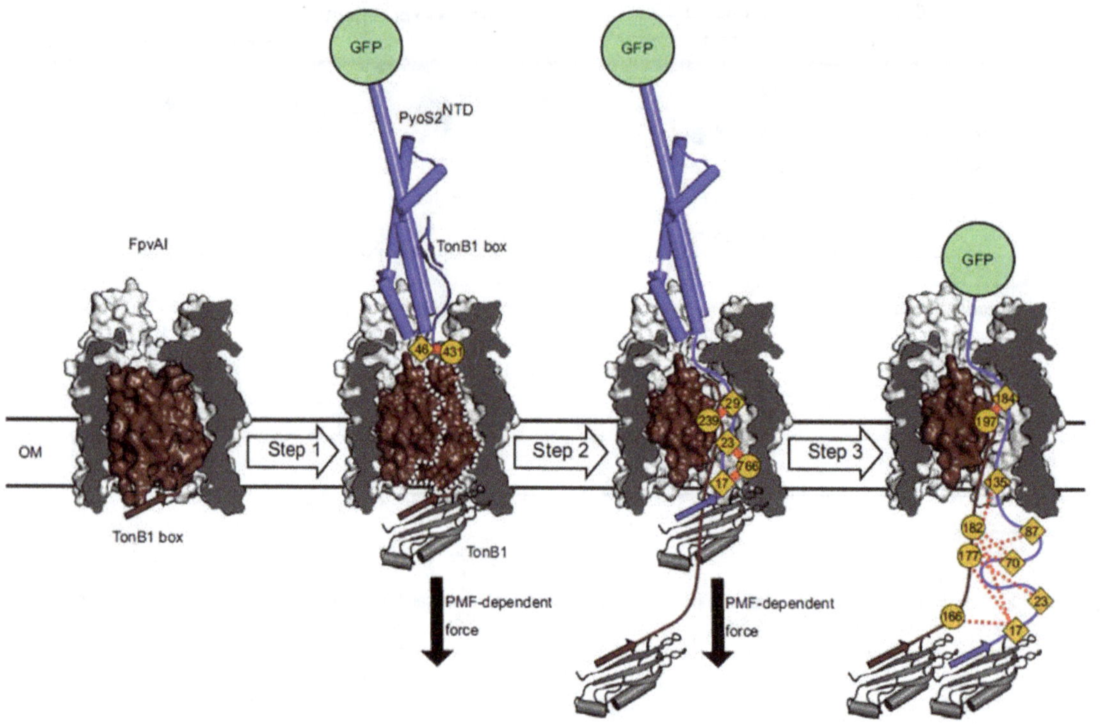

FIGURE 3 | *In vivo* cross-linking strategy developed by White et al. for dissecting the import pathway of pyocin S2 through the FpvAI receptor. Photoactivatable crosslinking data were used to establish a three-step model of translocation. In step 1, pyocin S2 binds to FpvAI and mimics its cognate ligand, ferro-pyoverdine. In step 2, a PMF-dependent mechanical force, applied via the ExbB–ExbD–TonB1 complex in the IM (not shown), drives unfolding of the labile half of the receptor plug domain and the N terminus of pyocin S2 enters the receptor lumen. In step 3, pyocin S2 binds to TonB1 and this interaction drives further passage of the pyocin through the receptor lumen. Complete translocation is blocked by the force-resistant GFP, which enables identification of translocation intermediates and mapping of interactions that govern pyocin S2 cell entry [image taken and used with permission from White et al. (2017), CC BY-NC-ND 4.0].

Another approach for receptor discovery is based on the isolation and characterization of *bacteriocin-resistant mutants*. A resistant mutant can lack a bacteriocin receptor; hence, picking up genetic differences between resistant and sensitive strains can pinpoint the receptor gene (**Figure 2**). When selecting for resistant mutants by use of lethal bacteriocin doses a major challenge is to distinguish between resistant and tolerant strains; only resistant strains bare mutations that specifically alter import machinery components. Therefore, it is always necessary to disregard tolerance by exposure to even higher bacteriocin doses than those used for selection and by checking if a mutant's growth kinetics is affected by the bacteriocin. Finally, resistance can be confirmed by checking if the mutant's OM has lost its bacteriocin binding properties by a neutralization assay or use of a fluorescently labeled bacteriocin to test for cell surface association (**Figure 3**; Rassam et al., 2015; White et al., 2017).

After isolating a resistant mutant, it is possible to compare its OM protein composition with the parental strain. A combination of electrophoresis and mass spectrometry can point out proteins absent in the OM of the resistant strain, but again, this has only been successful in cases where receptor genes are highly expressed (Ohkawa et al., 1980; Baysse et al., 1999). The advent of *whole-genome sequencing and comparative genomics* is now the preferred method of choice. Comparing a mutant's genome with a bacteriocin-sensitive reference strain can pinpoint potential receptor genes (McCaughey et al., 2014). This strategy has been successful in identifying bacteriocin receptors in Gram-positive bacteria (Cotter, 2014). The decreasing cost of DNA sequencing and continuous refinement of bioinformatics tools makes it likely that researchers in the field of Gram-negative bacteriocin import will increasingly turn to whole-genome sequencing. However, comparative genomics still has its limitations especially in the case of bacterial strains with a high rate of spontaneous mutations, where it can be difficult to filter out a mutation associated with bacteriocin resistance.

Receptor genes have also been identified by use of *cosmid libraries*. Genomic fragments from a bacteriocin-sensitive strain can be transformed into a bacteriocin-resistant background. The goal is to identify a fragment that can restore bacteriocin sensitivity and potentially carries a receptor gene (Pilsl et al., 1999; Smajs and Weinstock, 2001). An alternative approach is to construct *a library of transposon mutants* in a strain that is sensitive to the bacteriocin. Sequencing of genomic regions around the transposon insertion site in a resistant mutant can pinpoint genes linked to bacteriocin import (Baysse et al., 1999; de Chial et al., 2003; Elfarash et al., 2014; Ghequire et al., 2017). The power of this approach can be increased with the implementation of high-throughput transposon insertion sequencing techniques, such as TraDIS (Barquist et al., 2016), since the employment of a dense transposon library can give better genomic coverage and increase the probability of a resistance phenotype being detected. TraDIS has recently been used to show that LPSs bearing O-antigens shield bacteriocin receptors in uropathogenic *E. coli* but that this effect is modulated by growth conditions (Sharp et al., 2019). Nevertheless, if a receptor is an essential gene no transposon mutants will be obtained and a library search will fail to show the receptor. In this case, pull-down experiments or linkage analysis (see below) can be used.

Bacteriocin receptors can also be found by *linkage analysis*, as in the case of S-type pyocin receptors. S pyocins kill *P. aeruginosa* better under iron limiting conditions, which gave indications that their activity might be linked to the pyoverdine import system (Ohkawa et al., 1980; Smith et al., 1992). A collection of *P. aeruginosa* strains was screened for pyocin S2 sensitivity and ferripyoverdine receptor genes typed by multiplex PCR. All S2 sensitive strains had the type I ferripyoverdine *fpvAI* gene, indicating this was the S2 receptor (Denayer et al., 2007). The same approach was used to link pyocin S4 sensitivity to the *fpvAI* receptor gene (Elfarash et al., 2012). Another type of linkage analysis that was successful in bacteriocin receptor discovery was *metabolite analysis*, where pyoverdine production was compared between pyocin S3 resistant and sensitive strains. It was found that pyocin S3 kills only type II pyoverdine producers of *P. aeruginosa*, while type I and III producers were resistant to S3 (Govan, 1978; Baysse et al., 1999). This gave strong indications that pyocin S3 binds to the ferripyoverdine type II receptor, which was confirmed by subsequent studies (de Chial et al., 2003). A future challenge will be implementation of high-throughput linkage approaches, which can be used when there are no initial clues about the import mechanism. This could be achieved through *genome wide association studies*, if both a genome sequence database and a physical strain collection are available. One could then test bacteriocin sensitivity throughout the collection and conduct a gene linkage analysis for a collection of corresponding annotated genomic sequences (Brynildsrud et al., 2016). Genes that are present in a large number of sensitive, but absent in a large number of bacteriocin resistant strains, are then further tested for receptor coding activity. On the other hand, the development of new mass spectrometric approaches in high-throughput metabolomics (Zampieri et al., 2017) could enable full metabolome comparison between bacteriocin resistant and sensitive strains, where metabolites lacking in resistant strains could give hints about import mechanisms being hijacked by the bacteriocin.

The majority of bacteriocin receptors identified to-date are proteins; however, non-proteinaceous receptors have also been identified. Pyocin L1 is a lectin-like bacteriocin produced by *P. aeruginosa*. It consists of tandem MMBL domains and kills cells by targeting the CPA of *P. aeruginosa* LPS, which is predominantly a homopolymer of D-rhamnose. The widespread inclusion of D-rhamnose in the LPS of pseudomonads explains the unusual genus-specific activity of this lectin-like bacteriocin. The discovery of the pyocin L1 saccharide receptor was achieved through a combination of genetics, structural, and biophysical approaches (McCaughey et al., 2014). Alignment of the pyocin L1 protein sequence with other lectin-like bacteriocins revealed the presence of three conserved MMBL sugar-binding domains, giving the first indications that pyocin L1 might bind to polysaccharide rather than to a protein receptor. A *P. aeruginosa* strain sensitive to this pyocin was used to recover resistant mutants, the genome sequences of which showed a deletion in the *wbpZ* gene, which encodes a glycosyltransferase involved in the synthesis of the CPA component of LPS (Rocchetta et al., 1998). Subsequent immunoblotting with a CPA-specific antibody along with transposon insertions in genes *wzt* and *wzm*, which encode the ATP-binding and the membrane components of a CPA dedicated ABC transporter (Lam et al., 2011), confirmed that CPA on the cell surface is required for pyocin L1 killing. Direct binding of pyocin L1 to CPA and D-rhamnose was shown by ITC and NMR spectroscopy. Finally, X-ray crystallography defined the mode of binding of the D-rhamnose receptor to the C-terminal MMBL domain of pyocin L1. This study therefore provides an excellent example how a combination of genomics and mutational analysis combined with biophysics and structural data can identify non-proteinaceous bacteriocin receptors.

In summary, bacteriocin receptors come in many different types and so an equally varied toolkit is needed for their identification (**Figure 2**). Receptors with high expression levels can be pulled-down using a bacteriocin as bait. This might be the only viable approach if the receptor is essential. If non-essential, receptor coding genes can be discovered through isolation of bacteriocin-resistant mutants, either spontaneously generated or induced through transposon mutagenesis. Finally, the future development of high-throughput approaches based on whole-genome sequencing and comparative genomics will alleviate receptor discovery for an ever-growing number of newly identified bacteriocins (Sharp et al., 2017).

IDENTIFYING TRANSLOCON COMPONENTS DOWNSTREAM OF THE RECEPTOR

After binding to a specific receptor, bacteriocins translocate across the OM. The receptor itself can serve as a translocation pore, as for the group B pyocin S2 (White et al., 2017), or another protein can be recruited to the complex to serve as a translocator, as for the group A colicin ColE9 (Housden et al., 2013). Before establishing a translocation model, it is necessary to find all OM and periplasmic components of a bacteriocin's translocon.

Bacteriocin insensitive mutants can be used to find translocon components other than the receptor. Mutant library screens have been particularly useful in this regard. For example, a screen of the Keio collection library for mutants insensitive but still capable of binding colicin S4 showed that *ompF*, *tolA*, *tolB*, *tolQ*, and *tolR* genes are all linked to its translocation. In the same study, it was found that after binding to the receptor OmpW, colicin S4 recruits OmpF and the Tol–Pal system to translocate across the OM (Arnold et al., 2009). A complication of this approach, however, is that *tol* gene knock-outs have altered membrane stability and permeability; deletion of *tolA* in *E. coli* leads to a pleiotropic phenotype characterized by outer membrane blebbing, release of the periplasmic content, increased sensitivity to cholic acid and SDS, and defective O-antigen polymerization (Germon et al., 2001). Indeed, *P. aeruginosa tolQRA* knock-outs are lethal (Wei et al., 2009). Therefore, using *tol* deletion mutants to check if bacteriocin entry is Tol–Pal dependent is not always feasible.

Chimeric bacteriocins have been effectively used to separate the receptor binding and translocation phases of the import process, which can be important for finding translocon components downstream of the receptor. This approach was successfully used to show that colicin Ia uses two copies of the Cir protein for OM translocation - one copy is used as the receptor and the other copy is used for translocation. A chimeric colicin Ia, in which the receptor-binding domain was replaced by that from colicin E3, required BtuB, the colicin E3 receptor, but also a copy of Cir and TonB for its killing activity. This experiment gave indications that one copy of Cir interacts with the receptor-binding domain of colicin Ia to concentrate the protein on the cell surface, while the other copy of Cir interacts with the translocation domain of this colicin so it can pass through the OM and enter the periplasm (Buchanan et al., 2007; Jakes and Finkelstein, 2010). However, direct binding of the Cir translocator with colicin Ia has yet to be demonstrated biochemically. *Receptor bypass* experiments have also been used to find translocon components other than the receptor. In such experiments, the OM is first permeabilized, usually by osmotic shock, so the receptor binding step is bypassed (Thomas and Valvano, 1993). This can be useful when a receptor for a bacteriocin under investigation is not known or when suitable chimeras are not available.

Very little is known about *inner membrane translocation* of Gram-negative bacteriocins. However, mutational analysis successfully identified some IM proteins necessary for transport of nuclease colicins. Walker et al. (2007) used a Δ*ftsH E. coli* strain to show that the toxicity of all nuclease colicins (regardless of their Tol–Pal/Ton dependence) is dependent on FtsH, an inner membrane AAA+ ATPase/protease. This protease cleaves off the DNase domain during import to the cytoplasm (Chauleau et al., 2011; Mora and de Zamaroczy, 2014). In other studies, whole-genome sequencing of an *E. coli* mutant that is insensitive to colicin D gave indications that an inner membrane peptidase LepB is required for cell entry (de Zamaroczy et al., 2001). LepB is a key membrane component of the cellular secretion machinery, which releases secreted proteins into the periplasm by cleaving the inner membrane-bound leader. It was further shown that this protein binds to colicin D and probably directs it to the FtsH protease for cell entry (Mora et al., 2015).

Since IM translocation components are a part of protein translocation systems that are well conserved across different Gram-negative bacteria, it is possible to study the import of bacteriocins from other species using *E. coli* as a model system. The only limitation here is to bypass all the species-specific translocation steps that are mostly localized to the outer membrane. Hence, Mora et al. (2015) used a colicin D/klebicin D hybrid in which the N-terminal import domain of klebicin D was replaced with that of colicin D. Klebicin D targets *Klebsiella* species, but when fused to the receptor binding and the translocation domain of colicin D it can also kill *E. coli* obviating the need for a *Klebsiella* knock-out library. In this way, it was found that klebicin D, like colicin D, uses LepB for import (Mora et al., 2015).

DECONSTRUCTING THE PROTEIN–PROTEIN INTERACTIONS OF BACTERIOCIN TRANSLOCONS

Several approaches can be taken to define binding epitopes and binding induced conformational changes within bacteriocin translocons. PPIs between translocon components have to be first confirmed *in vitro* and *in vivo*. A common approach is *gene complementation* using a bacteriocin-resistant mutant or a bacteriocin-resistant species (Kjos et al., 2014), where the establishment of bacteriocin sensitivity can confirm the involvement of components in bacteriocin import (**Figure 2**). Apart from gene complementation assays, interactions between components can be assessed *in vivo* by *pull-down* experiments. A way to "freeze" the translocon in the assembly phase is by *in vivo* cross-linking (Masi et al., 2007; White et al., 2017) or by a disulphide locked bacteriocin (Housden et al., 2005, 2013). In both cases, a bacteriocin must be able to bind to its receptor and trigger translocon assembly without fully traversing the cell envelope and killing the target cell. Bacteriocin-bound protein complexes can further be extracted from the outer membrane by affinity chromatography using a bacteriocin or its immunity protein as bait. Pulldowns followed by limited proteolysis of the complex, and mass spectrometry of recovered protein fragments, can indicate which binding epitopes are involved in the translocon. For example, Housden et al. (2013) designed a disulphide lock that forms between the TolB-binding epitope of ColE9 and periplasmic TolB following recruitment of OmpF in the OM. A histidine tag on TolB enabled a heptameric assembly of the ColE9–Im9 complex, BtuB, OmpF trimer, and TolB to be purified and analyzed by mass spectrometry. Finally, limited proteolysis, in combination with planar lipid bilayer experiments and native mass spectrometry, demonstrated that within the translocon, ColE9's unstructured N-terminal region passes twice through its bound porin thereby presenting its TolB-binding epitope in a conformationally constrained orientation in the periplasm (Housden et al., 2013).

Calorimetric measurements have also been used extensively in colicin import studies (Housden and Kleanthous, 2011), in particular ITC. ITC parameters can provide evidence of conformational changes within the translocon (Housden et al., 2005). ITC has also been used to determine how a bacteriocin affects existing PPIs within the cell envelope. Changes in the heats of binding in presence of a bacteriocin can indicate if it abolishes or induces a certain PPI. In this way, it has been shown that ColE9 interacts with TolB when entering the periplasm, disrupting the TolB–Pal complex and stimulating formation of a TolA–TolB complex that traverses the periplasm (Bonsor et al., 2009). ITC combined with site-directed mutagenesis can map translocon-binding sites, as in the case of the ColE9 TolB-binding region. The favorable enthalpy and unfavorable entropy changes associated with ColE9-binding TolB correspond to a disorder-to-order transition that occurs when the intrinsically unstructured region of ColE9 folds and binds TolB (Loftus et al., 2006). In other words, ITC parameters can indicate not only which regions of bacteriocins and their translocon components interact, but also which regions undergo conformational changes and in which phases of the translocation process these conformational changes occur.

Stopped-flow FRET experiments demonstrated how a bacteriocin can remodel PPIs within the cell envelope during import. Papadakos et al. (2012a) used a series of pre-steady-state kinetic experiments utilizing FRET pairs of ColE9 TolB-binding epitope, TolB and Pal, to establish the kinetic basis for competitive recruitment of TolB by ColE9 during which Pal gets displaced from its TolB–Pal complex. Interactions between translocon components have also been investigated using *planar lipid bilayers*. For example, it has been shown that ColE1 occludes TolC channels and that ColE9 occludes OmpF channels in planar lipid bilayers, confirming previous findings that these OMPs are involved in bacteriocin translocation (Zakharov et al., 2004). This approach was also used to identify a TolC box in ColE1 (Zakharov et al., 2016).

ASSEMBLING THE TRANSLOCON

A major challenge in understanding protein bacteriocin import is to assemble their translocons for structural studies where, for the most part, only general import mechanisms have been described (Cascales et al., 2007; Ghequire and De Mot, 2014; McCaughey et al., 2016; White et al., 2017).

Since Gram-negative bacteriocins are large multi-domain proteins, it is thought they must unfold, either partially or completely, in order to translocate across the outer membrane. Introducing *disulphide bonds* to prevent conformational changes in certain regions of a bacteriocin has been a useful approach in delineating such structural changes (Penfold et al., 2004). Similarly, *protease cleavage sites* have been used to probe the accessibility of bacteriocin sequences within a translocon. Zhang et al. (2008) introduced unique EK cleavage sites in a disulphide-locked ColE9 at a number of locations to study the surface accessibility of colicin subdomains shortly after receptor binding. In this experiment, a disulphide-lock within the colicin was used to synchronize translocon assembly; disulfide bond reduction simultaneously triggers initiation of translocation in all bacterial cells. This enabled determination of EK cleavage site accessibility for different regions of the colicin, which gave important insight into the position of ColE9 in the assembled translocon (Zhang et al., 2008).

Studies are beginning to unravel the molecular mechanism(s) by which bacteriocins translocate across the OM. White et al. (2017) developed an *in vivo cross-linking strategy* to map the import of the pyocin S2 NTD through the FpvAI receptor (**Figure 3**). This approach depended on first blocking import of the NTD using a C-terminal GFP. GFP is able to withstand ~200 pN of force whereas the PMF can only deliver ~20 pN (Saeger et al., 2012). This strategy allowed the accumulation of translocation intermediates that would otherwise be undetectable by crosslinking. Variants of this GFP fusion were then generated in which benzoylphenylalanine was incorporated at different positions of the NTD using amber suppression and crosslinked following transport into *P. aeruginosa* cells. Detailed mass spectrometric analysis of crosslinked peptides demonstrated that the pyocin not only translocates through FpvAI but that it does so by a process which likely mimics that used by pyoverdine, the natural ligand for FpvAI (White et al., 2017).

An important aspect of nuclease bacteriocin import is the release of the tightly bound immunity protein. All nuclease bacteriocins are produced bound tightly ($K_d \sim 10^{-14}$ M at pH 7 and 25°C) to their immunity protein Papadakos et al. (2012b). The half-life for dissociation for this complex is several days yet killing occurs within minutes. Hence, it has been postulated that an energy transduction path exists that jettisons the immunity protein at the cell surface during import. Zhang et al. (2008) developed a sensitive *fluorescence assay* to investigate immunity release. The assay was based on release of a fluorescently labeled immunity protein into the cell supernatant. Bacteriocin import was synchronized using a disulfide-lock. In this way, fluorescently labeled Im9 was detected in the cell supernatant after the addition of a reducing agent and was dependent on the PMF across the inner membrane (Zhang et al., 2008; Vankemmelbeke et al., 2012), shown subsequently to be linked to global conformational changes within the colicin (Vankemmelbeke et al., 2013). How force might cause immunity dissociation has been investigated by *single molecule atomic force spectroscopy* (Farrance et al., 2013). These studies demonstrated that the ColE9 DNase–Im9 complex is exquisitely sensitive to mechanical deformation at the N-terminus of the nuclease, which could represent pulling into a cell, causing rapid dissociation of the immunity protein.

STRUCTURAL BIOLOGY APPROACHES FOR STUDYING BACTERIOCIN IMPORT

Structural studies are important in gaining a molecular understanding of the bacteriocin translocation process. To-date, there are only a few structures of intact Gram-negative bacteriocins (Wiener et al., 1997; Soelaiman et al., 2001; Helbig et al., 2011; Klein et al., 2016). More informative, in terms of translocation mechanism, are structures of bacteriocins or bacteriocin domains bound to their receptor or a component of the translocon assembly (Kurisu et al., 2003; Loftus et al., 2006; Buchanan et al., 2007; Sharma et al., 2007; Zhang et al., 2009; Housden et al., 2010; White et al., 2017). These structures give information about conformational changes that a bacteriocin induces and shed light on the import mechanism.

Crystallization of bacteriocins can often be challenging due to intrinsically disordered and flexible regions in these proteins. Flexibility can be reduced by deletion of these sequences or by the introduction of intramolecular disulfide bonds (Klein et al., 2016). To complete a structure of a bacteriocin it is often necessary to substitute missing X-ray diffraction data with results from other experiments. Modeling of data from *analytical ultracentrifugation* (Manon and Ebel, 2010) and *NMR experiments* (Collins et al., 2002; Hecht et al., 2009) can help in filling-in missing parts of a bacteriocin structure. Results from *SAXS* experiments can also be combined with diffraction data; a bacteriocin can be treated as a flexible system, namely by the ensemble optimization method, which enables a distribution of conformations to be included in the final model (Johnson et al., 2017).

Structures of *bacteriocin–receptor and bacteriocin–translocator complexes* are essential to understand bacteriocin import mechanisms. When compared to receptor–cognate ligand complexes, these structures can show to what extent a bacteriocin mimics the ligand (if at all) when traversing the cell envelope. For example, co-crystal structures for E-type colicins bound to the BtuB receptor (ColE2, ColE3) show that the colicins do not mimic the interactions of the ligand and do not induce conformational changes within the globular N-terminal plug domain of BtuB indicative of transport. This contrasts the situation of pyocin S2-NTD bound to its receptor FpvAI where the structure clearly supports a model (validated by crosslinking data) that the pyocin mimics the endogenous ligand, pyoverdine, and transports through the receptor in a TonB-dependent manner (White et al., 2017). For the E colicins (all of which require the Tol complex), entry to the periplasm requires OmpF or OmpC. These porins acts as translocators, which is supported by structures of OmpF in which fragments of E colicins are bound within its lumen (Yamashita et al., 2008; Housden et al., 2010) and by planar lipid bilayer experiments where colicin fragments block ion conductance (Zakharov et al., 2004).

The development of structure-prediction algorithms could broaden the understanding of bacteriocin translocons (Delarue and Koehl, 2018). For instance, protein fold predictions have already been employed in structure determination of a group A colicin translocon component, TolQ (Ovchinnikov et al., 2015). Additionally, future developments in translocon structures will undoubtedly involve cryo-EM methods. It may even be possible to eventually capture a bacteriocin in-transit and use cryo-tomography to map out its interactions within the cell envelope.

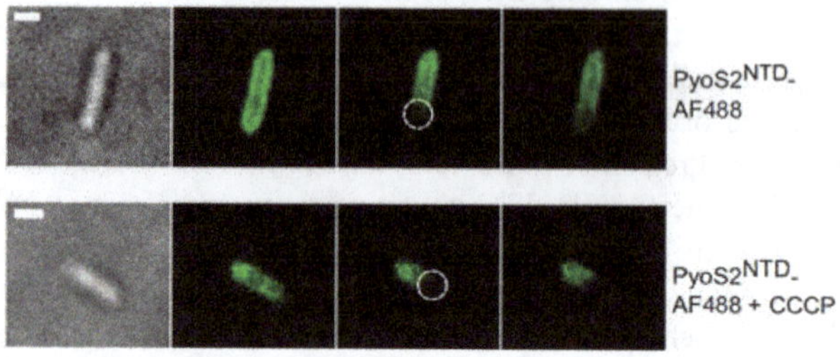

FIGURE 4 | FRAP experiments can be used to show that bacteriocin import is a PMF-dependent process. *P. aeruginosa* PAO1 cells are labeled with pyocin S2 AF488. The bleached region is highlighted (dashed circle). FRAP suggests pyoS2NTD-AF488 has translocated to the periplasm, where it can diffuse laterally. Absence of FRAP observed when cells are treated with 100 μM CCCP indicates that the pyocin remains bound to FpvAI in the OM and that the PMF is necessary for pyocin translocation. Scale bars, 1 μm [image taken and used with permission from White et al. (2017), CC BY-NC-ND 4.0].

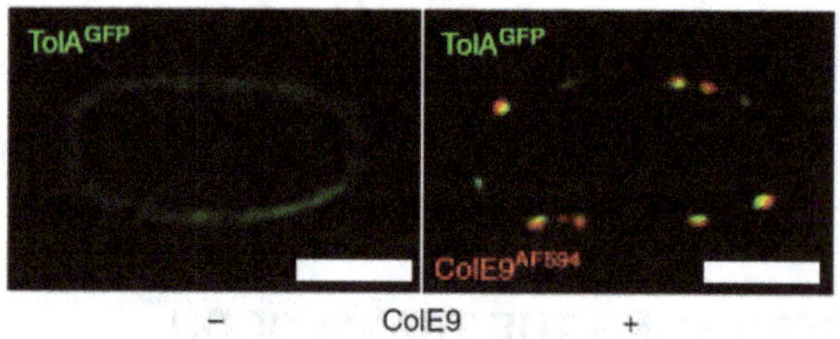

FIGURE 5 | Fluorescently labeled bacteriocins can be used to track outer and inner membrane protein clusters; used by Rassam et al. (2018) to show that bacteriocin-induced clustering of TolA in the IM mirrors that of OMPs in the OM. 2D-SIM z-slice showing significant co-clustering (yellow fluorescence) of GFP-TolA and ColE9AF594 in the IM and OM, respectively. Scale bars, 1 μm [image taken and used with permission from Rassam et al. (2018), CC BY-NC-ND 4.0].

VIEWING THE IMPORT PROCESS IN THE CONTEXT OF OUTER MEMBRANE ORGANIZATION

Bacteriocins have become valuable tools with which to investigate spatiotemporal organization in the cell envelope by fluorescence microscopy (Kleanthous et al., 2015). Fluorescently labeled bacteriocins have been used in conjunction with *single particle tracking TIRF microscopy* to show that OMPs display highly restricted mobility in the outer membrane due to the formation of supramolecular assemblies called OMP islands, which also explains the lack of fluorescence recovery for labeled OMPs in FRAP experiments (**Figure 4**). TIRF microscopy of bacteriocin-labeled OMPs has also shown that OMP islands move to the poles as new islands appear in the membrane (Rassam et al., 2015). Even more remarkably, the restricted mobility that is characteristic of OMPs within OMP islands becomes imprinted on inner membrane proteins when the bacteriocin forms its translocon across the two membranes (**Figure 5**; Rassam et al., 2018).

Fluorescently labeled bacteriocins have also been used for dissecting their import mechanism. GFP was deployed by White et al. (2017) to visualize association of pyocin S2 with *P. aeruginosa* cells, block translocation, and trap the pyocin within its receptor, FpvAI, for subsequent crosslinking studies. By switching to an organic dye (AF488), White et al. (2017) demonstrated import of the pyocin S2 domain since in contrast to GFP-labeled protein, fluorescence recovery was observed for AF488-pyocin S2-labeled cells in FRAP experiments. Imported fluorescent protein was also protected against exogenously added protease.

Live cell imaging can also be used to dissect the directionality of PPIs formed between bacteriocins and their translocators. Housden et al. (2018) used a combination of molecular dynamics simulations, fluorescence microscopy, and single channel recording planar lipid bilayer measurements to unambiguously demonstrate from which side of the OM different OBSs of

ColE9 associated with the lumen of the porin. The intrinsically unstructured N-terminal region of ColE9 houses two OBSs (OBS1 and OBS2) that reside within the pores of OmpF and that flank an epitope that binds periplasmic TolB. The studies revealed that OBS2 binds OmpF from the extracellular side, while the interaction of OBS1 occurs from the periplasmic face of OmpF, which ensures constrained presentation of the TolB epitope within the bacterial periplasm (Housden et al., 2018).

THE ENERGETICS AND KINETICS OF BACTERIOCIN IMPORT

The energetics of bacteriocin translocation are still controversial. Indeed, little is known about the energy dependence of individual translocation steps. Since bacteriocins are folded proteins, import is likely to rely on the input of energy, the main source being the PMF generated across the IM. However, some studies suggest that OM translocation is energy independent, as in the case of colicin A (Bourdineaud et al., 1990). Nevertheless, live cell imaging studies are beginning to show the link between PMF, Ton, Tol, and bacteriocin import (White et al., 2017; Rassam et al., 2018).

A way of testing if energy is necessary for a certain phase of bacteriocin import is to disrupt the PMF and then assess import with a suitable assay. Protonic ionophores have been used for this; for example, CCCP was used in FRAP experiments to show that PMF is necessary for import of pyocin S2 (**Figure 4**; White et al., 2017). Disulphide locked colicins and fluorescently labeled immunity proteins have been used to study the energy dependence of immunity protein release (Vankemmelbeke et al., 2012). A sensitive assay for detecting immunity protein release (described above) was used to confirm that both TolB and TolA are necessary for this process in ColE9 import and to define which regions of TolA are engaged. TolA is anchored in the cytoplasmic membrane via a single transmembrane region that interacts to TolQ and TolR and drives a TolA conformational change in response to PMF (Germon et al., 2001). Vankemmelbeke et al. (2009) focused on residue H22 of the TolA IM region that has been previously linked to energy-dependent conformational change of this protein (Larsen et al., 2007). They showed that an alanine mutation of this residue disrupts immunity protein release, which indicated that an energy-dependent conformational change of TolA is essential for nuclease colicin Im9 release at the cell surface. This points to a role for TolA in transducing cellular energy in a manner similar to that described for TonB (Postle and Larsen, 2007), but the mechanism remains unknown. Bonsor et al. (2009) went on to show that it is the contact between TolA and TolB within the periplasm that is the necessary energy-transduction step for nuclease colicin Im release. One model proposes that the rotation of Tol complex transmembrane helices is transduced into a conformational change in TolA that affects its interaction with the TolB–bacteriocin complex and triggers Im protein dissociation (Papadakos et al., 2012). New methodological approaches will be necessary to dissect how the electrochemical potential of the PMF is transduced by the Tol and Ton systems into the mechanical action of bacteriocin import.

Little is known of the kinetics of bacteriocin import beyond the onset of cellular changes these protein toxins induce. Early studies showed that conformational flexibility is a prominent bacteriocin trait, determining the kinetics of import (Duche et al., 1994). Additionally, bacteriocin charge (Walker et al., 2007) and cell envelope properties related to lipid composition are factors that influence the speed of import (Bourdineaud et al., 1990; Walker et al., 2007). In the case of pore forming colicins, measuring cytoplasmic potassium efflux caused by colicin A inner membrane insertion was used to show how inner membrane fluidity influences the kinetics of translocation (Bourdineaud et al., 1990). In the case of nuclease colicins, Walker et al. (2007) observed that inner membrane charge impacts the rate of import. In this study, a strain of *E. coli* in which the level of anionic phospholipids was regulated by isopropyl β-D-thiogalactopyranoside induction was used to show that both inner membrane and bacteriocin charge influence the rate of cell entry. Import kinetics were measured indirectly, through the efficiency of cell killing or DNA damage. Still, little is known about the kinetics of individual translocation steps and how PPIs between translocon components influence the rate of import. Therefore, to understand import kinetics in more detail, methods for direct measurement of individual translocation steps will have to be developed, most likely based on single molecule methods.

FUTURE PERSPECTIVES

As protein bacteriocins begin to be exploited as therapeutics for multidrug-resistant bacteria so our ability to understand their import mechanisms needs to develop (Behrens et al., 2017). Various approaches, ranging from classical biochemical methods to advanced molecular genetics, have been used over the years for translocon component discovery. The development of high-throughput approaches based on whole-genome sequencing and comparative genomics can speed up this process in the future. Calorimetric measurements have been used extensively to identify binding epitopes and to study the nature of interactions between translocon components. Moreover, implementation of various microscopy techniques, channel conductivity measurements, *in vivo* cross-linking, and disulphide locking of bacteriocins have been exploited for determining the directionality of PPIs within the translocon and for identifying entry paths that bacteriocins use when crossing the OM. Finally, *in vivo* imaging of cells bound to fluorescently labeled bacteriocins has enabled visualization of the import process for the first time at single cell level and provided new tools for probing the spatiotemporal organization of the cell envelope.

While substantial knowledge about OM translocation of bacteriocins has been gained over recent years, the IM component of translocation remains to be elucidated. Many questions remain unanswered - which proteins are involved in bacteriocin IM translocation, how is this process energized, which parts of a bacteriocin are necessary for IM translocation, and which parts enter the cytoplasm. Additionally, a clear link between the OM and IM components of bacteriocin translocons still has to be revealed. For example, are nuclease bacteriocins brought into the periplasm in their entirety before import across the cytoplasmic membrane begins? Finally, the study of bacteriocins in the context of cell envelope organization has breathed new life into bacteriocin research.

AUTHOR CONTRIBUTIONS

IA and CK contributed to the original manuscript and the editorial changes.

FUNDING

IA was funded by the Wellcome Trust Infection, Immunology and Translational Medicine Doctoral Training Centre. CK acknowledges funding from the ERC (OMPorg - 742555), Wellcome Trust (201505/Z/16/Z), MRC (MR/R009937/1), and BBSRC (BB/P009948/1).

ACKNOWLEDGMENTS

The authors would like to thank Ms. Hannah Behrens, Dr. Joanna Szczepaniak, Dr. Nathalie Reichmann, and Dr. Nick Housden for useful discussions and feedback on this manuscript.

REFERENCES

Arnold, T., Zeth, K., and Linke, D. (2009). Structure and function of colicin S4, a colicin with a duplicated receptor-binding domain. *J. Biol. Chem.* 284, 6403–6413. doi: 10.1074/jbc.M808504200

Barquist, L., Mayho, M., Cummins, C., Cain, A. K., Boinett, C. J., Page, A. J., et al. (2016). The TraDIS toolkit: sequencing and analysis for dense transposon mutant libraries. *Bioinformatics* 32, 1109–1111. doi: 10.1093/bioinformatics/btw022

Baysse, C., Meyer, J. M., Plesiat, P., Geoffroy, V., Michel-Briand, Y., and Cornelis, P. (1999). Uptake of pyocin S3 occurs through the outer membrane ferripyoverdine type II receptor of *Pseudomonas aeruginosa*. *J. Bacteriol.* 181, 3849–3851.

Behrens, H. M., Six, A., Walker, D., and Kleanthous, C. (2017). The therapeutic potential of bacteriocins as protein antibiotics. *Emerg. Top. Life Sci.* 1, 65–74. doi: 10.1042/ETLS20160016

Bindereif, A., Volkmar, B., and Klaus, H. (1982). The cloacin receptor of ColV-bearing *Escherichia coli* is part of the Fe3+-Aerobactin transport system. *J. Bacteriol.* 150, 1472–1475.

Bonsor, D. A., Hecht, O., Vankemmelbeke, M., Sharma, A., Krachler, A. M., Housden, N. G., et al. (2009). Allosteric β-propeller signalling in TolB and its manipulation by translocating colicins. *EMBO J.* 28, 2846–2857. doi: 10.1038/emboj.2009.224

Bourdineaud, J. P., Boulanger, P., Lazdunski, C., and Letellier, L. (1990). In vivo properties of colicin A: channel activity is voltage dependent but translocation may be voltage independent. *Proc. Natl. Acad. Sci. U.S.A.* 87, 1037–1041. doi: 10.1073/pnas.87.3.1037

Bowles, L. K., Miguel, A. G., and Konisky, J. (1983). Purification of the colicin I receptor. *J. Biol. Chem.* 258, 1215–1220.

Brynildsrud, O., Bohlin, J., Scheffer, L., and Eldholm, V. (2016). Rapid scoring of genes in microbial pan-genome-wide association studies with Scoary. *Genome Biol.* 17:238. doi: 10.1186/s13059-016-1108

Buchanan, S. K., Lukacik, P., Grizot, S., Ghirlando, R., Ali, M. M., Barnard, T. J., et al. (2007). Structure of colicin I receptor bound to the R-domain of colicin Ia: implications for protein import. *EMBO J.* 26, 2594–2604. doi: 10.1038/sj.emboj.7601693

Cascales, E., Buchanan, S. K., Duché, D., Kleanthous, C., Lloubès, R., Postle, K., et al. (2007). Colicin biology. *Microbiol. Mol. Biol. Rev.* 71, 158–229. doi: 10.1128/MMBR.00036-06

Chauleau, M., Mora, L., Serba, J., and de Zamaroczy, M. (2011). FtsH-dependent processing of RNase colicins D and E3 means that only the cytotoxic domains are imported into the cytoplasm. *J. Biol. Chem.* 286, 29397–29407. doi: 10.1074/jbc.M111.242354

Collins, E. S., Whittaker, S. B., Tozawa, K., MacDonald, C., Boetzel, R., Penfold, C. N., et al. (2002). Structural dynamics of the membrane translocation domain of colicin E9 and its interaction with TolB. *J. Mol. Biol.* 318, 787–804. doi: 10.1016/S0022-2836(02)00036-0

Cornforth, D. M., and Foster, K. R. (2013). Competition sensing: the social side of bacterial stress responses. *Nat. Rev. Microbiol.* 11, 285–293. doi: 10.1038/nrmicro2977

Cotter, P. D. (2014). An 'Upp'-turn in bacteriocin receptor identification. *Mol. Microbiol.* 92, 1159–1163. doi: 10.1111/mmi.12645

de Chial, M., Ghysels, B., Beatson, S. A., Geoffroy, V., Meyer, J. M., Pattery, T., et al. (2003). Identification of type II and type III pyoverdine receptors from *Pseudomonas aeruginosa*. *Microbiology* 149, 821–831. doi: 10.1099/mic.0.26136-0

de Zamaroczy, M., Mora, L., Lecuyer, A., Géli, V., and Buckingham, R. H. (2001). Cleavage of colicin D is necessary for cell killing and requires the inner membrane peptidase LepB. *Mol. Cell* 8, 159–168. doi: 10.1016/S1097-2765(01)00276-3

Delarue, M., and Koehl, P. (2018). Combined approaches from physics, statistics, and computer science for ab initio protein structure prediction: ex unitate vires (unity is strength)? *F1000Research* 7:F1000FacultyRev-1125. doi: 10.12688/f1000research.14870.1

Denayer, S., Matthijs, S., and Cornelis, P. (2007). Pyocin S2 (Sa) kills *Pseudomonas aeruginosa* strains via the FpvA type I ferripyoverdine receptor. *J. Bacteriol.* 189, 7663–7668. doi: 10.1128/JB.00992-07

Duche, D., Baty, D., Chartier, M., and Letellier, L. (1994). Unfolding of colicin A during its translocation through the *Escherichia coli* envelope as demonstrated by disulfide bond engineering. *J. Biol. Chem.* 269, 24820–24825.

Duquesne, S., Destoumieux-Garzon, D., Peduzzi, J., and Rebuffat, S. (2007). Microcins, gene-encoded antibacterial peptides from enterobacteria. *Nat. Prod. Rep.* 24, 708–734. doi: 10.1039/b516237h

Elfarash, A., Dingemans, J., Ye, L., Hassan, A. A., Craggs, M., Reimmann, C., et al. (2014). Pore-forming pyocin S5 utilizes the FptA ferripyochelin receptor to kill *Pseudomonas aeruginosa*. *Microbiology* 160, 261–269. doi: 10.1099/mic.0.070672-0

Elfarash, A., Wei, Q., and Cornelis, P. (2012). The soluble pyocins S2 and S4 from *Pseudomonas aeruginosa* bind to the same FpvAI receptor. *Microbiologyopen.* 1, 268–275. doi: 10.1002/mbo3.27

Farrance, O. E., Hann, E., Kaminska, R., Housden, N. G., Derrington, S. R., Kleanthous, C., et al. (2013). A force-activated trip switch triggers rapid dissociation of a colicin from its immunity protein. *PLoS Biol.* 11:e1001489. doi: 10.1371/journal.pbio.1001489

Germon, P., Ray, M. C., Vianney, A., and Lazzaroni, J. C. (2001). Energy-dependent conformational change in the TolA protein of *Escherichia coli* involves its N-terminal domain, TolQ, and TolR. *J. Bacteriol.* 183, 4110–4114. doi: 10.1128/JB.183.14.4110-4114.2001

Ghequire, M. G., and De Mot, R. (2014). Ribosomally encoded antibacterial proteins and peptides from *Pseudomonas*. *FEMS Microbiol. Rev.* 38, 523–568. doi: 10.1111/1574-6976.12079

Ghequire, M. G. K., Kemland, L., Anoz-Carbonell, E., Buchanan, S. K., and De Mot, R. (2017). A natural chimeric *Pseudomonas* bacteriocin with novel pore-forming activity parasitizes the ferrichrome transporter. *mBio* 8:e1961-16. doi: 10.1128/mBio.01961-16

Govan, J. R. W. (1978). Pyocin typing of *Pseudomonas aeruginosa*. *Methods Microbiol.* 10, 61–91. doi: 10.1016/S0580-9517(08)70660-3

Grinter, R., Milner, J., and Walker, D. (2012). Ferredoxin containing bacteriocins suggest a novel mechanism of iron uptake in *Pectobacterium* spp. *PLoS One* 7:e33033. doi: 10.1371/journal.pone.0033033

Héchard, Y., and Sahl, H. G. (2002). Mode of action of modified and unmodified bacteriocins from Gram-positive bacteria. *Biochimie* 84, 545–557. doi: 10.1016/S0300-9084(02)01417-7

Hecht, O., Ridley, H., Lakey, J. H., and Moore, G. R. (2009). A common interaction for the entry of colicin N and filamentous phage into *Escherichia coli*. *J. Mol. Biol.* 388, 880–893. doi: 10.1016/j.jmb.2009.03.035

Helbig, S., Patzer, S. I., Schiene-Fischer, C., Zeth, K., and Braun, V. (2011). Activation of colicin M by the FkpA prolyl cis-trans isomerase/chaperone. *J. Biol. Chem.* 286, 6280–6290. doi: 10.1074/jbc.M110.165274

Housden, N. G., Hopper, J. T., Lukoyanova, N., Rodriguez-Larrea, D., Wojdyla, J. A., Klein, A., et al. (2013). Intrinsically disordered protein threads through the bacterial outer-membrane porin OmpF. *Science* 340, 1570–1574. doi: 10.1126/science.1237864

Housden, N. G., and Kleanthous, C. (2011). Thermodynamic dissection of colicin interactions. *Methods Enzymol.* 488, 123–145. doi: 10.1016/B978-0-12-381268-1.00006-9

Housden, N. G., Loftus, S. R., Moore, G. R., James, R., and Kleanthous, C. (2005). Cell entry mechanism of enzymatic bacterial colicins: porin recruitment and the thermodynamics of receptor binding. *Proc. Natl. Acad. Sci. U.S.A.* 102, 13849–13854. doi: 10.1073/pnas.0503567102

Housden, N. G., Rassam, P., Lee, S., Samsudin, F., Kaminska, R., Sharp, C., et al. (2018). Directional porin binding of intrinsically disordered protein sequences promotes colicin epitope display in the bacterial periplasm. *Biochemistry* 57, 4374–4381. doi: 10.1021/acs.biochem.8b00621

Housden, N. G., Wojdyla, J. A., Korczynska, J., Grishkovskaya, I., Kirkpatrick, N., Brzozowski, A. M., et al. (2010). Directed epitope delivery across the *Escherichia coli* outer membrane through the porin OmpF. *Proc. Natl. Acad. Sci. U.S.A.* 107, 21412–21417. doi: 10.1073/pnas.1010780107

Jakes, K. S., and Finkelstein, A. (2010). The colicin Ia receptor, Cir, is also the translocator for colicin Ia. *Mol. Microbiol.* 75, 567–578. doi: 10.1111/j.1365-2958.2009.06966.x

Jamet, A., and Nassif, X. (2015). New players in the toxin field: polymorphic toxin systems in bacteria. *mBio* 6:e285-15. doi: 10.1128/mBio.00285-15

Johnson, C. L., Solovyova, A. S., Hecht, O., Macdonald, C., Waller, H., Grossmann, J. G., et al. (2017). The two-state prehensile tail of the antibacterial toxin colicin N. *Biophys. J.* 113, 1673–1684. doi: 10.1016/j.bpj.2017.08.030

Kim, Y. C., Tarr, A. W., and Penfold, C. N. (2014). Colicin import into *E. coli* cells: a model system for insights into the import mechanisms of bacteriocins. *Biochim. Biophys. Acta.* 1843, 1717–1731. doi: 10.1016/j.bpj.2017.08.030

Kjos, M., Oppegård, C., Diep, D. B., Nes, I. F., Veening, J.-W., Nissen-Meyer, J., et al. (2014). Sensitivity to the two-peptide bacteriocin lactococcin G is dependent on UppP, an enzyme involved in cell-wall synthesis. *Mol. Microbiol.* 92, 1177–1187. doi: 10.1111/mmi.12632

Kleanthous, C. (2010). Swimming against the tide: progress and challenges in our understanding of colicin translocation. *Nat. Rev. Microbiol.* 8, 843–848. doi: 10.1038/nrmicro2454

Kleanthous, C., Rassam, P., and Baumann, C. G. (2015). Protein-protein interactions and the spatiotemporal dynamics of bacterial outer membrane proteins. *Curr. Opin. Struct. Biol.* 35, 109–115. doi: 10.1016/j.sbi.2015.10.007

Klein, A., Wojdyla, J. A., Joshi, A., Josts, I., McCaughey, L. C., Housden, N. G., et al. (2016). Structural and biophysical analysis of nuclease protein antibiotics. *Biochem. J.* 473, 2799–2812. doi: 10.1042/BCJ20160544

Kurisu, G., Zakharov, S. D., Zhalnina, M. V., Bano, S., Eroukova, V. Y., Rokitskaya, T. I., et al. (2003). The structure of BtuB with bound colicin E3 R-domain implies a translocon. *Nat. Struct. Biol.* 10, 948–954. doi: 10.1038/nsb997

Lam, J. S., Taylor, V. L., Islam, S. T., Hao, Y., and Kocincova, D. (2011). Genetic and functional diversity of *Pseudomonas aeruginosa* lipopolysaccharide. *Front. Microbiol.* 2:118. doi: 10.3389/fmicb.2011.00118

Larsen, R. A., Deckert, G. E., Kastead, K. A., Devanathan, S., Keller, K. L., and Postle, K. (2007). His(20) provides the sole functionally significant side chain in the essential TonB transmembrane domain. *J. Bacteriol.* 189, 2825–2833. doi: 10.1128/JB.01925-26

Loftus, S. R., Walker, D., Maté, M. J., Bonsor, D. A., James, R., Moore, G. R., et al. (2006). Competitive recruitment of the periplasmic translocation portal TolB by a natively disordered domain of colicin E9. *Proc. Natl. Acad. Sci. U.S.A.* 103, 12353–12358. doi: 10.1073/pnas.0603433103

Lukacik, P., Barnard, T. J., Keller, P. W., Chaturvedi, K. S., Seddiki, N., Fairman, J. W., et al. (2012). Structural engineering of a phage lysin that targets gram-negative pathogens. *Proc. Natl. Acad. Sci. U.S.A.* 109, 9857–9862. doi: 10.1073/pnas.1203472109

Manon, F., and Ebel, C. (2010). "Analytical ultracentrifugation, a useful tool to probe intrinsically disordered proteins," in *Instrumental Analysis of Intrinsically Disordered Proteins*, eds V. Uversky and S. Longhi (Hoboken, NJ: John Wiley), 433–449.

Masi, D. R., White, J. C., Schnaitman, C. A., and Bradbeer, C. (1973). Transport of vitamin B12 in *Escherichia coli*: common receptor sites for vitamin B12 and the E colicins on the outer membrane of the cell envelope. *J. Bacteriol.* 115, 506–513.

Masi, M., Vuong, P., Humbard, M., Malone, K., and Misra, R. (2007). Initial steps of colicin E1 import across the outer membrane of *Escherichia coli*. *J. Bacteriol.* 189, 2667–2676. doi: 10.1128/JB.01448-06

McCaughey, L. C., Grinter, R., Josts, I., Roszak, A. W., Waløen, K. I., Cogdell, R. J., et al. (2014). Lectin-like bacteriocins from *Pseudomonas* spp. utilise D-rhamnose containing lipopolysaccharide as a cellular receptor. *PLoS Pathog.* 10:e1003898. doi: 10.1371/journal.ppat.1003898

McCaughey, L. C., Josts, I., Grinter, R., White, P., Byron, O., Tucker, N. P., et al. (2016). Discovery, characterization and in vivo activity of pyocin SD2, a protein antibiotic from *Pseudomonas aeruginosa*. *Biochem. J.* 473, 2345–2358. doi: 10.1042/BCJ20160470

Michel-Briand, Y., and Baysse, C. (2002). The pyocins of *Pseudomonas aeruginosa*. *Biochimie* 84, 499–510. doi: 10.1016/S0300-9084(02)01422-0

Mora, L., and de Zamaroczy, M. (2014). In vivo processing of DNase colicins E2 and E7 is required for their import into the cytoplasm of target cells. *PLoS One* 9:e96549. doi: 10.1371/journal.pone.0096549

Mora, L., Moncoq, K., England, P., Oberto, J., and de Zamaroczy, M. (2015). The stable interaction between signal peptidase LepB of *Escherichia coli* and nuclease bacteriocins promotes toxin entry into the cytoplasm. *J. Biol. Chem.* 290, 30783–30796. doi: 10.1074/jbc.M115.691907

Ohkawa, I., Shiga, S., and Kageyama, M. (1980). Effect of iron concentration in the growth medium on the sensitivity of *Pseudomonas aeruginosa* to pyocin S2. *J. Biochem.* 87, 323–331. doi: 10.1093/oxfordjournals.jbchem.a132740

Ovchinnikov, S., Kinch, L., Park, H., Liao, Y., Pei, J., Kim, D. E., et al. (2015). Large-scale determination of previously unsolved protein structures using evolutionary information. *eLife* 4:e09248. doi: 10.7554/eLife.09248

Papadakos, G., Housden, N. G., Lilly, K. J., Kaminska, R., and Kleanthous, C. (2012a). Kinetic basis for the competitive recruitment of TolB by the intrinsically disordered translocation domain of colicin E9. *J. Mol. Biol.* 418, 269–280. doi: 10.1016/j.jmb.2012.01.039

Papadakos, G., Wojdyla, J. A., and Kleanthous, C. (2012b). Nuclease colicins and their immunity proteins. *Q. Rev. Biophys.* 45, 57–103. doi: 10.1017/S0033583511000114

Penfold, C. N., Healy, B., Housden, N. G., Boetzel, R., Vankemmelbeke, M., Moore, G. R., et al. (2004). Flexibility in the receptor-binding domain of the enzymatic colicin E9 is required for toxicity against *Escherichia coli* cells. *J. Bacteriol.* 186, 4520–4527. doi: 10.1128/JB.186.14.4520-4527.2004

Pilsl, H., Smajs, D., and Braun, V. (1999). Characterization of colicin S4 and its receptor, OmpW, a minor protein of the *Escherichia coli* outer membrane. *J. Bacteriol.* 181, 3578–3581.

Postle, K., and Larsen, R. A. (2007). TonB-dependent energy transduction between outer and cytoplasmic membranes. *Biometals* 20, 453–465. doi: 10.1007/s10534-006-9071-76

Rassam, P., Copeland, N. A., Birkholz, O., Tóth, C., Chavent, M., Duncan, A. L., et al. (2015). Supramolecular assemblies underpin turnover of outer membrane proteins in bacteria. *Nature* 523, 333–336. doi: 10.1038/nature14461

Rassam, P., Long, K. R., Kaminska, R., Williams, D. J., Papadakos, G., Baumann, C. G., et al. (2018). Intermembrane crosstalk drives inner-membrane protein organization in *Escherichia coli*. *Nat. Commun.* 9:1082. doi: 10.1038/s41467-018-03521-24

Rocchetta, H. L., Burrows, L. L., Pacan, J. C., and Lam, J. S. (1998). Three rhamnosyltransferases responsible for assembly of the A-band D-rhamnan polysaccharide in *Pseudomonas aeruginosa*: a fourth transferase, WbpL, is required for the initiation of both A-band and B-band lipopolysaccharide synthesis. *Mol. Microbiol.* 28, 1103–1119. doi: 10.1046/j.1365-2958.1998.00871.x

Sabet, S. F., and Schnaitman, C. A. (1973). Purification and properties of the colicin E3 receptor of *Escherichia coli*. *J. Biol. Chem.* 248, 1797–1806.

Saeger, J., Hytönen, V. P., Klotzsch, E., and Vogel, V. (2012). GFP's mechanical intermediate states. *PLoS One* 7:e46962. doi: 10.1371/journal.pone.0046962

Sano, Y., Kobayashi, M., and Kageyama, M. (1993). Functional domains of S-type pyocins deduced from chimeric molecules. *J. Bacteriol.* 175, 6179–6185. doi: 10.1128/jb.175.19.6179-6185.1993

Sharma, O., Yamashita, E., Zhalnina, M. V., Zakharov, S. D., Datsenko, K. A., Wanner, B. L., et al. (2007). Structure of the complex of the colicin E2 R-domain and its BtuB receptor. The outer membrane colicin translocon. *J. Biol. Chem.* 282, 23163–23170. doi: 10.1074/jbc.M703004200

Sharp, C., Boinett, C., Cain, A., Housden, N., Kumar, S., Turner, K., et al. (2019). O-antigen dependent colicin insensitivity of uropathogenic *Escherichia coli*. *J. Bacteriol.* 201:e00545-18. doi: 10.1128/JB.00545-18

Sharp, C., Bray, J., Housden, N. G., Maiden, M. C. J., and Kleanthous, C. (2017). Diversity and distribution of nuclease bacteriocins in bacterial genomes revealed using hidden markov models. *PLoS Comput. Biol.* 13:e1005652. doi: 10.1371/journal.pcbi.1005652

Smajs, D., and Weinstock, G. M. (2001). The iron- and temperature-regulated cjrBC genes of *Shigella* and enteroinvasive *Escherichia coli* strains code for colicin Js uptake. *J. Bacteriol.* 183, 3958–3966. doi: 10.1128/JB.183.13.3958-3966.2001

Smith, A. W., Hirst, P. H., Hughes, K., Gensberg, K., and Govan, J. R. (1992). The pyocin Sa receptor of *Pseudomonas aeruginosa* is associated with ferripyoverdin uptake. *J. Bacteriol.* 174, 4847–4849. doi: 10.1128/jb.174.14.4847-4849.1992

Soelaiman, S., Jakes, K., Wu, N., Li, C., and Shoham, M. (2001). Crystal structure of colicin E3: implications for cell entry and ribosome inactivation. *Mol. Cell* 8, 1053–1062. doi: 10.1016/S1097-2765(01)00396-3

Thomas, J. A., and Valvano, M. A. (1993). Role of tol genes in cloacin DF13 susceptibility of *Escherichia coli* K-12 strains expressing the cloacin DF13-aerobactin receptor IutA. *J. Bacteriol.* 175, 548–552. doi: 10.1128/jb.175.2.548-552.1993

Vankemmelbeke, M., Housden, N. G., James, R., Kleanthous, C., and Penfold, C. N. (2013). Immunity protein release from a cell-bound nuclease colicin complex requires global conformational rearrangement. *Microbiologyopen* 2, 853–861. doi: 10.1002/mbo3.122

Vankemmelbeke, M., Shea, O. P., James, R., and Penfold, C. N. (2012). Interaction of nuclease colicins with membranes: insertion depth correlates with bilayer perturbation. *PLoS One* 7:e46656. doi: 10.1371/journal.pone.0046656

Vankemmelbeke, M., Zhang, Y., Moore, G. R., Kleanthous, C., Penfold, C. N., and James, R. (2009). Energy-dependent immunity protein release during *tol*-dependent Nuclease Colicin Translocation. *J. Biol. Chem.* 284, 18932–41. doi: 10.1074/jbc.M806149200

Walker, D., Mosbahi, K., Vankemmelbeke, M., James, R., and Kleanthous, C. (2007). The role of electrostatics in colicin nuclease domain translocation into bacterial cells. *J. Biol. Chem.* 282, 31389–31397. doi: 10.1074/jbc.M705883200

Wei, Y., Li, Z., Chen, B., Liang, H., and Duan, K. (2009). Characterization of the orf1-tolQRA operon in *Pseudomonas aeruginosa*. *Microbiol. Immunol.* 53, 309–318. doi: 10.1111/j.1348-0421.2009.00130.x

Weltzien, H. U., and Jesaitis, M. A. (1971). The nature of the cilicin K receptor of *Escherichia coli* Cullen. *J. Exp. Med.* 133, 534–553. doi: 10.1084/jem.133.3.534

White, P., Joshi, A., Rassam, P., Housden, N. G., Kaminska, R., Goult, J. D., et al. (2017). Exploitation of an iron transporter for bacterial protein antibiotic import. *Proc. Natl. Acad. Sci. U.S.A.* 114, 12051–12056. doi: 10.1073/pnas.1713741114

Wiener, M., Freymann, D., Ghosh, P., and Stroud, R. M. (1997). Crystal structure of colicin Ia. *Nature* 385, 461–464. doi: 10.1038/385461a0

Yamashita, E., Zhalnina, M. V., Zakharov, S. D., Sharma, O., and Cramer, W. A. (2008). Crystal structures of the OmpF porin: function in a colicin translocon. *EMBO J.* 27, 2171–2180. doi: 10.1038/emboj.2008.137

Zakharov, S. D., Eroukova, V. Y., Rokitskaya, T. I., Zhalnina, M. V., Sharma, O., Loll, P. J., et al. (2004). Colicin occlusion of OmpF and TolC channels: outer membrane translocons for colicin import. *Biophys. J.* 87, 3901–3911. doi: 10.1529/biophysj.104.046151

Zakharov, S. D., Wang, X. S., and Cramer, W. A. (2016). The colicin E1 TolC-binding conformer: pillar or pore function of TolC in colicin import? *Biochemistry* 55, 5084–5094. doi: 10.1021/acs.biochem.6b00621

Zampieri, M., Sekar, K., Zamboni, N., and Sauer, U. (2017). Frontiers of high-throughput metabolomics. *Curr. Opin. Chem. Biol.* 36, 15–23. doi: 10.1016/j.cbpa.2016.12.006

Zhang, Y., Li, C., Vankemmelbeke, M. N., Bardelang, P., Paoli, M., Penfold, C. N., et al. (2009). The crystal structure of the TolB box of colicin A in complex with TolB reveals important differences in the recruitment of the common TolB translocation portal used by group A colicins. *Mol. Microbiol.* 75, 623–636. doi: 10.1111/j.1365-2958.2009.06808.x

Zhang, Y., Vankemmelbeke, M. N., Holland, L. E., Walker, D. C., James, R., and Penfold, C. N. (2008). Investigating early events in receptor binding and translocation of colicin E9 using synchronized cell killing and proteolytic cleavage. *J. Bacteriol.* 190, 4342–4350. doi: 10.1128/JB.00047-8

Permissions

All chapters in this book were first published by Frontiers; hereby published with permission under the Creative Commons Attribution License or equivalent. Every chapter published in this book has been scrutinized by our experts. Their significance has been extensively debated. The topics covered herein carry significant findings which will fuel the growth of the discipline. They may even be implemented as practical applications or may be referred to as a beginning point for another development.

The contributors of this book come from diverse backgrounds, making this book a truly international effort. This book will bring forth new frontiers with its revolutionizing research information and detailed analysis of the nascent developments around the world.

We would like to thank all the contributing authors for lending their expertise to make the book truly unique. They have played a crucial role in the development of this book. Without their invaluable contributions this book wouldn't have been possible. They have made vital efforts to compile up to date information on the varied aspects of this subject to make this book a valuable addition to the collection of many professionals and students.

This book was conceptualized with the vision of imparting up-to-date information and advanced data in this field. To ensure the same, a matchless editorial board was set up. Every individual on the board went through rigorous rounds of assessment to prove their worth. After which they invested a large part of their time researching and compiling the most relevant data for our readers.

The editorial board has been involved in producing this book since its inception. They have spent rigorous hours researching and exploring the diverse topics which have resulted in the successful publishing of this book. They have passed on their knowledge of decades through this book. To expedite this challenging task, the publisher supported the team at every step. A small team of assistant editors was also appointed to further simplify the editing procedure and attain best results for the readers.

Apart from the editorial board, the designing team has also invested a significant amount of their time in understanding the subject and creating the most relevant covers. They scrutinized every image to scout for the most suitable representation of the subject and create an appropriate cover for the book.

The publishing team has been an ardent support to the editorial, designing and production team. Their endless efforts to recruit the best for this project, has resulted in the accomplishment of this book. They are a veteran in the field of academics and their pool of knowledge is as vast as their experience in printing. Their expertise and guidance has proved useful at every step. Their uncompromising quality standards have made this book an exceptional effort. Their encouragement from time to time has been an inspiration for everyone.

The publisher and the editorial board hope that this book will prove to be a valuable piece of knowledge for researchers, students, practitioners and scholars across the globe.

List of Contributors

Sarah Wettstadt, Thomas E. Wood, Selina Fecht and Alain Filloux
MRC Centre for Molecular Bacteriology and Infection, Department of Life Sciences, Imperial College London, London, United Kingdom

Sachith D. Gunasinghe, Chaille T. Webb, Iain D. Hay and Trevor Lithgow
Infection and Immunity Program, Department of Microbiology, Biomedicine Discovery Institute, Monash University, Clayton, VIC, Australia

Kirstin D. Elgass
Monash Micro Imaging, Monash University, Clayton, VIC, Australia

Bailey Milne-Davies, Carlos Helbig, Stephan Wimmi, Dorothy W. C. Cheng, Nicole Paczia and Andreas Diepold
Department of Ecophysiology, Max Planck Institute for Terrestrial Microbiology, Marburg, Germany

Janie Liaw, Geunhye Hong, Cadi Davies, Abdi Elmi, Brendan W. Wren, Ozan Gundogdu and Nick Dorrell
Faculty of Infectious and Tropical Diseases, London School of Hygiene & Tropical Medicine, London, United Kingdom

Filip Sima and Alexandros Stratakos
Bacteriology Branch, Veterinary Sciences Division, Agri-Food and Biosciences Institute, Belfast, United Kingdom

Lavinia Stef and Ioan Pet
Bioengineering of Animal Science Resources, Banat University of Agricultural Sciences and Veterinary Medicine - King Michael the I of Romania, Timisoara, Romania

Abderrahman Hachani
Faculty of Infectious and Tropical Diseases, London School of Hygiene & Tropical Medicine, London, United Kingdom
The Peter Doherty Institute for Infection and Immunity, Department of Microbiology and Immunology, University of Melbourne, Melbourne, VIC, Australia

Nicolae Corcionivoschi
Bacteriology Branch, Veterinary Sciences Division, Agri-Food and Biosciences Institute, Belfast, United Kingdom
Bioengineering of Animal Science Resources, Banat University of Agricultural Sciences and Veterinary Medicine - King Michael the I of Romania, Timisoara, Romania

Hsiao-Han Lin
Institute of Plant and Microbial Biology, Academia Sinica, Taipei, Taiwan
Institute of Biotechnology, National Taiwan University, Taipei, Taiwan

Manda Yu and Erh-Min Lai
Institute of Plant and Microbial Biology, Academia Sinica, Taipei, Taiwan
Molecular and Biological Agricultural Sciences Program, Taiwan International Graduate Program, National Chung Hsing University and Academia Sinica, Taipei, Taiwan
Biotechnology Center, National Chung Hsing University, Taichung, Taiwan

Manoj Kumar Sriramoju and Shang-Te Danny Hsu
Institute of Biological Chemistry, Academia Sinica, Taipei, Taiwan

Chi-Te Liu
Institute of Biotechnology, National Taiwan University, Taipei, Taiwan
Agricultural Biotechnology Research Center, Academia Sinica, Taipei, Taiwan

Natalya B. Zakharzhevskaya, Anna A. Vanyushkina, Anna M. Varizhuk, Daria V. Rakitina, Victor V. Podgorsky, Daria D. Kharlampieva and Valentin A. Manuvera
Federal Research and Clinical Centre of Physical-Chemical Medicine Federal Medical Biological Agency, Moscow, Russia

Vladimir B. Tsvetkov
Federal Research and Clinical Centre of Physical-Chemical Medicine Federal Medical Biological Agency, Moscow, Russia
Department of Polyelectrolytes and Surface-Active Polymers, Topchiev Institute of Petrochemical Synthesis, Moscow, Russia
Department of Molecular Virology, FSBI Research Institute of Influenza, Ministry of Health of the Russian Federation, Saint Petersburg, Russia

Innokentii E. Vishnyakov
Lab of Genome Structural Organization, Institute of Cytology, Russian Academy of Sciences, Saint Petersburg, Russia
Institute of Nanobiotechnologies, Peter the Great St. Petersburg Polytechnic University, Saint Petersburg, Russia

Fedor V. Lisitsyn and Elena A. Gushina
N.F. Gamalei Federal Research Centre for Epidemiology and Microbiology, Ministry of Health Russian Federation, Moscow, Russia

Vassili N. Lazarev
Federal Research and Clinical Centre of Physical-Chemical Medicine Federal Medical Biological Agency, Moscow, Russia
Lab of Systems Biology, Moscow Institute of Physics and Technology, Dolgoprudny, Russia

Vadim M. Govorun
Federal Research and Clinical Centre of Physical-Chemical Medicine Federal Medical Biological Agency, Moscow, Russia
Lab of Systems Biology, Moscow Institute of Physics and Technology, Dolgoprudny, Russia
Department of Proteomics, Shemyakin-Ovchinnikov Institute of Bioorganic Chemistry of the Russian Academy of Sciences, Moscow, Russia

Alexander Wagner, Colin Tittes and Christoph Dehio
Biozentrum, University of Basel, Basel, Switzerland

Jeremy Guérin and Susan K. Buchanan
Laboratory of Molecular Biology, National Institute of Diabetes and Digestive and Kidney Diseases, National Institutes of Health, Bethesda, MD, USA

Sarah Bigot
Cell Biology of Bacterial Pathogenicity Team, Laboratory of Molecular Microbiology and Structural Biochemistry, CNRS UMR 5086, University of Lyon, Lyon, France
Cell to Cell DNA Transfer Team, Laboratory of Molecular Microbiology and Structural Biochemistry, CNRS UMR 5086, University of Lyon, Lyon, France
Molecular Microbiology and Structural Biochemistry, Centre National de La Recherche Scientifique UMR 5086-Université Lyon 1, Institute of Biology and Chemistry of Proteins, Lyon, France

Robert Schneider
NMR and Molecular Interactions, Université de Lille, Centre National de La Recherche Scientifique, UMR 8576-Unité de Glycobiologie Structurale et Fonctionnelle, Lille, France

Françoise Jacob-Dubuisson
Université de Lille, Centre National de La Recherche Scientifique, Institut National de La Santé et de La Recherche Médicale, CHU Lille, Institut Pasteur de Lille, U1019-UMR 8204-Centre d'Infection et d'Immunité de Lille, Lille, France

Morgane Roussin, Sedera Rabarioelina, Laurence Cluzeau and Suzana P. Salcedo
Cell Biology of Bacterial Pathogenicity Team, Laboratory of Molecular Microbiology and Structural Biochemistry, CNRS UMR 5086, University of Lyon, Lyon, France

Julien Cayron and Christian Lesterlin
Cell to Cell DNA Transfer Team, Laboratory of Molecular Microbiology and Structural Biochemistry, CNRS UMR 5086, University of Lyon, Lyon, France

Ina Meuskens
Section for Evolution and Genetics, Department of Biosciences, University of Oslo, Oslo, Norway
Interfaculty Institute for Biochemistry, Eberhard Karls University, Tübingen, Germany

Marcin Michalik, Nandini Chauhan, Dirk Linke and Jack C. Leo
Section for Evolution and Genetics, Department of Biosciences, University of Oslo, Oslo, Norway

Mary Nia M. Santos
Institute of Plant and Microbial Biology, Academia Sinica, Taipei, Taiwan
Molecular and Biological Agricultural Sciences Program, Taiwan International Graduate Program, National Chung Hsing University and Academia Sinica, Taipei, Taiwan
Graduate Institute of Biotechnology, National Chung Hsing University, Taichung, Taiwan

Shu-Ting Cho, Chih-Feng Wu and Chun-Ju Chang
Institute of Plant and Microbial Biology, Academia Sinica, Taipei, Taiwan

Chih-Horng Kuo
Institute of Plant and Microbial Biology, Academia Sinica, Taipei, Taiwan
Molecular and Biological Agricultural Sciences Program, Taiwan International Graduate Program, National Chung Hsing University and Academia Sinica, Taipei, Taiwan
Biotechnology Center, National Chung Hsing University, Taichung, Taiwan

Anna M. Lasica
Department of Oral Immunology and Infectious Diseases, University of Louisville School of Dentistry, Louisville, KY, United States
Department of Bacterial Genetics, Faculty of Biology, Institute of Microbiology, University of Warsaw, Warsaw, Poland

Miroslaw Ksiazek and Jan Potempa
Department of Oral Immunology and Infectious Diseases, University of Louisville School of Dentistry, Louisville, KY, United States

Mariusz Madej
Department of Microbiology, Faculty of Biochemistry, Biophysics, and Biotechnology, Jagiellonian University, Krakow, Poland

Germán G. Sgro, Gabriel U. Oka, Diorge P. Souza, William Cenens, Ethel Bayer-Santos, Bruno Y. Matsuyama, Natalia F. Bueno, Thiago Rodrigo dos Santos, Roberto K. Salinas and Chuck S. Farah
Departamento de Bioquímica, Instituto de Química, Universidade de São Paulo, São Paulo, Brazil

Cristina E. Alvarez-Martinez
Departamento de Genética, Evolução, Microbiologia e Imunologia, Instituto de Biologia, University of Campinas (UNICAMP), Campinas, Brazil

Jesús Arenas, Patricia Rodríguez-Castaño, Sara Cano-Crespo and Jan Tommassen
Department of Molecular Microbiology and Institute of Biomembranes, Utrecht University, Utrecht, Netherlands

Fernanda L. Paganelli
Department of Medical Microbiology, University Medical Center Utrecht, Utrecht, Netherlands

Arie van der Ende
Department of Medical Microbiology, Academic Medical Center, Amsterdam, Netherlands

Jos P. M. van Putten
Department of Infectious Diseases and Immunology, Faculty of Veterinary Medicine, Utrecht University, Utrecht, Netherlands

Charlotte Lombardi, Luca Signor, Daphna Fenel, Jean-Marie Teulon, Juliane Brock and Jean-Luc Pellequer
Univ. Grenoble Alpes, CEA, CNRS, Institut de Biologie Structurale (IBS), Grenoble, France
James Tolchard, Birgit Habenstein and Antoine Loquet
Institute of Chemistry and Biology of Membranes and Nanoobjects, Institut Européen de Chimie et Biologie (CBMN), UMR5248 CNRS, University of Bordeaux, Pessac, France

Stephanie Bouillot, Caroline Gebus, David Liebl, Eric Faudry and Ina Attrée
Univ. Grenoble Alpes, Bacterial Pathogenesis and Cellular Responses Group, U1036 INSERM, ERL5261 CNRS, CEA, Grenoble, France

Andréa Dessen
Univ. Grenoble Alpes, CEA, CNRS, Institut de Biologie Structurale (IBS), Grenoble, France
Brazilian Biosciences National Laboratory (LNBio), Centro Nacional de Pesquisa em Energia e Materiais (CNPEM), Campinas, Brazil

Viviana Job
Univ. Grenoble Alpes, CEA, CNRS, Institut de Biologie Structurale (IBS), Grenoble, France
Univ. Grenoble Alpes, Bacterial Pathogenesis and Cellular Responses Group, U1036 INSERM, ERL5261 CNRS, CEA, Grenoble, France

Iva Atanaskovic and Colin Kleanthous
Department of Biochemistry, University of Oxford, Oxford, United Kingdom

Index

O

P

Q

R

S

T

V

X

Y